# CHEMISTRY OF
# SYNAPTIC TRANSMISSION

## *Essays and Sources*

Zach W. Hall
John G. Hildebrand
Edward A. Kravitz

*Harvard Medical School*

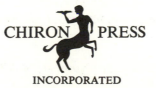

CHIRON PRESS

INCORPORATED

Newton, Massachusetts
1816 S.W. Hawthorne Terrace
Portland, Oregon

Library of Congress Catalog Card Number 73-92880

ISBN 0-913462-03-9

To Steve Kuffler

Who saw the need to combine biochemistry with neurophysiology
and neuroanatomy and created an environment that made it possible.

# CONTENTS

# Contents

# Contents

## Contents

# PREFACE

We have designed this collection of essays and research papers as a resource for students in elementary and advanced courses in neurobiology. We have also attempted to make it a useful introduction to synaptic chemistry for practicing scientists: for example, for the biochemist who wishes to find out what all the recent fuss over the nervous system is about, or for the electrophysiologist who wishes to discover what chemical techniques have revealed about synaptic transmission.

A particular attraction of research on the nervous system is that it often transcends the boundaries traditionally defined by experimental disciplines. We hope that our book will clearly illustrate this point. Chemical processes of synaptic transmission are best understood within physiological and anatomical contexts. Therefore, many of the papers reprinted and referred to in the book require knowledge of the basic principles of neurophysiology and neuroanatomy as well as those of general biochemistry. In that sense, this is not an introductory text.

The book follows the organizational framework of an advanced seminar course that we offer at Harvard Medical School for graduate students, medical students, and advanced undergraduates. For each of eleven topics, we have written a short essay to provide a general background and have reprinted several papers in an attempt to convey the experimental texture of the field. Papers were selected either because they represent landmarks in the field, or because they introduce or support a key idea or a promising approach to a problem. In each case we have tried to choose articles of lasting interest and usefulness. Yet many of the areas covered here are developing vigorously, so that the reader may find papers of equal or greater importance in current journals. In addition, a list of readings follows each chapter and offers a broad, but not comprehensive, entry to the current literature for each subject. Here, we have selected certain research reports, both historical and contemporary, and a few recent reviews, in order to assemble a representative and manageable reading list for each topic.

We are indebted to our colleagues and especially our students, past and present, who have helped us to formulate our ideas and to design this book and the course on which it is based. We owe a particular debt of gratitude to Delores Cox who, with exceptionally good cheer, typed the numerous revisions of our essays. Our thanks go also to Patricia Schubert, Shirley Wilson, Joseph Gagliardi, and Katherine Auerbach. The work on this book by one of us (JGH) was done during the tenure of an Established Investigatorship of the American Heart Association. Finally, we wish to thank the authors whose papers are reproduced in this book for permission to use their papers and for their kindness in providing reprints.

ZWH
JGH
EAK

Boston
October, 1973

# LIST OF ABBREVIATIONS

| | |
|---|---|
| Å | Ångström unit ($10^{-10}$ meter) |
| ACh | Acetylcholine |
| AMP (5'-AMP) | Adenosine 5'-monophosphate |
| ATP | Adenosine 5'-triphosphate |
| cAMP | Adenosine 3',5'-cyclic phosphate |
| cGMP | Guanosine 3',5'-cyclic phosphate |
| CNS | Central nervous system |
| CoA | Coenzyme A |
| COMT | Catechol-O-methyl transferase |
| DFP | Diisopropylfluorophosphonate |
| DNA | Deoxyribonucleic acid |
| DOPA | 3-Hydroxytyrosine |
| dopamine | 3-Hydroxytyramine |
| GABA | Gamma-aminobutyric acid |
| 5-HT | 5-Hydroxytryptamine (serotonin) |
| MAO | Monoamine oxidase |
| mm | Millimeter ($10^{-3}$ meter) |
| mV | Millivolt ($10^{-3}$ Volt) |
| NAD$^+$, NADH | Nicotinamide adenine dinucleotide (oxidized and reduced forms) |
| SIF cells | Small, intensely fluorescent cells |

# INTRODUCTION

A limited number of chemical substances, called neurotransmitters, mediate information transfer between cells within the nervous system and between the nervous system and the rest of the organism. These substances exert their physiological actions through the process of synaptic transmission.

Arrival of an action potential in the most distal processes of a neuron (the presynaptic nerve terminals) triggers release of a neurotransmitter. This substance diffuses across the synaptic cleft between cells and combines with specific receptor sites in the post-synaptic cell membrane. Transmitter binding results in opening or closing of highly specific ionic permeability channels in the membrane. The ions that move, the charges that they carry, and the directions of their movement determine whether the effect of the transmitter is excitatory or inhibitory. The direction of movement of each ion, in turn, is determined by the transmembrane concentration gradient of that ion and the electrical potential difference across the membrane. (The potential at which there is no net ionic movement in either direction is called the equilibrium potential, and can be defined by the Nernst equation. At different synapses, the ions involved, either singly or in combinations, are: potassium, sodium, calcium, and chloride. See Katz, 1966, for details.) Finally, a specific inactivation mechanism removes the transmitter from its sites of action. The entire process of synaptic transmission is brief and can be repeated up to several hundred times per second for short periods.

This book focuses on the biochemical events underlying synaptic transmission. These are shown schematically in Figure 1.

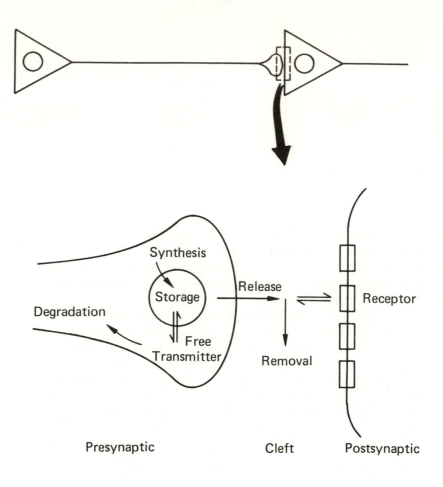

Figure 1

*Note:* Readers not familiar with the physiology and anatomy of neurons and synapses will find the following books helpful.

Cooke, I. and M. Lipkin, Jr. (Eds.) (1972). *Cellular Neurophysiology—A Source Book,* New York: Holt, Rinehart and Winston, Inc.

Katz, B. (1966). *Nerve, Muscle, and Synapses,* New York: McGraw-Hill Book Co.

Peters, A., S.L. Palay, and H. de F. Webster (1970). *The Fine Structure of the Nervous System,* New York: Harper and Row.

*Chapter 1*

# HISTORY

In 1904, T.R. Elliot, enlarging the scope of earlier observations of M. Lewandowsky and J.N. Langley, completed an exhaustive comparison of the effects of sympathetic nerve stimulation and of adrenaline (epinephrine) on various tissues. Impressed by the similarity of effects, he wrote in a preliminary communication of the work (1904, reprinted here) that epinephrine "might then be the chemical stimulant liberated on each occasion when the [nerve] impulse arrives at the periphery." This was the first published suggestion of the idea of chemical transmission at synapses. Elliot himself apparently regarded the hypothesis as so tentative that when a full account of the work was published the following year, he made only oblique reference to the idea in connection with a discussion of epinephrine inactivation.

Although by 1910 it was well known that the effects of sympathetic nerve stimulation could be closely mimicked by epinephrine and those of parasympathetic nerve stimulation, by acetylcholine (ACh), the idea of chemical transmission virtually disappeared from the literature until 1921. Then the simple, elegant experiments of Otto Loewi (1921), using techniques that had been available for many years, provided direct experimental support for the hypothesis. Loewi reasoned that if a transmitter were released from a nerve ending, some portion of the material released might be collected in the fluid bathing the preparation. Accordingly a frog heart was cannulated and filled with Ringer's solution, and the cardioinhibitory (vagus) nerve was stimulated. After stimulation, the fluid from within the heart was transferred to a second heart, whereupon the effect of inhibitory nerve stimulation was duplicated. In an analogous experiment, the solutions from hearts in which cardioacceleratory nerves were stimulated increased the rates of contraction in control (unstimulated) hearts. These experiments left little doubt that nerve stimulation caused the release of substances that could reproduce the effects of the stimu-

1

lation. The inhibitory substance was called "Vagusstoff"; partial characterization in the next few years suggested that it was ACh. Within the decade following the Loewi experiment, there grew a large body of work to support the idea that ACh served as a chemical transmitter at synapses of parasympathetic nerves on glands and smooth muscle.[1]

From the vantage point of the present, when the idea of chemical transmission forms a fundamental part of our understanding of how the nervous system works, the broad significance of Loewi's early experiments is clear. At the time, however, extension of the hypothesis to other synapses met strong resistance, particularly on the part of electrophysiologists who noted several difficulties. For instance, autonomic nerve stimulation of target tissues produces a relatively slow and long-lasting response; at ganglionic synapses and at the neuromuscular junction, however, each presynaptic impulse causes a postsynaptic action potential with very little delay. Transmission at these synapses seemed too rapid to be mediated by a chemical transmitter, and it appeared reasonable to assume that some continuous electrical process was responsible. Nevertheless, ACh produced postsynaptic responses at these synapses, leading H.H. Dale and others to investigate the possibility of chemical transmission. Supporting evidence was soon obtained by W. Feldberg and A. Vartiainen (1934) who showed that ACh was released from autonomic ganglia during stimulation.

But the most decisive and influential experiments by far were those of Dale and his colleagues on the neuromuscular junction. H.H. Dale, W. Feldberg, and M. Vogt (1936, reprinted here) demonstrated the liberation of ACh upon stimulation of motor nerves. ACh release was observed in several preparations, and these investigators were careful to exclude the possibility that autonomic or sensory fibers might have served as the source of ACh. Direct electrical stimulation of denervated muscles did not cause ACh release, nor did curare affect the release caused by nerve stimulation, indicating that ACh liberation did not depend on muscle excitation. These experiments rigorously demonstrated ACh release from active motor nerves.

Evidence that ACh could cause a physiological response in muscle similar to that elicited by nerve stimulation followed quickly. Earlier investigations had shown that ACh, introduced into the bathing solution, could stimulate skeletal muscles, but the response was a slow contracture unlike the rapid twitch produced by nerve stimulation. In an effort to mimic the sudden increase in ACh concentration

1. For an interesting personal account of these experiments see Loewi (1960).

2

that would be caused by liberation from an active nerve terminal, G.L. Brown, H.H. Dale, and W. Feldberg (1936) rapidly and synchronously applied high concentrations of ACh to the muscle fibers by arterial injection of small doses of ACh close to the muscle. A short, rapid contraction followed, similar to that normally seen after nerve stimulation.

With these two papers Dale and his colleagues showed that ACh was released by nerve stimulation and produced an effect similar to that of nerve stimulation at the skeletal neuromuscular junction. They concluded that the most reasonable explanation of their findings was that ACh is the chemical mediator of the interaction between nerve and muscle. In spite of these clear and direct experiments, controversy persisted, and it was not until the early 1950's that the idea of electrical transmission at the neuromuscular junction was completely abandoned. Tribute should be paid to the skill and insight of Dale and his coworkers, who throughout this long period were instrumental in developing and establishing the idea of chemical transmission. One of our colleagues, E.J. Furshpan, has observed aptly, "Dale had the ability to walk through a cow pasture and step only on the daisies."[2]

During the next twenty years, intracellular recording techniques allowed further definition of the physiological effect of nerve stimulation on postsynaptic muscle cells, thereby providing a basis, more rigorous than speed of contraction, for comparison of the effects of applied ACh and of nerve stimulation. Both ACh and nerve stimulation cause a depolarizing potential by increasing the permeability of the muscle membrane to sodium and potassium ions. Antagonists of the transmitter-receptor interaction, such as curare, block the effects of applied ACh, and acetylcholinesterase inhibitors prolong the effects of both ACh and the natural transmitter released by nerve stimulation. In addition, the development of the technique of applying ACh by iontophoresis from the tip of a microelectrode permits an even closer approximation to the natural release process. It is thus possible to make a nearly precise comparison between the amount of ACh released by a nerve terminal and the amount required to mimic the natural physiological response of the muscle. The next two papers reprinted in this section deal with the effort to achieve this accurate comparison.

K. Krnjevic and R. Miledi (1958, reprinted here) demonstrated that in the rat diaphragm careful positioning of an ACh micropipette allows one to obtain iontophoretically induced potentials similar in

2. Dale (1938) gives an excellent account of the development of the idea of chemical transmission and the evidence supporting it.

rise time (about one-half as fast) and duration to neurally evoked potentials. An estimate of the amount of ACh required to produce the potentials can be made, based on the amount of current passed through the micropipette. But, because an assumption must be made about the fraction of current carried by ACh, the estimate must be regarded as-rough. ACh pulses as small as $1.5 \times 10^{-17}$ moles evoked detectable responses, but a pulse of $10^{-16}$ moles elicited a rapid potential, ten mV in amplitude.

K. Krnjevic and J.F. Mitchell (1961, reprinted here) used the same preparation to determine the amount of ACh released per impulse per nerve ending. At low stimulation frequencies they obtained a value of $10^{-17}$ moles, a figure that is remarkably similar to that calculated by Dale some 25 years earlier, although he did not give the details of his calculation (Dale, 1938). Krnjevic and Mitchell estimated that under the conditions of their experiment the average quantal content was about twenty, giving an endplate potential of about ten mV. Thus the ACh actually released and that required to reproduce the observed response did correspond within an order of magnitude.

The evidence supporting the idea that ACh is a chemical transmitter has been presented here in some detail, not only because it was the first transmitter to be identified, but also because that evidence is most complete for the vertebrate neuromuscular junction. Even in this case, however, no one has demonstrated a rigorously quantitative correspondence between the amount of ACh released and that required to produce the observed response. At other cholinergic synapses, such as those formed by preganglionic sympathetic fibers, ACh has been identified as the transmitter solely on the basis of experiments showing that it is released and has the required qualitative effects. Comparable evidence supports the identification of two other neurotransmitters, norepinephrine and GABA, and the remainder of the chapter will deal with them. A number of other substances are suspected of being neurotransmitters. These include glutamate, glycine, 5-hydroxytryptamine (serotonin), dopamine, ATP, octopamine, and substance P (a polypeptide). Most of these substances have been shown to be contained within nervous tissue and to produce physiological effects, but their release with nerve stimulation has not been adequately demonstrated.

The development of our understanding of synaptic transmission between sympathetic nerves and their target organs proceeded almost as slowly as our understanding of cholinergic junctions, although for entirely different reasons. After the demonstration by Loewi and others that sympathetic nerve stimulation caused the release of a substance (called sympathin by W.B. Cannon and his colleagues) capable of exerting sympathomimetic effects when applied to a target organ, the idea that transmission was mediated by a chemical substance was easily accepted. The difficulty lay in identifying the active substance. Although Elliot's early experiments had shown that the effects of epinephrine were similar to those of sympathetic nerve stimulation, it later became clear that there were important differences. For example, while epinephrine was known to excite some tissues and inhibit others, the inhibitory effects of sympathin were never very prominent and seemed to vary with the source. Cannon attempted to reconcile these observations with a complicated theory. He proposed that an epinephrine-like compound was released from sympathetic nerves and combined with a substance in the postsynaptic cell to produce the active agent, which was either sympathin E (excitatory) or sympathin I (inhibitory).

The difficulties were resolved in a series of experiments in the late 1940's. The key observation was that of U.S. von Euler (1946), who showed by careful pharmacological and chemical studies that the active constituent of sympathetic nerve extracts most closely resembled norepinephrine, not epinephrine. This was the first clear indication that norepinephrine is a naturally occurring compound, and the idea that it is the transmitter immediately followed. The decisive experiment was performed by W.S. Peart (1949), who showed that the predominant active substance collected after splenic nerve stimulation was norepinephrine.

The confusing array of postsynaptic actions of the catecholamines was clarified by R.P. Ahlquist (1948) when he showed that two classes of responses were defined by their pharmacological specificities. He suggested that two different types of receptor mediated the effects of catecholamines. One, called $\alpha$, is associated mainly with excitatory effects, such as vasoconstriction of the vessels in the skin and viscera, but is also involved in relaxation of intestinal smooth muscle. $\beta$-receptors, the second type, mediate excitation of the heart, inhibition of the uterus and bronchi, and dilation of certain blood vessels. The previous distinction between excitatory and inhibitory effectors was a spurious one, which caused much of the confusion. After norepine-phrine had been identified as the transmitter, intensive investigation of its synthesis and storage began, and studies in the last twenty years have provided a detailed picture of presynaptic biochemistry at noradrenergic terminals (see Chapter 3).

The history of the identification of gamma-aminobutyric acid (GABA) as a transmitter is much more brisk than that of ACh or norepinephrine. Isolated from nervous tissue in 1950, its physiological activity was unrecognized for several years. The initial observations that led to the idea that GABA might be a transmitter were made in 1957 by A.W. Bazemore, K.A.C. Elliott, and E. Florey, who observed that extracts of mammalian brain reversibly inhibited the firing of a crayfish stretch receptor neuron. The active substance in the extracts was purified and identified as GABA. In a later publication Florey suggested that GABA might be the transmitter released by the inhibitory nerves innervating the stretch receptor neuron.

More extensive studies, both on the crayfish stretch receptor and on crustacean exoskeletal muscle, which receives inhibitory as well as excitatory innervation, revealed a detailed correspondence between the action of GABA and that of the natural inhibitory transmitter (Kuffler, 1960; Takeuchi and Takeuchi, 1965). Both caused inhibition by increasing the permeability of the postsynaptic membrane to chloride ions and shifted the membrane potential toward the same reversal potential. Picrotoxin blocked both responses. Studies in which GABA was applied to crayfish muscle by iontophoresis indicated that sensitivity to GABA was confined to discrete sites on the muscle surface that coincided with the sites of inhibitory nerve terminals. In 1961, J. Dudel and S.W. Kuffler provided physiological evidence that branches of the inhibitory neurons innervating crustacean muscle also made synapses with excitatory nerve terminals, where they acted to decrease the amount of transmitter released. The process was called presynaptic inhibition, and it could also be mimicked by application of GABA. Thus, GABA resembled the inhibitory transmitter in all respects.

Despite these clear indications that GABA acted like the crustacean neuromuscular inhibitory transmitter, GABA was considered not to be a transmitter because of the failure of initial efforts to detect it and its biosynthetic enzyme in crustacean tissues. Moreover, although GABA was found in large concentrations in the mammalian central nervous system (CNS), it was not thought to be a transmitter there because the effects of applied GABA and of inhibitory nerve stimulation in the spinal cord were not exactly the same. As we will describe in Chapter 9 the technical difficulties of identifying CNS transmitters are formidable. Nevertheless, it appeared that where GABA was found, it did not mimic the natural transmitter, and where GABA mimicked the transmitter, no GABA could be found.

Later investigations, more fully discussed in Chapter 4, were successful in isolating both GABA and its biosynthetic enzyme (glutamic decarboxylase) from inhibitory nerves innervating exoskeletal muscles in Crustacea. The demonstration of the release of GABA by stimulated inhibitory nerves (Otsuka, Iversen, Hall, and Kravitz, 1966) decisively established GABA as the transmitter at the crustacean inhibitory neuromuscular junction. The amount of GABA released was proportional to the frequency of stimulation, and release was prevented when the calcium ion concentration of the bath was lowered enough to block inhibitory neuromuscular transmission. Further studies on lobster inhibitory and excitatory neurons, on the mechanism of GABA inactivation, and on the role of GABA in the mammalian brain are discussed in later chapters.

The history we have outlined in this chapter spans seventy years. As often happens during the emergence of new scientific ideas, experimental clues have appeared at one time or another only to disappear again for many years, either because the field was not ready for them or because dominant personalities were unreceptive to them. In times of confusion, an occasional experimenter was able to see straight to the heart of a problem and to test his ideas with simple and direct experiments. Today, when we can often duplicate the decisive experiments in a few hours or days, we sometimes find it difficult to understand why the idea of chemical transmission developed so slowly. But hindsight has a way of removing the obstacles to insight.

What has emerged from these studies is an idea fundamental to our understanding of how the nervous system works: that neurons communicate with each other chiefly by means of chemical transmitters. Three of these transmitters have been identified at readily accessible peripheral synapses. Now a more challenging and ultimately more interesting problem stands before us: to define the transmitters that function at the myriad synapses of the mammalian CNS.

## READING LIST

*Reprinted Papers*

1. Elliot, T.R. (1904). On the action of adrenalin. *J. Physiol.* 31: xx (Proc.).
2. Dale, H.H., W. Feldberg, and M. Vogt (1936). Release of acetylcholine at voluntary motor nerve endings. *J. Physiol.* 86: 353–380.
3. Krnjevic, K. and R. Miledi (1958). Acetylcholine in mammalian neuromuscular transmission. *Nature* 182: 805–806.
4. Krnjevic, K. and J.F. Mitchell (1961). The release of acetylcholine in the isolated rat diaphragm. *J. Physiol.* 155: 246–262.

*Selected Personal Accounts*

5. Dale, H.H. (1938). The William Henry Welch Lectures, 1937:

Acetylcholine as a chemical transmitter of the effects of nerve impulses. 1. History of ideas and evidence. Peripheral autonomic actions. Functional nomenclature of nerve fibers. 2. Chemical transmission at ganglionic synapses and voluntary motor nerve endings. Some general considerations. *J. Mount Sinai Hosp.* 4: 401–429.

6. Loewi, O. (1960). An autobiographic sketch. *Perspectives in Biol. Med.* 4: 3–25.

*Other Selected Papers*

7. Loewi, O. (1921). Über humorale Übertragbarkeit der Herznervenwirkung. I. Mitteilung. *Pflügers Archiv.* 189: 239–242. *Note:* an English translation of this article can be found in I. Cooke and M. Lipkin (Eds.), *Cellular Neurophysiology: A Source Book,* New York: Holt, Rinehart, and Winston, Inc., 1972, pp. 464–466.

8. Feldberg, W. and A. Vartiainen (1934). Further observations on the physiology and pharmacology of a sympathetic ganglion. *J. Physiol.* 83: 103–128.

9. Brown, G.L., H.H. Dale, and W. Feldberg (1936). Reactions of the normal mammalian muscle to acetylcholine and eserine. *J. Physiol.* 87: 394–424.

10. von Euler, U.S. (1946). A specific sympathomimetic ergone in adrenergic nerve fibers (sympathin) and its relation to adrenaline and noradrenaline. *Acta Physiol. Scand.* 12: 73–97.

11. Ahlquist, R.P. (1948). A study of the adrenotropic receptors. *Am. J. Physiol.* 153: 586–600.

12. Peart, W.S. (1949). The nature of splenic sympathin. *J. Physiol.* 108: 491–501.

13. Bazemore, A.W., K.A.C. Elliott, and E. Florey (1957). Isolation of factor I. *J. Neurochem.* 1: 334–339.

14. Brown, G.L. and J.S. Gillespie (1957). The output of sympathetic transmitter from the spleen of the cat. *J. Physiol.* 138: 81–102.

15. Kuffler, S.W. (1960). Excitation and inhibition in single nerve cells. *The Harvey Lectures,* 1958–59: 176–218.

16. Dudel, J. and S.W. Kuffler (1961). Presynaptic inhibition at the crayfish neuromuscular junction. *J. Physiol.* 155: 543–562.

17. Takeuchi, A. and N. Takeuchi (1965). Localized action of gamma-aminobutyric acid on the crayfish muscle. *J. Physiol.* 177: 225–238.

18. Otsuka, M., L.L. Iversen, Z.W. Hall, and E.A. Kravitz (1966). Release of gamma-aminobutyric acid from inhibitory nerves of lobster. *Proc. Nat. Acad. Sci.* 56: 1110–1115.

# ON THE ACTION OF ADRENALIN

*T.R. Elliott*

## Preliminary Communication

In further illustration of Langley's generalisation that the effect of adrenalin upon plain muscle is the same as the effect of exciting the sympathetic nerves supplying that particular tissue, it is found that the urethra of the cat is constricted alike by excitation of the hypogastric nerves and by the injection of adrenalin. The sacral visceral nerves, on the other hand, relax the urethra of the cat. But while the hypogastric nerves relax the tension of the bladder wall in the cat, they do not cause any similar change in the dog, monkey, or rabbit: and though, as is well known[1], adrenalin inhibits the cat's bladder, this reaction is the exception in the mammalian bladder, for adrenalin does not produce any change in those of the three animals named above.

I have repeated the experiment of clean excision of the suprarenal glands and find that the animal, when moribund, exhibits symptoms that are referable to a hindrance of the activities of those tissues especially that are innervated by the sympathetic. They lose their tone; and may even fail to respond to electrical stimulation of the sympathetic nerves. The blood-pressure falls progressively, and the heart-beat is greatly weakened. And at the latest stage previous to death, though the nerves of external sensation and those controlling the skeletal muscles are perfectly efficient, the sympathetic nerves exhibit a partial paralysis of such a nature that nicotine, when injected, is unable to effect through them a rise of blood-pressure or to cause dilatation of the pupil.

This marked functional relationship of the suprarenals to the sympathetic nervous system harmonises with the morphological evidence that their medulla and the sympathetic ganglia have a common parentage.[2] And the facts suggest that the sympathetic axons cannot

Reprinted from *The Journal of Physiology* 31, XX (Proc.) (1904) by permission of the publisher.

excite the peripheral tissue except in the presence, and perhaps through the agency, of the adrenalin or its immediate precursor secreted by the sympathetic paraganglia.

Adrenalin does not excite sympathetic ganglia when applied to them directly, as does nicotine. Its effective action is localised at the periphery. The existence upon plain muscle of a peripheral nervous network, that degenerates only after section of both the constrictor and inhibitory nerves entering it, and not after section of either alone, has been described.[3] I find that even after such complete denervation, whether of three days' or ten months' duration, the plain muscle of the dilatator pupillae will respond to adrenalin, and that with greater rapidity and longer persistence than does the iris whose nervous relations are uninjured.[4]

Therefore it cannot be that adrenalin excites any structure derived from, and dependent for its persistence on, the peripheral neurone. But since adrenalin does not evoke any reaction from muscle that has at no time of its life been innervated by the sympathetic,[5] the point at which the stimulus of the chemical excitant is received, and transformed into what may cause the change of tension of the muscle fibre, is perhaps a mechanism developed out of the muscle cell in response to its union with the synapsing sympathetic fibre, the function of which is to receive and transform the nervous impulse. Adrenalin might then be the chemical stimulant liberated on each occasion when the impulse arrives at the periphery.

1. Lewandowsky. *Centralblatt f. Physiol.* p. 433, 1900.
2. Kohn. *Arch. Mikr. Anat.* LXII, 1903.
3. Fletcher. *Proc. Physiol. Soc. The Journal of Physiology*, XXII, 1898.
4. Cp. S.J. Meltzer and Clara Meltzer Auer, who obtained a like result after excising the superior cervical ganglion alone. *Amer. Journ. Physiol.* XI, 1904.
5. Cp. Brodie and Dixon, this *Journal* XXX, 1904, regarding its absence of action on the muscle of the bronchioles and of the pulmonary blood vessels; and also experiments quoted above on the bladder.

# RELEASE OF ACETYLCHOLINE AT VOLUNTARY MOTOR NERVE ENDINGS

## H. H. DALE, W. FELDBERG[1] and M. VOGT[1]

*From the National Institute for Medical Research, London, N.W.3*

IN a note published some time ago [Dale and Feldberg, 1934], two of us gave a preliminary description of experiments which indicated that something having the properties of acetylcholine (ACh.) is liberated, when impulses in motor nerve fibres excite contraction of a voluntary, striated muscle. Several earlier observers had recorded observations of this kind, but their significance had not been clear. Geiger and Loewi [1922] estimated the choline present in extracts from frog's voluntary muscle, and observed an apparent large increase (five- to tenfold) after prolonged direct and indirect stimulation. Plattner and Krannich [1932] and Plattner [1932, 1933] found that the substance present in such extracts was rapidly inactivated by fresh blood, like acetylcholine, and that the quantity present had a general correspondence to the wide differences in sensitiveness of different muscles to the stimulating action of acetylcholine. Faradic stimulation of the nerve increased the yield; but Plattner associated the apparent presence of the acetylcholine in the muscle, and its increase on mixed nerve stimulation, with a " parasympathetic " innervation of the blood vessels. In the tongue, excised from a cat treated with eserine, and divided longitudinally into halves, he found that stimulation of the chorda-lingual nerve caused increase of acetylcholine in the extract from one half, while stimulation of the hypoglossal nerve did not significantly increase the yield of the other.

Hess [1923], Brinkman and Ruiter [1924, 1925] and Shimidzu [1926], all perfused the muscles of a frog's hindlimbs and tested the effluent Ringer's solution on isolated preparations sensitive to acetylcholine, with some variations of method. All found evidence of the liberation, when the nerves supplying the muscles were stimulated, of something acting like acetylcholine. Brinkman and Ruiter observed that the liberation still occurred, when curare was present in sufficient amount to prevent the motor impulses from causing contractions.

It will be seen that these different observations, though suggestive, are not clear in significance. Something like acetylcholine was apparently liberated, when the mixed nerves to voluntary muscles were stimulated; but the identification of the substance was incomplete, and there was little to indicate what kind of nerve fibres were responsible for its liberation. There is no real evidence, indeed, for a secondary " parasympathetic " nerve supply to the voluntary muscle fibres them-

[1]Rockefeller Foundation Fellow.

Reprinted from *The Journal of Physiology* 86: 353–380 (1936) by permission of the publisher.

11

selves, responsible for maintenance and variation of tone, such as Frank and his co-workers have assumed [Frank and Katz, 1921; Frank, Nothmann and Hirsch-Kauffmann, 1922]. There is evidence, however, that the sympathetic nerve supply to the blood vessels of the leg muscles contains a cholinergic component in the cat [Hinsey and Cutting, 1933] and in the dog [Bülbring and Burn, 1935]; and the same might be the case in the frog. As regards the vaso-dilator action of sensory axon branches, the mode of its chemical transmission is still in doubt; it is still possible, though in the light of recent evidence no longer probable, that it may also be cholinergic. It is clear, in any case, that the liberation of acetylcholine in a voluntary muscle, as the result of stimulating a mixed nerve containing sensory and sympathetic as well as motor fibres, could not be regarded as having any necessary connection with motor nerve impulses, and the transmission of their excitatory action to the voluntary muscle fibres.

Our object has been to discover whether stimulation of the motor nerve fibres innervating voluntary muscles fibres, to the complete exclusion of the autonomic or sensory fibres running with them in a mixed nerve, causes the liberation of acetylcholine in appreciable quantities; and, if so, to endeavour to obtain evidence as to the site of such liberation.

Such an enquiry formed a natural sequel to the experiments which, during the past few years, have produced evidence of the liberation of acetylcholine when a nerve impulse reaches the ending of a preganglionic fibre of the autonomic system, whether that ending makes contact with a cell of the suprarenal medulla [Feldberg, Minz and Tsudzimura, 1934] or with a nerve cell in a ganglion [Feldberg and Gaddum, 1934; Feldberg and Vartiainen, 1934; Barsoum, Gaddum and Khayyal, 1934]. The acetylcholine is, in these cases, liberated in contact with cells which are responsive to that aspect of its activity in which it resembles nicotine [Dale, 1914]. The direct stimulant action of acetylcholine on certain voluntary muscles after degeneration of their motor nerve supply, also belongs to its " nicotine " action, and not to its "muscarine" action [Dale and Gasser, 1926]. It had been further shown long ago, by Langley and Anderson, that voluntary motor nerve fibres and preganglionic autonomic fibres are functionally interchangeable in crossed regeneration; so that, as evidence for a cholinergic function of preganglionic fibres accumulated, the presumption of a cholinergic function for the motor fibres to voluntary muscle increased [cf. Dale, 1935a, b]. On the other hand, it was clear that the task of demonstrating the liberation of acetylcholine by nerve impulses reaching the endings of motor nerve fibres in a voluntary muscle, would be attended with difficulties of a different kind from those involved in the experiments on a ganglion. For the small substance of the ganglion is closely packed with the synaptic endings of preganglionic fibres; so that if acetylcholine were liberated by impulses arriving at the synapses, it might be expected to appear in relatively high concentration in the slow-dropping venous effluent; and this expectation had been realized in experiment. In a voluntary muscle, on the other hand, the bulk of the tissue, requiring effective perfusion to maintain its functional activity, is relatively enormous in relation to the motor nerve endings. If acetylcholine were liberated by the arrival of impulses at these endings, it could not, therefore, be expected to appear in the perfusion fluid in more than a very low concentration. This expectation has again been realized in our experiments, but we have, nevertheless, been able with regularity to detect the appearance of a substance having the recognizable characters of acetylcholine, when the purely motor nerve supply to a voluntary muscle has been stimulated under the conditions of our experiments.

Most of our experiments have been made on the muscles of cats and dogs. These mammalian muscles are usually regarded as completely insensitive to the action of acetylcholine when their motor nerve supply is intact. Recent evidence, to be discussed later, shows that they are not, in fact, indifferent to acetylcholine in relatively large doses, applied through the circulation or directly; but their response, under such conditions, is by twitches or fibrillation, and they do not exhibit the slow contracture with which many muscles of the frog and other lower vertebrates respond to acetylcholine in low dilutions. It was accordingly of special importance to discover whether acetylcholine was liberated when motor impulses, causing only quick contractions, passed down the motor nerve fibres to such normal, mammalian muscles. A few experiments were also made on frog's muscles, with stimulation of motor fibres separately from the other components of the mixed nerve.

## METHODS

All our successful experiments on mammalian muscles have been made by perfusing them with Locke's solution at 37° C., pre-oxygenated to saturation, and containing 1 part of eserine in $5 \times 10^5$. Perfusion was carried out with the Dale-Schuster pump. In a few experiments the attempt was made to demonstrate the liberation of acetylcholine during stimulation of motor nerve fibres to a muscle with normal circulation, eserine being given to the whole animal with sufficient atropine to prevent excessive circulatory depression. Feldberg [1933a], who under such conditions had readily detected acetylcholine in blood of the lingual vein of the dog when the vaso-dilator chorda-lingual nerve was stimulated, had failed to find any when he stimulated the motor hypoglossal nerve. We had a like failure in experiments with natural circulation on the tongue and on the gastrocnemius, stimulating only motor fibres. Franel [1935], in experiments apparently suggested by our preliminary account, also failed in most cases to detect acetylcholine in venous blood from a leg, the muscles of which were thrown into contraction by stimulating the whole limb. The same author, had, indeed, no greater proportion of success when eserinized Locke's solution was used for perfusion. The conditions of these experiments, however, so differed from those of our own that we cannot profitably discuss the cause of their mostly negative results. Our own success in perfusion experiments, with Locke's solution containing eserine, was regular, in contrast to our failure in the few experiments made with normal circulation.

It may be that the relatively low concentration of acetylcholine released by motor stimulation cannot be protected from the blood esterase by eserine in doses insufficient, by themselves, to cause general twitchings of the voluntary muscles. It is possible, on the other hand, that the artificial conditions of saline perfusion in some other way facilitate the escape of the acetylcholine from the site of its origin into the blood vessels. Whatever the reason, artificial perfusion with an eserine-containing saline fluid has been necessary for success. This has caused a limitation of the period of an experiment in which success was possible. Perfusion must be continued long enough to wash the blood thoroughly out of the vessels; on the other hand, if it is continued too long, the muscle becomes more quickly insensitive to motor nerve impulses. In our few experiments on the frog, the skinned hindlimbs were perfused with Ringer's solution containing eserine at the room temperature. Mammals, after preliminary anæsthesia with ether, were given a stable anæsthesia with chloralose, administered intravenously, before the dissection was begun.

*Cat's tongue.* All branches of both common carotid arteries and all tributaries of both external jugular veins were tied, excepting only the lingual arteries and veins respectively. The transverse vein connecting the jugulars at the hyoid level was left open, small tributaries to it being tied, so that the effluent from both lingual veins could later be collected from one jugular, the other being then tied. Both hypoglossal nerves were tied as near as possible to their exits from the skull, cut and dissected free from the accompanying lingual arteries up to the point of their entry into the tongue muscles. As soon as these dissections had been completed, an injection of " Chorazol Fast Pink " was given intravenously, to render the blood incoagulable, and thus facilitate its complete removal by perfusion. Cannulæ, united by a **Y**-junction to the tube leading from the perfusion pump, were then tied into the peripheral ends of both common carotid arteries, the perfusion was begun, and the fluid collected from one jugular vein, as above described. It is, of course, impossible to isolate the vascular system of the tongue from anastomatic communications. While the heart it still beating the perfusion fluid does not become free from blood, unless the pump is so adjusted as to give a comparatively high perfusion pressure and rapid perfusion rate. Our procedure was to cut down the throw of the pump until the venous outflow was about 1-3 c.c. per minute, and then to kill the animal by incising the heart. The last traces of blood then quickly disappeared from the venous fluid. Only an uncertain part of the perfusion fluid pumped into the lingual arteries was thus recovered from the outflow through the lingual veins, a substantial proportion passing by arterial and venous anastomoses and flowing from the open heart cavities into the chest. This unavoidable and unmeasured loss prevented any calculation of the total quantity of acetylcholine liberated in the tongue muscles during stimulation, and restricted observation to a comparison of the acetylcholine contents of the fluid from the lingual veins, when the tongue was at rest and when it was stimulated through its motor nerve. In most of the experiments on the cat's tongue the hypoglossal nerves had been freed from their sympathetic component by aseptic removal of both superior cervical ganglia, under ether anæsthesia, a few weeks before the experiment was made.

*Gastrocnemius.* In experiments on the gastrocnemius muscle of the cat and dog, the stimulation was in most cases through ventral spinal roots. In the animal under chloralose the sympathetic chain, on the side chosen for experiments, was first removed, through an abdominal incision, from the fourth lumbar to the first sacral ganglion. The muscles covering the lumbar vertebræ were then dissected away, and the neural arches removed from as many vertebræ as necessary, for later exposure of the required roots, with careful hæmostasis at each stage.  The popliteal artery and vein were then prepared, all branches except those to and from the gastrocnemius being tied.  The Achilles tendon was isolated and a strong ligature passed under it, round the whole of the other tissues of the leg above the ankle.  The saphena veins were separately tied.  Mass ligatures were also tied round the thigh muscles above the knee, leaving the main vessels and the sciatic nerve free.  The crural nerve was cut at the groin.  A stout steel rod was pushed through a hole drilled in the lower end of the femur, enabling that bone to be fixed by a clamp, so that muscular contractions would not drag on the popliteal vessels and interfere with the perfusion.  The roots to be stimulated were now exposed by opening the *dura mater*.  The dorsal roots were separated, and, unless required for control stimulation, were completely removed, so as to leave good lengths of ventral roots for stimulation, without danger of stimulating dorsal roots by escape of current.  The ventral roots of the side not under experiment were similarly removed.  The last lumbar and the first two sacral roots on the experimental side were then tied with fine ligatures close to the cord.  These roots were separately tested with short faradic stimuli, those being kept which caused contractions of the gastrocnemius.  These were tied together for stimulation, or, in some cases, left attached to a segment of the cord, which could be raised with them for stimulation.  The cannulæ were then tied into the popliteal vessels and the perfusion begun.  If the exclusion of collateral circulation had not been sufficient to render the venous effluent free from blood, this was effected by lowering the blood-pressure by bleeding.  It was not considered desirable, in this case, to deprive the whole nervous pathway, from the roots to the gastrocnemius, completely of its blood supply by killing the animal.  In a few experiments, however, in which the whole sciatic nerve was stimulated, or in which the gastrocnemius muscle was stimulated directly, the preparation was isolated completely after the perfusion had been started, by killing the animal and cutting through the femur.

*Quadriceps extensor femoris.*  To exclude by degeneration the sympathetic nerve endings on the blood vessels, which could not easily be effected with the gastrocnemius, a few experiments were made on the quadriceps extensor mass of the dog's thigh.  By aseptic operation under ether, the sympathetic chain, from the third lumbar to the first or second sacral ganglion on the experimental side, together with the first sacral ganglion of the other side, was removed some weeks beforehand.  At the experiment the quadriceps was isolated by dividing all the other muscles of the thigh, the ilio-psoas and the glutæal muscles between ligatures.  The leg was amputated at the knee joint.  The perfusion cannulæ were tied into the femoral artery and vein, all branches except those to the quadriceps being tied.  Further to minimize collateral circulation, a ligature was tied round the quadriceps mass above the entry of the vessels and nerves supplying it.  Stimulation was through the appropriate lumbar ventral roots, or, in some cases, through the crural trunk.

*Frog's Legs.*  Large specimens of Hungarian *R. esculenta* were used.  The frog was killed by decapitation and skinned.  The abdominal sympathetic chains of both sides were removed.  Perfusion was through the abdominal aorta and the anterior abdominal vein, the renal portal veins being tied.  The roots of the lumbosacral plexus were exposed in the spinal canal, dorsal and ventral roots being tied separately and prepared for stimulation. The perfusion fluid was oxygenated Ringer's solution, containing 1 part of eserine in $3\text{-}5 \times 10^5$. A perfusion pressure of 25-35 c.c. of solution was found to give a convenient rate of outflow of about 1 c.c. per minute.

*Stimulation.* For stimulation the nerves or roots were laid across a suitable pair of chlorided silver electrodes. Direct stimulation of muscles was made through electrodes in the forms of chlorided silver pins, one impaling the muscle near its tendon of insertion, and the other, of several pins, penetrating the muscle near its origin. The stimuli used were maximal break shocks from a secondary coil, Lewis's rotating interruptor being used so as to give from 5 to 15 shocks per second. This method, causing a rhythmic series of twitches, was chosen in preference to tetanization, so as to avoid impediment to the perfusion during the activity of the muscle.

*Rate of perfusion.* As explained above, the unknown and irregular escape of some of the venous fluid by collateral channels made impossible a strict adjustment of the rate of flow to the size of the muscle perfused. A rough adjustment, however, had to be made; and it has already been indicated that venous fluid was collected from a cat's tongue at about 1-3 c.c., and from the hind legs of a large frog at about 1 c.c. per minute. For a cat's gastrocnemius the rate of collection was 3-8 c.c., and for the quadriceps femoris of a large dog, sometimes as high as 25 c.c. per minute. An estimate of total output rate being impracticable, our main concern was to ensure that an increased liberation of acetylcholine was not masked, on the one hand, by accelerated perfusion, or simulated, on the other, by retarded perfusion during the period of stimulation. Failing adjustment, the rate of perfusion was, in fact, always accelerated during a period of the rhythmic stimulation employed, especially during its latter part. This acceleration was approximately corrected by an assistant, who watched the rate of dropping from the vein cannula, and reduced the throw of the pump as required, so as to ensure that the rate was not unduly accelerated during stimulation, but not, in any case, to retard it below the control rate.

*Tests for acetylcholine.* Tests were made as usual on the preparation of leech muscle sensitized by eserine. The preparations used usually responded well to acetylcholine in a dilution of 1 in $5 \times 10^8$. The tonicity of the mammalian Locke's solution had to be adjusted to that used for the leech by adding distilled water, and was then further diluted, if necessary, in accordance with its activity. The samples as collected were placed on ice and tested with as little delay as possible. In a number of experiments tests were also made on the blood-pressure of cats under chloralose, the sensitiveness of which to small doses of acetylcholine was, when necessary, increased by injecting eserine, and by restricting the circulation volume by removal of the abdominal viscera. For such tests the samples as collected were made acid to congo red by adding a drop of HCl solution, and then kept cold till the perfusion experiment was finished. The stability of the active substance could be tested by either method, and the test on the cat further enabled its sensitiveness to atropine to be demonstrated.

## RESULTS

### (1) *Stimulation of purely motor fibres to voluntary muscles*

#### (a) *Tongue of the cat*

The perfusion being started, the rate adjusted, and a bloodless effluent obtained, control samples were tested on the leech. The earlier samples, after the rather prolonged dissection and manipulation, usually showed detectable amounts of a substance acting like acetylcholine, as Hess [1923] observed in his perfusions of frog muscle. The activity might be such as to correspond to an ACh. content of 1 in $4 \times 10^8$ of the undiluted fluid. This activity diminished rapidly, however, with successive samples, and, after perfusion for about half an hour, was no longer perceptible by the very delicate test. The hypoglossal nerves were then stimulated rhythmically, the tongue muscles responding with rhythmic contractions. The perfused muscles show rapid fatigue to the effects of such stimuli, the initially vigorous contractions rapidly becoming weaker, until, at the end of a stimulation period of 2-3 min. they have practically ceased. The stimulation was not continued when the muscles showed signs of this failure. The fluid collected during the stimulation showed a pronounced activity, in comparison with the inactive control. The contrast is illustrated in Fig. 1 A and C. All the fluids in this experiment were

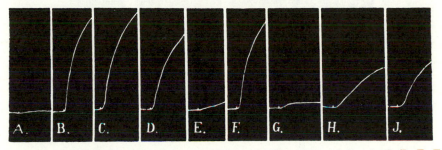

Fig. 1. Leech preparation; eserine 1 in $3 \times 10^5$ (same in Figs. 3, 4 and 5). A, C, D, E, F, G, H, venous fluids from cat's tongue, 50 p.c. dilutions (details in text). B and J, control ACh. dilutions; B, 1 in $10^8$, J, 1 in $4 \times 10^8$.

tested in 50 p.c. dilutions. The control fluid, at A, has no significant action. At C the fluid collected during a first period of stimulation at 5 shocks per sec. was applied and produced an effect closely similar to that of a control solution of ACh. 1 in $10^8$, applied at B; so that the undiluted effluent during stimulation would correspond in activity to ACh. 1 in $5 \times 10^7$. The rate of outflow being 3 c.c. per min., the amount of ACh. actually collected in 1 min., apart from what escaped by anastomotic channels, was $0.06\gamma$. The active substance was still present in fluid collected after the stimulation period, but in rapidly diminishing concentration in successive samples. Fig 1 D shows the effect of fluid collected in the 2 min. after the end of stimulation, and E that of fluid collected 20 min. later. A second period of stimulation was then given, again causing vigorous contractions of the tongue at its commencement but with a more rapid onset of fatigue. The fluid collected during this second period, applied at F, was still highly active; and again the stimulating substance had almost disappeared from a further sample, applied at G,

17

which was collected 20 min. after the end of the stimulation. Further periods of stimulation, after the second, were usually progressively ineffective, as regards both the contractile activity evoked in the tongue muscle and the concentration of stimulant substance in the venous fluid. Fig. 1 H shows the effect of the venous fluid collected during a third and less effective period of stimulation. The 50 p.c. dilution at this stage is rather less active than ACh. 1 in 4 × 10⁸, applied as a control at J.

In the later period of the experiment, the tongue gradually becomes œdematous with the prolonged perfusion; and this not only lowers the activity of the fluid collected during stimulation, but causes the activity to disappear more slowly from successive subsequent samples. Eventually, after four, five or more periods of stimulation, the tongue muscles fail to respond further, and the " stimulation " fluid is then not perceptibly more active than the control.

*Identity of substance released.* The action on the leech muscle, though closely similar to that of acetylcholine, would not by itself identify it. In several cases, when the concentration in the stimulation effluent was sufficiently high, it was directly tested on the blood-pressure of the cat under chloralose, and the activity again

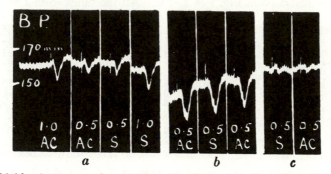

Fig. 2. Carotid blood-pressure of cat under chloralose. Injections (i.v.) of S=concentrated venous effluent from tongue (see text), and AC=acetylcholine in dilution matching S in the leech test. *a*, before eserine; *b*, after eserine; *c*, after atropine.

matched against known doses of acetylcholine. In every case the match so obtained was identical with that obtained in the comparison made on the leech muscle. In every case also, the effect on the blood-pressure was completely annulled by a small dose of atropine. In one experiment a larger volume of the effluent was collected, during several periods of stimulation, stabilized by acidification, and evaporated to complete dryness under reduced pressure. The residue was extracted with dry alcohol, and this was evaporated again to dryness, its residue being finally taken up in saline. This solution was then accurately matched against acetylcholine on the eserinized leech preparation, and a solution of acetylcholine corresponding with it in activity, as so determined, was prepared, the actual concentration required being 1 in 2 × 10⁷. These solutions (S and AC) were then compared against one another on the blood-pressure of a cat under chloralose, the record of the comparison being shown in Fig. 2. It will be seen that in doses of 1 and 0·5 c.c. the two solutions gave indistinguishable effects. The cat was then given 0·15 mg. of eserine per kg.

intravenously, and after 15 min. the comparison of the two solutions was repeated (Fig. 2b). It will be seen that 0·5 c.c. of the concentrated effluent again accurately matches 0·5 c.c. of the ACh. solution, the effect of both being intensified to the same extent, in comparison with their earlier effects. Finally, after 1 mg. of atropine, the effects of both solutions were annulled (Fig. 2c).

If the effluent was made alkaline by adding one-tenth of its volume of $N/10$ NaOH, allowed to stand for 20 min. at the room temperature and then reneutralized with HCl, its actions on the leech and the blood-pressure were found to have disappeared. Since the perfusion fluid contained eserine, it was not possible to test directly the sensitiveness to esterase of the active substance after collection. Indirectly, however, its liability to esterase was demonstrated by an experiment in which the tongue was perfused with Locke's solution containing no eserine. Under these conditions the muscles responded as usual to hypoglossal stimulation, but no trace of stimulant action on the previously eserinized leech muscle was acquired by the effluent. The stimulation was repeated several times, with a similarly negative result, until the tongue muscle ceased to respond. The perfusion fluid remained throughout free from any trace of a substance acting like acetylcholine. Eserine was then added to the perfusion fluid in the usual concentration of 1 in $5 \times 10^5$. In the subsequent period of stimulation there was an obvious renewed response of the tongue muscles to the nerve impulses, and the venous fluid now acquired the usual stimulant action on the leech muscle. The revival of muscular response is of interest, but it would not be proper to emphasize its significance on the basis of one observation. For our present purpose the point of importance is the appearance of the stimulant substance in the venous effluent, whereas without eserine it had been consistently absent, even when the muscle contracted well. The substance is normally destroyed on the way from the site of its liberation to the perfusion fluid, but is protected from this destruction by eserine. We are dealing, then, with a substance stable in acid and rapidly destroyed in dilute alkali; protected by eserine from destruction in the tissues; equivalent to the same doses of acetylcholine when tested on the eserinized leech muscle and on the cat's blood-pressure, before and after eserine; and having its action on the cat's blood-pressure annulled by atropine in parallel with that of acetylcholine. There can be no real ground for doubting that it is acetylcholine itself.

*Nerve fibres concerned.* The tongue muscles and the hypoglossal nerve were chosen, in the first instance, because of the readiness with which this motor nerve could be freed, by degeneration, from sympathetic fibres joining it from the superior cervical ganglion. In most of the experiments above described, both ganglia had been aseptically removed some weeks before the experiment. The hypoglossal nerve has the further advantage that the sensory supply to the tongue runs separately in the lingual nerve and is not stimulated. Langworthy [1924], has shown, however, that the cat's hypoglossal nerve often contains a vestigial sensory ganglion, in the form of a few cells of sensory type embedded among its fibres. There is no evidence that these are connected with sensory fibres from the tongue; the available evidence indeed, connects them rather with fibres from the infrahyoid muscle[1], not

[1]Personal communication from Dr. D. H. Barron.

included in our perfusion.  There was little likelihood, in any case, that this trival and inconstant sensory component of the hypoglossal nerve would be responsible for the regular liberation of acetylcholine from the tongue, in the significant amounts which we obtained on stimulating the nerve.  The exclusion of all sensory elements, however, was even more complete in the later experiments on leg muscles.  Another possibility which gave us some concern was that of a mechanical stimulation, by the muscular contractions, of the fibres and endings of the cholinergic chorda tympani, in connection with the blood vessels of the tongue and the glands in its mucous membrane.  In several experiments, accordingly, the chorda tympani was also cut by aseptic operation, at a point before its junction with the lingual nerve, and allowed to degenerate completely before the experiment, without affecting the result; stimulation of the hypoglossal, freed from sympathetic fibres, still caused liberation of acetylcholine from the parasympathetically denervated tongue.  In another experiment the whole chorda-lingual nerve was cut on one side by previous operation and allowed to degenerate.  The margin of the insensitive half of the tongue had been indented by biting before the experiment was performed.  The two halves of the tongue were perfused separately on this occasion, and there was no significant difference in their yields of acetylcholine in response to stimulation of their respective hypoglossal nerves.

We shall see later that the mechanical stimulation of chorda-lingual fibres, together with other possibilities, can be more easily excluded by the use of curarine.  At the present stage we had established a very strong presumption that the observed liberation of acetylcholine was due to the impulses passing along motor nerve fibres to excite voluntary muscle fibres.  For the further testing of this presumption we turned to other muscles.

## (b)  Gastrocnemius

*Cat.*  The experiments on the cat's gastrocnemius were less successful than those on the tongue.  After the rather long preliminary preparation, and the further period required to obtain a bloodless perfusate, we found, in several cases, that the muscle failed to respond to maximal stimulation of the ventral roots, or responded very weakly.  In such cases we failed to observe any liberation of acetylcholine during the stimulation.  The sciatic nerve was then isolated in the thigh, cut and stimulated peripherally, and the resulting contractions of the gastrocnemius were accompanied by the appearance of acetylcholine in the venous fluid.  This latter form of stimulation, however, involved the sympathetic and sensory fibres running in the nerve, and the result was not beyond criticism for our purpose.  We may confine attention, therefore, to two experiments in which the roots remained satisfactorily sensitive, the muscle responding when they were stimulated.  As in the tongue perfusion, the first samples of perfusion fluid, after it had become free from blood, still contained perceptible traces of acetylcholine.  These, however, rapidly disappeared with continued perfusion.  When blank controls had been obtained, the roots were stimulated for a period, and with the contractions of the gastrocnemius acetylcholine appeared in the venous fluid, rapidly disappearing again with continued perfusion after the stimulation was stopped.  The concentration reached during the stimulation was never high, being about 1 in $4 \times 10^8$; on the other hand, the response of this muscle to the root stimulation was never vigorous, even in the most successful experiments.

*Dog.* The sensitiveness of the dog's roots, as shown by the response of the muscle to their stimulation, survived the conditions of the experiment much better. The first samples of clear venous fluid showed a weak activity on the leech muscle, but practically inactive controls were soon obtained with continued perfusion. Before the motor roots were stimulated, in some experiments, a further control sample was collected during a period of stimulation of the corresponding sensory roots. Fig. 3 shows the record from such an experiment. In all cases the venous fluid was applied in 75 p.c. dilution. A shows the negative effect of a blank control, B that of the fluid collected during stimulation of the sensory roots, and C the response of the leech muscle to ACh. 1 in $10^9$, given for calibration. At D a further resting control sample was applied, and at E the venous fluid collected during a period of stimulation of the motor roots, causing contractions of the gastrocnemius. At F a sample collected 2 min. after the end of stimulation was tested, and at G a sample collected after a further 20 min. perfusion, by which time the effluent was again practically inactive. The sequence could be repeated with a second period of

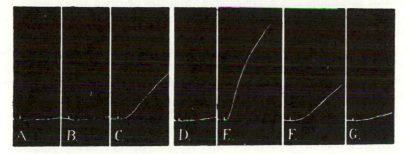

Fig. 3. A, B, D, E, F, G, venous fluids from dog's gastrocnemius, in 75 p.c. dilution (see text). C, ACh. 1 in $10^9$.

stimulation, but with later periods the response of the muscle, and the concurrent output of acetylcholine, declined together. As with the tongue, if perfusion was continued till the muscle had become visibly œdematous, the appearance in the effluent, of the acetylcholine liberated during stimulation, was delayed and prolonged. Results like the above could be obtained regularly in experiments on the dog's gastrocnemius, stimulated through the motor roots. The concentration of acetylcholine in the stimulation effluent did not rise above about 1 in $2 \times 10^8$, and was accordingly lower than that observed in successful experiments on the tongue. On the assumption that the acetylcholine is liberated by the arrival of impulses at the motor nerve endings, for which evidence will be given later, it may be suggested that the leg muscles, with their relatively long fibres and consequently large mass perfused in relation to the number of nerve endings, might be expected to yield a lower concentration in the venous fluid than the comparatively short-fibred muscles of the tongue. The crude adjustment of the perfusion rate to the size of the muscle, however, forbids any attempts at calculation.

*Identification.* The substance from the gastrocnemius, like that from the tongue, behaved like acetylcholine in its instability to alkali, and its action on the cat's arterial pressure, abolished by atropine. It was further shown in one experiment, that an effluent, active on the leech muscle previously sensitized by eserine, had no immediate action on a control strip which had not been so treated.

### (c) *Quadriceps extensor femoris (dog)*

As mentioned earlier, a few experiments were performed on this muscle mass because it could be freed from sympathetic nerve endings, by degeneration following removal of the abdominal sympathetic chain at a preliminary operation. The results obtained by stimulating the appropriate ventral nerve roots were closely similar to those obtained with the gastrocnemius, acetylcholine in 1 in 4 $\times$ $10^8$ appearing in the venous effluent, during contractions of the muscle evoked by such stimulation. The mechanical stimulation of cholinergic sympathetic fibres and endings could, therefore, be excluded as a possible source. In one experiment the dorsal roots were also stimulated, with negative result.

### (d) *Hind leg muscles of the frog*

The object of these experiments was to identify the nerve fibres, responsible for the output of something like acetylcholine from the perfused frog's muscles, which Hess [1923] and others had observed with stimulation of the mixed nerve supply. The results were very similar to those we had already obtained with mammalian muscles. At the beginning of the perfusion, perceptible amounts of acetylcholine appeared in the venous fluid from the unstimulated muscles, and these disappeared as the perfusion was continued. Stimulation of the ventral roots, the sympathetic chain being extirpated, then regularly caused the appearance of acetylcholine in the venous fluid. The concentrations were low, 1 in 2 $\times$ $10^8$ being the maximum obtained. The activity of the fluid, as in the mammalian experiments, slowly disappeared with continued perfusion, and reappeared on renewed stimulation. In two experiments the sympathetic chain was preserved and directly stimulated, causing vaso-constriction, as shown by retarded perfusion; but no acetylcholine appeared. In several experiments the dorsal roots were stimulated with completely negative results. In one experiment only, a perceptible quantity of something acting on the leech like acetylcholine appeared in the venous fluid at an interval of 10 min. after a period of sensory root stimulation. This result cannot properly be regarded as related to the stimulation, and it is only recorded as a presumably accidental, and obviously doubtful exception to otherwise completely negative results. Fig. 4 shows tests, on the eserine treated leech preparation, of a control fluid at A, fluid collected during

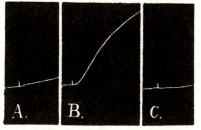

Fig. 4. Venous fluids from skinned hind-limbs of frog. A, before; B, during stimulation of motor roots; C, same fluid as B, after treatment with alkali.

effective motor root stimulation at B, and a portion of the same fluid after standing with alkali and reneutralization, at C. These experiments show that the substance detected by previous observers, as liberated during the stimulation of the mixed nerve supply, is produced by stimulation of the motor fibres to voluntary muscle, and has the instability to alkali of acetylcholine.

### (2) *Direct stimulation of muscles*

We have seen that, when stimulation of the motor fibres failed to produce contractions of the muscle, acetylcholine was no longer liberated. It was possible, therefore, that it might come from the muscle fibres themselves, as a by-product of the contractile process. It was further possible that fluid collecting in inadequately perfused areas, or in the tissue between the muscle fibres, might acquire acetyl-choline from some source, and that contractions might mechanically press some of it into the perfusion stream. To test these possibilities we first studied the effects of producing contractions of the muscle by direct stimulation. A normally innervated muscle cannot be effectively stimulated without stimulating, at the same time, the branches and endings of motor nerve fibres in its substance. We accordingly made comparative experiments on normal muscles, and on corresponding muscles denervated by degeneration. The muscles chosen were again the gastrocnemius of the cat and the dog and the quadriceps extensor femoris of the dog, the sciatic or crural nerve on one side having been divided aseptically under ether 10 days previously.

The results with direct stimulation of the normally innervated muscles were not different from those produced by stimulating a similar muscle through its motor nerve supply. The first samples of venous effluent contained some acetylcholine, which disappeared with further perfusion. Stimulation of the muscle then caused acetylcholine to appear, as with motor nerve stimulation, and it disappeared as usual with further perfusion. With the denervated muscle the results were entirely different. In the first place, even the earliest samples of venous fluid, after it had become free from blood, showed no significant activity on the most sensitive leech

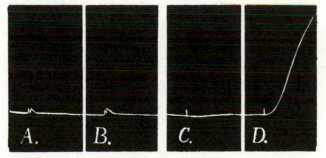

Fig. 5. Venous fluids from gastrocnemius muscles of cat, in 75 p.c. dilution. A and B from denervated muscle, A resting, B during stimulation; C and D from normal muscle, C resting, D during stimulation.

preparation. Further, though the muscle contracted powerfully in response to direct stimulation, no trace of activity was shown by the fluid collected during or after the stimulation period. A comparison between the results obtained with a normal cat's gastrocnemius and the denervated gastrocnemius of the other leg, similarly perfused and tested in succession, is illustrated in Fig. 5. The venous fluids were tested in 75 p.c. dilutions. At A the control fluid from the denervated muscle was tested, and at B the fluid collected while the muscle was contracting vigorously in response to direct stimulation. In neither case is any trace of activity to be detected. (The small and brief rises of the writing point are accidental mechanical effects of emptying the testing bath and refilling with the test fluid.) At C the control fluid from the normal muscle was tested, and at D that collected during direct stimulation of that muscle.

An experiment on a dog's quadriceps, deprived of its sympathetic supply by degeneration but otherwise normally innervated, showed that it gave the usual yield of acetylcholine to direct stimulation. Another experiment on a sympathetically denervated quadriceps gave a result of special interest. This muscle had initially responded normally by contractions, with output of acetylcholine, to motor nerve stimulation. With continued perfusion successive periods of such stimulation had been progressively less effective, till finally the muscle no longer contracted or yielded acetylcholine, with renewed stimulation of the nerve. Direct stimulation being now applied, the muscle contracted vigorously, but no trace of acetylcholine appeared in the venous fluid. The mechanism concerned with transmission of the excitatory process from the nerve to the muscle fibres being exhausted, acetylcholine was no longer liberated, though the muscle contracted well. The muscle, in this respect, behaved now like one which had been denervated.

### (3) *Curarine*

Some of the results described in the foregoing section might still find a conceivable explanation in the passage of acetylcholine from some source into stagnant fluid in the muscle, and the mechanical expression of some of this into the circulation by the contractions. It would be necessary then to assume, indeed, that this source disappeared with degeneration of the nerves and their endings, and that it could be exhausted with repeated stimulation of the nerve to the perfused muscle. It was important, however, to find conditions under which the effects of motor nerve stimulation could be tested, in the complete absence of muscular response. The use of curarine provided the required condition, and gave a decisive result.

Experiments were made on the perfused cat's tongue, stimulated through the hypoglossal nerves, deprived by degeneration of their sympathetic fibres. A little difficulty was experienced in adjusting the dose of curarine, in the necessary presence of eserine in the perfusion fluid, since eserine is well known to be an antagonist of the paralytic action of curare. With our usual concentration of eserine (1 in $5 \times 10^5$) curarine even in tenfold concentration (1 in $5 \times 10^4$) did not always produce an immediate complete paralysis to the onset of a series of maximal break shocks, applied to the hypoglossal nerves. The experimental stimulation, however, for collection of the venous sample was not carried out until all trace of such initial response had disappeared, the tongue remaining completely passive during the whole period of stimulation. A venous sample was collected, as usual, during a control period, and another during the ineffective stimulation. The presence of curarine made it difficult to test the fluids accurately on the leech muscle, the response of which to acetylcholine is slowly paralysed by curarine. Their activity on the blood-pressure of a cat under chloralose, however, could be readily determined with some accuracy, in comparison with those of known concentrations of acetylcholine. The Locke's solution, containing eserine and curarine in the indicated concentrations, had by itself no perceptible effect on the blood-pressure. Fig. 6 shows a comparison of the depressor effects of the venous effluents collected in such an experiment, with those of two dilutions of acetylcholine. The volume injected was in each case 2 c.c. At A the control venous fluid, collected just before stimulation, was injected; at B the fluid collected during hypoglossal stimulation; at C and D acetylcholine in dilutions of 1 in $2 \times 10^8$ and 1 in $10^8$ respectively. It will be seen that the stimulation effluent is slightly less active than ACh. 1 in $10^8$ and much more active than ACh. 1 in $2 \times 10^8$. That is to say, its activity in terms of acetylcholine is not different from that of a venous effluent obtained during hypoglossal stimulation from the

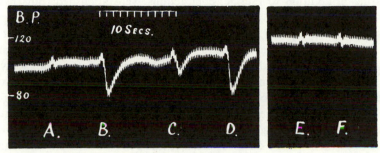

Fig. 6. Carotid blood-pressure of cat, eviscerated under chloralose. Eserine. A and B, 2 c.c. (i.v.) of venous fluids from cat's tongue under curarine. A before, B during motor nerve stimulation. C and D, 2 c.c. of ACh. dilutions; C, 1 in $2 \times 10^8$, D, 1 in $10^8$. E and F, same as at B and D, after 1·75 mg. atropine.

uncurarized and actively contracting tongue, in an average successful experiment. Between D and E 1 mg. of atropine was given, at E acetylcholine 1 in $10^8$ and at F the stimulation effluent.

The leech muscle is not rendered immediately insensitive to acetylcholine by curarine, so that, although no comparison can be obtained between different fluids containing curarine applied in succession to the same preparation, a qualitative contrast was easily demonstrated by applying them to two symmetrical strips of leech, previously sensitized by eserine. A preliminary test with acetylcholine showed that one strip was slightly more sensitive than the other. The control venous fluid from the tongue before stimulation was then tested on the more sensitive strip, and produced no perceptible effect, while the fluid collected during the period of hypoglossal stimulation caused prompt contraction of the other, less sensitive strip. A further application of the same fluid, however, was ineffective, the muscle being now affected by the curarine.

Brinkman and Ruiter [1924] had already shown that curare did not prevent the liberation from the frog's muscles, during nerve stimulation, of the substance stimulating the plain muscle of the cloaca. They stimulated the mixed nerves, however, and it seemed desirable to repeat the observation with stimulation of voluntary motor fibres only, through the ventral roots, and with a different physiological test for acetylcholine. The fluids were therefore compared on symmetrical leech strips, as above described, the hindlimbs of the frog being perfused with Ringer's solution containing both eserine and curarine. As with the tongue, the fluid collected before stimulation was inactive on one strip, while that collected during motor root stimulation, without contraction of the leg muscles, caused the usual contraction of the other leech preparation.

The experiments on the curarized tongue gave opportunity for a passing observation on another point. In the experiments with eserine but without curarine, we had always observed a conspicuous acceleration of the venous outflow when the hypoglossal nerves, freed from sympathetic fibres, were rhythmically stimulated. We had suspected that vaso-dilatation due to acetylcholine had some part in this effect; but we could not exclude mechanical action of the rhythmically contracting muscles, or the action of products of the contractile metabolism. In the experiments with curarine in addition to eserine, contractions were abolished, but the outflow was still accelerated, though only to the extent of 10 p.c., when the hypoglossal nerve was stimulated. When Locke's solution containing curarine, without eserine, was used for perfusion, no vaso-dilatation was caused by hypoglossal stimulation, just as we had earlier found that, if eserine was not present, no acetylcholine appeared in the venous effluent. We may safely attribute this residual vaso-dilator effect, therefore, to acetylcholine leaking from the motor nerve endings and, if eserine is present, reaching the blood vessels, where it causes arterial dilatation and diffuses into the fluid passing through the capillaries. It should be pointed out that, in the absence of heavy doses of eserine, this action could play no part in the vasodilatation which accompanies the contraction of a muscle with normal circulation.

These experiments with curarine show quite definitely that the appearance of acetylcholine in the perfusion fluid is not directly or indirectly connected with contraction of the muscle fibres. Feldberg and Vartiainen, in their experiments on the vagus and sympathetic ganglia, failed to find evidence for the liberation of acetylcholine by impulses passing along uninjured nerve fibres in continuity. We have had the privilege of reading in advance a forthcoming paper by Gaddum and Khayyal, who have observed the liberation of a small quantity of a substance acting on the leech like ACh., when faradic stimulation is applied to the end of a longer stretch of vagosympathetic (preganglionic) nerve. Without anticipating the details of this publication, we may say that, if the intramuscular portions of motor nerves liberated acetylcholine at the maximum rate observed by Gaddum and Khayyal, it would not make a significant contribution to the amount which we have obtained from the tongue during motor nerve stimulation. The only supposition which accords with our facts is that a motor nerve impulse, on reaching the nerve ending, there liberates a small charge of acetylcholine, in close proximity to the motor end plate or other structure immediately subjacent to the nerve ending; and that this liberation is not affected by curarine, in a dose sufficient to prevent the response of the muscle fibre to excitation by the nerve impulse.

## DISCUSSION

There is an obvious analogy between the release of acetylcholine by impulses arriving at motor nerve endings in voluntary muscle, for which evidence has been here presented, and its release by impulses reaching the endings of preganglionic fibres in ganglionic synapses. In both cases the chief interest of the phenomenon centres in the question of its relation to the transmission of the excitatory process, with very little delay, across the anatomical discontinuity usually regarded as existing between the nerve terminal, on the one hand, and the ganglion cell or muscle fibre on the other. It may be noted that Samojloff [1925] concluded, from its high temperature coefficient (Av. = 2·37), that the conduction of excitation from motor nerve ending to voluntary muscle involved a chemical process of some kind. He even suggested that a stimulant substance might be liberated at the nerve endings, and drew an analogy from Loewi's observations on the nervous control of the heart.

In the case of the sympathetic ganglion, the direct excitatory effect upon the cells exhibited by acetylcholine with artificial application is of the " nicotine " type [Dale, 1914], being annulled by the secondary, depressant effect of nicotine itself, or by curarine in sufficient concentration [Brown and Feldberg, 1936], but resistant to atropine. It has been shown [Feldberg and Gaddum, 1934; Feldberg and Vartiainen, 1934] that acetylcholine may escape into the fluid perfusing a ganglion, during preganglionic stimulation, in a concentration which excites the cells to the output of impulses, when it is artificially injected into the perfused ganglion; and it has been argued that this indicates its release at the synapses in a concentration which cannot be without excitatory effect. In the case of the voluntary muscle the position is less clear, owing to the relatively low concentration of acetylcholine in the perfusion effluent during motor stimulation, the reason for which has been already discussed, and to the more complex nature of the stimulant actions of acetylcholine, when artificially applied to various types of voluntary muscle. Striated, involuntary muscle fibres can, indeed, be found, such as the outer, striated muscle coat of the intestine in certain fishes [Méhes and Wolsky, 1932], and the sphincter of the pupil in birds, innervated by parasympathetic nerve fibres and responding to the application of acetylcholine with a type of contraction closely simulating the effects of impulses in those nerves; and in such cases the effects of acetylcholine and of parasympathetic impulses differ from those on analogous layers of plain muscle, only in the quickness of the contractile response and in its suppression by curare instead of by atropine.

The reactions to acetylcholine shown by the voluntary striated muscles of different vertebrates, on the other hand, are complex and variable, and it is necessary to consider them in some detail. In the first place, certain normal muscles of the frog, the tortoise and the bird exhibit a prolonged type of contracture, of low tension, in response to nicotine and to various bases which resemble it in action. Riesser and Neuschlosz [1921] first showed that acetylcholine produced this type of effect in relatively low concentrations. It was subsequently shown [Sommerkamp, 1928; Wachholder and Ledebur, 1930] that there are wide differences in the sensitiveness of different muscles of the frog and the tortoise to this action of acetylcholine, corresponding to differences in the prominence of contracture in their natural functions; and, according to Plattner and Krannich [1932], the same muscles show corresponding differences in the amounts of acetylcholine which they yield to artifical extraction. This contracture is relatively resistant to curare, and somewhat sensitive to atropine [Riesser and Neuschlosz, 1921]. Although it seems likely that this type of response has some relation to the normal, functional contractures exhibited by such muscles, it would be difficult to make a case for a participation of acetylcholine in the excitation of voluntary muscle fibres to quick contractions by motor nerve impulses, if this were the only detectable type of reaction shown by skeletal muscle to its artificial application. There is, however, another type of reaction, which the predominant interest given to muscles showing the contracture has been apt to obscure.

Langley [1907], in his experiments with nicotine on the frog's sartorius, showed that it first produced twitches, and a quick type of contraction resembling a short tetanus, prior to the slowly developing contracture. He made the significant observation that, with punctiform application of the alkaloid in low concentrations, the quick reactions could only be elicited from the neighbourhood of the nerve endings, from which the excitation was apparently propagated, whereas the contracture, while it could be produced in any part of the muscle fibres, usually remained localized to the region of application. Sommerkamp [1928] found that some frog's muscles give only quick contractions when immersed in acetylcholine, while others respond mainly by contracture. In the ilio-fibularis muscle the contracture was limited to a small part of the muscle, separable by dissection; the remainder, freed from it, gave only a quick evanescent contraction, when immersed in ACh. 1 in $10^5$. The normally innervated voluntary muscles of the mammal, with the exception of the small muscles moving the eyeball [Duke-Elder, 1930], are often regarded as insensitive to acetylcholine. They do, indeed show a striking contrast in this respect, under ordinary experimental conditions, to muscles denervated by motor fibre degeneration, which respond to very small injections of acetylcholine with a slow type of contraction. Feldberg and Minz [1931] and Feldberg [1933b], however, observed quick contractions and fibrillation of normal mammalian muscles when acetylcholine was injected in moderate doses (0·01-0·2 mg.) into the arteries supplying them. According to the Simonarts [1935a] the response of normal mammalian muscles to acetylcholine is very readily depressed by ether. In rabbits and cats in the early stages of anæsthesia by a barbiturate, or in spinal preparations freed from the preliminary ether by prolonged ventilation, they observed quick contractions of the muscles, unaffected by fresh section of the nerve supply, when doses of acetylcholine of the order of 1 mg. were injected intravenously. The reaction was unaffected by atropine, which, indeed, had to be given in advance, to eliminate the effects of such doses of acetylcholine on the heart and the blood vessels. On the other hand, the Simonarts found them to be suppressed by a quaternary ammonium salt having a curare action. Acetylcholine solutions applied to the bared surface of a muscle, or injected by a fine needle into its substance, caused brisk and fugitive contractions of fibres, or of whole bundles, localized to the neighbourhood of the application. In a more recent paper A. Simonart [1935b] describes results obtained with the more effective method of arterial injection. As was to be expected, the threshold dose of ACh. for normal cat's muscle was much lower by this method, and the tensions recorded with larger doses were of the order of those obtained with maximal indirect faradization. Curare readily abolished these effects. We hope to deal further with this aspect of our problem in a later paper.

Admittedly there are points still requiring further investigation. The relation of the reaction of denervated mammalian muscle to the quicker but less sensitive reaction of normal mammalian muscle, on the one hand, and to the persistent contracture of low tension shown by certain frog muscles on the other, does not seem to be adequately defined by the present evidence. In the case of the mammalian muscles, the facts still suggest that the presence of the normal nerve ending in some way hinders the access, to the sensitive point on the muscle fibre, of acetylcholine applied from without; just as we found that, with normal circulation, there appears to be some hindrance to the escape of acetylcholine from the neighbourhood of the motor nerve endings, where it is liberated by nerve impulses. It may be remarked that such restriction would not be unexpected, in a muscle consisting of fibres which can act as independent physiological units. However that may be, the point requiring emphasis for our purpose is the distinction between the quick contractions elicited by acetylcholine, apparently, on Langley's evidence, by excitation of the structures immediately subjacent to the motor nerve endings, and the persistent contractures produced in certain amphibian and other muscles.

As in the case of the ganglion synapses, the failure of eserine under normal conditions to facilitate or to prolong the excitatory effect of a motor nerve impulse, appears to have been regarded as evidence against the participation of acetylcholine in the transmission of the excitatory process [Kruta, 1935]. In neither case does the argument appear to us well founded. The motor nerve ending is in such immediate contact with the nucleated end plate or other structure, from which the excitatory process in the muscle fibre must start, that there is no room for destruction of acetylcholine during diffusion to its points of action, from which eserine might protect it. On the other hand, when acetylcholine has to reach muscle fibres by diffusion from a solution in which the whole muscle is immersed, the effect of low dilutions in producing contracture should be enchanced by eserine, as Kruta found it to be; just as we have found that eserine is necessary to protect acetylcholine during diffusion from the points of its release into the blood vessels.

The transmission of the effects of nerve impulses by a chemical substance, reaching the effector cells by diffusion, is now an accepted fact in the case of simpler types of contractile cells and tissues, usually displaying an automatic activity which the nerve impulses may modify in either direction. Such transmission by a diffusible stimulant can now be traced in the nervous control of most involuntary muscle, including, as we have seen, some which is striated and relatively quick in contraction. The question which here concerns us is whether in voluntary striated muscle, specialized for the quick contraction of individual fibres in response to nerve impulses, and normally at rest in their absence, this more primitive, chemical method of transmission has been superseded by an entirely different one, in which the chemico-physical disturbance constituting the nerve impulse passes, by continuous propagation, on to the muscle fibre; or whether, on the other hand, the required specialization has been effected by concentrating the release and the action of the chemical stimulant at the point of immediate contact of the nerve ending with the muscle fibre. An analogous question has already arisen in connection with the response to nerve impulses of more than one plain muscle structure. Henderson and Roepke [1934] find that stimulation of the pelvic nerve causes two kinds of reaction of the plain muscle of the urinary bladder—a quick contraction and a maintained tonus. They find that atropine readily abolishes the maintained tonus, just as it abolishes the response to acetylcholine applied from without, leaving the quick contraction. Similarly Bacq and Monnier [1935] distinguish a quick and a slow component in the response to stimulation of the cervical sympathetic nerve of the plain muscle retracting the nictitating membrane. They find that a synthetic substance " F. 933 " depresses the slow component, and with it the response to adrenaline, leaving the quick reaction unaffected, or even apparently enhanced. In both cases the observers suggest that the slower reaction is due to chemical transmission, but that this form of control is supplemented by the presence of certain nerve fibres ending directly in plain muscle cells, the propagated change constituting the nerve impulse being directly continued from these to the plain muscle, without chemical intervention. The number of nerve endings in such sheets of plain muscle is known to be small, in relation to the number of muscle cells. It appears to us that the quick reactions, in both these cases, may equally well be explained by the liberation of the transmitter in high concentration in immediate relation to, possibly within the limiting membranes of, the directly innervated cells; the slow reaction being then evoked by its escape and secondary diffusion on to other cells, in a manner analogous to its artifical application through the blood stream or from the surface. In the case of the vaso-dilator effect of the chorda tympani on the blood vessels of the tongue, which is typically resistant to atropine, there is direct evidence of such escape by diffusion of a chemical transmitter with all the properties of acetylcholine, causing contracture of adjacent voluntary muscle fibres if these have been denervated [Bremer and Rylant, 1924; Dale and Gaddum, 1930], and appearing in the blood or perfusion fluid flowing from the tongue [Feldberg, 1933a; Bain, 1933].

If Henderson and Roepke, Bacq and Monnier were right in postulating a supplementary, direct transmission of nerve impulses to plain muscle, when quick contraction is required, we should expect it to supersede entirely the chemical method of transmission, for nerve impulses causing excitation of the very rapid and individually reacting fibres of skeletal muscle, giving a single twitch, with minimal transmission delay, in response to each impulse. Similarly we should expect such a direct method of transmission at a ganglionic synapse, where each preganglionic impulse can evoke a single postganglionic impulse, again with minimal transmission delay. Such a conception, however, leaves us with no explanation of the release of acetylcholine at the preganglionic and the motor nerve endings. This can hardly be the survival of an archaic form of transmission, no longer having any function. In the ganglion acetylcholine has been shown to be liberated in a concentration which effectively stimulates ganglion cells; while in the muscle we have shown that, when the liberation of acetylcholine fails by exhaustion, the excitation of the muscle no longer occurs. There seem to be two possibilities.

30

(1) That the propagated disturbance in the nerve fibre is directly transmitted to the effector cell, but that the latter cannot accept it for further propagation unless sensitized by the action of the acetylcholine, which appears with its arrival at the nerve ending. Such an hypothesis might be stated in terms of Lapicque's well-known conception, by supposing that the action of acetylcholine shortens the chronaxie of the nerve cell, or of the motor end plate of the muscle fibre, so that it is momentarily attuned to that of the nerve. H. Fredericq [1924] has observed, indeed, a shortening of the chronaxie of heart muscle by acetylcholine.

(2) That the acetylcholine, in these as in other cases, acts as the direct stimulant of nerve cell or muscle end plate, releasing an essentially new propagated wave of excitation in postganglionic nerve or muscle fibre, which, however, may so resemble that in the preganglionic or motor nerve fibre as to simulate an unbroken propagation. On this view there is no introduction of a new form of transmission, in evolution from the slowest and most primitive to the most rapid and specialized. The required rapidity of transmission is attained by concentrating the release of the chemical transmitter on the actual surface of the responsive structure.

Of the two possibilities, the latter appears to us to be more easily reconciled with the facts yet available concerning transmission at ganglionic synapses. The former would provide an explanation, alternative to that which we have considered earlier, for the apparently low sensitiveness of some normal muscles to stimulation by acetylcholine. The shortness of the delay in transmission appears to cause no greater difficulty for one conception than the other. The action of curare is explicable, in either case, as rendering the receptive element resistant to the action of acetylcholine, whether this may be merely to sensitize or directly to stimulate. On the existing evidence we favour the second conception, while admitting that further facts are required for the exclusion or the establishment of either.

As in the case of transmission at the ganglionic synapse [cf. Feldberg and Vartiainen, 1934], either of the above conceptions of the function of acetylcholine, in the transmission of excitation to the voluntary muscle fibre, would require not only its liberation in immediate relation to the excitable structure, but presumably its very rapid disappearance when the excitatory wave in the muscle had been started. The known extreme liability of acetylcholine to the action of an esterase naturally comes to mind in that connection; but there is no direct experimental evidence to justify an assumption that this esterase is, in fact, responsible for removing acetylcholine from the site of its action in this case, and that eserine would, therefore, increase its persistence at that site. Nor can we predict the effect of such persistence on the transmission under particular conditions, if it could be proved to occur. All that our evidence shows is, that acetylcholine which has escaped from the sites of its liberation requires protection by eserine to enable it to diffuse into a fluid perfused through the blood vessels.

## SUMMARY

1. Stimulation of the motor nerve fibres to perfused voluntary muscle causes the appearance of acetylcholine in the venous fluid.

2. Direct stimulation of a normal muscle, or of one deprived only of its

autonomic nerve supply, has a similar result; but when the muscle is completely denervated no acetylcholine appears in response to effective stimulation.

3. When transmission of excitation from the nerve to the perfused muscle is prevented by curarine, stimulation of the motor nerve fibres causes the usual release of acetylcholine.

4. When conduction from motor nerve fibres to perfused muscle fails from exhaustion, after repeated stimulation, acetylcholine is no longer released by stimulation of either nerve or muscle.

5. The function of acetylcholine in the transmission of excitation from nerve to voluntary muscle is discussed.

We are indebted to Dr H. King for the supply of pure curarine, and to Dr H. Schriever for kind assistance in certain experiments.

## REFERENCES

Bacq, Z. M. and Monnier, A. M. (1935). *Arch. int. Physiol.*, **40**, 467, 485.

Bain, W. A. (1933). *Quart. J. exp. Physiol.*, **23**, 381.

Barsoum, G., Gaddum, J. H. and Khayyal, M. A. (1934). *J. Physiol.*, **82**, 9P.

Bremer, F. and Rylant, P. (1924), *C.R. Soc. Biol.*, Paris, **90**, 982.

Brinkman, R. and Ruiter, M. (1924). *Pflüger's Arch.*, **204**, 766.

Brinkman, R. and Ruiter, M. (1925). *Ibid.*, **208**, 58.

Brown, G. L. and Feldberg, W. (1936). *J. Physiol.*, **86**, 10P.

Bülbring, E. and Burn, J. H. (1935). *Ibid.*, **83**, 483.

Dale, H. H. (1914). *J. Pharmacol.*, Baltimore, **6**, 147.

Dale, H. H. (1935a). *Proc. R. Soc. Med.*, **28**, 15.

Dale, H. H. (1935b). *Nothnagelvorträge*, Nr. 4. Wien: Urban u. Schwarzenberg.

Dale, H. H. and Feldberg, W. (1934). *J. Physiol.*, **81**, 39P.

Dale, H. H. and Gaddum, J. H. (1930). *Ibid.*, **70**, 109.

Dale, H. H. and Gasser, H. S. (1926). *J. Pharmacol.*, Baltimore, **29**, 53.

Duke-Elder, W. S. and Duke-Elder, P. M. (1930). *Proc. Roy. Soc.*, **107**, 332.

Feldberg, W. (1933a). *Pflüger's Arch.*, **232**, 88.

Feldberg, W. (1933b). *Ibid.*, **232**, 75.

Feldberg, W. and Gaddum, J. H. (1934). *J. Physiol.*, **81**, 305.

Feldberg, W. and Minz, B. (1931). *Arch. exp. Path. Pharmak.*, **163**, 66.

Feldberg, W., Minz, B. and Tsudzimura, H. (1934). *J. Physiol.*, **81**, 286.

Feldberg, W. and Vartiainen, A. (1934). *Ibid.*, **83**, 103.

Franel, L. (1935). *Arch. int. Physiol.*, **41**, 256.

Frank, E. and Katz, R. A. (1921). *Arch. exp. Path. Pharmak.*, **90**, 149.

Frank, E., Nothmann, M. and Hirsch-Kauffmann, H. (1922). *Pflüger's Arch.*, **197**, 270.

Fredericq, H. (1924). *C. R. Soc. Biol.*, Paris, **91**, 1171.

Geiger, E. and Loewi, O. (1922). *Biochem. Z.*, **127**, 66.

Henderson, V. E. and Roepke, M. H. (1934). *J. Pharmacol.*, Baltimore, **51**, 97.

Hess, W. R. (1923). *Quart. J. exp. Physiol.* (Suppl.), p. 144.

Hinsey, J. C. and Cutting, C. C. (1933). *Amer. J. Physiol.*, **105**, 535.

Kruta, V. (1935). *Arch. int. Physiol.*, **41**, 187.

Langley, J. N. (1907). *J. Physiol.*, **36**, 347.

Langworthy, O. R. (1924). *Johns Hopk. Hosp. Bull.*, **35**, 239.

Méhes, J. and Wolsky, A. (1932). *Arb. Ung. Biol. Forsch.*, **5**, 139.

Plattner, F. (1932). *Pflüger's Arch.*, **130**, 705.

Plattner, F. (1933). *Ibid.*, **232**, 342.

Plattner, F. and Krannich, E. (1932). *Ibid.*, **229**, 730; **230**, 356.

Riesser, O. and Neuschlosz, S. M. (1921). *Arch. exp. Path. Pharmak.*, **91**, 342.

Samojloff, A. (1925). *Pflüger's Arch.*, **208**, 508.

Shimidzu, K. (1926). *Ibid.*, **211**, 403.

Simonart, A. and Simonart, E. F. (1935a). *Arch. int. Pharmacodyn.*, **49**, 302.

Simonart, A. (1935b). *Ibid.*, **51**, 381.
Sommerkamp, H. (1928). *Arch. exp. Path. Pharmak.*, **128**, 99.
Wachholder, K. and Ledebur, J. (1930). *Pflüger's Arch.*, **225**, 627.

## Acetylcholine in Mammalian Neuromuscular Transmission

AFTER reviewing experimental results described in the literature, Acheson[1] came to the conclusion in 1948 that the amount of acetylcholine liberated by a single impulse at a presynaptic nerve terminal in muscle and sympathetic ganglia is probably of the order of $1 \cdot 5 \times 10^{-16}$ gm. ($10^{-18}$ moles). He pointed out the large discrepancy between this quantity and the relatively large amounts ($3 \times 10^{-14}$ moles) hitherto found necessary for excitation when applied directly to the muscle. This discrepancy has been much reduced in recent years by the electrophoretic application of acetylcholine from micropipettes[3,7], and spikes have been produced in frog muscle fibres by this method with as little as $5 \cdot 5 \times 10^{-16}$ moles[7].

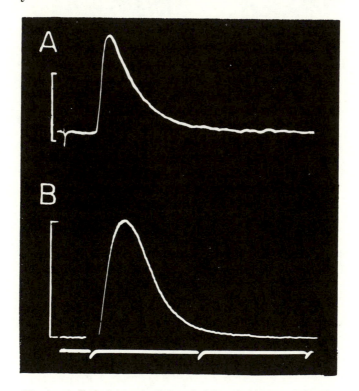

Fig. 1. *A*, End-plate potential evoked by stimulation of phrenic nerve at 2 c./s. The muscle was paralysed by $15 \cdot 0$ m$M$ magnesium. *B*, Acetylcholine potential evoked in another muscle by a 1 msec. pulse of current ($3 \cdot 5 \times 10^{-8}$ amp.) at a rate of 1 c./s. In both cases, muscles were rat diaphragms, at 24–25° C.; the potentials were recorded with intracellular electrodes. Voltage scale: 5 mV. in *A* and 10 mV. in *B*. Common time scale: 10 msec.

Reprinted from *Nature* 182: 805–806 (1958) by permission of the publisher.

However, there still remained a substantial difference, and most of the potentials obtained by this method have not been strictly comparable with end-plate potentials elicited by nerve stimulation since they have a much slower time-course. For example, the quickest potential published by del Castillo and Katz[3] rose to its maximum in 13 msec. These authors concluded that much faster potentials, and even greater sensitivity to acetylcholine, would be expected in the case of nervous release of acetylcholine, where the diffusion distance is less than $1\mu$ ; in their experiments, the distance of the acetylcholine pipette from the end-plate was estimated to be $10-20\mu$ (in a later paper[4], they mention potentials with a rise time of 2–5 msec.).

By the use of a similar technique, we have found that acetylcholine potentials could be produced in the rat diaphragm with amounts as small as $1.5 \times 10^{-17}$ moles (assuming a transport number of $0.3$ for ACh+). The experiments were performed *in vitro*, at room temperature (24–25° C.), with an intracellular recording electrode (filled with 3 $M$ potassium chloride) in the end-plate region of a muscle fibre ; jets of acetylcholine were delivered from an external micro-pipette filled with 2–4 $M$ acetylcholine (as chloride, Roche Products) by square outward current pulses lasting $0.1$ to $1.0$ msec. The lowest values were obtained with $0.1$ msec. pulses. No allowance was made for the appreciable loss of current to be expected with such short pulses in view of the relatively high pipette resistance and capacitance to earth.

The amplitude and time course of the fastest acetylcholine potentials were extraordinarily sensitive to the slightest disturbance. The fastest potentials had a time course comparable with that of end-plate potentials evoked by nerve stimulation. Fig. 1 shows on the same time scale the potential produced with a 1 msec. pulse of acetylcholine ($3.5 \times 10^{-11}$ coulombs or $10^{-16}$ moles) and a typical end-plate potential in another diaphragm paralysed by $15.0$ m$M$ magnesium (the voltage scales differ by about 15 per cent). The rise time to the maximum of the acetylcholine potential is approximately twice as long as the corresponding time for the end-plate potential ($1.3$ msec.). A time lag of about 3 msec. is consistent with a diffusion distance of about $4\mu$. The peak of the acetylcholine potential is somewhat more rounded than that of the end-plate potential, but its rate of fall is fairly similar, so that the total durations of the two potentials differ by relatively little.

It seems that with the present technique an even closer approximation to nervous transmission is likely to be limited by the width of the end plate (19–28$\mu$ in the rat diaphragm[2]). The rounded peak of the acetylcholine potential might well be caused by saturation of the receptors closest to the pipette.

Although some discrepancy may therefore be expected to remain, the value computed somewhat indirectly by Acheson ($10^{-18}$ moles) is quite likely to be too small by a factor of at least 10, as suggested by Acheson himself, since most experimental errors would tend to reduce it. As a further source of error, presynaptic failure of nerve conduction may well occur during repetitive stimulation[5]; it is particularly likely under conditions of reduced oxygen supply[6] such as would be expected during the perfusion of muscle with Locke solution as in the experiments reviewed by Acheson.

K. Krnjević
R. Miledi*

Physiology Department,
Australian National University,
Canberra.

* Rockefeller Foundation Fellow.

[1] Acheson, G. H., *Fed. Proc.*, **7**, 447 (1948).
[2] Cole, W. V., *J. Comp. Neurol.*, **108**, 445 (1957).
[3] del Castillo, J., and Katz, B., *J. Physiol.*, **128**, 157 (1955).
[4] del Castillo, J., and Katz, B., *J. Physiol.*, **132**, 630 (1956).
[5] Krnjević, K., and Miledi, R., *J. Physiol.*, **140**, 440 (1958).
[6] Krnjević, K., and Miledi, R., *J. Physiol.*, (in the press).
[7] Nastuk, W. L., *Fed. Proc.*, **12**, 102 (1953).

# THE RELEASE OF ACETYLCHOLINE IN THE ISOLATED RAT DIAPHRAGM

By K. KRNJEVIĆ AND J. F. MITCHELL

*From the A.R.C. Institute of Animal Physiology, Babraham, Cambridge*

(*Received* 17 *June* 1960)

It is generally believed that acetylcholine (ACh) is responsible for the transmission of activity from nerve to muscle in vertebrates. This belief is based principally on a large amount of evidence that ACh has a powerful specific stimulating action on the muscle end-plate and that various agents which interfere with, or promote, its action have a corresponding effect on neuromuscular transmission (Riesser & Neuschlosz, 1921; Brown, 1937; Rosenblueth, 1950; Eccles, 1953; Fatt, 1954; Katz, 1958). There is very much less evidence that ACh is in fact released by the motor nerve endings. Since the classical experiments of Dale, Feldberg & Vogt (1936), comparatively little work has been published dealing with this problem. With few exceptions (e.g. Emmelin & MacIntosh, 1956) recent studies of the factors that influence release of ACh have been confined to experiments on sympathetic ganglia.

As a result, a large discrepancy has remained between the amounts of ACh known to be released in muscle, and the amounts needed for stimulation (cf. Acheson, 1948). There are, of course, many reasons why such a discrepancy might be expected (cf. Rosenblueth, 1950; Fatt, 1954; del Castillo & Katz, 1956), and the gap has tended to diminish in recent years, thanks to the more efficient application of ACh to end-plates from micropipettes (Nastuk, 1953; del Castillo & Katz, 1956; Krnjević & Miledi, 1958c). Nevertheless, even the smallest effective amount of ACh has been at least 15 times greater than the amount estimated to be released by a nerve ending.

In the experiments about to be described we have studied the release of ACh in the isolated diaphragm. This muscle seemed particularly suitable for such an investigation because much is already known about its behaviour during repetitive stimulation and about the amounts of ACh needed to produce end-plate activity (Krnjević & Miledi, 1958b, c). It is also convenient for various technical reasons: it has a long nerve, and only single innervation of its muscle fibres, and as it is flat and thin the inward diffusion of $O_2$ and the outward diffusion of ACh take place under relatively favourable conditions. We have shown in a previous paper (Krnjević &

Mitchell, 1960*b*) that one half of the extracellular ACh can diffuse out in $1\frac{1}{2}$ min.

Failure of neuromuscular transmission tends to occur rather quickly during sustained repetitive stimulation of the nerve, and this is accompanied by a marked reduction in the release of ACh (Dale *et al.* 1936). We have therefore endeavoured to keep the rate and duration of stimulation to a minimum determined by the sensitivity of the methods of bioassay. Our results show that ACh (or some very similar substance) can be collected in amounts which would be sufficient to produce appreciable depolarization if applied directly to the end-plate. A preliminary report of some of these results has already appeared (Krnjević & Mitchell 1960*a*). A comprehensive study of the release of ACh in the rat diaphragm during prolonged stimulation at various frequencies and temperatures has been published recently by Straughan (1960).

### METHODS

Albino rats (Wistar strain) weighing between 200 and 400 g were used exclusively. They were anaesthetized with ether, and the left hemidiaphragm and phrenic nerve were removed and placed in cold (15° C) Ringer–Locke solution thoroughly aerated with 5 % $CO_2$ in $O_2$. The period during which the diaphragm was without an extra supply of oxygen (after opening the chest and before completing the dissection), varied between 3 and 5 min. The composition of the Ringer–Locke solution is given in the previous paper (Krnjević & Mitchell, 1960*b*).

*Muscle holder.* In most cases the hemidiaphragm was cut from its costal insertion and after trimming off excess connective tissue was tied to a rectangular Perspex frame at each corner. This operation was performed in Ringer–Locke solution at room temperature, with a fast stream of oxygen bubbles keeping the solution well stirred and aerated. The Perspex holder had a central turret with five platinum electrodes over which the phrenic nerve could be drawn when the muscle was to be stimulated (Fig. 1). The top of the turret was closed by a disk of Perspex, sealed with tap grease; under these conditions, the nerve remained moist for periods of at least $\frac{1}{2}$ hr, but, for safety, the nerve was left in the solution except during the periods of stimulation. Two types of frame were used, the second being somewhat smaller and lighter, and trapezoid in shape.

*Collecting chamber.* The muscle holder, with the muscle stretched out, fitted accurately into shallow rectangular (or trapezoid) chambers in a Perspex slab. When 5 ml. of solution was added the depth of fluid in the chamber was sufficient to keep the diaphragm well immersed. (For the lighter frames smaller chambers were used and only 3 ml. of solution.) There were several such chambers adjacent in the slab, and the holder, with the diaphragm attached, could conveniently be transferred from one to another without disconnecting the flexible leads of the electrodes. To maintain an adequate $O_2$ supply a fine polythene cannula was attached to the frame and a constant stream of $O_2$ (with 5 % $CO_2$) bubbles was directed at the muscle throughout (cf. Creese, 1954). Although most experiments were done at room temperature, the chamber could be kept at a higher temperature by placing the slab on a special warm water-bath.

*Electrical stimulation and recording.* With five electrodes it was possible to monitor continuously the spike potential of the phrenic nerve during stimulation. The second recording electrode was very close to the entrance of the nerve into the diaphragm; as long as the recorded spike was adequately diphasic, one could be sure that impulses were being transmitted to the intramuscular branches. The stimulating pulses had a duration of 10 $\mu$sec and their intensity was usually kept at 1·5–3 times maximal for the fastest A fibres, except during a high-frequency tetanus when it was raised to 5 times maximal.

### Procedure

The muscle was placed in one of the collecting chambers and stimulated for a given period. It was allowed to remain in the chamber for a further period of either 2 or 4 min, and then replaced in a large volume of aerated Ringer–Locke solution; as a rule there was no further stimulation for 30–60 min. When studying the release of ACh after a tetanus, the muscle was stimulated at a rate of 100–250/sec for 15–20 sec in a second chamber, and after 45–60 sec was shifted to a third chamber in which the standard period of stimulation at a lower frequency was repeated. The solutions were removed with a pipette and either assayed for ACh immediately, or kept on ice if the assay was delayed by an hour or so; they were in any case assayed within 2–3 hr of collection.

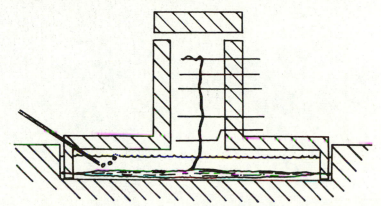

Fig. 1. Diagrammatic cross-section of rat diaphragm frame and chamber. Rat diaphragm is tied across the bottom of the frame, in Ringer–Locke solution bubbled continuously with $O_2 + CO_2$ mixture. Phrenic nerve passes over stimulating, earthing and recording electrodes. Top of frame is sealed with a greased Perspex disk.

*Preservation of ACh.* The hydrolysis of ACh was minimized by adding $1·5 \times 10^{-5}$ M eserine sulphate to the solution in which the diaphragm was soaked for about 30 min before stimulating. In some experiments di-*iso*-phosphorofluoridate (DFP) was injected into the rats intraperitoneally in doses of 1–2 μmole/100 g body weight. This normally caused the animals to die after a period of some 3–5 min, when the diaphragm was removed as usual. As a further precaution, in a number of experiments, we used a solution rendered somewhat acid (pH 6·2–6·7 instead of 7·3–7·4) by reducing the bicarbonate content.

### Assay of ACh

Since it was important to stimulate the diaphragm preparations as little as possible, only very small amounts of ACh were available for assay. It was therefore essential to use methods of assay which were highly sensitive, as well as reasonably specific. Since the frog rectus was too insensitive, a number of other preparations were tried in turn, with varying degrees of success. A few attempts at assaying with the frog lung (Corsten, 1940), were not very profitable, because of enormous variations in sensitivity. In four experiments longitudinal muscles from the locally available sea-cucumber (*Holothuria forscali*) were not found to be any more sensitive to ACh than the frog rectus, unlike longitudinal muscles of other sea-cucumbers which have a very low threshold to ACh (Bacq, 1939; Florey, 1956). The following methods were more successful (Fig. 3) although each had its disadvantages. The accuracy of the assays varied with different preparations; it is estimated that the error of the best assays did not exceed ± 20 %, and that of the poorest ± 50 %.

*Cat blood pressure.* The samples were injected intravenously into eviscerated cats under chloralose anaesthesia (80 mg/kg), as in the method described by MacIntosh & Perry (1950). Although this was not a particularly sensitive method, it was little affected by moderate variations in the ionic concentration and pH of samples, and regularly gave predictable results.

*Isolated rat duodenum.* A short length of duodenum (2–2·5 cm) was taken from immediately below the stomach of a small rat (100–200 g), and after washing suspended in a 1 ml. Perspex bath through which oxygen was bubbled. The solution in the bath (De Jalon, Bayo &

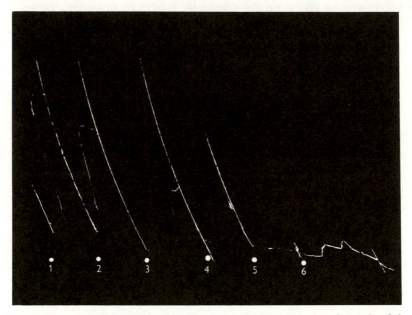

Fig. 2. Part of assay of ACh released from rat diaphragm on dorsal muscle of the leech with curare control. (1) 55 nM-ACh; (2) test solution (3 stim/sec for 5 min); (3) 2·8 nM-ACh; (4) 55 nM-ACh 7 min after tubocurarine ($1·5 \times 10^{-5}$ M); (5) 55 nM-ACh 11 min after curare; (6) test solution 15 min after curare. After prolonged rinsing in curare-free solution, sensitivity to ACh returned.

De Jalon, 1945) was run through continuously (4–6 ml./min), except when test solutions were added. The volume of the fluid in the bath was kept constant at 1·0 ml. and the temperature maintained at 32° C. Movement of the gut was recorded by a balanced lever on a kymograph. ACh could be detected in concentrations as low as $5 \times 10^{-11}$ M, although the usual threshold was at $1–3 \times 10^{-10}$ M. The test solutions were added to the bath (after equilibration at the correct temperature) in volumes of 0·1–0·4 ml.; larger volumes gave misleading results owing to insufficient dilution of the Ringer–Locke with De Jalon's solution. Although this preparation was very sensitive to ACh it deteriorated rather quickly, becoming more and more sensitive to slight changes in temperature, ionic composition (especially $Ca^{2+}$), pH or rate of flow of solution. It could only be used as a reliable method of assay for a rather small number of samples.

*Dorsal muscle of the leech.* The dorsal muscle was set up as described by MacIntosh &

Perry (1950), but in an 0·3 ml. Perspex bath and, on some occasions, with the addition of morphine sulphate ($1·5 \times 10^{-5}$ M) to all solutions to facilitate relaxation (Murnaghan, 1958).

*Heart of Mya arenaria (Hughes, 1955).* The heart was suspended by the ventricles in 1 ml. artificial sea water (Tower & McEachern, 1948) at 16° C. The heart beat was recorded on a smoked drum. Although this preparation can be extremely sensitive, with threshold concentrations as low as $2 \times 10^{-13}$ M, it is highly unpredictable, and the very sensitive hearts are not common. Furthermore, it has the great drawback that ACh often causes the beat to become not only weaker but slower; assaying can then be done only over a very small range of concentrations, since an amount 5–10 times threshold is likely to stop the beat altogether for a time. In this respect it is evidently unlike the heart of *Venus mercenaria* (Welsh & Taub, 1948). Its use would seem to be limited to cases in which very high sensitivity is absolutely essential and it can hardly be recommended for routine use.

*ACh controls.* The amounts of solution available were always too small for a really exhaustive series of control tests. However, whenever conditions were suitable, at least one control test was performed (this happened on the average once in every three assays). The most convenient procedure was to destroy the ACh in the sample by adding one-tenth volume of N/3-NaOH, letting the solution stand for 20 min at room temperature, and then neutralizing it with N/3-HCl. Specific antagonism by such drugs as curare (Fig. 2) or atropine was only used occasionally as a terminal experiment, the effects being too slowly reversible to allow useful assays to be performed again.

In several experiments the diaphragm was soaked initially in Ringer–Locke solution containing no anticholinesterase. No ACh could be detected under these conditions, even after prolonged stimulation.

*Counts of fibres in the rat diaphragm.* The counts were made in histological sections of diaphragms used in the experiments described above. The muscles were fixed in 10% formol saline and embedded in paraffin, and sections which included the entire width of the hemidiaphragm were cut at right angles to the fibres.

## RESULTS

Most of the experiments were done at room temperature (19–23° C), because neuromuscular transmission in the isolated diaphragm persists for a longer period at lower temperatures (cf. Krnjević & Miledi, 1959). In fifteen experiments the temperature was kept at 37° C.

Only those experiments in which appreciable amounts of ACh were collected could be considered as yielding really useful information. The rejection of other experiments was based mostly on evidence that adequate excitation of the nerve endings was not taking place for various technical reasons, such as short-circuiting or displacement of stimulating electrodes, or because of obvious injury to the phrenic nerve or one of its main branches. Contraction of the diaphragm was not in itself very informative, since twitches of relatively few fibres may give the impression of widespread activity. However, in a substantial number of cases we failed to detect any ACh at all (this means less than about one tenth of the usual amount); sometimes this turned out to be because our anticholinesterases had lost their potency, but in other cases there was no obvious explanation.

*ACh release at room temperature.* On the basis of previous experiments with the phrenic-diaphragm preparation it was decided that there was a reasonable chance of avoiding presynaptic failure of propagation if stimulation was effected at a rate not greater than 5/sec or did not last more than 5 min, arbitrarily limiting the number of impulses in one sequence of stimulation to 1500 or less. Results of experiments in which these limits were exceeded are considered separately. Clearly, even more moderate stimulation was preferable whenever the assay preparations were sufficiently sensitive; in several cases it was possible to obtain sufficient ACh while stimulating at 2/sec for 2–5 min. A few hearts of *Mya arenaria*

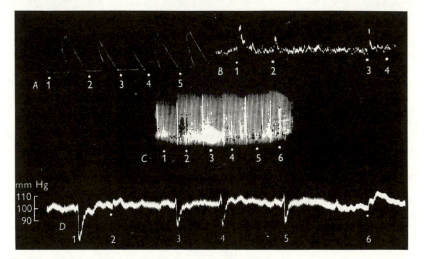

Fig. 3. Assay of ACh released from rat diaphragm during stimulation. Examples shown do not necessarily include complete assay. *A* Dorsal muscle of leech: (1) Test solution (5 stim/sec for 20 min); (2) 28 nM-ACh; (3) Test solution, alkali-treated; (4) Test solution; (5) 33 nM-ACh. *B* Rat duodenum: (1) Test solution (5 stim/sec for 5 min); (2) 11 nM-ACh; (3) 22 nM-ACh; (4) test solution, alkali-treated. Test solutions were diluted 5 times. *C* Heart of *Mya arenaria*: (1) 5·5 nM-ACh; (2) test solution (1·8 stim/sec for 15 min); (3) 4·3 nM-ACh; (4) test solution; (5) test solution, alkali-treated; (6) 5·5 nM-ACh. Test solutions were diluted 3 times. *D* Cat blood pressure: (1) 0·25 nmole ACh; (2) 1·0 ml. Ringer–Locke solution; (3) 0·1 nmole ACh; (4) 1·0 ml. test solution (5 stim/sec for 5 min); (5) 0·1 nmole ACh; (6) 1·0 ml. test solution, alkali-treated.

were so sensitive that we tried to stimulate even at 1/sec for only 2 min; the results were not very satisfactory, partly because such sensitive hearts tended to respond irregularly in the presence of solutions which had been in contact with the muscle, and partly because the yield seemed to be reduced, perhaps as a result of destruction by minimal amounts of cholinesterases or because of binding in the tissue (cf. Krnjević & Mitchell, 1960*b*).

The mean release of ACh from the hemidiaphragm, in twenty-four experiments at temperatures of 19–23° C, was 0·12 pmole (S.D. ± 0·079) per impulse. These results were obtained by assaying the collected ACh either on the heart of *Mya arenaria*, the rat duodenum or the cat blood pressure (Fig. 3). Although these three methods of assay gave comparable answers, the mean result of assays on the rat duodenum was somewhat larger (0·19 pmole/impulse) than the mean value of assays on the heart of *Mya arenaria* (0·064 pmole), and the mean value of assays on the cat blood pressure which had an intermediate position (0·098 pmole). There was much overlap of individual results and the general scatter was such that no statistical significance can be attached to these deviations from the over-all mean (the greatest difference between mean values obtained with different preparations has a probability of just $> 0.05$, and the other differences have probabilities $> 0.25$ on the null-hypothesis, as determined by the $t$ test).

*ACh release at 37° C.* No systematic study was made of the release of ACh from the same muscle at different temperatures. The mean release in six muscles excited at 2–3/sec for 5 min at 37° C was 0·15 pmole/impulse. The ACh was assayed on leeches and the rat duodenum. These results overlapped those at a lower temperature; it does not seem that there is a very pronounced change in the amount liberated at the higher temperature.

### ACh release under other conditions

*Release during faster and longer stimulation.* The mean yield of ACh during activity at 37° C in a group of seven muscles stimulated at frequencies of 10–20/sec for 10–20 min was 0·025 pmole (range 0·011–0·033), i.e. one-sixth of the yield in a comparable series of six muscles during stimulation at 2–5/sec for 5 min. Similar differences were observed in experiments at room temperature. If the preparation was stimulated tetanically (at 100–200/sec) for 10–20 sec, the total number of impulses being greater than when stimulating at a slow rate for 5 min, the yield of ACh was as a rule below threshold amounts for assay.

*Release of ACh in the presence of curare.* In ten experiments a comparison was made of the yield of ACh during ordinary activity and activity during paralysis by curare. After the preliminary control series the muscle was soaked for 30–60 min in $3 \times 10^{-5}$ M tubocurarine chloride, and then stimulated as before in $3 \times 10^{-6}$ M tubocurarine (with the usual amount of anticholinesterase also present). In two experiments there was no marked change in the yield of ACh per impulse. Figure 4 shows the assay on the heart of *Mya arenaria* of solutions obtained during indirect stimulation of a hemidiaphragm before and after soaking in tubocurarine. It can be seen that the sensitivity of the preparation to ACh was reduced by the presence of tubocurarine in the solution. However, the assay could be performed satisfactorily by adding the same amount of tubocurarine to the standard ACh solution used for comparison. There was clearly no appreciable increase in the release of ACh in the presence of tubocurarine. In two other experiments the ACh release apparently rose by 50 and 100 %, respectively, and in one experiment it diminished by 15 %. In the five remaining experiments various technical difficulties in assaying prevented any accurate quantitative comparison, but it was evident that there was no marked change after curare: any difference could not have exceeded a factor of 2–3.

When simple solutions of ACh were compared with those in which the muscle had contracted, it was often found that the latter caused irregular

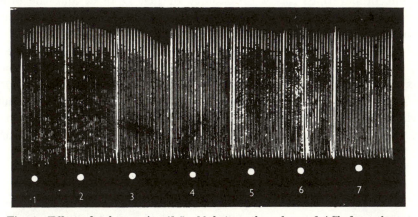

Fig. 4. Effect of tubocurarine ($1.5 \times 10^{-5}$ M) on the *release* of ACh from the rat diaphragm. Assay on heart of *Mya arenaria*: (1) Test solution (2 stim/sec for 5 min) alkali-treated; (2) test solution; (3) 2·8 nM-ACh; (4) test solution, alkali-treated; (5) 2·8 nM-ACh + tubocurarine ($1.5 \times 10^{-5}$ M); (6) test solution from curarized diaphragm; (7) 1·7 nM-ACh. Test solutions were diluted 3 times.

variations in base line, and also in ACh sensitivity. There was some evidence that solutions which had bathed muscles paralysed by curare were less likely to give rise to such effects, suggesting that disturbing factors are released mainly during contraction of the muscle fibres.

*Spontaneous release of ACh.* In some experiments the diaphragm was allowed to soak in the collecting chamber in the presence of anticholinesterase, but without stimulating the nerve. The period of soaking was usually 5–7 min, as in most experiments. In the majority of cases no ACh was found in the solution (i.e. less than $10^{-10}$–$10^{-9}$ M, depending upon the sensitivity of the assay). In several cases, however, there was an appreciable quantity of ACh in the solution, equivalent to a spontaneous release of about 1 pmole per hemidiaphragm per minute (at room temperature). The lower limit of the range of estimates was set, as always, by the threshold concentration for assay, and values of 0·5 pmole/min or less were mainly seen when the period of soaking was extended to 30–60 min. The upper limit was reached in one experiment, in which the very high, apparently spontaneous, release of 9 pmole/min was seen twice out of four trials with one muscle; in the other two trials there was no detectable release. The high apparent rate of release in this case may conceivably have resulted from contamination with ACh.

*Post-tetanic release of ACh.* In seven experiments we were able to compare the yield of ACh before and after short tetani at a high frequency. Altogether fourteen such comparisons were made, as it was possible to repeat this procedure several times with some preparations.

It was clearly preferable to use the lowest possible rate of stimulation during the periods before and after tetanus. Unfortunately, it is important

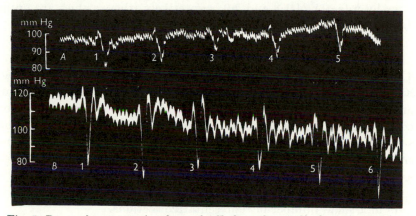

Fig. 5. Pre- and post-tetanic release of ACh from the rat diaphragm assayed on cat blood pressure. *A* (1) 0·023 nmole ACh; (2) 1·0 ml. test solution (5 stim/sec for 4 min); (3) 0·02 nmole ACh; (4) 1·0 ml. test solution (5 stim/sec for 4 min 50 sec after end of tetanus); (5) 0·023 nmole ACh. *B* (1) 1·0 ml. test solution (5 stim/sec for 5 min); (2) 0·03 nmole ACh; (3) 1·0 ml. test solution; (4) 0·025 nmole ACh; (5) 1·0 ml. test solution (5 stim/sec for 5 min, 60 sec after end of tetanus); (6) 0·03 nmole ACh.

to be able to analyse several samples quickly and reliably in this kind of experiment whereas the most sensitive methods of assay proved often very erratic, and seldom gave results at the highest level of sensitivity for very long. We were therefore only able to perform satisfactorily two experiments stimulating at 1 or 2/sec. The most stable conditions for assaying were available when using the cat blood pressure, which was relatively insensitive and required stimulation at 5/sec.

The periods of stimulation before and after the tetanus lasted 4 or 5 min and the second one usually began 45–60 sec after the end of the tetanus (120–250/sec for 10–20 sec), to allow at least some of the ACh which might have accumulated during the tetanus to diffuse out. In fact only very small amounts of ACh were usually found after such tetanization, and three control experiments, in which the muscle was returned to the original chamber 45–60 sec after the end of the usual short tetanus and left there without further stimulation for 7 min, did not give a higher final concentration of ACh. These controls are in any case only of somewhat academic interest, since the twelve experiments performed when stimulating at 5/sec did not show a significant change in the release of ACh. The mean value of the twelve ratios of post-tetanic to pre-tetanic release was 1·08, with a standard error of $\pm 0·05$. Examples of assays of solutions obtained in these experiments are shown in Fig. 5. On the other hand, two experiments performed at a low rate of stimulation (1 and 2/sec) suggested that more ACh was released after the tetanus, the yields being greater by a factor of 1·8 and 2·0, respectively (these values are unlikely to be incorrect by more than $\pm 0·3$ and $\pm 0·5$).

## Counts of fibres in the rat diaphragm

The numbers of muscle fibres counted by one observer in histological sections of 3 hemidiaphragms came to 7896, 10,384 and 11,407, the mean count being 9896. As there is always some degree of arbitrary selection in deciding what is and what is not a 'fibre' in such sections, three other observers also counted independently the fibres in the first specimen; their estimates were 7094, 8016 and 8294. All four counts differed from the mean value by less than 10 %. These results confirm an estimate of 10,000 ($\pm 20 \%$) made by Krnjević & Miledi (1958a) on the basis of fibre counts in a small number of representative sections.

### DISCUSSION

*Identification of ACh.* The amounts of substance released from the diaphragms were always so small that it was not possible to identify ACh with an extremely high degree of certainty by performing a series of parallel assays on different preparations (cf. Chang & Gaddum, 1933). However, if we consider that the active substance was only obtained in the presence of anticholinesterase, that it was destroyed in alkaline solutions, that different methods of bioassays gave approximately the same estimate in terms of ACh, and that such specific antagonists as curare and atropine had the expected action, notwithstanding the fact that these observations were made at different times, we can conclude that the substance in question is very likely to be ACh, or at least a similar choline ester.

*Site of release.* We have not excluded the possibility that ACh is released by antidromic activation of sensory nerve fibres in the diaphragm, but it is very unlikely that so much could be released by sensory fibres in view of the observations of Dale *et al.* (1936) and Brecht & Corsten (1941). It is clear that autonomic nerve fibres were not involved, since stimuli just maximal for the fast A fibres were adequate for the release of ACh.

### Amounts collected

As the muscles were bathed in 3 or 5 ml. of solution, the external concentration of ACh could never be greater than 1 or 2 % of that in the extracellular space of the muscle (the free ACh space in the diaphragm is 25 ml./ 100 g (Krnjević & Mitchell, 1960*b*); i.e. 0·05 ml. in a typical hemidiaphragm weighing 200 mg). If we assume that ACh released during stimulation is free to diffuse out, and to simplify matters, that the rate of outward movement is simply proportional to the amount already present, we can calculate approximately what fraction ($f$) of the total ACh released can be expected to remain in the muscle at a given time.

$$f = \frac{T}{ts} \left\{ \exp - \frac{(t - ts)}{T} - \exp - \frac{t}{T} \right\},$$

where $T$ is the time constant of outward movement, $ts$ the period of stimulation, and $t$ the total period in the bath from the beginning of stimulation. It was found in previous experiments (Krnjević & Mitchell, 1960*b*) that one half of the 'extracellular' ACh leaves the diaphragm in 1·5 min, and that the remainder moves out with a time constant of 3·6 min. Taking therefore a value of 2·9 min for $T$, the amount of ACh collected during a 7 min period, which includes a 5 min period of stimulation (our usual procedure), would come to 76 % of the total ACh released. It seems reasonable to conclude that our method would enable us to collect some 3/4 of the ACh in the muscle which was free to diffuse out.

### Release of ACh per impulse

Previous authors who have made observations on the release of ACh in the rat diaphragm have tended to use a standard technique in which the diaphragm is stimulated at 50/sec for 20 min (e.g. Burgen, Dickens & Zatman, 1949; Brownlee, 1957). It is very unlikely that the nerve endings would be capable of releasing ACh in anything like the normal amount at such a frequency and for such a long time. In any case it is certain that most phrenic nerve fibres would very soon begin to fail to transmit impulses at such a frequency, so that the over-all effective contribution of the nerve endings would be at a much lower rate (Krnjević & Miledi, 1958*b*, 1959). Hence it is not surprising that the yield of ACh per impulse in such experiments (about 0·006 pmole per hemidiaphragm) is considerably less than we have found when stimulating at 2–5/sec for periods of 2–5 min (0·12 pmole). In our own experiments faster and longer periods of stimulation yielded substantially less ACh per impulse. Even more significant are the observations made recently by Straughan (1960), who has analysed systematically the release of ACh from the rat diaphragm during 20 min periods of stimulation at frequencies varying between 6/sec and 100/sec. He has found that increasing the rate of stimulation causes only a relatively small increase in total ACh release, which reaches a maximum at about 25/sec with little further change up to 100/sec.

The highest relative yield obtained by Straughan (1960) during stimulation at 6/sec for 20 min was about one quarter of the average amounts which we collected. Most of this difference can be ascribed to the shorter periods and lower rates of stimulation in our experiments, although other experimental factors such as temperature and methods of assay may have tended to exaggerate it.

It should not be thought surprising that comparatively small variations in the frequency of stimulation may lead to marked changes in the release of ACh at the nerve endings. In the curarized rat diaphragm the amplitude of the end-plate potential is very sensitive to the frequency of stimulation: Lundberg & Quilish (1953) have shown that an impulse is followed by a period of presynaptic depression lasting at least 3 sec, during which a second end-plate potential is appreciably reduced, presumably because of a smaller release of ACh. According to our own observations the end-plate potential in the curarized diaphragm is almost immediately reduced to about one third when the frequency of nerve stimulation is changed from 1/10 sec to 2–5/sec. It is highly probable that much lower rates of stimulation than we were able to use would be required to demonstrate the maximal release of ACh.

*Spontaneous release of ACh.* The finding of a spontaneous release of ACh in a number of unstimulated diaphragms confirms the observations of Straughan (1960), although the typical amounts were smaller by about one half, perhaps because of the lower temperature (cf. Liley, 1956). Such a small release is equivalent to 1/20–1/30 of the usual rate of release during stimulation, and would not as a rule be detected after soaking the muscle for only 5–7 min. It is most unlikely that injury discharge of the phrenic nerve could contribute appreciably to the spontaneous release, since no spontaneous twitching could be observed. To liberate this amount of ACh, one quarter of all the fibres would have to twitch at a mean rate of 1/sec.

The release of about 1 pmole/min can probably be correlated with the spontaneous miniature electrical activity recorded at the end-plate. The relatively small size of the end-plate potential during stimulation at 2–5/sec suggests that its quantum content may not be much more than 20. Taking our figure of 0·12 pmole for the release of ACh per impulse, a quantum of ACh would correspond to about 0·006 pmole (per hemidiaphragm). It follows that a spontaneous quantal release at 3/sec (well within the common frequency range of miniature end-plate potentials in the diapragm; Liley, 1956) would be sufficient to give 1 pmole/min. However, it is difficult to associate single presynaptic vesicles (cf. del Castillo & Katz, 1956) with this release, which is equivalent to $3.6 \times 10^5$ molecules per quantum at a single nerve ending and would require an improbably high concentration of ACh (10M) within the 500 Å vesicles. Furthermore, the total bound ACh in the rat phrenic nerve endings (about 300 pmole according to preliminary observations by C. O. Hebb and K. Krnjević) would be accounted for by only 50,000 vesicles per nerve ending; if the density of vesicles is $1000/\mu^3$ of axon terminal, as in the frog (Birks, Huxley & Katz, 1960), the total volume of terminal would be only $50 \mu^3$, compared with $3000 \mu^3$ in frog muscle. Such a small volume seems unlikely if one considers that the motor ending spreads over an area with a diameter of some $20\mu$ on the diaphragm fibres (Cole, 1957).

*Yield of ACh in the presence of tubocurarine.* Our results confirm previous evidence that curare does not prevent the release of ACh in muscle (Dale *et al.* 1936; Emmelin & MacIntosh, 1956); they also show that under its influence there is no marked increase in the amounts of ACh which can be collected, presumably because the reaction between ACh and the receptor is so rapid (cf. del Castillo & Katz, 1957) that formation of a relatively stable receptor–curare compound does not displace any appreciable amount of fixed ACh. This is in contrast with the action of dibenamine on sympathetic transmission in the spleen (Brown & Gillespie, 1957).

*ACh release during post-tetanic potentiation (PTP).* It is unfortunate that it was not possible to perform most of the experiments on PTP under conditions more likely to give a conclusive answer. In most cases stimulation had to be at 5/sec, at which frequency PTP is not nearly so marked as, for instance, at 0·5/sec. We have found in the curarized rat diaphragm that PTP does clearly occur at 5/sec (Fig. 6), although its duration was shorter than during stimulation at lower frequencies, when appreciable PTP may be detected for over 6 min. The enormous apparent potentiation of the end-plate immediately after the end of the tetanus was probably largely caused by a short gap of 2–5 sec between the end of the tetanus and the resumption of stimulation at 5/sec.

It can be seen from the second curve in Fig. 6 that if one waited some 45–60 sec before resuming stimulation after the tetanus there was a much more rapid decline of PTP when testing is resumed, so that the curve soon joined and then followed that obtained by the usual procedure. This behaviour, which has been seen at other frequencies of testing stimuli, suggests that the rate of decay of PTP depends upon time rather than on the discharge of impulses.

Inspection of such PTP curves obtained during stimulation at 5/sec shows that if there is an increased post-tetanic release of ACh (Hutter, 1952) the mean increment over a period of 4–5 min is unlikely to exceed 10 % of the pre-tetanic release (assuming a simple relation between height of end-plate potential and ACh release). Our results are consistent with

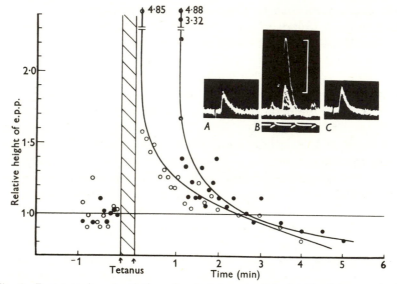

Fig. 6. Post-tetanic potentiation of end-plate potentials (at 5/sec) in curarized rat diaphragm, recorded beginning 5 sec (O—O) and 60 sec (●—●) after the end of tetanic stimulation of the phrenic nerve (250/sec for 20 sec). Inset, examples of intracellular potentials actually recorded: *A*, before tetanus; *B*, 10 sec after tetanus; *C*, 30 sec after tetanus; vertical scale 1 mV, horizontal scale 10 msec.

such a change, but they are too variable to be conclusive evidence one way or the other. On the other hand, the two results obtained during stimulation at a lower frequency can only be considered as suggestive evidence that appreciably more ACh may be released after a tetanus. The ephemeral nature of PTP during activity at 5/sec supports previous evidence that PTP may not be of great significance for normal function (Ström, 1951).

### Release of ACh per nerve ending

With a mean number of 10,000 muscle fibres in the hemidiaphragm, we can take the release of ACh by an average ending to be about $10^{-17}$ mole per impulse (fibres in the diaphragm only extremely rarely show evidence of multiple innervation (Lundberg & Quilish, 1953; Liley, 1957; and personal observations)). This amount of ACh is 10–20 times greater than previous estimates, calculated rather indirectly (e.g. Acheson, 1948; R. I. Birks, quoted by MacIntosh, 1959). It has been shown previously (Krnjević & Miledi, 1958c) that substantial end-plate potentials can be produced iontophoretically in the diaphragm with as little as $10^{-17}$–$10^{-16}$ mole of ACh; very short pulses of current were used, and under these conditions the ACh potentials were practically indistinguishable from normal end-plate potentials. We have already mentioned reasons for believing that the number of quanta released by impulses is likely to be reduced in our experiments, so that the amounts of ACh released can be compared directly with the amounts needed to produce 5–10 mV ACh potentials without gross error. It is clear that, although there is overlap of extreme values, a small gap remains between typical values; this is not surprising, since the liberation of ACh from a point source at the tip of a micropipette is inherently less efficient than the release of a similar amount spread over the whole area of the end-plate; the amounts which we have collected are likely to be substantially short of the maximal release for various reasons already mentioned. One can conclude that for the rat diaphragm the quantitative agreement between the effectiveness of applied ACh and its release during stimulation is about as satisfactory as could be expected.

### SUMMARY

1. Estimations have been made by bioassay methods of the release of ACh in the isolated rat hemidiaphragm caused by not more than 1500 maximal impulses in the phrenic nerve (at frequencies of 2–5/sec). The mean release in twenty-four experiments was 0·12 pmole per impulse at room temperature.

2. The rate of release was substantially less during stimulation at a higher frequency and for longer periods.

3. The yield of ACh during low-frequency stimulation was not increased to any pronounced extent in experiments performed at 37° C, or in the presence of tubocurarine.

4. Post-tetanic potentiation during stimulation at 1–2/sec (in two experiments) was associated with a greater release of ACh; at 5/sec, although the mean increase was of the order expected, there was too much variation for the change to be significant.

5. Spontaneous release of ACh was seen in some cases, in amounts which are not incompatible with those expected from the spontaneous activity at the end-plate.

6. The calculated mean release of ACh in the rat diaphragm from a single nerve ending ($10^{-17}$ mole) during low-frequency stimulation is of

the same order of magnitude as the smallest amounts of ACh which have previously been found to be effective when applied directly to the end-plate in the rat diaphragm.

## REFERENCES

ACHESON, G. H. (1948). Physiology of neuromuscular junctions: chemical aspects. *Fed. Proc.* **7**, 447–457.

BACQ, Z. M. (1939). Un test marin pour l'acétylcholine. *Arch. int. Physiol.* **49**, 20–24.

BIRKS, R., HUXLEY, H. E. & KATZ, B. (1960). The fine structure of the neuromuscular junction of the frog. *J. Physiol.* **150**, 134–144.

BRECHT, K. & CORSTEN, M. (1941). Acetylcholin in sensiblen Nerven. *Pflüg. Arch. ges. Physiol.* **245**, 160–169.

BROWN, G. L. (1937). Transmission at nerve endings by acetylcholine. *Physiol. Rev.* **17**, 485–513.

BROWN, G. L. & GILLESPIE, J. S. (1957). The output of sympathetic transmitter from the spleen of the cat. *J. Physiol.* **138**, 81–102.

BROWNLEE, G. (1957). The action of Polymyxin E on the neuromuscular junction. *J. Physiol.* **136**, 19–20P.

BURGEN, A. S. V., DICKENS, F. & ZATMAN, L. J. (1949). The action of botulinum toxin on the neuro-muscular junction. *J. Physiol.* **109**, 10–24.

CHANG, H. C. & GADDUM, J. H. (1933). Choline esters in tissue extracts. *J. Physiol.* **79**, 255–285.

COLE, W. V. (1957). Structural variations of nerve endings in the striated muscles of the rat. *J. comp. Neurol.* **108**, 445–464.

CORSTEN, M. (1940). Bestimmung kleinster Acetylcholinmengen an Lungenpräparat des Frosches. *Pflüg. Arch. ges. Physiol.* **244**, 281–291.

CREESE, R. (1954). Measurement of cation fluxes in rat diaphragm. *Proc. Roy. Soc.* B, **142**, 497–513.

DALE, H. H., FELDBERG, W. & VOGT, M. (1936). Release of acetylcholine at voluntary motor nerve endings. *J. Physiol.* **86**, 353–380.

DE JALON, P. G., BAYO, J. B. & DE JALON, M. G. (1945). Sensible y nuevo metodo de valoracion de adrenalina en utero aislado de rata. *Farmacoterap. actual.* **11**, 313–318.

DEL CASTILLO, J. & KATZ, B. (1956). Biophysical aspects of neuro-muscular transmission. *Progr. Biophys.* **6**, 121–170.

DEL CASTILLO, J. & KATZ, B. (1957). A comparison of acetylcholine and stable depolarizing agents. *Proc. Roy. Soc.* B, **146**, 362–368.

ECCLES, J. C. (1953). *The Neurophysiological Basis of Mind.* Oxford: Clarendon Press.

EMMELIN, N. & MACINTOSH, F. C. (1956). The release of acetylcholine from perfused sympathetic ganglia and skeletal muscles. *J. Physiol.* **131**, 477–496.

FATT, P. (1954). Biophysics of junctional transmission. *Physiol. Rev.* **34**, 674–710.

FLOREY, E. (1956). The action of Factor I on certain invertebrate organs. *Canad. J. Biochem. Physiol.* **34**, 669–681.

HUGHES, B. (1955). The isolated heart of *Mya arenaria* as a sensitive preparation for the assay of acetylcholine. *Brit. J. Pharmacol.* **10**, 36–38.

HUTTER, O. F. (1952). Post-tetanic restoration of neuromuscular transmission blocked by D-tubocurarine. *J. Physiol.* **118**, 216–227.

KATZ, B. (1958). Microphysiology of the neuromuscular junction. A physiological 'quantum of action' at the myoneural junction. *Johns Hopk. Hosp. Bull.* **102**, 275–295.

KRNJEVIĆ, K. & MILEDI, R. (1958a). Motor units in the rat diaphragm. *J. Physiol.* **140**, 427–439.

KRNJEVIĆ, K. & MILEDI, R. (1958b). Failure of neuromuscular propagation in rats. *J. Physiol.* **140**, 440–461.

KRNJEVIĆ, K. & MILEDI, R. (1958c). Acetylcholine in mammalian neuromuscular transmission. *Nature, Lond.,* **182**, 805–806.

KRNJEVIC, K. & MILEDI, R. (1959). Presynaptic failure of neuromuscular propagation in rats. *J. Physiol.* **149**, 1–22.

KRNJEVIĆ, K. & MITCHELL, J. F. (1960a). Release of acetylcholine in rat diaphragm. *Nature, Lond.*, **186**, 241.

KRNJEVIĆ, K. & MITCHELL, J. F. (1960b). Diffusion of acetylcholine in agar gels and in the isolated rat diaphragm. *J. Physiol.* **153**, 562–572.

LILEY, A. W. (1956). An investigation of spontaneous activity at the neuromuscular junction of the rat. *J. Physiol.* **132**, 650–666.

LILEY, A. W. (1957). Spontaneous release of transmitter substance in multiquantal units. *J. Physiol.* **136**, 595–605.

LUNDBERG, A. & QUILISH, H. (1953). Presynaptic potentiation and depression of neuro-muscular transmission in frog and rat. *Acta physiol. scand.* **30**, Suppl. 111, 111–120.

MacINTOSH, F. C. (1959). Formation, storage and release of acetylcholine at nerve endings. *Canad. J. Biochem. Physiol.* **37**, 343–356.

MacINTOSH, F. C. & PERRY, W. L. M. (1950). Biological estimation of acetylcholine. *Methods med. Res.* **3**, 78–92.

MURNAGHAN, M. F. (1958). The morphinized-eserinized leech muscle for the assay of acetylcholine. *Nature, Lond.*, **182**, 317.

NASTUK, W. L. (1953). Membrane potential changes at a single muscle end-plate produced by transitory application of acetylcholine with an electrically controlled microjet. *Fed. Proc.* **12**, 102.

RIESSER, O. & NEUSCHLOSZ, S. M. (1921). Physiologische und kolloidische Untersuchungen über den Mechanismus der durch Gifte bewirkter Kontraktur quergestreifter Muskeln. *Arch. exp. Path. Pharmak.* **91**, 342–365.

ROSENBLUETH, A. (1950). *The Transmission of Nerve Impulses at Neuro-effector Junctions and Peripheral Synapses.* New York: John Wiley and Sons, Inc.

STRAUGHAN, D. W. (1960). The release of acetylcholine from mammalian motor nerve endings. *Brit. J. Pharmacol.* **15**, 417–424.

STRÖM, G. (1951). Physiological significance of post-tetanic potentiation of the spinal monosynaptic reflex. *Acta physiol. scand,* **24**, 61–83.

TOWER, D. B. & McEACHERN, D. (1948). Experiences with the 'Venus' heart method for determining acetylcholine. *Canad. J. Res. Zool.* **26**, 183–187.

WELSH, J. H. & TAUB, R. (1948). The action of choline and related compounds on the heart of *Venus mercenaria. Biol. Bull., Woods Hole*, **95**, 346–353.

*Chapter 2*

# ACETYLCHOLINE
*Storage and Metabolism*

As the field of synaptic neurochemistry has developed over the last half century, acetylcholine (ACh) has been the prototypic neurotransmitter. Despite the fact that specific differences in detail have emerged between synapses that release ACh and those that release other transmitters, investigations involving cholinergic junctions have had broad physiological significance. As examples, studies of cholinergic synapses led to the first demonstration of chemical synaptic transmission, generated the idea that transmitters are stored in vesicles, and recently opened up promising approaches to the investigation of receptors in membranes.

Given this perspective, it is perhaps not surprising that the early experiments of W. Feldberg and T. Mann (1945, 1946) and of D. Nachmansohn (Nachmansohn and Machado, 1943; Nachmansohn and Berman, 1946) on the biosynthesis of ACh led to the discovery of a cofactor of fundamental importance for biochemistry. These investigators showed that synthesis of ACh in brain extracts required a metabolic precursor of acetate (such as pyruvate or citrate), choline, adenosine triphosphate, and an unidentified cofactor. About the same time, F. Lipmann and N. Kaplan (1946) discovered a cofactor requirement for another enzymatic acetylation reaction in which sulfanilamide was the acetyl-acceptor. Lipmann showed that the two cofactors were identical, and the new acetylation cofactor was called coenzyme A (CoA). The discovery of CoA quickly led to the realization that acetylation of choline, catalyzed by choline acetyltransferase, requires only two substrates: the acetylated cofactor (acetyl-CoA) and choline (Korkes, *et al.*, 1952).

$$\text{Acetyl-CoA + Choline} \xrightleftharpoons{\text{choline acetyltransferase}} \text{ACh + CoA}$$

55

The source of acetyl-CoA in neurons, as in other cells, is oxidative metabolism. The choline required for transmitter synthesis, however, ultimately must be provided by extracellular sources. Hemicholinium compounds block choline uptake into nerve terminals, and the *in vitro* biosynthesis of ACh cannot be maintained for long periods in the absence of an exogenous source of choline or in the presence of hemicholinium.

Hydrolysis of ACh to acetate and choline, catalyzed by the enzyme acetylcholinesterase, completes the pathway of metabolism.

$$ACh + H_2O \xrightarrow{\text{acetylcholinesterase}} Acetate + Choline$$

This enzyme is responsible for the destruction of extracellular ACh released during synaptic transmission (see Chapter 6). Pharmacological evidence (see below) indicates that acetylcholinesterase is also active presynaptically and plays a role in regulating ACh levels in cholinergic nerve terminals. The classical studies of I.B. Wilson (1960) elucidated many mechanistic details of ACh hydrolysis by acetylcholinesterase. His experiments indicated that ACh binds to the enzyme at two sites, one specific for the quaternary ammonium moiety of ACh and the other for its esteratic group. Acyl transfer then occurs through nucleophilic attack on the ester carbonyl by a serine residue in the enzyme, releasing choline and forming an acyl-enzyme intermediate. Hydrolysis of the acyl-enzyme, the rate-limiting step, completes the over-all reaction. Organophosphorus compounds, such as diisopropyfluorophosphonate (DFP) and several nerve gases, are powerful and irreversible acetylcholinesterase inhibitors, which form stable acyl-enzyme intermediates, thus inactivating the enzyme.

Within the presynaptic nerve terminals a large part of the ACh is contained in vesicles, as first indicated by the findings of V. Whittaker, I. Michaelson, and J. Kirkland (1964, reprinted here). Vesicles that are 300 to 800 Å in diameter and enclosed by membrane were first observed in nerve terminals in 1954–55, shortly after the demonstration of the quantal release of ACh from the presynaptic nerve. This prompted several investigators to propose that the transmitter is stored in vesicles and released directly from them into the synaptic cleft (see Chapter 5).

In order to demonstrate directly that vesicles contain ACh, V. Whittaker and E. De Robertis independently attempted to isolate synaptic vesicles from nervous tissue and to characterize them chemically. They found that gentle homogenization of brain in isotonic sucrose, followed by fractionation of the homogenate by differential and density gradient sedimentation, yielded a particulate fraction containing ACh. Electron microscopic examination of the fraction, however, revealed that the main component was not vesicles, but pinched-off nerve terminals, which were named synaptosomes. These were identified on the basis of the mitochondria and vesicles that they contained and the bits of postsynaptic membrane adhering to many of the synaptosomes.

Whittaker, Michaelson, and Kirkland (1964) demonstrated that synaptosomes can be lysed by osmotic shock and further fractionated by sucrose density gradient centrifugation. One of the fractions containing ACh consisted largely of vesicles. These experiments also illustrated the usefulness of such preparations for subcellular localization of the enzymes of transmitter synthesis and metabolism. Choline acetyltransferase was present largely in the soluble cytoplasmic fraction, and acetylcholinesterase was associated with membranous fractions. ACh itself was found in both cytoplasmic and vesicular fractions. Whether the ACh found outside vesicles is actually cytoplasmic or is derived from vesicles disrupted during homogenization is not clear.

R. Birks and F. MacIntosh (1961, reprinted here) investigated the factors controlling ACh synthesis in physiological situations. It was well known before these studies were initiated that levels of ACh in tissues are maintained over long periods despite widely varying degrees of nervous activity. Clearly, transmitter that is released must be replaced, and the question is: how is this accomplished? Three general models can be proposed. First, the amount of ACh released, even under the most extreme physiological conditions, might be small in comparison with the stores present in the terminals. If so, then presynaptic transmitter levels would not change during activity, and alteration of the rate of ACh synthesis would be unnecessary. Second, release could alter the presynaptic level of ACh, but cause no compensatory increase in synthesis. According to this model, as the level of ACh fell, so also the amount released per impulse might fall. Hence the amount of transmitter released at any time would depend on the previous history of activity of the releasing nerve ending. Third, the amount released could be a significant portion of the stored ACH, but the rate of its synthesis would be coupled to the rate of release so that released transmitter would be replaced immediately.

Model three received strong support from the detailed and elegant experiments of Birks and MacIntosh (1961) on a perfused sympathetic ganglion from the cat. Only the preganglionic axons and terminals in the ganglion are cholinergic; the postsynaptic cells contain norepine-phrine or dopamine. Therefore studies on ACh synthesis and turnover in the whole ganglion provide an accurate index of the events in preganglionic cells.

The experiments of Birks and MacIntosh led to several important conclusions about ACh synthesis under physiological conditions. First, during physiological activity, the presynaptic neurons release much more ACh than is normally present in the resting ganglion, and the dif-ference is provided by increased rates of synthesis during stimulation. Stimulation produces no deficit in the amount of ACh in the ganglion. Second, in order to maintain adequate rates of ACh synthesis during stimulation, the neurons require an external source of choline. Finally, a two-fold increase in the steady-state ACh content of the ganglion results from administration of the cholinesterase inhibitor, eserine. This increase suggests that, even in the resting terminal, ACh normally turns over continually, owing to the action of acetylcholinesterase. More recent experiments on cholinergic terminals in a neuromuscular preparation strengthened this interpretation by showing that a charged cholinesterase inhibitor (which presumably does not enter cells) does not cause an increase in ACh content (Potter, 1970). It is inter-esting to note that Birks and MacIntosh observed that the amount of ACh released per impulse did not change when the ACh content of the ganglion increased. Thus changes in the level of transmitter in a tissue may have no effect on its release from nerve terminals.

Other experiments on ACh synthesis in intact tissue, using incorpor-ation of radioactive choline to measure synthetic rates (Collier and MacIntosh, 1969; Potter, 1970), have confirmed the basic findings of Birks and MacIntosh. The methods used in these later experiments have also demonstrated that a considerable portion of the choline arising from hydrolysis of released ACh by acetylcholinesterase can be taken up and reused for ACh synthesis.

All these experiments, showing that ACh synthesis is coupled to release, raise the question of how ACh synthesis is regulated. A mech-anism involving feedback inhibition—such as may regulate the synthesis of norepinephrine (in Vertebrates) and GABA (in Crustacea)—appears unlikely, because *in vitro* studies have shown that only very high levels of ACh inhibit isolated choline acetyltransferase (Glover and Potter, 1971). Such concentrations presumably would occur only in vesicles, whereas the studies of V. Whittaker and of F. Fonnum (1968) suggest that choline acetyltransferase is largely localized to the soluble cyto-plasm. Other investigators have proposed an alternative model in which the rate of synthesis of ACh is limited by mass action: as ACh is released from the terminal by impulses, the resulting drop in cyto-plasmic ACh concentration would accelerate synthesis simply by displacement of equilibrium (Glover and Potter, 1971; Bennett and McLachlan, 1972b). Although the mechanism regulating ACh synthesis is unclear, these studies demonstrate that in cholinergic nervous tissue, transmitter metabolism is closely linked to neuronal activity, and responds dramatically and exquisitely with enhanced or diminished rates of synthesis to the physiological demands of altered cell stimulation.

## READING LIST

*Reprinted Papers*

1. Birks, R.I., and F.C. MacIntosh (1961). Acetylcholine metabolism of a sympathetic ganglion. *Can. J. Biochem. Physiol.* 39: 787–827.
2. Whittaker, V.P., I.A. Michaelson, and R.J.A. Kirkland (1964). The separation of synaptic vesicles from nerve-ending particles ('synaptosomes'). *Biochem J.* 90: 293–303.

*Historical Papers*

3. Dale, H.H., W. Feldberg, and M. Vogt (1936). Release of acetyl-choline at voluntary motor nerve endings. *J. Physiol.* 86: 353–380.
4. Nachmansohn, D. and A.L. Machado (1943). The formation of acetylcholine. A new enzyme: "choline acetylase." *J. Neuro-physiol.* 6: 397–403.
5. Feldberg, W. and T. Mann (1945). Formation of acetylcholine in cell-free extracts from brain. *J. Physiol.* 104: 8–20.
6. Feldberg, W. and T. Mann (1946). Properties and distribution of the enzyme system which synthesizes acetylcholine in nervous tissue. *J. Physiol.* 104: 411–425.
7. Lipmann, F. and N.O. Kaplan (1946). A common factor in the enzymatic acetylation of sulfanilamide and of choline. *J. Biol. Chem.* 162: 743–744.
8. Nachmansohn, D. and M. Berman (1946). Studies on choline acetylase. III. On the preparation of the coenzyme and its effect on the enzyme. *J. Biol. Chem.* 165: 551–563.
9. Korkes, S., A. del Campillo, S.R. Korey, J.R. Stern, D. Nachman-

sohn, and S. Ochoa (1952). Coupling of acetyl donor systems with choline acetylase. *J. Biol. Chem.* 198: 215–220.

10. Wilson, I.B. (1960). "Acetylcholinesterase," in P. Boyer, H. Lardy, and K. Myrbäck (Eds.), *The Enzymes,* Vol. 4, pp. 501–520. New York: Academic Press.

*Other Selected Papers*

11. Fonnum, F. (1968). Choline acetyltransferase binding to and release from membranes. *Biochem. J.* 109: 389–398.

12. Marchbanks, R.M. (1968). Exchangeability of radioactive acetylcholine with the bound acetylcholine of synaptosomes and synaptic vesicles. *Biochem. J.* 106: 87–95.

13. Collier, B. and F.C. MacIntosh (1969). The source of choline for acetylcholine synthesis in a sympathetic ganglion. *Can. J. Physiol. Pharmacol.* 47: 127–135.

14. Potter, L.T. (1970). Synthesis, storage and release of [$^{14}$C] acetylcholine in isolated rat diaphragm muscles. *J. Physiol.* 206: 145–166.

15. Glover, V.A.S. and L.T. Potter (1971). Purification and properties of choline acetyltransferase from ox brain striate nuclei. *J. Neurochem.* 18: 571–580.

16. Bennett, M.R. and E.M. McLachlan (1972a). An electrophysiological analysis of the storage of acetylcholine in preganglionic nerve terminals. *J. Physiol.* 221: 657–668.

17. Bennett, M.R. and E.M. McLachlan (1972b). An electrophysiological analysis of the synthesis of acetylcholine in preganglionic nerve terminals. *J. Physiol.* 221: 669–682.

18. Whittaker, V.P., W.B. Essman, and G.H.C. Dowe (1972). The isolation of pure cholinergic synaptic vesicles from the electric organs of Elasmobranch fish of the family Torpedinidae. *Biochem. J.* 128: 833–846.

# ACETYLCHOLINE METABOLISM OF
# A SYMPATHETIC GANGLION[1]

R. Birks and F. C. MacIntosh

## Abstract

The synthesis, storage, and release of acetylcholine (ACh) were studied in perfused and intact superior cervical ganglia of cats. ACh was determined by bio-assay in ganglion extracts and in the venous effluent from ganglia perfused with fluid containing an anticholinesterase drug. Of the extractable ACh in a normal ganglion, about 85% is "depot ACh" available for release by nerve impulses. This must be located in the nerve endings; most of the remainder is in the intraganglionic portions of the preganglionic axons. The depot ACh exists as two fractions, of which one, the smaller, is the more readily available for release by nerve impulses. ACh synthesis and release go on at a measurable low rate in the absence of nerve impulses; both are greatly accelerated by activity. Under physiological conditions of excitation and perfusion, ACh release does not outrun ACh synthesis; but synthesis is slowed, with consequent depletion of depot ACh and reduction in ACh release, if choline is absent from the extracellular fluid, or if the hemicholinium base HC-3 is present. The latter compound specifically inhibits ACh synthesis by competing with choline; as a result it produces delayed block in repetitively activated cholinergic pathways. For efficient synthesis of ACh during experiments lasting an hour or so, a ganglion need be supplied with no substances other than choline and the constituents of Locke's solution; for the efficient release of ACh, the perfusion fluid must also contain $CO_2$ and an unidentified factor present in plasma. ACh accumulates above the resting level in a ganglion whose cholinesterase has been inactivated, provided that the perfusing fluid is one that supports ACh synthesis; the additional ACh is not immediately available for release by nerve impulses. Under physiological conditions of perfusion the amount of ACh set free by each maximal preganglionic volley is highest in a ganglion that has been at rest, and is then independent of stimulation frequency; after repetitive activation for several minutes the volley output is lower and is only frequency-independent at rates of excitation below 20/second. Consideration is given to the probable intracellular locations of the several fractions of the ganglionic ACh, and to their interrelationship.

## Introduction

The metabolism of acetylcholine (ACh) at active nerve endings was first studied quantitatively by Brown and Feldberg (1). In their procedure the superior cervical ganglion of a cat was perfused with eserinized Locke's solution and subjected to prolonged repetitive stimulation by way of its preganglionic trunk; the ACh released from the activated nerve endings diffused into the perfusion fluid, and could be estimated in successive samples of the venous effluent; and finally the ganglion and its unstimulated fellow were extracted with trichloroacetic acid and the ACh content of each was determined. In such experiments Brown and Feldberg found regularly that the rate of ACh liberation was high at the beginning of stimulation, but fell off progressively to reach, after 20–30 minutes, a much lower level, which was then maintained with little further decline. It might have been expected that the ganglion would be found at this point to have lost most of its initial store of ACh, especially as the total

[1]Manuscript received October 12, 1960.
Contribution from the Department of Physiology, McGill University, Montreal, Que.

amount it had released exceeded the amount it had contained to start with. In fact no such loss was found: the stimulated ganglion and the control, when extracted, yielded about the same amount of ACh. Thus, although degeneration experiments (2, 3) showed clearly that most of the extractable ACh of the ganglion must be in the nerve endings, it remained in doubt how far this ACh could be taken to represent the depot from which the transmitter is discharged when nerve impulses arrive at the synapses.

Other workers have confirmed the findings of Brown and Feldberg, and on the basis of their own experiments have tried to explain the paradoxical association of a declining ACh output with a well-maintained store of ganglionic ACh. Thus Kahlson and MacIntosh (4) suggested that stimulation did deplete the ACh depots, but that the deficit went unobserved because ACh was rapidly reformed in the short interval between removal of the ganglion and its disintegration in the extracting medium. Perry (5) advanced the hypothesis that only part of the extractable ACh of a ganglion is readily available for release by nerve impulses, and that while the ACh released by stimulation (under the usual conditions of perfusion with eserinized Locke's solution) is quickly replenished by synthesis, the newly formed ACh only becomes 'available' at a relatively slow rate, which is equal to the steady rate of ACh output after prolonged stimulation.

In the present study we have again measured, with some improvements in technique, the ACh output and content of ganglia perfused with eserinized Locke's solution, and we have obtained results that help to account for those of Brown and Feldberg. We have also done parallel experiments with perfusion fluids of altered composition, and have found that the synthesis and the release of ACh are to some degree independent processes for which the rate-controlling factors are different. Our results have enabled us to identify several of these factors, and appear to throw light on some of the processes involved in the turnover of ACh at nerve endings.

Some of our findings have already been presented briefly (6, 7, 8).

## Methods

The experiments were carried out on cats. Medium-sized healthy animals of either sex were chosen. Anaesthesia was induced with ethyl chloride followed by ether, and maintained with chloralose.

### Perfusion

The superior cervical ganglion, usually on the right side, was prepared for perfusion essentially by the method of Kibjakow (9) as modified by Feldberg and Gaddum (10). The main postganglionic trunk was left intact in order that the response of the nictitating membrane could be recorded. Particular care was taken to separate this trunk from accompanying arterial twigs through which reflux of blood into the perfusion stream might occur: with this precaution the perfusion pressure could nearly always be kept well below 100 mm Hg.

Since oedema and leakage were thus minimized the pressure-flow characteristics of the preparation usually changed little during an hour or more of perfusion, and little adjustment of the pressure was needed to keep the flow
within the range 0.2–0.4 ml/minute. The perfusion fluid had previously been
filtered through sintered glass and equilibrated with $O_2$ or a $CO_2$–$O_2$ mixture.
It was placed in a separatory-funnel reservoir, which was connected to a tank
containing the same gas at the desired perfusion pressure, and was led to the
ganglion by fine-bore polyethylene tubing, in which it was warmed to body
temperature ($38 \pm 1°$ C) in the way described by Emmelin and MacIntosh (11).
The arterial cannula had a capacity of less than 0.1 ml and was closed by a
rubber stopper; the tubing from the reservoir was fitted to the ground-down
butt of a fine hypodermic needle whose point was thrust through the stopper.
When more than one perfusion fluid was to be used in an experiment, each was
put into a similar reservoir and was led to the cannula in the same way. The
perfusion could then be switched over to a fluid of different composition without
losing time or disturbing the preparation, merely by turning the stopcocks of
the appropriate reservoirs. Samples of venous effluent were collected in chilled
tubes and stored at $0°$ until they were assayed not more than 3 hours later.

*Perfusion Fluids*

Locke's solution was freshly prepared and in most of the experiments had
practically the same composition as that used by Brown and Feldberg (1) and
by Perry (5); in g/l., NaCl 9.0, $KHCO_3$ 0.56, $CaCl_2$ 0.24, glucose 1.0, eserine
sulphate 0.005 ($8 \times 10^{-6}$ $M$). It was usually oxygenated at room temperature,
and its pH was then about 8.5. In a few experiments in which it was equilibrated
(at $20°$) with 3.5% $CO_2$ in $O_2$, the bicarbonate was raised to $2.5 \times 10^{-2}$ $M$ by
addition of $NaHCO_3$ and the NaCl was reduced correspondingly: the pH after
treatment with $CO_2$ was then $7.4 \pm 0.1$ (at $38°$).

Plasma was obtained on the day of the experiment by arterial bleeding of
lightly etherized cats and was made incoagulable with heparin sodium
(Connaught, 0.5 mg/ml). Plasma from human donors was obtained by veni-
puncture, the blood being drawn under negative pressure into bottles containing
heparin, with sterile precautions. In either case eserine sulphate ($2 \times 10^{-5}$ g/ml;
$3 \times 10^{-5}$ $M$) was added, and the plasma was gassed with $O_2$ or $CO_2$–$O_2$ in a large
tonometer.

Plasma dialyzates were prepared by dialyzing 50-ml quantities of plasma
overnight at $4°$, with stirring, against 500 ml of distilled water. They were
lyophilized and reconstituted to give an isotonic solution for perfusion.

HC-3 (hemicholinium compound No. 3 (12)), as the dibromide, was generously supplied by Dr. F. W. Schueler. Its concentration when added to Locke
or plasma was $2 \times 10^{-5}$ $M$. Tetraethyl pyrophosphate (TEPP) solutions were
made up by dilution of sealed stock of the pure fluid (Eli Lilly & Co., Albright
& Wilson Ltd.) immediately before use. A stock solution of eserine sulphate
(Merck, $3 \times 10^{-3}$ $M$) was made in saline and kept in the cold for not more than

a week; this was added in the required volume to the perfusion fluid just before each experiment. The molecular weight of the salt was taken as 648.5.

## Stimulation

Stimulation of the preganglionic trunk was always begun 15 minutes after the start of the perfusion. The stimuli were rectangular voltage pulses of 1.0 millisecond duration and appropriate frequency, delivered through agar–saline pore electrodes via chlorided silver wires. The electrodes were transformer-coupled to the stimulator and the animal was grounded. During periods of prolonged high-frequency stimulation the electrodes were moved along the nerve towards the ganglion every 5 minutes: in spite of this precaution the stimuli sometimes fell temporarily below maximal, as was indicated by the nictitating-membrane record. Random irregularities of the ACh output curve could usually be attributed to this cause; but this source of error could not have been serious when conclusions were based on the pooled data from several experiments. It should be noted that the nictitating-membrane record in experiments of this kind is not always a reliable guide to the effectiveness of stimulation. This was particularly true in ganglia whose cholinesterase was inactivated and whose ACh output was high: under these conditions, repetitive stimulation floods the ganglion with free ACh (1); synaptic transmission is partly or wholly blocked although the ganglion cells may be firing rapidly and asynchronously (13); as an after-effect of their prolonged depolarization, asynchronous firing may persist for a long time after stimulation is over (cf. Emmelin and MacIntosh (11)).

## Ganglion Extracts

It has been shown that cold trichloroacetic acid efficiently extracts ACh from nervous tissue (14, 15, 16, 17). Extracts were made with 2-ml portions of 10% acid. Particular care was taken to establish a fixed routine for removing the ganglion. The rostral end of the ganglion was freed first and the last step was to cut the preganglionic trunk, so that in stimulation experiments the ganglion remained active until the last possible moment. The time from the beginning of the dissection until the immersion of the ganglion in the ice-cold extractive was regularly $45 \pm 15$ seconds. Each ganglion was then finely minced without delay and the suspension was kept at $0°$ C for 90 minutes. At the end of this time, the fluid was transferred with the aid of 1 ml of saline to a 15-ml centrifuge tube (filtration was unnecessary) and extracted 5 times with 10-ml portions of water-saturated ether. The remaining ether was removed by aeration and the supernatant was used directly for the assay. Control experiments showed that added ACh was quantitatively recovered and that the extracts contained no material other than ACh that affected the assay preparation.

## Estimation of Plasma Choline

Free choline in cat plasma was extracted essentially by Bligh's (18) method and acetylated with acetyl chloride as described by Emmelin and MacIntosh

(11). Added choline was found to be quantitatively converted to ACh. Results were expressed in terms of choline chloride. HC-3 when present did not interfere with the estimation of choline.

### Assay of ACh

Ganglion extracts, samples of venous effluent, and acetylated plasma extracts were assayed against freshly prepared solutions of ACh chloride (Hoffmann-LaRoche) by the cat's blood pressure method as described by MacIntosh and Perry (16). Each sample was injected at two or more dose levels bracketed by ACh standards. The results of duplicate assays generally agreed to within 10%. Standard solutions of ACh for the assay of perfusates were always made up in the perfusion fluid itself, and the volume injected was always about the same for standard and unknown. These precautions were particularly important in the case of plasma samples, since plasma tended to depress the response to simultaneously injected ACh. When the assay preparation deteriorated, as it often did after prolonged testing, it could usually be resuscitated by maintaining a constant infusion of adrenaline hydrochloride (2-3 $\mu$g/kg minute) in isotonic glucose. All values for ACh are given in terms of the chloride.

### Time Course of ACh Release

ACh set free at the nerve endings of a perfused ganglion reaches the collecting vessel after a short delay, representing the time required for it to diffuse into the vessels and be carried to the venous cannula. This lag tends to obscure somewhat the time course of ACh release when the efflux rate is changing rapidly. Thus when successive 1-minute samples of effluent were collected at the beginning of a stimulation period, the ACh output usually showed a peak in the second minute and then declined (cf. Perry (5)). Control experiments with brief periods of stimulation indicated that with our perfusion routine the mean lag between release and collection was about ½ minute. In plotting the data for ACh output during prolonged stimulation, therefore, it was assumed that the mean output rate during each period of collection after the first minute indicated the rate at which ACh was being released at a time ½-minute before the mid-point of the collection period: thus the measured output rate during the second minute was plotted as the instantaneous output rate at the end of 1 minute. Since ACh output changed most rapidly at the outset of stimulation, it was found convenient to collect the earlier samples over shorter periods; the routine adopted in experiments where stimulation lasted an hour was to collect 1-minute samples during the first 5 minutes, then one 5-minute sample, two 10-minute samples, and two 15-minute samples. When the ACh output during a brief period of stimulation was to be determined, the effluent was collected for the duration of stimulation and for an additional 2 minutes to ensure that practically all the released ACh had been washed out.

### Synthesis of ACh

The amount of ACh synthesized by a perfused ganglion must be equal to the total quantity of ACh it discharges into the perfusion fluid corrected for the change in its extractable ACh, on condition that no ACh has been lost by leakage of perfusion fluid or by hydrolysis. We have satisfied ourselves that under the conditions of our experiments no correction need be made for loss by leakage. Emmelin and MacIntosh (11) have shown, further, that in experiments of this sort the enzymatic hydrolysis of released ACh must be small. A little non-enzymatic hydrolysis, however, may occur through the action of H ions when ganglia are being extracted with trichloroacetic acid at 0° or through the action of OH ions when bicarbonate-containing perfusates are stored at 0° before being assayed. The errors arising from either source could hardly be more than a few per cent and would affect the calculated synthesis rate in opposite directions: they have therefore been disregarded. Further evidence that the estimates of ACh content and output are reliable is supplied by the satisfactory agreement between output and loss of ganglionic ACh in experiments in which synthesis was prevented. We have therefore calculated the ACh synthesized by a perfused ganglion by adding its residual ACh content to the total output of ACh (as determined by assay of the successive samples of effluent) and subtracting the ACh content of the unperfused control ganglion.

*Cholinesterase Inactivation In Vivo*

Some experiments were undertaken with the purpose of measuring changes in the ACh content of unstimulated ganglia whose cholinesterase was inactivated as completely as possible for periods of up to 1–2 hours while the natural blood supply was maintained. More satisfactory results were obtained with TEPP than with eserine. Each animal was placed on artificial respiration and given atropine sulphate (1 mg/kg) and gallamine triethiodide (5 mg/kg); the control ganglion was then removed, and the preganglionic trunk supplying the test ganglion was cut or kept in contact with procaine hydrochloride (1%). Treatment with TEPP by vein was then started; the priming dose was 2 mg/kg and a further 1 mg/kg was given every 5 minutes. ACh appeared in the blood of animals so treated and rose within 30 minutes to $10^{-8}$ g/ml or higher; most of this presumably came from the alimentary canal, since in eviscerated animals similarly treated the blood ACh level stayed below $10^{-9}$ g/ml. In either case, although blood flow through the ganglion of such an animal was only 0.04–0.10 ml/minute, its rate of ACh release during preganglionic stimulation was about the same, in $m\mu g$/minute, as for ganglia perfused with eserinized plasma. Transmission through a ganglion so treated and repetitively stimulated failed within a minute, no doubt because of the very high concentration of free ACh ($>10^{-7}$ g/ml) which must have been present in its extracellular fluid. These results were considered to justify the assumption that almost complete inactivation of ganglionic cholinesterase had been achieved by treatment with TEPP.

# Results

## 1. ACh METABOLISM OF RESTING GANGLIA

### (A) ACh Content of Resting Ganglia

The ganglia of different cats vary rather widely in ACh content. In a series of 50 resting ganglia we found a mean of 266 m$\mu$g with a standard deviation of 41 m$\mu$g. Left and right ganglia from the same cat, however, agree within a few per cent (15). A resting unperfused ganglion may therefore be taken without serious error to contain the same amount of ACh as its fellow did before being perfused.

On this basis resting ganglia perfused for 1 to 2 hours with *eserine-free Locke* or plasma were found to show no important change in their ACh content. This also happened in one experiment in which the hemicholinium base HC-3 ($2 \times 10^{-5}$ $M$) was present in the perfusion fluid. It is possible that in some of these cases a change did occur but was disregarded as falling within experimental error: if so it could hardly have exceeded 10%.

Perfusion of a ganglion with *eserinized* ($8 \times 10^{-6}$ $M$) *Locke*, however, regularly increased the yield of extractable ACh by about 25% (Table I). The effect appeared to be independent of the duration of the perfusion over the range

TABLE I

Effect of perfusion on ACh content of unstimulated ganglion

| Perfused with: | ACh as % of ACh in control ganglion | | |
|---|---|---|---|
| | Perfused for: | | |
| | 5 min | 60 min | 120 min |
| Locke | — | 100 | — |
| Locke + HC-3 | — | 100 | — |
| Plasma | — | 96 | — |
| Locke + eserine | 123 ± 8 (6) | — | 134, 123 |
| Locke + HC-3 + eserine | 125 ± 8 (4) | — | — |
| Plasma + eserine | 129 ± 13 (3) | 193 ± 11 (3) | 202 |
| Locke + eserine at 0° C | *102 ± 5 (4) | 104 | — |
| Plasma + eserine, followed by 15 minutes with plasma alone | — | 114, 102 | — |

NOTE: ( ) Number of observations.
*Perfusion for 5 minutes with eserine-free Locke followed by 15 minutes with eserine–Locke.

5 minutes to 2 hours, and was also seen when HC-3 was present. Brief (5 minutes) perfusion with eserinized plasma had a similar effect. This effect of eserine could be explained in either of two ways. First, the ACh content of the uneserinized control ganglion would be underestimated if the extraction procedure allowed some destruction of ACh by cholinesterase before that enzyme could be inactivated by the extracting fluid. Alternatively, the ACh content of the perfused and eserinized ganglion would increase if ACh were formed in it during the first few minutes of perfusion and were preserved from enzymatic

destruction. (The absence of a further increase during continued perfusion of eserinized Locke could then be ascribed either to the exhaustion of some material necessary for the rapid synthesis of ACh, or to saturation of the sites in which the additional ACh was held.) The first alternative seems unlikely because enzymatic destruction of ACh at 0° is a slow process, and because extraction of brain with trichloroacetic acid even at room temperature has been found to yield about the same amount of ACh as extraction at a temperature below 0° (17). Furthermore we have found that if a ganglion is perfused for 15 minutes with ice-cold Locke containing eserine, it yields no more ACh on extraction than its unperfused and uneserinized control (Table I). We conclude therefore that when a ganglion is eserinized at body temperature its extractable ACh is rapidly increased through synthesis by about 25%, and that the ACh extractable by our method from a control ganglion gives a valid measure of normal ACh level at rest.

When *eserinized plasma* was used for perfusion, the ACh content was again increased through synthesis, and during the first 5 minutes to about the same degree as when eserinized Locke was used (Table I). Continued perfusion with eserinized plasma led, however, to a further rise in ACh content: in three experiments the increment in an hour was $93 \pm 11\%$ (mean $\pm$ standard deviation). A similar increase of bound ACh, $93 \pm 20\%$ in an hour, was observed in four ganglia with intact blood supply when TEPP was given repeatedly by vein in large doses (see Methods). The time course of the ACh accumulation is shown in Fig. 1, in which the upper curve is derived from the data of both plasma-perfusion and intact-circulation experiments. In both cases the ACh content, after the rapid initial ascent, rose linearly for an hour and then became steady. This secondary rise of ACh content was not seen in the ganglia of animals treated with both TEPP and HC-3. In this case (as with eserine–Locke perfusion) only the small initial rise appeared, as the lower curve of Fig. 1 shows. It will be shown later that both HC-3 and perfusion with Locke interfere with the ganglion's ability to maintain a high rate of ACh synthesis. In animals treated with HC-3 alone, there was a moderate fall in ACh which became significant ($28 \pm 12\%$) in three experiments lasting 2 hours.

The extra ACh, which accumulates in a ganglion whose cholinesterase has been inactivated, will be referred to as "surplus ACh", and its significance will be discussed later. We may note here, however, that it cannot be free in the ganglion's extracellular spaces, for in that case it would certainly diffuse into the eserinized plasma perfusing the ganglion in amounts that could easily be assayed; and moreover its local concentration would exceed $10^{-5}$ g/ml, more than enough to produce a complete depolarization block: but there is no block in ganglia so treated, nor do they leak ACh except in minute amounts. A further significant fact is the following. When, after an hour of perfusion with eserine-containing plasma, the perfusion is continued for 15 minutes with eserine-free plasma, most of the surplus ACh is found to have disappeared (Table I). Surplus ACh thus accumulates in some intracellular compartment

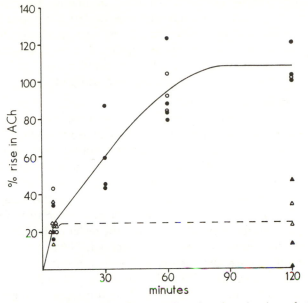

FIG. 1. ACh accumulation in resting ganglia after inactivation of cholinesterase.
●, TEPP, natural circulation; ○, eserine, plasma perfusion; △, TEPP + HC-3, natural
circulation; ▲, eserine, Locke perfusion.

where it would have been exposed to enzymatic destruction if the cholinesterase
there had not been inactivated. It must be separated in some way from the
resting ganglion's normal ACh stock, which is not exposed to the action of the
enzyme. The formation of surplus ACh must take place in the region of the
nerve endings, rather than in the intraganglionic parts of the cholinergic
axons, for the ACh content of the undissected preganglionic trunk was found
to increase much less ($22 \pm 10\%$ in nine experiments) than the ACh content
of the ganglia, in the experiments in which the whole animal was kept for
$\frac{1}{2}$ to 2 hours under the influence of large doses of TEPP.

### (B) ACh Release by Resting Ganglia

Earlier workers (10, 19, 20) have stressed their finding that the venous fluid
leaving an eserinized perfused ganglion normally contains very little ACh, and
we can confirm this. The rate at which a ganglion perfused with eserinized
plasma, for example, discharges ACh at rest is very small compared with the
rate at which it can accumulate surplus ACh, or can discharge ACh when its
preganglionic fibers are excited. There is, however, a continuous discharge of
ACh from the eserinized resting ganglion. It amounts to about 0.15–0.5 mμg/
minute, and so can only be detected when the pooled effluent from several
minutes' perfusion is injected into a sensitive assay cat. This minute trickle
of ACh is observed also in Locke-perfused ganglia, and continues with little
change during at least 2 hours of perfusion. It may well represent a spon-

taneous "quantal" release of the transmitter, analogous to that occurring at the neuromuscular junction (21), but we have not tried to prove that it originates from the axonal endings. The rapidly waning discharge of ACh, occasionally observed at the outset of perfusion in previous studies (1), and attributed (19) to the leaching of ACh from severed nerve trunks, was seldom, if ever, seen in our experiments on plasma-perfused ganglia.

*(C) ACh Turnover in Resting Ganglia*

There is thus, in a ganglion perfused with eserinized plasma, a considerable metabolism of ACh, even when no nerve impulses are arriving. A little ACh is being released into the perfusate, and a larger amount (in the first hour of perfusion) is being synthesized and retained within the ganglion as surplus ACh. It seems reasonable to suppose that this ACh metabolism is associated with the preganglionic endings, which contain most of the ganglion's choline acetylase (15, 22, 23). The amount of ACh formed per minute (except for the first few minutes when the rate is faster) is of the order of 1 to 2% of the resting content, and of this perhaps a tenth is released. Such a rate of release, if maintained, would require the resting nerve endings to replace their bound ACh every 8 to 16 hours. It will be shown that a stimulated ganglion under optimal conditions may turn over its bound ACh in about 10 minutes. (These statements refer to ganglia that are perfused with plasma, or retain their natural blood supply. Resting ganglia perfused with Locke form less surplus ACh, but they appear to release ACh at about the same very slow rate.)

In these experiments, synthesis and release of ACh by resting nerve endings were studied in ganglia whose cholinesterase had been inactivated. It seems likely that the same processes occur at similar rates in ganglia not so treated, but cannot then be detected by direct assay because the newly formed or released ester is immediately hydrolyzed.

## 2. ACH METABOLISM OF ACTIVE GANGLIA

*(A) ACh Release by Active Perfused Ganglia*

In a series of 20 experiments, four perfusion fluids were compared for their ability to support the ACh metabolism of ganglia subjected to prolonged stimulation. These fluids were: Locke's solution of the usual formula, containing glucose, bicarbonate as the only buffer, and eserine sulphate ($8 \times 10^{-6}$ $M$); the same solution with the addition of HC-3 ($2 \times 10^{-5}$ $M$); heparinized cat plasma containing eserine sulphate ($3 \times 10^{-5}$ $M$); and similar plasma containing HC-3 ($2 \times 10^{-5}$) as well as eserine. Each fluid had been equilibrated with $O_2$, according to the practice of earlier workers, and its pH was therefore about 8.5, or that of an aqueous bicarbonate solution; errors due to enzymatic hydrolysis of ACh in the collected effluent were minimized by chilling the samples and assaying them within 1 to 2 hours. The perfusion fluids were assigned to the experiments on the basis of a randomized block design, with five experiments for each fluid; the procedures for perfusion, stimulation, and assay were kept constant throughout the series.

In each experiment a control sample of effluent, which never contained more than the trace of ACh that corresponds to the resting output, was collected for a 5-minute period before the start of stimulation. The preganglionic trunk was then excited maximally at 20/second for 60 minutes, during which time the whole of the effluent was collected in successive samples and assayed. At the end of stimulation the perfused ganglion was quickly removed and minced in the chilled extracting medium; lastly the opposite ganglion was also removed and similarly extracted. From the assay values, ACh output rates and ganglion contents were calculated, as described under Methods.

The results within each group of five experiments were in good agreement. The time course of ACh output is shown in Fig. 2. The rate of output was

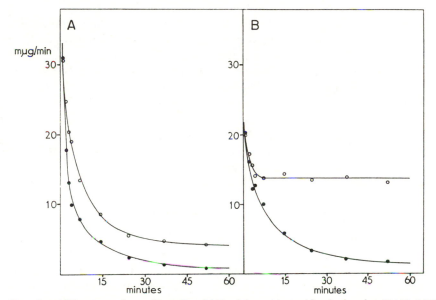

FIG. 2. ACh output of ganglia perfused (A) with oxygenated Locke (eserine $6 \times 10^{-6}\ M$), (B) with oxygenated plasma (eserine $3 \times 10^{-5}\ M$). Preganglionic stimulation at 20/second throughout. In each case upper curve is mean of five experiments without HC-3; lower curve is mean of five experiments with HC-3 ($2 \times 10^{-5}\ M$).

nearly always highest in the sample collected during the 2nd minute of stimulation, and lowest in the sample collected during the last 15 minutes of stimulation. Mean values for these two samples and for the total output, with the corresponding standard deviations, are given in Table II.

*(a) Ganglia Perfused with Locke* (Table II, A)

The five experiments of this group gave results very much like those obtained by previous workers (1, 4, 5). The ACh output rose steeply to a peak (usually for the second 1-minute sample) of $31 \pm 2$ m$\mu$g/minute and then fell off gradually towards a much lower level, almost, but not quite, reached during the last 15-minute sample, for which the rate was $4.3 \pm 0.7$ m$\mu$g/minute. When the data were plotted against time (Fig. 2), allowance was made for the time taken for released ACh to reach the collecting vessel, as described under Methods. The above figures for ACh output agree very well with those in a series of experiments by Perry (5), who found $34 \pm 4$ and $4.0 \pm 1.2$ m$\mu$g/minute for the peak and final output rates. Perry stimulated at 10/second as against 20/second in our tests; but under these conditions of perfusion, as he was able to show, the minute output is nearly independent of the frequency of stimulation, at least over the range 5–100/second.

The total amount of ACh released by these five ganglia during an hour's stimulation averaged 464 m$\mu$g. This was about double the average initial content, as determined by extraction of the control ganglia.

*(b) Ganglia Perfused with Locke Containing HC-3* (Table II, B)

The ganglia perfused with this fluid discharged ACh, when stimulated, at the same initial rate as the ganglia perfused with Locke. They showed, however, even less ability to maintain a high rate of ACh output (Fig. 2A). The minute output fell off more steeply than in the Locke experiments to a final mean value of 0.9 m$\mu$g/minute, significantly lower ($P < 0.01$) than the figure for the unpoisoned ganglia, and indeed not much above the threshold for assay. The ability of ganglia poisoned with HC-3 to transmit impulses runs parallel to their ability to release ACh. At the outset of stimulation impulses are transmitted normally; after prolonged stimulation there is little or no transmission, even though eserine is present.

The total quantity of ACh released by these ganglia averaged 246 m$\mu$g, which was significantly less ($P < 0.01$) than in the experiments with Locke alone, and was only slightly less than the initial store of ACh in the ganglia.

*(c) Ganglia Perfused with Plasma* (Table II, F)

The ganglia of this group did not behave like those perfused with Locke. Their peak rate of ACh output averaged 20 m$\mu$g/minute, which was significantly ($P < 0.01$) lower than that of the Locke-perfused ganglia (Fig. 2B). The output, however, was better maintained than in the Locke experiments. It fell off by only about one-third, and this fall was complete within the first 5 minutes, after which the rate remained practically steady. The output for the final sample, 13 m$\mu$g/minute, was significantly higher ($P < 0.01$) than in the Locke experiments.

The total output of ACh from these ganglia was 852 m$\mu$g, significantly ($P < 0.01$) greater than in either of the preceding series, and more than 3 times the initial ACh content of the ganglia.

Emmelin and MacIntosh (11) compared the ACh output rates of Locke- and plasma-perfused ganglia during 3-minute periods of stimulation and found that they were about the same. In fact, they reported somewhat higher figures for their Locke than for their plasma experiments, and though they did not regard the difference as significant, their results are clearly in satisfactory agreement with our own.

### (d) Ganglia Perfused with Plasma Containing HC-3 (Table II, G)

The five ganglia perfused with this fluid released ACh at the same initial rate as those in the preceding series (Fig. 2B). Thereafter they behaved like the ganglia perfused with Locke containing HC-3. Their ACh output fell off steeply and continued to fall: the mean rate for the final sample, 1.8 m$\mu$g/minute, though significantly ($P < 0.05$) above the mean for the experiments with Locke containing HC-3, was far below the mean for the experiments with Locke alone.

The total output of ACh from these ganglia, 285 m$\mu$g, was a little higher than their mean initial content, but not significantly greater than the total output from ganglia perfused with Locke containing HC-3.

Thus, with prolonged stimulation, plasma-perfused ganglia release at the outset less ACh than Locke-perfused ganglia; but this is true for only a few minutes: thereafter their ACh output stabilizes at a much higher level, unless HC-3 is present. The effects of HC-3 are the same with either fluid: the initial rate of ACh output is not altered; but the output, instead of declining only to a characteristic steady level, falls almost to zero. It is clear that these findings can be most simply explained by supposing (a) that ACh is more readily released, from the preformed stock at the axon endings, when Locke rather than plasma is used for perfusion; but that (b) in the presence of plasma this stock (and therefore the ACh output rate) is better maintained during stimulation, because ACh can be synthesized faster; while (c) HC-3 prevents ACh synthesis, so that both stock and output fall to low levels if stimulation is prolonged. The correctness of these suppositions is proved by the observations described in the next section.

### (B) ACh Turnover in Active Perfused Ganglia

Each of the 20 ganglia whose ACh output was followed during an hour's stimulation was excised at the end of that time, and its ACh content was compared with that of its unperfused control. The difference between these two values, combined with the output of ACh into the perfusate, gave the amount of ACh synthesized by the perfused ganglion. The data are summarized in Table II.

### (a) Ganglia Perfused with Locke

The five ganglia perfused with Locke (Table II, A) were found to have lost about half (53 ± 11%) of their preformed ACh as a result of being stimulated for an hour. In view of the waning ACh output in these experiments the loss would not have been surprising, were it not that previous workers failed to obtain it. Brown and Feldberg (1), who did four experiments of this sort, found no significant change in ACh content: their stimulated ganglia appeared sometimes to lose, and sometimes to gain, ACh. Kahlson and MacIntosh (4) in three tests did find a loss but it was only 24%. Our lack of agreement with the earlier workers on this point is the more puzzling, since our figures for ACh output are so similar to theirs. It is true that they stimulated at rather lower

TABLE II

ACh turnover in perfused ganglia
(mean ±S.D.)

| Group | Perfusion fluid | No. of expt. | Gas | Eserine ($M \times 10^{-6}$) | ACh output 1-2 min (mμg/min) | ACh output 45-60 min (mμg/min) | ACh output Total (mμg) | ACh content Initial (mμg) | ACh content Final mμg | ACh content Final % of initial | ACh synthesis Total (mμg) | ACh synthesis Rate (mμg/min) |
|---|---|---|---|---|---|---|---|---|---|---|---|---|
| A | Locke | 5 | O₂ | 8 | 30.6 ±2.4 | 4.3 ±0.7 | 464 ±61 | 241 ±26 | 111 ±22 | 47 ±11 | 334 ±67 | 5.6 ±0.9 |
| B | Locke + HC-3 ($2 \times 10^{-5}$ M) | 5 | O₂ | 8 | 31.0 ±4.6 | 0.9 ±0.4 | 246 ±47 | 250 ±85 | 48 ±14 | 19 ±3 | 44 ±72 | 0.7 ±1.2 |
| C | Locke | 3 | O₂ + CO₂ | 8 | 30.7* ±7.0 | 7.2 ±1.0 | 610 ±57 | 310 ±22 | 170 ±46 | 55 ±13 | 470 ±80 | 7.8 ±1.3 |
| D | Locke + choline ($3.5 \times 10^{-5}$ M) | 3 | O₂ + CO₂ | 8 | 26.3* ±5.5 | 11.8 ±0.7 | 733 ±89 | 238 ±35 | 493 ±97 | 207 ±35 | 988 ±131 | 16.5 ±2.1 |
| E | Locke | 5 | O₂ | 40 | 31.8 ±3.7 | 2.5 ±0.8 | 367 ±67 | 321 ±89 | 166 ±81 | 51 ±15 | 212 ±68 | 3.5 ±1.1 |
| F | Plasma | 5 | O₂ | 40 | 20.0 ±4.5 | 13.2 ±3.5 | 852 ±114 | 265 ±8 | 593 ±101 | 224 ±43 | 1180 ±141 | 19.7 ±2.4 |
| G | Plasma + HC-3 ($2 \times 10^{-5}$ M) | 5 | O₂ | 40 | 20.4 ±5.7 | 1.8 ±0.5 | 285 ±103 | 237 ±56 | 61 ±20 | 26 ±7 | 109 ±98 | 1.8 ±1.6 |
| H | Plasma | 5 | O₂ + CO₂ | 40 | 31.0 ±6.6 | 27.8 ±7.7 | 1591 ±438 | 267 ±51 | 397 ±105 | 151 ±35 | 1721 ±344 | 28.7 ±6.8 |

*In experiments of groups C and D, peak outputs sometimes occurred in 0- to 1-minute sample.

frequency than we did, 10–17/second as against 20/second, but in view of Perry's results (5) it seems quite unlikely that this difference can account for the discrepancy. It is easier to suppose that in the present experiments we were more successful in continuing to stimulate the ganglion effectively right up to the moment of its excision and immersion in extracting fluid: for there is evidence (4, 24) that the ACh stores of nervous tissue when depleted by activity can be made good by a brief period of rest. Whether or not this is the explanation of our failure to confirm the older results, we feel sure that the present observations cannot be seriously in error. We have repeated our experiments, using a higher frequency of stimulation, or a different anticholinesterase drug, or one of several modifications of the Locke's solution formula, and have always obtained the same result.

We can, however, confirm the finding of Brown and Feldberg (1) that the Locke-perfused ganglion synthesizes ACh during preganglionic stimulation. The total amount formed when the stimulation lasted an hour exceeded the initial ACh content of the ganglion; it was less than the total amount discharged into the perfusate, since some of this total was accounted for by expenditure of the ganglion's ACh stores. Figure 3 presents the balance sheet in diagrammatic form, with the results for Locke perfusion on the left. If it is assumed that synthesis proceeded at a constant rate throughout the period of stimulation, one would have expected the calculated rate of synthesis to be about equal to the rate of ACh discharge observed at the end of the period, at a time when synthesis and release have come nearly into balance. This expectation was only approximately realized: the mean rate of synthesis as derived from the data for ACh output and change in ACh content was $5.6 \pm 0.9$ m$\mu$g/minute, significantly higher ($P < 0.05$) than the mean output rate for the last 15-minute sample ($4.3 \pm 0.7$ m$\mu$g/minute), which was itself no doubt a little higher than the final asymptotic rate of release. Several possible explanations may be suggested for this small but real discrepancy. In the first place, it may be noted that each ganglion at the beginning of stimulation must have contained some 55 m$\mu$g of ACh that was not present at the beginning of perfusion: this was the surplus ACh formed during the 15 minutes in which the ganglion was perfused with eserinized fluid but not stimulated. The amount of surplus ACh present at the end of the experiment is not known: it might have been higher, as a result of continued formation, or lower, as a result of dissipation. If the same amount were present at the end of stimulation as at the beginning the calculated rate of ACh synthesis would have been 4.7 m$\mu$g/minute, not much above the observed final rate of ACh release. Alternatively, there may have been some falling-off in the rate of ACh synthesis during the hour of stimulating, for instance because of a diminishing supply of free choline. Or a little ACh may have been formed during the unavoidable delay between the excision of the ganglion and its fixation in the cold extracting fluid. In any case it seems reasonable to suppose, on the basis of the data presented above, that the final steady rate of ACh release, in a Locke-perfused ganglion subjected to prolonged stimulation, is a measure of the rate at which the ganglion is synthesizing ACh.

Perry (5) found that a Locke-perfused ganglion, which had been stimulated for a long time in the absence of eserine, could on being eserinized release as much ACh as if it had not been active. On the basis of this and other evidence he concluded that although the nerve endings cannot recapture the ACh they have released, they can take up the choline derived from its hydrolysis and use it to manufacture new ACh. If this can happen one would expect that when two ganglia, one eserinized and one not, were perfused with Locke and stimulated for the same time, the eserinized ganglion would show a greater loss of bound ACh. Experiments to test this idea did not give a conclusive answer. Three ganglia perfused with eserine-free Locke and stimulated for an hour lost $38 \pm 15\%$ of their ACh. The loss was significant ($P < 0.05$), but not significantly smaller ($P > 0.1$) than the $53 \pm 11\%$ lost by the five ganglia stimulated during perfusion with eserine–Locke. Further testing might have shown the difference to be a genuine one. It is also possible that some of the ACh remaining in the eserinized ganglion at the end of stimulation was surplus ACh formed earlier in the experiment: the presence of surplus ACh would tend to obscure any greater depletion of the regular stock of ACh that might have occurred under the influence of eserine. It seems clear, in any case, that even in the absence of eserine a Locke-perfused ganglion cannot synthesize ACh as fast as it can release it, and consequently suffers some diminution of its transmitter stocks. It will be shown later that this deficiency of ACh synthesis, characteristic of the Locke-perfused ganglion, can be corrected by adding choline to the perfusion fluid.

### (b) Ganglia Perfused with Locke Containing HC-3

The five ganglia perfused with this fluid lost on the average 81% of their ACh during an hour's stimulation (Table II, B). This was a significantly greater loss ($P < 0.01$) than that found in the ganglia perfused with Locke without the drug. It was accounted for, within the limits of experimental error, by the ACh that appeared in the perfusate (Fig. 3): the calculated mean rate of synthesis, $0.7 \pm 1.2$ m$\mu$g/minute, though about equal to the mean final rate of ACh discharge, was not significantly different from zero. Thus the inability of these ganglia to replace their lost ACh was reflected both by the greater depletion of their ACh stores as compared with Locke-perfused ganglia, and also by the almost complete cessation of ACh discharge by the end of the experiment.

Since stimulation of a ganglion perfused with eserinized Locke, especially in the presence of HC-3, can lead to so great a loss of its ACh, it seems clear that the extractable ACh of the ganglion, or at any rate the greater part of it, must represent the depots from which ACh is set free when nerve impulses reach the synapses. It is unnecessary to consider, as Brown and Feldberg (1) felt obliged to do, the possibility that each impulse brings about the synthesis of the ACh it releases. But although most of the ganglion's preformed ACh can be set free by sufficiently prolonged excitation, it must be pointed out that we have never been able in this way to deplete a ganglion completely of its ACh. The residual content, after an hour's stimulation in the presence of HC-3 had reduced the ACh output to a very low level, was $48 \pm 14$ m$\mu$g, or about 19% of the original amount. Still longer stimulation might have reduced it a little further, say to 40 m$\mu$g, but hardly to below that figure.

It might have been thought that this residual ACh represented some of the surplus ACh which must have been formed in these experiments during the 15 minutes of perfusion with eserinized fluid that preceded the hour of stimulation. On the basis of our results with unstimulated ganglia (Table I) there should have been some 55 m$\mu$g of ACh in this fraction at the end of perfusion, more than enough to account for the 48 m$\mu$g actually found in the ganglia. We have, however, found in parallel experiments, in which ganglia were stimulated for an hour while being perfused with Locke containing HC-3 but no eserine, that the residual ACh was not significantly less than when eserine was present: the final contents in two trials were 36 and 45 m$\mu$g. It must therefore be concluded that surplus ACh disappears, even in the presence of eserine, where ACh synthesis is defective. The ACh left in a ganglion, during prolonged stimulation under such conditions, must constitute a different fraction of the ganglion's extractable ACh. Since the ACh in this fraction is not releasable by stimulation, we shall designate it 'stationary ACh', in contrast to the 'depot ACh' which accounts for most of the ganglion's resting content and represents the stock available for synaptic transmission.

The ACh of the preganglionic trunk behaves like stationary ACh. Its concentration (average 35 $\mu$g/g wet weight) is not appreciably altered by prolonged stimulation of the trunk in the whole animal, even when HC-3 has been given in massive dosage. The intraganglionic portions of the preganglionic fibers must compose at least 4% of the bulk of the ganglion, and more than that if the total cross section of these fibers increases with their branching. If the axonal ACh concentration were the same inside as outside the ganglion, the intraganglionic portions would account for at least 20 m$\mu$g of the 40 m$\mu$g in the stationary fraction. A little ACh is doubtless present also in cholinergic axons originating within the ganglion. It seems reasonable to conclude that nearly all the stationary ACh is extrasynaptic.

### (c) Ganglia Perfused with Plasma

We have shown that ganglia perfused with eserinized plasma, and not poisoned by HC-3, can maintain a relatively high rate of ACh output however long they are stimulated. It would therefore be expected that their ACh stores would remain at a correspondingly high level. This has been confirmed. In fact, as Table II, F, shows, such ganglia actually accumulate ACh during prolonged stimulation: the mean percentage increase of ACh content in the five experiments amounted to $124 \pm 43$. This increase was not significantly different from the $93 \pm 11$% found for resting ganglia perfused for the same time with eserinized plasma, and, like it, must be thought to represent 'surplus' ACh, held in some location other than the depots in which releasable ACh is normally stored. Because in plasma-perfused ganglia the ACh output remains steady while the ganglion is nearly doubling its ACh content, we must conclude that surplus ACh does not contribute substantially to the ACh output during synaptic activity.

ACh was synthesized in these experiments (Fig. 3) at an average rate of about 20 m$\mu$g/minute, 3 or 4 times as fast as in parallel trials with Locke perfusion. Since, however, the plasma-perfused ganglia had a significantly lower initial rate of ACh output, they must have been less efficient in releasing their stored ACh. It will be shown later that this is an abnormality that can be corrected by raising the $CO_2$ tension of the perfused plasma.

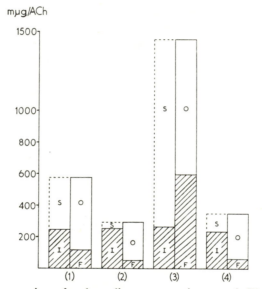

FIG. 3. ACh turnover in perfused ganglia: same experiments as in Fig. 2. I, initial ACh content; F, final ACh content; O, total output of ACh during stimulation for 1 hour; S (= F+O−I), ACh synthesized during experiment.
(1) Ganglia perfused with Locke. (2) Ganglia perfused with Locke + HC-3. (3) Ganglia perfused with plasma. (4) Ganglia perfused with plasma + HC-3.

### (d) Ganglia Perfused with Plasma Containing HC-3

These ganglia, like the Locke-perfused ganglia exposed to HC-3 in the same concentration, were found to have lost most of their ACh during an hour's stimulation (Table II, G). The mean loss, 74±7%, was somewhat, but not significantly, less than in the experiments with Locke and HC-3, and the calculated rate of synthesis, 1.8±1.6 m$\mu$g/minute, was not significantly greater than zero ($P > 0.05, < 0.1$). Thus even in ganglia perfused with plasma, which in the absence of HC-3 supports ACh synthesis so much better than Locke does, the effect of HC-3 was to inhibit ACh synthesis almost completely.

There is a suggestion, however, that a little more ACh was manufactured than in the experiments with Locke and HC-3.

*(C) ACh Turnover in Active Ganglia with Intact Blood Supply*
*(a) Effect of Prolonged Stimulation on ACh Content*

The high steady rate of ACh discharge in plasma-perfused ganglia subjected to prolonged stimulation suggested that the depot ACh under these conditions also stayed at a high steady level. The correctness of this idea could be tested by measuring the ACh content of ganglia supplied with blood or plasma and stimulated in the absence of any anticholinesterase drug, since any change in the depot ACh should then not be obscured by the accumulation of surplus ACh. Three experiments of this sort have been done. When one of a pair of ganglia, both with their blood supply intact was stimulated for 1–2 hours at 20/second while the other remained at rest, their ACh content at the end of the period differed by less than 5%. No indication was found of the sequences of changes described by Rosenblueth, Lissák, and Lanari (25) in the ACh content of ganglia subjected to prolonged repetitive excitation; but we stimulated at a lower frequency and did not try to reproduce their experimental conditions exactly. Our own data thus show that ganglia stimulated repetitively at frequencies up to 20/second maintain their depot ACh at close to its resting level for at least an hour or two, provided that they are supplied with the normal blood (or plasma) necessary for efficient ACh synthesis.

*(b) Effect of HC-3 on ACh Content and Release*

In the experiments with HC-3 that have been described above (B, (b) and (d)), the ganglia could be considered abnormal both because they were perfused and because they were under the influence of eserine. But the effect of HC-3 on ACh synthesis does not depend on the existence of such abnormal conditions, for we have found that ganglia that were neither perfused nor eserinized behaved similarly, in that they lost their stored ACh when they were stimulated in the presence of HC-3. In five experiments on cats that had been given no drug but chloralose, and were maintained on artificial respiration, the preganglionic trunk of one side was stimulated at 20/second for 20 minutes and the ganglion was immediately removed for extraction. HC-3 (1 mg/kg) was then given by vein and the second ganglion was similarly stimulated. All the unpoisoned control ganglia were found to contain the usual amount of ACh, but the ganglia stimulated after injection of HC-3 contained only $29 \pm 9\%$ as much as their fellows. In these experiments the percentage loss of ACh was a little less than in the earlier experiments in which HC-3 was added to the perfusion fluid, but in the earlier tests the stimulation had lasted 3 times as long.

*(c) Delayed Ganglion Block after HC-3*

In the experiments just described the ACh output of the stimulated ganglia could not be measured directly, but indirect evidence was obtained that the output fell off under the influence of HC-3, just as it had done in ganglia that were perfused and eserinized. At the outset of preganglionic stimulation, the

retraction of the nictitating membrane, when the drug had been given, matched
the retraction that had previously been obtained from the opposite membrane.
But while the latter had responded maximally right through the 20 minutes of

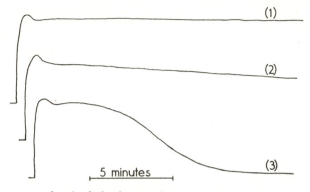

FIG. 4.   Responses of cat's nictitating membrane to continued sympathetic stimulation
at 20/second: (1) before HC-3, preganglionic stimulation; (2) after HC-3 (1 mg/kg), postganglionic stimulation; (3) after HC-3, preganglionic stimulation.

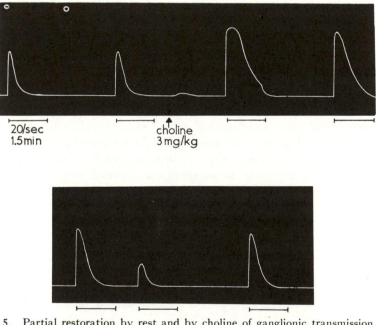

FIG. 5.   Partial restoration by rest and by choline of ganglionic transmission in cat
poisoned by HC-3.  Nictitating membrane: bars indicate maximal preganglionic stimulation
for 1.5 minutes at 20/second; except in penultimate case, interval between stimulation
periods was 2.5 minutes.  Before the record started, the cat had been given HC-3 (3 mg/kg)
and placed on artificial respiration, and complete ganglionic block had been produced by
stimulating the preganglionic trunk for 20 minutes.  At arrow, choline chloride (3 mg/kg)
by vein.

stimulation, the response in the poisoned animal always began to fall off within a few minutes and eventually disappeared almost completely. With post-ganglionic stimulation, on the other hand, a nearly maximal retraction of the membrane could be maintained in the poisoned animal for at least an hour (Fig. 4). In further experiments it was shown that the response to preganglionic stimulation, when it had failed, could be partially restored either by rest, or by lowering the frequency of stimulation, or by injecting a small dose of choline chloride (1–4 mg/kg). Such a dose of choline, in the absence of HC-3, produces no more than a small and fleeting effect either on ganglionic transmission or on the nictitating membrane itself (Fig. 5).

The possibility that HC-3 might possess slowly developing ganglion-blocking activity, or might be converted in vivo into a ganglion-blocking agent, was eliminated by the observation that even after repeated large doses of the compound had been given the ganglion transmitted impulses normally when it was first subjected to preganglionic stimulation, and failed to transmit only when it was stimulated repetitively for several minutes. HC-3 has been found to possess some activity as a neuromuscular blocking agent (12), but if it has any ganglion-blocking power this must be weak: in one test on a perfused uneserinized ganglion we found that it actually sensitized the ganglion cells to the action of exogenous ACh. So far as our observations go, HC-3 has no important effect on autonomically innervated structures that cannot be explained by its ability to inhibit ACh synthesis, and thus to produce delayed failure of transmission at repetitively activated cholinergic junctions.

### 3. Substances that Influence the ACh Metabolism of Perfused Ganglia

It has been shown above that ganglia perfused with plasma synthesize ACh more efficiently but release it less readily than ganglia perfused with Locke. This difference of behavior could not have been due to differences in $O_2$ tension, perfusion pressure, or flow rate, since these were similar for the two fluids. It is explained at least in part by the experiments described below, which show that ACh turnover in a perfused ganglion may be affected by altering the concentration in the perfusion medium of $CO_2$, choline, and (or) an unidentified factor (or factors) present in plasma. The effects of eserine and of adrenaline have also been examined in this connection.

### (A) Carbon Dioxide

The Locke and plasma used in the perfusion experiments so far described had been gassed with $O_2$ and were unphysiologically alkaline (pH up to 8.5). It was thought that in plasma so alkaline there might be a significant reduction of ionized calcium, which is known to be required for the release of ACh at ganglionic (26, 27) and neuromuscular junctions (cf. 28). Such an effect would be greater with plasma perfusion than with Locke perfusion for two reasons: first, the protein and phosphate (and perhaps the heparin) of plasma would tend to bind calcium ions (29, 30); and secondly, in the presence of plasma the endogenous $CO_2$ produced by neuronal activity would be less effective in lowering the pH locally, since plasma is better buffered than Locke. A new series of experiments was therefore carried out, in which the pH of each fluid was lowered to $7.4 \pm 0.1$ (at $38°$ C) by equilibrating it with $O_2$ to which the required concentration of $CO_2$ had been added.

Plasma so treated was used for perfusion in five experiments (Table II, H). In these the initial rate of ACh release was found to be higher than in the earlier experiments with $CO_2$-free plasma, and not significantly different from the initial rate in the experiments with Locke. Some decrease of the output rate occurred as usual during the first 5 minutes, but in this case it amounted to only about 10%; and for the remainder of the experiment the output was nearly constant and higher than in any other series of experiments (Fig. 6). The total amount of ACh discharged was 87% greater, and the mean rate of synthesis was 46% greater, than in the tests with $CO_2$-free plasma: the difference in both cases was significant ($P < 0.01$ and $P < 0.05$). The ACh content of each ganglion rose during the experiment, but not so far as in the experiments without $CO_2$: this difference was also significant ($P < 0.05$). It follows from these observations that the more rapid output of ACh, when $CO_2$ is present, does not depend on a corresponding elevation of the depot ACh; the primary effect of $CO_2$ must rather be to facilitate the release of ACh. The more rapid release of ACh is accompanied by an increase in its rate of synthesis, so that the stock of available transmitter is well maintained. But this is a secondary effect. Some mechanism must exist by which synthesis is kept in step with release, as is illustrated by the fact that in an active ganglion the rate of synthesis is higher than in a resting ganglion. In the present experiments, at least, there is nothing to suggest that $CO_2$ has any important direct action on ACh synthesis.

Experiments to test the effect of $CO_2$ on the ACh metabolism of Locke-perfused ganglia led to similar conclusions (Table II, C). In these trials the bicarbonate content of the Locke was raised to $2.5 \times 10^{-2}$ $M$ with a corresponding reduction of chloride; the solution was then better buffered and its $CO_2$ tension was about the same as that of the $CO_2$-treated plasma. The ACh output of the three ganglia perfused with this fluid was initially about the same as that of the ganglia perfused with $CO_2$-free Locke; thereafter it was somewhat better maintained and the total output was significantly ($P < 0.01$) larger, though it was still significantly below the output from the plasma-perfused ganglia even when these latter were not supplied with $CO_2$ (Fig. 7). The reduction in ganglionic ACh was about the same as when $CO_2$ was omitted from the medium. The effects of $CO_2$ in these experiments on Locke-perfused ganglia, like the more striking effects seen with plasma perfusion, support the idea that $CO_2$ exerts its action mainly by promoting ACh release rather than by speeding ACh synthesis. It is plausible to suppose, but remains to be proved, that this action depends mainly on increased ionization of calcium.

An apparently similar effect of $CO_2$ (or the $CO_2$–bicarbonate system) in promoting ACh turnover was observed by Quastel, Tennenbaum, and Wheatley

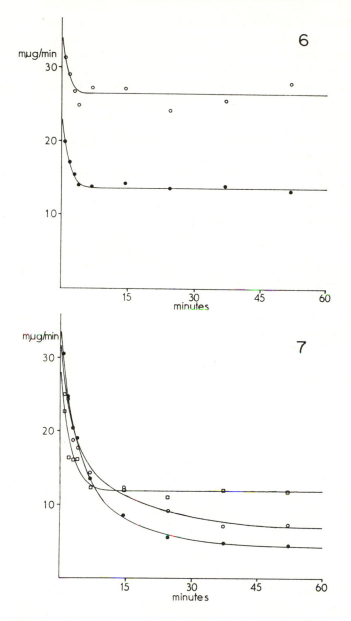

FIG. 6.   ACh output of plasma-perfused ganglia.  Eserine $(3 \times 10^{-5}\ M)$; preganglionic stimulation at 20/second throughout.  Upper curve, mean of five experiments in which plasma had been gassed with $CO_2$–$O_2$ mixture and was at pH 7.4; lower curve, mean of five experiments in which plasma had been gassed with $O_2$ only (cf. Fig. 2B).

FIG. 7.   ACh output of Locke-perfused ganglia.  Eserine $(6 \times 10^{-6}\ M)$; preganglionic stimulation at 20/second throughout.  ●, mean of five experiments with Locke of original formula, gassed with $O_2$ (cf. Fig. 2A); ○, mean of three experiments with high-bicarbonate Locke, gassed with $CO_2$–$O_2$ to pH 7.4; □, mean of three experiments with Locke of latter composition supplemented with choline $3.5 \times 10^{-5}\ M$.

(31) and analyzed by McLennan and Elliott (32), in experiments on brain slices. McLennan and Elliott showed that the effect of $CO_2$ is a specific one and does not depend merely on lowering the pH of the medium. Emmelin and MacIntosh (11) also concluded from their experiments on Locke-perfused ganglia that the rate of ACh release is little affected by changes in pH over the range 7.4–8.5.

### (B) Choline

Brown and Feldberg (1) suspected that choline might be a rate-limiting factor for ACh synthesis in Locke-perfused ganglia. They therefore tested the effect of adding choline to the perfusion fluid at a time when the ACh output had been reduced to a low level by prolonged stimulation. In 5 out of 10 trials they got positive results; and in another experiment, in which choline ($1.4 \times 10^{-5}\ M$) had been present from the start, the ACh output appeared to fall off more slowly than it usually did. We have done three further experiments of the latter sort. The concentration of choline was $3.5 \times 10^{-5}\ M$, and the Locke to which it was added contained extra bicarbonate and was equilibrated with $CO_2$–$O_2$ to bring its pH to 7.4, as described in the last section.

The effect of adding choline was unambiguous (Table II, D). The ACh output from the stimulated ganglia began at the usual rate and showed the usual early decline, but became steady within 10 minutes at a level significantly ($P < 0.01$) higher than in the experiments with $CO_2$–Locke, though well below the steady level obtained with $CO_2$–plasma (Fig. 7). Even more striking was the effect of choline on the ACh content of the stimulated ganglia. Instead of being reduced by 40–60% as in all the other experiments with Locke perfusion, it rose by 107%, significantly further than in the experiments with $CO_2$-treated plasma, and nearly as far as in the experiments with $CO_2$-free plasma. These ganglia, therefore, were able to synthesize ACh at a perfectly adequate rate: in this respect they resembled ganglia perfused with plasma. They were, however, unable to release it at the maximal rate: in this respect, and also in their tendency to accumulate a great deal of surplus ACh, they behaved very much like ganglia perfused with $CO_2$-free plasma, but unlike ganglia perfused with $CO_2$-treated plasma. Since, however, these ganglia were exposed to $CO_2$ at the same tension as the ganglia perfused with $CO_2$–plasma, which were efficient releasers of ACh, we must conclude that plasma contains a factor (or factors) necessary for optimal ACh release, and different from $CO_2$. The superiority of $CO_2$-treated plasma over Locke containing choline, as a medium for the support of ACh release, must be due to the presence of this unknown material. But the superiority of plasma over ordinary Locke, as a medium for the support of ACh synthesis, must be due at least in large part to the presence of choline. Bligh (18) found that cat plasma contains about $5 \times 10^{-6}\ M$ choline, and we have obtained similar values. While this is only one-seventh of the concentration in our choline-enriched Locke, it is apparently enough for optimal ACh synthesis, for we have found that the addition of extra choline to the perfusing plasma does not appreciably increase the output of ACh during prolonged high-frequency stimulation.

Even in a ganglion perfused with Locke, some free extracellular choline is probably available to the nerve endings for ACh synthesis. Such a ganglion continues to discharge choline at the rate of 10–50 m$\mu$g/minute, even after long perfusion without stimulation, and whether eserine is present or not (5, 11). This choline may not all come from the region of the synapses, but that some of it does is made likely by an observation of Perry (5). He found that during preganglionic stimulation in the absence of eserine the choline output first rose and then fell: the rise, as he pointed out, might be due to the appearance of hydrolyzed ACh (cf. 1, 11) and the fall, to uptake of extracellular choline for ACh synthesis. Some results of our own also suggest that the active ganglion may draw on a store of endogenous choline. In two experiments we added HC-3 at the usual concentration to the plasma perfusing a ganglion that was being stimulated, and observed, in addition to the expected fall in ACh output, a sharp but temporary increase in the output of choline: the peak rate of discharge, after allowing for the choline originally present in the plasma, was 200–400 m$\mu$g/minute. HC-3 may perhaps have released this choline through some kind of base–exchange reaction. It seems not unlikely, however, that in the active ganglion choline released from some cellular store is available for the synthesis of ACh, and perhaps also of phospholipid, unless its uptake is prevented by HC-3.

*(C) Antagonism of HC-3 by Choline*

Schueler (12) showed that choline is an effective antidote to the toxic action of HC-3 in mice. It has since been found that HC-3 does not inhibit ACh synthesis by minced brain if the choline concentration of the medium is raised (6, 33, 34). Choline can also antagonize HC-3 at ganglionic synapses, as we have shown in the experiments already described, in which choline restored transmission through ganglia that had become blocked as a result of stimulation in the presence of HC-3.

Experiments on perfused ganglia gave further evidence that choline acts as an antidote to HC-3 because it supports ACh synthesis, and consequently allows ACh output to be maintained. The perfusion fluid was eserinized Locke or plasma containing HC-3 ($2 \times 10^{-5}$ $M$), and the preganglionic trunk was stimulated at 20/second. When choline was added to the fluid before stimulation began, the ACh output was better maintained than in its absence, and the ganglion lost less of its ACh; when choline was added after the effect of HC-3 was well developed, the ACh output of the stimulated ganglion rose to a higher level and remained there. The degree of restoration of synthesis depended on the choline:HC-3 ratio. When the molar ratio was 5:1 or 50:1 the inhibitory effect of HC-3, though reduced, was still present; when it was 1000:1 the normal rate of synthesis was restored and the ganglia gained ACh while they were being stimulated.

### (D) Eserine

Shelley (35) found that eserine in high concentration $(2.7 \times 10^{-3}\ M)$ reduces the rate at which brain slices form ACh. She showed that the effect can be antagonized by choline, and concluded that eserine can compete with choline at the active centers of choline acetylase. Perry (5) also concluded, as we have noted, that eserine inhibits ACh synthesis in perfused ganglia, but he explained its action somewhat differently: he considered that choline, but not ACh, can be taken up by the nerve endings and that eserine affects synthesis by preventing the hydrolysis of released ACh.

We have found that Locke-perfused ganglia synthesize less ACh during stimulation when the concentration of eserine is raised (Table II, A and E). In five experiments eserine was added to the oxygenated Locke at 5 times the usual level: its concentration was then the same $(3 \times 10^{-5}\ M)$ as in the plasma experiments. The initial ACh output matched the output found in the experiments with Locke containing the lower concentration of eserine, but the final output rate and the rate of synthesis were both significantly lower $(P > 0.05)$. These results suggest that the inhibitory effect of eserine on ACh turnover was in fact due to an action on ACh synthesis, as Shelley and Perry have proposed, rather than on ACh release. The suggestion would have been verified if the ganglia treated with the higher eserine concentration had lost more of their ACh during stimulation, but in fact the loss was about the same as for ganglia exposed to the lower level of eserine. A less equivocal result might have been found if we had used eserine in 100-fold higher concentration, as Shelley did. In her in vitro experiments, as well as in those of Mann, Tennenbaum, and Quastel (36) on the ACh metabolism of brain slices, the distribution of ACh between tissue and medium was not affected by raising the eserine concentration. As Shelley points out, this finding argues against an important inhibitory effect of the drug on ACh release. It seems probable, on the whole, that eserine can interfere with ACh synthesis in two different ways: first, as Perry suggested, merely by preventing the hydrolysis of released ACh to choline; and secondly, by competing with choline in some process necessary for ACh synthesis. One might expect that the first effect would be more prominent at low levels of eserine, and would only be significant in experiments where the perfusion fluid carried no exogenous choline to the ganglion; the second effect would become more important as the concentration of eserine was raised: excess of choline would antagonize either effect. Further work is needed to decide these points. The present experiments at least show that the superiority of plasma over Locke as a medium favoring ACh turnover, in the perfusion experiments described earlier, could not be due to the higher eserine content of the plasma.

### (E) Adrenaline

The effect of adrenaline was tested because of the possibility that the plasma used for perfusion contained significant amounts of adrenaline set free by pressor reflexes in the donor animals. Paton and Thompson (37) have already shown that adrenaline diminishes ACh release in Locke-perfused ganglia. Their finding was confirmed in one experiment, in which the concentration of adrenaline was $5 \times 10^{-8}$ g/ml and the reduction of output during prolonged stimulation at 20/second was about 50%; no effect was detected when the concentration was $10^{-8}$. The opposite result was obtained in some experiments with plasma. After a steady level of ACh release had been established, the addition of adrenaline ($10^{-8}$ g/ml) to the perfusion fluid reversibly increased the output. This effect of adrenaline was not due to vasoconstriction, which was slight or absent: it seemed to be greater when the output rate was low, and was not seen at all in one experiment when the rate was higher than usual. Adrenaline opposes the action of ACh on ganglion cells (37), and most workers have agreed with Marrazzi (38) that it inhibits ganglionic transmission, although it may under some conditions facilitate neuromuscular transmission. A facilitatory action on ganglia may, however, appear under some conditions, especially when the concentration is low (39, 40) and the present observations suggest that this may be due to an increased release of ACh. It is unlikely that the increased release is due to a more rapid synthesis of ACh, for in the plasma-perfused ganglion synthesis is already adequate to maintain the depots fully stocked.

## (F) A Plasma Factor that Promotes ACh Release

It has already been seen that the higher rate of ACh output maintained in ganglia perfused with plasma must be ascribed to the presence in plasma of a factor (or factors), other than $CO_2$, that promotes ACh release. The experiments described in the last paragraph suggested that the plasma factor might be adrenaline. Some experiments on ganglia perfused with eserinized human plasma did not support this idea. Blood was obtained in small quantities (<100 ml) from experienced donors: it was thought unlikely that such blood would contain appreciable amounts of adrenaline. Heparin was used as anticoagulant and the separated plasma was gassed with a $CO_2$–$O_2$ mixture as in the experiments with cat plasma. The plasma choline level is about the same in the two species (18). The results for ACh release and synthesis, when human plasma was perfused through cat ganglia, were indistinguishable from those obtained with cat plasma. It is therefore unlikely that the plasma factor is adrenaline.

A dialyzate of plasma, concentrated so that the diffusible constituents would be present in their original concentration, was eserinized and used as the perfusion fluid in three experiments. Although it was not treated with $CO_2$ it was as effective in supporting ACh release and synthesis as the plasma from which it was prepared. Further tests showed that the dialyzate retained its activity during 48 hours of storage at 5° C, and in one experiment it lost most or all of its effect when heated to 90° for 10 minutes. It thus appears that the plasma factor (or factors) must be diffusible through cellophane and heat-labile.

Speculation as to its identity would hardly be profitable.

### (G) Plasma from Patients with Myasthenia Gravis

Since human plasma was found to be a satisfactory perfusion fluid for cat ganglia, the opportunity was taken, with the kind cooperation of Dr. Reuben Rabinovitch, to see whether or not the plasma of patients with severe myasthenia gravis would support ACh release and synthesis equally well. This was found to be the case with three plasma samples which had been stored overnight before being tested. The experiments thus show that myasthenic plasma is not deficient in plasma factor, since this is not lost during overnight storage, nor does it contain a stable inhibitor of ACh synthesis that can act like HC-3 on ganglia. The choline content of one plasma sample was also tested and found to be within the normal range. The possibility that a labile or a slowly acting inhibitor of synthesis might be present in myasthenic blood or muscle (cf. 41) has not been formally excluded.

### 4. Time Course of ACh Release during Repetitive Stimulation

### (A) ACh Release during Prolonged Stimulation

Earlier workers have suggested that when a ganglion is stimulated for a long time, ACh is released from a depot of preformed ACh, and that when this depot is depleted by stimulation the final steady efflux is equal to the rate at which the depot can be restocked, either by synthesis (1, 4) or by transformation of synthesized ACh into an available form (5). Our present results are in conformity with this general scheme. They show in addition (a) that most of the ganglion's extractable ACh is in the depot available for release, and (b) that the rate at which the depot can be depleted, or replenished, depends on the composition of the perfusion fluid. We have thought it worth while to see how far the observed facts can be fitted by a simple formula in which the variables are the size of the ACh depot and the rates of ACh release and synthesis.

We shall make the simplifying assumptions that the rate of ACh output at any moment during the stimulation period is proportional to the amount of ACh in the depot, and that ACh is synthesized at a constant rate throughout the period. If these assumptions are correct, then whenever the rate of release exceeds the rate of synthesis the depot ACh must decay exponentially toward a final value that is proportional to the rate of synthesis. For if $Y$ is the depot ACh in $m\mu g$, which is being released at the fractional rate $b$/minute, and $s$ is the rate of synthesis in $m\mu g$/minute, then in any short time $dt$ minutes, $dY/dt = -bY + s$. On integration this gives the amount of ACh in the depot after $t$ minutes of stimulation as

$$[1] \qquad\qquad Y_t = \frac{C_b}{b} e^{-bt} + \frac{s}{b}$$

where $s/b$ is the final level toward which $Y$ falls, and $C_b$ is constant for any one experiment and is equal to the initial rate of depletion of the depot in $m\mu g$/minute. The momentary output rate of ACh output at time $t$ minutes is then and

[2]
$$Qt = bY_t = C_b e^{-bt} + s,$$

if the final steady output rate $s$ is subtracted from the successive observed output rates the values of log $(Q_t - s)$ so obtained should give a linear plot against time.

This hypothesis has been tested with the results shown in Fig. 8, where the ordinates are the mean values of $Q_t - s$ obtained from each of five groups of experiments (Table II, A, B, C, E, G) in which the perfusion fluid did not adequately support ACh synthesis. It was assumed that the asymptotic output rate $s$, which was not quite reached in an hour's stimulation, would have been 0.5 m$\mu$g/minute below the mean output rate for the last 15-minute sample. The values for the last 15 minutes were not plotted since they formed the basis for calculating $s$. The plotted points show some scatter about their means: this is not surprising in view of the uncertainties introduced by variation between ganglia, assay error, and the varying deficiency of the perfusion fluids in the factors that support ACh release. Nevertheless, most of the points are fitted tolerably well by a straight line. The points for the first 4–5 minutes are an exception, lying on a curve of significantly steeper slope. The relationship is shown more clearly in Fig. 9, in which the over-all mean values of $Q_t - s$ are plotted for each time interval. With the addition of another exponential term to take account of the steeper decay in the first few minutes, equation [2] becomes

[3]
$$Qt = C_a e^{-at} + C_b e^{-bt} + s.$$

The continuous line of Fig. 9 represents equation [3] with fitted values for the constants: 28 and 14 m$\mu$g/minute for $C_a$ and $C_b$, and 0.8 and 0.075 for the rate constants $a$ and $b$. In the experiments with Locke and HC-3, $s$ may be taken as zero. The output $Q_0$ at the start of stimulation must then be derived wholly from the original depot, which according to equation [3] consists of two portions: a smaller one $D_a$ $(= C_a/a)$ amounting to 35 m$\mu$g, which is more readily released by stimulation and therefore tends to be soon depleted; and a larger one $D_b$ $(= C_b/b)$ amounting to 187 m$\mu$g. The depot ACh would thus amount to 222 m$\mu$g and the total extractable ACh of the ganglion to 262 m$\mu$g if one adds the 40 m$\mu$g of 'stationary ACh' found experimentally (cf. 2(B), (b)) not to be available for release. This calculated value for the resting ACh content agrees, as it should, with the observed mean for the control ganglia, which was 266 m$\mu$g. From equation [3] it also follows that the final ACh content of a ganglion, in which the depot ACh suffers depletion during 60 minutes of stimulation, should be $(Q_{60}/b - 40)$ m$\mu$g, the 40 m$\mu$g being the stationary ACh as before. ($Q_{60}$ was not directly measured but could only be a little, say 0.2 m$\mu$g/minute, less than the mean output for the last 15 minutes as given in Table II.) The expected final content of the ganglion in each group of such experiments has been calculated from this formula. The values in m$\mu$g, with the corresponding observed values in parentheses, are as follows: $O_2$–Locke, 95 (111); Locke + HC-3, 49 (48); $CO_2$–Locke, 134 (170); $O_2$–Locke with high eserine, 71 (166); plasma + HC-3, 61 (61). The agreement in most cases is as good as could be

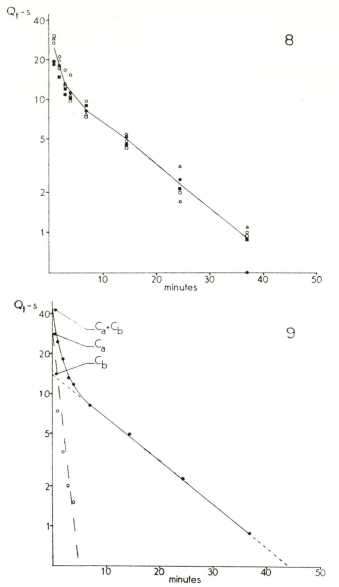

FIG. 8. Time course of ACh release: combined data for all experiments in which depot ACh was depleted by stimulation. $Q_t - s$ is output rate minus final output rate. O, $O_2$–Locke; △, $O_2$–Locke with raised eserine; □, $O_2$–Locke + HC-3; ●, $CO_2$–$O_2$–Locke; ■, $O_2$–plasma + HC-3. For explanation see text.

FIG. 9. Time course of ACh release: combined data for all experiments. For explanation see text.

expected, but the tendency of the calculated values to lie below the observed ones suggests that some surplus ACh was still present at the end of stimulation in many cases, especially when the eserine level was high. To a first approximation, then, the behavior of depot ACh in these depletion experiments conformed satisfactorily with equation [3]. (It should be noted, however, that the ratios $C_a/a$ and $C_b/b$ give a measure of the two portions of the depot only if these release ACh independently of each other. It is, however, possible that one portion is derived from the other, and in that case the respective sizes of the two portions would be different from the figures of 35 and 187 m$\mu$g given above. This possibility will be discussed later.)

In the experiments in which the ACh depot was kept well stocked throughout the stimulation, because the perfusion fluid was one that supported ACh synthesis, the output declined only during the first 5 minutes and then remained high and steady. Such a finding would be expected if the formation of $D_a$, the more readily releasable fraction, could not keep pace with the demand although the larger fraction $D_b$ was being well maintained by synthesis. Under these conditions $C_b$ of equation [3] becomes zero and the time course of ACh output should be given by

[4] $$Qt = C_a e^{-at} + s$$

with $C_a$ and $a$ having their former values. The expected time course of $Q_t - s$ is shown by the steep broken line at the left of Fig. 9. It agrees well with the plotted points representing the mean values of $Q_t - s$ for all those experiments (perfusion with plasma or with choline–Locke, Table II, D, F, H) in which ACh synthesis was adequate, $s$ in each case being taken as the mean output during the last 50 minutes of stimulation. The final steady rate of release in these experiments, according to theory, should be $s = bD_b$, or 14 m$\mu$g/minute if $b = 0.075$ as before and $D_b$ is maintained at its maximum value of 187 m$\mu$g. The observed values of $s$ were 13 m$\mu$g/minute for $CO_2$–choline–Locke (Table II, D) and 12 m$\mu$g/minute for $O_2$ plasma (Table II, F). The above value for $b$, however, was derived from experiments in which the perfusion fluid was deficient in one or other of the constituents, $CO_2$ and plasma factor, necessary for optimal ACh release. Under the more physiological conditions of perfusion with $CO_2$–plasma, depot ACh was more readily liberated, and the observed steady-state output was 28 m$\mu$g/minute, corresponding to a value of 0.15 for $b$. Too few data were obtained to decide whether $a$, the rate constant for depletion of the readily releasable fraction $D_a$, was also higher when this fluid was used for perfusion.

The time course of ACh output during prolonged stimulation at 20/second can now be seen to depend, to a first approximation, on four variables. The first of these is the amount of depot ACh in the ganglion. It varies considerably from animal to animal but averages about 230 m$\mu$g, or 85% of the total extractable ACh. In a resting ganglion the depot ACh is composed of two fractions of which one, the smaller, contains ACh in a more readily releasable form than the other. The other variables depend on the composition of the perfusion fluid. One of these is the rate at which ACh can be synthesized: this is a limiting factor for ACh output if the perfusion fluid is deficient in choline, or if it contains an inhibitor of ACh synthesis such as HC-3; in earlier work (4) the rate of synthesis was found to depend also on the extracellular glucose level. The remaining two variables are the rates at which ACh can be released by stimulation from either fraction of the depot. The rate of ACh discharge from the smaller fraction was not obviously affected by changes in the composition of the perfusion fluid in our experiments, but from earlier work (26, 27) it is known to depend on the extracellular levels of calcium and magnesium. The rate of ACh discharge from the larger fraction—or alternatively, the rate of ACh transfer from the larger to the smaller fraction—has been shown to depend on the extracellular levels of $CO_2$ and an unidentified plasma factor, and may also be sensitive to the levels of calcium and magnesium.

The quantity of ACh released by each maximal volley may be calculated from the data discussed above. With the ganglion in its most nearly physiological state (perfusion with plasma equilibrated with $CO_2$–$O_2$) the initial volley output, as determined by extrapolation to zero time, averaged 35 $\mu\mu g$; the steady-state volley output established after 5 minutes of stimulation averaged 23 $\mu\mu g$. These figures were derived from experiments in which the preganglionic trunk was stimulated at 20/second. Whether the volley output is altered by changing the frequency of stimulation was investigated in the experiments described below.

*(B) ACh Release as a Function of Stimulation Frequency*
  *(a) Plasma Perfusion*

In the four experiments whose results are shown in Table III the frequency of stimulation was systematically varied. In each case the perfusion fluid was cat plasma equilibrated with a $CO_2$–$O_2$ mixture to bring its pH close to 7.4, and the preganglionic trunk was stimulated maximally at seven frequencies, 1, 2, 4, 8, 16, 32, and 64/second, taken in random order with 500 volleys at each trial and with 12 minutes of rest between trials. Samples of effluent were collected during and for 2 minutes after each series of volleys, and were assayed against matching dilutions of ACh made up in the perfusion fluid. A small correction, 0.3 m$\mu g$/minute, was subtracted from each measured output to allow for the ACh released from the ganglion during rest. The four experiments gave similar results. The volley output was nearly the same at every frequency, and its mean value, 35 $\mu\mu g$, was the same as the initial volley output (determined by extrapolation) in the experiments with ganglia stimulated for an hour at 20/second. Under these conditions, liberated ACh comes mainly from the smaller and more readily releasable fraction of the depot, and the figure of 35 $\mu\mu g$ may be regarded as a fair estimate of the volley output from a ganglion in which this fraction has not been depleted by a prior stimulation.

Such a level of volley output cannot be maintained indefinitely in a repetitively stimulated ganglion. Table IV presents the results of three experiments in which stimuli of varying frequency were applied for a longer time. In each experiment the perfusion fluid was plasma equilibrated with $CO_2$ and $O_2$ as before, and the preganglionic trunk was stimulated maximally at 4, 16, and 64/second for 20 minutes with 30 minutes of rest between each period of stimulation. The ACh output in these trials was found to fall off as usual

TABLE III

Release of ACh from plasma-perfused ganglia:
brief stimulation

| Volleys/second | Volley output, μμg | | | | |
|---|---|---|---|---|---|
| | 1 | 2 | 3 | 4 | Mean |
| 1 | 32 | 29 | 52 | 44 | 39 |
| 2 | 17 | 28 | 47 | 28 | 30 |
| 4 | 26 | 24 | 52 | 32 | 34 |
| 8 | 30 | 30 | 52 | 32 | 36 |
| 16 | 23 | 34 | 47 | 34 | 34 |
| 32 | 30 | 34 | 49 | 38 | 38 |
| 64 | 23 | 28 | 54 | 38 | 36 |

TABLE IV

Release of ACh from plasma-perfused ganglia: prolonged stimulation

| Volleys/second | Volley output, μμg | | | | Minute output, mμg | | | |
|---|---|---|---|---|---|---|---|---|
| | 1 | 2 | 3* | Mean | 1 | 2 | 3* | Mean |
| 4 | 22 | 37 | 19 | 26 | 5.3 | 9 | 4.6 | 6.3 |
| 16 | 24 | 37 | 19 | 27 | 23 | 36 | 19 | 26 |
| 64 | 5.5 | 9.6 | 5.4 | 6.8 | 22 | 37 | 21 | 27 |

*Choline added.

during the first 5 minutes, but it remained practically steady while the last three 5-minute samples were being obtained. The mean output per volley and per minute for each of these 15-minute periods of steady discharge are given in the table. It can be seen that in every experiment the volley output was about the same at 16/second as at 4/second, but was only one-fourth as great at 64/second. On the other hand, the minute output was about the same at 16/second and 64/second but was only one-fourth as great at 4/second. It follows from the combined results that under these conditions of perfusion, when the readily releasable ACh had been depleted by prior stimulation, the volley output was independent of frequency of stimulation for frequencies up to 16/second and with more rapid stimulation fell off in inverse ratio to the frequency. The maximum volley output for an average ganglion under these conditions was about 27 μμg; the maximum minute output, in agreement with figures presented earlier (Table II, H), was about 27 μμg. In one of the experiments of this series the choline content of the perfused plasma had been raised about 100-fold, to $7 \times 10^{-4}$ $M$, by the addition of choline chloride. Since this enrichment with choline did not increase the rate of ACh output, the extracellular choline level cannot be a rate-limiting factor for ganglia perfused with plasma.

93

### (b) Locke Perfusion

Perry (5) has shown that the time course of ACh release during prolonged excitation of a Locke-perfused ganglion is substantially independent of stimulation frequency over the range 5–100/second and amounts to about 4 m$\mu$g/minute. We have not thought it necessary to duplicate his observations, but in two experiments we tested the relationship between stimulation frequency and ACh output for brief periods of stimulation in ganglia perfused with $O_2$–Locke. As in the corresponding trials with plasma perfusion, bursts of 500 volleys were fired down the preganglionic trunk at seven different frequencies over the range 1–64/second. The results differed from those with plasma-perfused ganglia in that the volley output was somewhat higher for the medium frequencies than for the higher and lower ones. It does not seem profitable to speculate on the reasons for the shape of the frequency-output curve under these unphysiological conditions. No evidence was obtained in these experiments, or in those with plasma perfusion, that the volley output at low frequencies or at the outset of stimulation may approach or exceed 100 $\mu\mu$g as has been reported by several authors (19, 27, 42, 43). It is of course probable that the first few volleys of a series may discharge more ACh than the later ones. Indeed, electrophysiological studies strongly suggest that this happens at neuromuscular junctions (44, 45). The possibility cannot, however, be verified by direct measurement of the released ACh, since the quantity involved would be below the threshold for assay.

## Discussion

We have confirmed the finding of Brown and Feldberg (1) that a Locke-perfused ganglion stimulated for a long time through its preganglionic trunk releases ACh at a rate that falls off to reach a steady low level. But unlike them we have found that this fall in ACh output is accompanied by an important depletion in the ganglion's content of extractable ACh. The discrepancy between their results and ours on this point is probably to be ascribed to differences in technique. Unless special care is taken to continue maximal stimulation until the moment when the ganglion is removed and placed in the extracting medium, and to prevent any reflux of blood into the ganglion (through vessels accompanying the postganglionic trunk) when perfusion is shut off, it is easy to obtain misleadingly high values for the final ACh content. Some of the data recorded by Brown and Feldberg (1) (and also by Kahlson and MacIntosh (4), who did some similar tests) suggest that these sources of error may have been present in their experiments. Both pairs of workers did, indeed, obtain some evidence for a decrease of ganglionic ACh as a result of prolonged stimulation when the conditions of perfusion were similar to our own: this happened in two of three experiments by Brown and Feldberg (the third experiment gave the opposite result), and in all three experiments by Kahlson and MacIntosh. The mean fall in ACh in these five experiments was 27%, as against 53% in five experiments by us.

Even in our own experiments the observed decrease in ACh content appears at first sight too small to account for the decline in ACh output, averaging over 80%, found in our Locke-perfusion experiments. The explanation for this finding is that even in a normal ganglion a proportion of the ACh is not releasable by nerve impulses, and in a ganglion whose cholinesterase has been inactivated the proportion is higher. The nature of unreleasable ACh is discussed below.

*Storage of ACh*

We have designated as 'stationary ACh' that fraction of the total store that remains in a ganglion whose ACh has been maximally depleted by prolonged stimulation in the presence of the drug HC-3, which blocks ACh synthesis. It amounts to about 40 m$\mu$g, or 15% of the total extractable ACh, and apparently can only be set free by procedures that destroy the structural integrity of the ganglion. We have argued that stationary ACh is for the most part located in the extrasynaptic portions of the preganglionic axons; if so, it is presumably separated spatially from the cholinesterase which is also present in these axons. It is attractive to suppose that this fraction is situated in subcellular particles of some kind, in association with the choline acetylase by which it was formed. From the experiments of Hebb, Krause, and Silver (46) on ventral root homogenates it can be concluded that axonal choline acetylase is located in subcellular particles, but whether the same particles contain the axonal ACh is not known. In homogenates of brain, most of the enzyme and most of the ACh sediment together (47), but such homogenates, as Gray and Whittaker (48) have shown, contain intact nerve endings. Their plausible suggestion, that both substances are located in a single kind of particle within these endings has therefore, as they point out, still to be proved. It seems not unlikely, then, that both stationary ACh and releasable ACh are contained within specific subcellular particles, but, as yet, one cannot confidently identify such particles with any of the structures that have been recognized in axons or axonal terminals.

In a ganglion whose cholinesterase remains active the whole of the ACh not included in the stationary fraction is available for release by nerve impulses, as is shown by its disappearance from active ganglia in which synthesis has been prevented by HC-3. This fraction has been denoted 'depot ACh'. It must be located in the nerve terminals, since the preganglionic axons are not depleted of their ACh by stimulation in the presence of HC-3. In an average ganglion the depot ACh amounts to 220 m$\mu$g, or about 85% of the extractable total. Our analysis of the time course of ACh discharge during prolonged stimulation has shown that depot ACh is composed of two subfractions, one of which is smaller and more readily liberated than the other. In that analysis we assumed, for simplicity, that the two subfractions responded independently to stimulation, each releasing a characteristic proportion of its ACh in response to each arriving volley until the smaller fraction was exhausted. Another interpretation is, however, equally possible and in some ways more attractive. This is to suppose that the two reservoirs of depot ACh are connected, as it were, in series rather than in parallel, and that ACh from the larger one must pass into the smaller before it can finally be discharged. The two hypotheses account equally well for the time course of ACh release during prolonged stimulation; they also account equally well for the high and constant volley output found when a ganglion that has been rested is briefly stimulated at any frequency over the range 1–64/second, and for the somewhat lower, though still constant, volley output during prolonged stimulation at any frequency up to 16/second. One set of results, however, appears to favor the "series" as against the "parallel" hypothesis. With prolonged stimulation at frequencies above 16/second, the volley output falls off in inverse ratio to the frequency. This fall is not due to depletion of the main ACh depot, for extraction of the ganglion reveals no such depletion; nor can it be due to a progressive failure of some part of the release mechanism, for the volley output, though low, can be maintained indefinitely without further reduction. At the higher frequencies it is the minute output, rather than the volley output, that is independent of frequency; and there must therefore be some process, independent of both the speed of ACh synthesis and the spacing of the incoming volleys, that limits the rate at which ACh can be discharged. This process is most simply imagined, in terms of the "series" hypothesis, as the movement of depot ACh from the larger into the smaller, more readily releasable fraction; in terms of the "parallel" hypothesis one would have to postulate either a further subdivision of the larger fraction, or else that the effectiveness of closely spaced impulses in releasing ACh declines as a precise inverse function of their frequency. Further work, however, will be needed before one hypothesis can be strongly preferred to the other.

It may be noted here that the "series" hypothesis is similar to one proposed by Perry (5), to account for the paradox of a declining ACh output from Locke-perfused ganglia whose ACh stores were supposedly well maintained. Perry suggested, in explanation, that newly synthesized depot ACh could only be made "available" at the rate of about 4 m$\mu$g/minute. On the basis of our own experiments it seems clear, however, that ACh release under the conditions of his tests must have been limited by the speed of synthesis, rather than by the speed with which synthesized ACh could be made available for release.

In recent years it has been strongly argued that the minute vesicles which abound in the presynaptic axoplasm represent the transmitter depot. Our findings are obviously compatible with this idea. It has been observed with several kinds of synapse (49, 50, 51) that vesicles are not uniformly distributed within nerve endings but show some tendency to be grouped close to the presynaptic membrane. The vesicles so located might be thought to contain the readily releasable fraction of the depot ACh.

Besides stationary and depot ACh, we have described a third kind of intracellular ACh, which is present only in ganglia whose cholinesterase has been inactivated. This we have called "surplus" ACh. It is formed rather slowly, but may rise to a level above that of the depot ACh. Since it quickly disappears when the enzyme is reactivated, it must be located in a compartment where it would have been destroyed in the presence of the active enzyme. It cannot make an important contribution to the ACh released by stimulation, since the volley output from an eserinized ganglion remains constant while surplus ACh is accumulating. We have pointed out (52) that the formation of surplus ACh, and also the steady release of ACh in minute quantity from the eserinized resting ganglion, are evidence that depot ACh undergoes a continuous slow turnover even when no nerve impulses are arriving at the terminals. It is plausible to suppose that the continuous release during rest may represent a quantal discharge of depot ACh into the extracellular space, such as is known to occur at motor nerve endings in striated muscle, while the continuous formation of surplus ACh may represent a concurrent discharge of depot ACh into the presynaptic axoplasm. But other explanations for these phenomena are conceivable, and it is even possible that surplus ACh is held in structures other than the nerve endings.

Whittaker (53) has recently demonstrated the existence of two forms of bound ACh in a particular subfraction of homogenized brain: one form is readily, one much less readily, set free by simple physical procedures. Since this fraction contained many intact nerve endings (48), and was eserinized, it seems quite likely that the more labile form represented our surplus ACh.

*Synthesis of ACh*

Although we have confirmed the finding of earlier workers (1, 4) that Locke-perfused ganglia can manufacture important quantities of ACh during stimulation, our experiments emphasize that ACh synthesis in such ganglia is much less efficient than under physiological conditions. The abnormality of synthesis can be completely corrected by adding choline to the Locke; when this is done the ACh turnover of a ganglion can be maintained at a high level as long as stimulation is continued. Normal plasma contains enough choline (about $7 \times 10^{-7}$ g/ml) to support ACh turnover at the maximum level. A simple calculation shows that the nerve endings must be remarkably efficient in extracting choline from the extracellular fluid. The superior cervical ganglion preparation of the cat when perfused with plasma at our usual rate of 0.3 ml/minute will continue to release ACh at the rate of about 28 m$\mu$g/minute during an indefinitely long period of preganglionic stimulation. This ACh must be derived from the plasma choline, which is therefore esterified at the rate of about 21 m$\mu$g/minute. About half the perfusion fluid flows through structures adjacent to the ganglion, which, if the plasma choline is 700 m$\mu$g/ml (18), is supplied with choline at the rate of 100 m$\mu$g/minute. The nerve endings are therefore able to take up and acetylate some 20% of the choline supplied to the ganglion during the few seconds required for the plasma to pass through the ganglionic vessels. Since choline as a quaternary base diffuses slowly into most cells, and since the nerve endings can form only a small part of the bulk of the ganglion, this fact is rather remarkable. It suggests that the endings (or perhaps the teloglial elements that embrace them) must be provided with some special mechanism for the entry of choline ions.

We have already (7, 8, 52) recapitulated the evidence that the remarkably specific and potent action of the base HC-3 as an inhibitor of ACh synthesis is to be ascribed to its ability to compete with choline for transport by just such a mechanism. It seems very likely that some sort of choline carrier, located in a membrane lying between the extracellular fluid and the sites of ACh formation, is a constant feature of cholinergic mechanisms. Most of the effects that have been described for HC-3 (6, 12, 54, 55, 56) in the whole animal can be attributed with some confidence to its ability to prevent the synthesis of ACh at cholinergic nerve endings. Blockade of transmission in cholinergic pathways occurs only in the presence of repetitive activity in such pathways, and after an appreciable latency; it is intensified by increasing the frequency of stimulation and it is antagonized by choline. The present paper provides some illustrative examples in the case of the pathway through the superior cervical ganglion: a comparison of the time course of transmission failure with that of ACh release suggests that the volley output must be reduced by about 80% for transmission to be blocked by 50%.

Other bases besides HC-3 can depress ACh synthesis; and we have confirmed earlier reports (35) that eserine in high dosage has such an effect: its mode of action is not necessarily identical with that of HC-3. The possibility that a failure of ACh synthesis at the neuromuscular junction is the basic defect in myasthenia gravis has been raised by Desmedt (45), and prompted us to examine the ability of myasthenic plasma to support synthesis in perfused ganglia. No evidence was found that a circulating inhibitor was present, but either a labile or a slowly acting material might have escaped detection.

*Release of ACh*

Previous work has emphasized the necessity of external calcium (26, 27, 57) for the release of ACh by the nerve impulse and the antagonistic action of magnesium (27, 57). The concentrations of these ions have not been deliberately varied in our experiments, but we have shown that two other factors must be present in the external fluid for optimal ACh release, even in the case of ganglia whose depot ACh is well maintained. These factors are dissolved $CO_2$ and an unknown material present in plasma. We have suggested that $CO_2$ may act by promoting the ionization of calcium, and it is possible that the plasma factor may also be concerned in some way with the uptake or action of calcium.

The amount of ACh released by any series of preganglionic volleys will depend not only on the concentrations of the factors listed above, but also on the amount of depot ACh present in the ganglion at the time and on its partition between the two fractions we have identified. In terms of the "series" hypothesis for which we have expressed a preference, namely that the readily releasable fraction is the immediate source of all released ACh, this fraction in a normal resting ganglion will contain about 50 m$\mu$g of ACh and there will be about 170 m$\mu$g in the remainder of the depot. If the extracellular factors for release are maintained at the physiological level, each arriving volley will discharge about 1/1200 of the ACh in the smaller fraction: the proportion discharged will be the same, to a first approximation, whatever the frequency of stimulation, and whether or not the readily releasable fraction has undergone depletion. The ACh lost from that fraction will be replenished from the larger fraction, but the rate of replenishment cannot exceed 28 m$\mu$g/minute, and will be proportionately smaller if the larger fraction has been depleted or if the smaller fraction has undergone only a small depletion. The transfer of ACh from the larger to the smaller fraction may correspond to a movement of depot ACh towards the synaptic membrane. The larger fraction, in its turn, will be replenished at a rate determined by the conditions for ACh synthesis. (On the basis of the "parallel" hypothesis, the proportion of depot ACh in the readily releasable fraction of a resting ganglion will be somewhat smaller than on the basis of the "series" hypothesis, and that fraction will be reduced to a low level by a few minutes of high-frequency stimulation in the way suggested by equation [3] of Section 4($A$).) It should be re-emphasized that the volley output from a ganglion remains high at physiological frequencies of excitation, however long the excitation may last. Thus it may be doubted whether failure of transmission, at unpoisoned cholinergic junctions, is ever due to failure of ACh liberation. If prolonged high-frequency stimulation leads to junctional block, the block must be due to lowered sensitivity of the postsynaptic structures to ACh, or to an excess of free ACh, or to asynchronous release of ACh, rather than to a reduction of volley output.

### Relationship of ACh Synthesis to ACh Release

A ganglion supplied with a fluid that supports ACh synthesis has a considerable turnover of ACh even when it is at rest, as is revealed when its cholinesterase is inactivated. In such a ganglion ACh is manufactured at the rate of about 4 m$\mu$g/minute and released into the circulation at about 1/10th that rate. During prolonged stimulation at high frequency the rate of release goes up by a factor of perhaps 70 and the rate of synthesis by a factor of 7, the increase in synthesis being somewhat more than is needed to keep pace with the accelerated release. But even under the most favorable conditions of repetitive activity, the choline acetylase of the ganglion is working at only a fraction of its capacity, as is shown by the ability of the enzyme after it has been extracted from a ganglion to form ACh 4 times as fast (22). Synthesis in the intact ganglion may therefore be limited either by the supply of substrate (choline and acetyl-coenzyme A) or by accumulation of the product, ACh, in the vicinity of the synthesizing enzyme. It is unlikely that choline is a limiting factor for synthesis either in the resting or in the active ganglion, unless a drug like HC-3

CANADIAN JOURNAL OF BIOCHEMISTRY AND PHYSIOLOGY. VOL. 39, 1961

is present. When a resting ganglion is eserinized, its ACh content rises by about 25% in the first 5 minutes even in the presence of HC-3, so that there must have been some choline available for ACh synthesis in the nerve endings; and in an active ganglion perfused with plasma, the ACh output cannot be raised by adding more choline to the plasma. The possibility that acetyl-coenzyme A is a limiting factor cannot be excluded, but it is not obvious how synaptic activity could determine the rate at which it is supplied to the enzyme. A more attractive hypothesis is to suppose that the rate-controlling factor for synthesis is the concentration of ACh in the vicinity of the synthesizing enzyme. We have referred to the possibility that the ACh and choline acetylase of brain are contained within the same subcellular particle, which may be the synaptic vesicle; and it can be calculated (7, 58) that if the vesicles do indeed represent the ACh store the concentration of ACh in the vesicular fluid must be very high, even approaching isotonicity. If newly synthesized ACh remains associated with choline acetylase within a vesicle, further synthesis should be retarded so long as the vesicle remains intact, but would be resumed after ACh has been released by an effective collision between the vesicle and the presynaptic membrane. The formation of surplus ACh, on this hypothesis, would suggest that some ACh can escape from the vesicles into the surrounding axoplasm, where it can accumulate if cholinesterase has been inhibited, this accumulation, in turn, ceasing when the concentration of ACh outside the vesicles approaches that inside.

## Acknowledgments

This work was generously supported by grants from the National Research Council of Canada and the Defence Research Board (Grant No. 8950–18). We are indebted to Mr. Karl Holeczek for his technical assistance.

## References

1. G. L. BROWN and W. FELDBERG. J. Physiol. **88**, 265 (1936).
2. G. L. BROWN and W. FELDBERG. J. Physiol. **86**, 290 (1936).
3. F. C. MACINTOSH. J. Physiol. **99**, 436 (1941).
4. G. KAHLSON and F. C. MACINTOSH. J. Physiol. **96**, 277 (1939).
5. W. L. M. PERRY. J. Physiol. **119**, 439 (1953).
6. F. C. MACINTOSH, R. I. BIRKS, and P. B. SASTRY. Nature, **178**, 1181 (1956).
7. F. C. MACINTOSH. Can. J. Biochem. and Physiol. **37**, 343 (1959).
8. F. C. MACINTOSH, R. I. BIRKS, and P. B. SASTRY. Neurology, **8**, Suppl. 1, 90 (1958).
9. A. W. KIBJAKOW. Pflüger's Arch. ges. Physiol. **232**, 432 (1933).
10. W. FELDBERG and J. H. GADDUM. J. Physiol. **81**, 305 (1934).
11. N. EMMELIN and F. C. MACINTOSH. J. Physiol. **131**, 477 (1956).
12. F. W. SCHUELER. J. Pharmacol. Exptl. Therap. **115**, 127 (1955).
13. R. I. BIRKS. Rev. can. biol. **14**, 235 (1955).
14. H. C. CHANG and J. H. GADDUM. J. Physiol. **79**, 255 (1933).
15. W. FELDBERG. J. Physiol. **101**, 432 (1943).
16. F. C. MACINTOSH and W. L. M. PERRY. Biological estimation of acetylcholine. *In* Methods of medical research. Vol. 3. The Year Book Publishers, Inc., Chicago. 1950. p. 78.
17. J. CROSSLAND, H. M. PAPPIUS, and K. A. C. ELLIOTT. Am. J. Physiol. **183**, 27 (1955).
18. J. BLIGH. J. Physiol. **117**, 234 (1952).
19. W. FELDBERG and A. VARTIAINEN. J. Physiol. **83**, 103 (1934).
20. F. C. MACINTOSH. J. Physiol. **94**, 155 (1938).

21. P. Fatt and B. Katz. J. Physiol. **117**, 109 (1952).
22. J. Banister and M. Scrase. J. Physiol. **111**, 437 (1950).
23. C. O. Hebb and G. M. H. Waites. J. Physiol. **132**, 667 (1956).
24. D. Richter and J. Crossland. Am. J. Physiol. **159**, 247 (1949).
25. A. Rosenbleuth, K. Lissak, and A. Lanari. Am. J. Physiol. **128**, 31 (1939).
26. A. M. Harvey and F. C. MacIntosh. J. Physiol. **97**, 408 (1940).
27. O. F. Hutter and K. Kostial. J. Physiol. **124**, 234 (1954).
28. J. del Castillo and B. Katz. Progr. in Biophys. and Biophys. Chem. **6**, 121 (1956).
29. L. M. Dillman and M. B. Visscher. J. Biol. Chem. **103**, 291 (1933).
30. T. Hopkins, J. E. Howard, and H. Eisenberg. Bull. Johns Hopkins Hosp. **91**, 1 (1952).
31. J. H. Quastel, M. Tennenbaum, and A. H. M. Wheatley. Biochem. J. **30**, 1668 (1936).
32. H. McLennan and K. A. C. Elliott. Am. J. Physiol. **163**, 605 (1950).
33. P. B. Sastry. The functional significance of acetylcholine in the brain. Ph.D. Thesis, McGill University, Montreal, Que. 1956.
34. J. E. Gardiner. J. Physiol. **138**, 13P (1957).
35. H. Shelley. J. Physiol. **131**, 329 (1956).
36. P. J. G. Mann, M. Tennenbaum, and J. H. Quastel. Biochem. J. **32**, 243 (1938).
37. W. D. M. Paton and J. W. Thompson. (Abstr.) Intern. Physiol. Congr. XIXth Congr. 664 (1953).
38. A. S. Marrazzi. Am. J. Physiol. **127**, 738 (1939).
39. E. Bulbring and J. H. Burn. J. Physiol. **101**, 289 (1942).
40. E. Bulbring. J. Physiol. **103**, 55 (1944).
41. J. E. Desmedt. Federation Proc. **18**, 36 (1959).
42. O. F. Hutter and K. Kostial. J. Physiol. **129**, 159 (1955).
43. K. Kostial and V. B. Vouk. J. Physiol. **132**, 239 (1956).
44. O. F. Hutter. J. Physiol. **118**, 216 (1952).
45. J. E. Desmedt. Nature, **182**, 1673 (1958).
46. C. O. Hebb, M. Krause, and A. Silver. J. Physiol. **148**, 69P (1959).
47. C. O. Hebb and V. P. Whittaker. J. Physiol. **142**, 187 (1958).
48. E. G. Gray and V. P. Whittaker. J. Physiol. **153**, 7P (1960).
49. G. A. Edwards, H. Ruska, and E. de Harven. J. Biophys. Biochem. Cytol. **4**, 107 (1958).
50. S. L. Palay. Exptl. Cell Research, Suppl. **5**, 275 (1958).
51. R. Birks, H. E. Huxley, and B. Katz. J. Physiol. **150**, 134 (1959).
52. R. I. Birks and F. C. MacIntosh. Brit. Med. Bull. **13**, 157 (1957).
53. V. P. Whittaker. Biochem. J. **72**, 694 (1959).
54. N. L. Reitzel and J. P. Long. Arch. intern. pharmacodynamie, **119**, 20 (1959).
55. H. Wilson and J. P. Long. Arch. intern. pharmacodynamie, **120**, 343 (1959).
56. V. G. Longo. Arch. intern. pharmacodynamie, **119**, 1 (1959).
57. J. del Castillo and B. Katz. J. Physiol. **124**, 560 (1954).
58. R. I. Birks. Acetylcholine turnover in sympathetic ganglia. Ph.D. Thesis, McGill University, Montreal, Que. 1957.

# The Separation of Synaptic Vesicles from Nerve-Ending Particles ('Synaptosomes')

By V. P. WHITTAKER, I. A. MICHAELSON* AND R. JEANETTE A. KIRKLAND

*Biochemistry Department, Agricultural Research Council Institute of Animal Physiology, Babraham, Cambridge*

(*Received 24 June 1963*)

When brain tissue is homogenized in media iso-osmotic to plasma, the club-like presynaptic nerve endings resist disruption and are snapped or torn off from their attachments to form discrete particles (nerve-ending particles) in which all the main structural features of the nerve ending are preserved. For these particles we propose the name 'synaptosomes' in order to emphasize their relative homogeneity and their resemblance in physical properties to other subcellular organelles. They can be separated as a distinct fraction by differential and density-gradient centrifuging (Gray & Whittaker, 1960, 1962; Whittaker, 1960). This fraction contains most of the particle-bound acetylcholine (Hebb & Whittaker, 1958; Whittaker, 1959), choline acetyltransferase (choline acetylase) (Hebb & Whittaker, 1958), hydroxytryptamine (Whittaker, 1959; Michaelson & Whittaker, 1962, 1963) and noradrenaline (Chruściel, 1960) of the tissue. Since acetylcholine is now well established, by all the classical criteria, as a central as well as a peripheral transmitter (for a review see Gaddum, 1961), it seems reasonable to conclude that the particle-bound acetylcholine and choline acetyltransferase of the fraction represent acetylcholine and enzyme localized within synaptosomes derived from cholinergic neurones. Similarly, the 5-hydroxytryptamine and noradrenaline in this fraction are probably due to the presence of synaptosomes derived from neurones containing these amines. This view has been strengthened by the findings of Carlsson, Falck & Hillarp (1962), who have obtained histochemical evidence for the neuronal localization of these amines in the brain.

The nerve endings and the synaptosomes derived from them have a complex fine structure when examined under the electron microscope with positive staining and thin sectioning (see review by Whittaker & Gray, 1962) or negative staining (Horne & Whittaker, 1962). They are seen to consist (Plate 1d) of thin-walled bags containing cytoplasm packed with synaptic granules or vesicles (Sjöstrand, 1953; Palay & Palade, 1954;

* Present address: Laboratory of Chemical Pharmacology, National Heart Institute, National Institutes of Health, Bethesda 14, Md., U.S.A.

Robertson, 1956; De Robertis & Bennett, 1955; Morán, 1957); frequently (though not in this example) one or more mitochondria are also present. The region of the post-synaptic membrane immediately adjacent to the ending is thickened; on homogenization it may remain adherent and accompany the synaptosome through the various steps of the fractionation procedure. Synaptic vesicles appear to be of at least three main kinds: 'hollow', 'dense-cored' and 'compound' (Plate 1d). They have been proposed as the actual binding sites of transmitters within the nerve endings (De Robertis & Bennett, 1955; del Castillo & Katz, 1955, 1956; De Robertis, 1958) and as the morphological counterpart of the 'quantized' release of acetylcholine detected electrophysiologically (Fatt & Katz, 1952). The dense-cored vesicles are numerous in peripheral adrenergic nerve endings, and have there been proposed as the binding sites of noradrenaline.

We have for some time been studying the disruption of synaptosomes with the object of obtaining, as separate fractions, synaptic vesicles, intraneuronal mitochondria, external and post-synaptic membranes and the soluble constituents of the nerve-ending cytoplasm for biochemical and pharmacological analysis (Whittaker, 1961). For the morphological control of the various disruptive procedures in the electron microscope, negative staining was found to avoid many of the limitations inherent in conventional methods of positive staining, embedding and thin sectioning when applied to this kind of material (Horne & Whittaker, 1962; Whittaker, 1963a).

Suspension of synaptosomes in media hypo-osmotic to plasma was found to result in the bursting of about 80% of the synaptosomes with the survival of intact synaptic vesicles and about 50% of the bound acetylcholine. By contrast, frozen-and-thawed preparations contained fewer ruptured synaptosomes and almost no intact synaptic vesicles unconfined by an external membrane (Johnson & Whittaker, 1962, 1963). In this work, lactate dehydrogenase was used as a marker for the easily-diffusible water-soluble components of the nerve-ending cytoplasm.

Reprinted from *The Biochemical Journal* 90: 293–303 (1964) by permission of the publisher.

It was therefore decided, in the current series of experiments, to use suspension in water as a means of releasing the vesicles. To separate the vesicles from membrane fragments, mitochondria and incompletely disrupted synaptosomes, a density-gradient procedure was devised. The tendency of vesicles to remain clumped together after release as though embedded in a sticky cytoplasm (Whittaker, 1961, 1963 a) proved troublesome and decreased the yield of free vesicles. Preliminary accounts of this work have already been given (Whittaker, 1963 b; Whittaker, Michaelson & Kirkland, 1963).

While this work was in progress, De Robertis, Arnaiz & de Iraldi (1962), De Robertis, Salganicoff, Zieher & Arnaiz (1963 b) and De Robertis, Arnaiz, Salganicoff, de Iraldi & Zieher (1963 a) claimed to have isolated synaptic vesicles by a simpler procedure than ours. Reasons are given, in the Results section of the present paper, for believing that the preparations of De Robertis and co-workers are heterogeneous and are heavily contaminated with small membrane fragments and intact and partially disrupted synaptosomes. We consider that their electron-microscopic methods greatly underestimate the amount of this contamination and that their conclusions on the biochemical make-up of the isolated vesicles are therefore open to question.

## METHODS

### Preparation of tissue fractions

*Primary fractions.* All operations were conducted at 0–4°, with analytical-grade reagents and freshly prepared glass-distilled water. Guinea-pig forebrains were homogenized in 0·32M-sucrose and separated into fractions $P_1$ (nuclei, large myelin fragments, tissue debris), $P_2$ (mitochondria, synaptosomes, small myelin fragments, some microsomes) and $S_2$ (microsomes, some small mitochondria and synaptosomes) as described by Gray & Whittaker (1962), except that, to speed preparation and to diminish microsomal contamination, $P_1$ was not washed and $P_2$ was separated at 10000g for 20 min. instead of at 17000g for 60 min. This resulted in a lower yield of synaptosomes (and therefore of acetylcholine and choline acetyltransferase) in fraction $P_2$ but this was immaterial for our purposes. In some experiments the $P_2$ pellet was washed by resuspension in 0·32M-sucrose and recentrifuging at 10000g for 30 min. In other experiments the resuspended $P_2$ pellet was further fractionated into subfractions A (myelin, some synaptosomes and microsomes), B (synaptosomes and some microsomes) and C (mitochondria) by means of a discontinuous density gradient consisting of equal volumes of 0·8M- and 1·2M-sucrose as described by Gray & Whittaker (1962). The A and B fractions were diluted with equal volumes of water and centrifuged at 40000 rev./min. (100000g) for 60 min. to give well-packed pellets.

For comparison, fractions were prepared under identical conditions from guinea-pig liver.

*Disruption of fractions.* The $P_2$ or B pellets were dis-rupted (1) by freezing-and-thawing ten times, or (2) by suspending in water (2 ml./g. of original tissue). When the latter method was used, the water suspension, $W$, was usually centrifuged at 10000g for 20 min. to remove the larger mitochondria and myelin fragments as a loosely packed pellet, $W_p$, leaving a cloudy supernatant, $W_s$, for further fractionation. In some experiments the water contained eserine sulphate (0·2%). This had the effect of preserving the 50% of the acetylcholine originally present in the $P_2$ fraction which was released into the free state by the water treatment (Whittaker, 1959) and which was otherwise destroyed by the cholinesterase present in the preparation.

In a few experiments, $CaCl_2$ (0·001–0·1%) was added to the sucrose or the water, or both, used in the fractionations. Concentrations of $CaCl_2$ less than about 0·01% had no effect, but concentrations greater than this tended to cause particulate material to form coacervates, thereby decreasing yields.

*Density-gradient separation of disrupted fractions.* Suspensions of disrupted material (5–6 ml., corresponding to 1·5–2·5 g. of tissue/tube) were transferred to discontinuous density gradients usually consisting of five successive layers (5 ml./tube) of sucrose differing in concentration by 0·2M at the top to 1·2M at the bottom of the gradient. In an abbreviated procedure, when only the lightest fractions were required, the gradient consisted of 0·4M-sucrose (5 ml./tube) layered over 20 ml. of 0·6M-sucrose. The gradients were set up about 1 hr. before use in Lustroid tubes of the SW25 head of the Spinco model L preparative ultracentrifuge. After centrifuging at 25000 rev./min. (53500g) for 2 hr. the tubes and contents were sliced in a tube cutter to give a number of separate fractions. Volume recoveries were 85–92%.

### Analysis of fractions

*Total nitrogen.* This was determined by the micro-Kjeldahl method and expressed in milligrams.

*Potassium.* This was kindly determined by Dr M. W. Smith, using an EEL model A flame photometer. Results are expressed in micrograms.

*Lactate dehydrogenase.* This was determined spectrophotometrically as described by Johnson (1960) by following the change in extinction at 340 mµ, accompanying the transfer of hydrogen from $NADH_2$ to sodium pyruvate, with a Unicam SP. 700 recording spectrophotometer. Lactate dehydrogenase has been shown to be a soluble cytoplasmic enzyme in brain; the portion of the enzyme associated with particles is a marker for the soluble cytoplasm of synaptosomes (Johnson & Whittaker, 1962, 1963). Enzyme activities are expressed as the change in extinction at 340 mµ ($\Delta E_{340}$)/min.

*Succinate dehydrogenase.* This was used as a mitochondrial marker and was determined manometrically with potassium ferricyanide as the electron acceptor, as described by Whittaker (1959). The enzyme activity is expressed as µmoles of succinate oxidized/hr.

*Choline acetyltransferase.* This was determined after activation with ether (Hebb & Smallman, 1956) by the procedure of Berry & Whittaker (1959). The enzyme activity is expressed as µmoles of acetylcholine formed/hr.

*Cholinesterase.* This was determined manometrically by the method of Ammon (1933), with acetylcholine as substrate in a final concentration of 10 mM. A decrease in activity was observed with higher concentrations of acetylcholine, indicating that the enzyme was mainly acetylcholinesterase. The enzyme activity is expressed as $\mu$moles of acetylcholine hydrolysed/hr.

*Acetylcholine.* The acetylcholine content of fractions was assayed on a small (8 mm. $\times$ 0·25 mm.) slip of the dorsal muscle of the leech mounted in a horizontal organ bath of 0·05 ml. capacity as described by Szerb (1962), except that eserine (1 mg./100 ml.) added to the medium was used to sensitize the preparation instead of a short exposure to sarin. Contractions were isotonic. The thickness of the muscle slip was found to be fairly critical; slips thicker than 0·5 mm. did not relax well. The threshold was usually 0·5–2 $\mu\mu$moles of acetylcholine (i.e. about 0·1–0·4 $\mu$mg. of acetylcholine chloride)/ml. Sucrose fractions were heated at pH 4 and 100° for 10 min. to release any bound acetylcholine, diluted 1:10 or more with medium and neutralized, if necessary, with 0·33 N-NaOH before assay. That muscle responses were due to acetylcholine (or a related ester) was shown by tests in which the activity was abolished by the addition of erythrocyte cholinesterase. G. Dowe & V. P. Whittaker (unpublished work) have shown that at least 95 % of the acetylcholine-like activity of guinea-pig brain is due to acetylcholine itself.

*Expression of results.* Activities of fractions are expressed (1) in units/vol. of fraction equivalent to 1 g. of original tissue (units/g.), (2) as a percentage of the total recovered activity, and (3) as relative specific activity, i.e. as (2) divided by the nitrogen content of the fraction expressed as a percentage of the total recovered nitrogen.

Nitrogen rather than protein content was used to calculate relative specific activities because the protein content of fractions consisting mainly of phospholipid membranes may be extremely low. Relative specific activities determined on a protein basis may be subject to considerable error. Relative specific activities of fractions low in nitrogen into which soluble active material may have diffused are also misleading.

Percentage recoveries were corrected for losses of material during tube slicing.

### Electron microscopy

Samples were prepared for examination in the Siemens Elmiskop I ÜM 11 electron microscope by using the technique of negative staining as adapted for mammalian subcellular fractions by Horne & Whittaker (1962). Dilute suspensions of particles were usually fixed by the addition of an equal volume of ice-cold 10 % (w/v) formaldehyde in 0·32 M-sucrose previously neutralized to pH 7·4 with 0·33 N-NaOH. A drop of the fixed suspension was placed on a collodion–carbon-coated specimen grid grasped in forceps and most of the liquid withdrawn with a piece of filter paper lightly applied to the side of the grid. A drop of 1–2 % (w/v) phosphotungstic acid previously neutralized to pH 7·4 with 2 N-NaOH was then placed on the grid and similarly almost completely removed. Some grids were found to be markedly hydrophobic and withdrawal of most of the droplet did not leave the thin film of liquid evenly deposited over the surface of the grid which was essential for successful negative staining. Such grids were rejected. Prior coating of the grids with a thin film of aqueous 1 % (w/v) bovine serum albumin promoted spreading but reduced resolution. Interference by sucrose was occasionally troublesome. If not diluted out sufficiently by phos-

photungstate it disrupted the negative-staining pattern, forming hard-edged patches of light contrast. When present in low concentrations it sometimes gave rise, in regions of thick phosphotungstate deposition, to a pattern of small regular white patches superficially similar to small membrane fragments. With practice, however, such patches could be readily distinguished from biological structures by their locus and hard contrast.

Negatively stained preparations of free synaptic vesicles were found to be unstable and were best examined as soon as possible after preparation. Larger structures (e.g. mitochondria) were stable for several days.

### RESULTS

#### Fractionation of water-treated synaptosomes on a density gradient

When the supernatant of the water-treated $P_2$ fraction, $W_s$, was submitted to density-gradient separation, the appearance of the tubes after centrifuging was as shown in Fig. 1.

The tube and contents were separated into seven fractions in a manner dictated by the distribution of material in the gradient. Fraction $O$ was the water-clear topmost zone, corresponding to the position of fraction $W_s$ at the beginning of the run. Fraction $D$ corresponded approximately to the

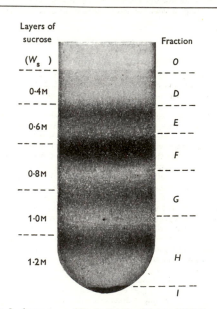

Fig. 1. Appearance of Lustroid tube of Spinco SW 25 head after centrifuging the 10000*g* supernatant of water-treated $P_2$ fraction (fraction $W_s$) at 25000 rev./min. (53500*g*) for 2 hr. The gradient was separated into seven fractions as shown.

Table 1. *Morphology of fractions prepared from water-treated* $P_2$ *fractions of guinea-pig brain by density-gradient separation*

For nomenclature of the fractions see the text and Fig. 1. The density of the particles of the fractions is expressed as the concentrations of sucrose in molar units whose density is equal to that of the particles after centrifuging.

| Fraction | Particle density | Morphological identification |
|---|---|---|
| O | <0·4 | No organized structures |
| D | 0·4 | Synaptic vesicles, occasional microsomes |
| E | 0·4–0·6 | Microsomes, some synaptic vesicles, often in clumps, occasional myelin fragments |
| F | 0·6–0·8 | Synaptosome ghosts, myelin fragments, non-vesicular membrane fragments |
| G | 0·8–1·0 | Synaptosome ghosts, membrane fragments |
| H | 1·0–1·2 | Damaged synaptosomes |
| I | >1·2 | Small mitochondria, some shrunken synaptosomes |

layer of 0·4 M-sucrose immediately below the initial position of fraction $W_s$ and had a faintly-hazy bluish appearance such as would be caused by light-scattering by extremely small particles. Fractions E, F, G and H corresponded to well-marked cream-coloured bands of particulate material floating between 0·4 M- and 0·6 M-sucrose, 0·6 M- and 0·8 M-sucrose, 0·8 M- and 1·0 M-sucrose, and 1·0 M- and 1·2 M-sucrose respectively. Fraction H included all the 1·2 M-sucrose layer. Fraction I was the tan-coloured pellet of particles denser than 1·2 M-sucrose which had sedimented to the bottom of the tubes, and was resuspended in 0·32 M-sucrose for analysis.

*Morphology of fractions.* Each fraction was examined by negative staining in the electron microscope. The results are summarized in Table 1; representative electron-micrographs are reproduced in Plates 1 (a)–1 (c), 2 (a)–2 (d) and 3 (a).

Fraction O contained no organized structures. The pattern of phosphotungstate deposition was not entirely uniform and was broken up in patches. This could have been caused by the presence of soluble protein or lipid deposited in amorphous masses on drying.

Fraction D (Plates 1a–1c) consisted almost entirely of small vesicular structures about 500Å in diameter together with a few larger oval membrane fragments of a kind that were abundant in the next fraction E. The small vesicles were identical in size and shape with the synaptic vesicles seen within negatively-stained nerve-ending particles when these had been sufficiently disrupted to permit the ingress of phosphotungstate (Plate 1d), and all the various types were represented.

The mean diameter (± S.D.) of 351 small vesicles of the preparation shown in Plates 1 (a) and 1 (b) was 469 ± 110Å, close to the value of 451 ± 108Å (406) calculated from Fig. 84A of Andersson-Cedergren (1959) for whole-tissue sections and to the value of 439 ± 137Å (70) for the small sample represented by the synaptosome in Plate 1 (d).

Fraction E (Plate 2a) consisted mainly of circular or oval membrane fragments about 0·1–0·3 μ in diameter similar to those seen in the microsomal fraction of brain homogenates by Gray & Whittaker (1962). Synaptic vesicles were, however, also present, sometimes in small clumps, and there were occasional myelin fragments.

Fractions F and G (Plates 2b and 2c) were similar. They contained membrane fragments of various shapes and sizes, from microsomal dimensions to those of intact synaptosomes. Occasionally synaptic vesicles could be seen within the larger fragments which are probably the outer membranes of synaptosomes with some cytoplasm and synaptic vesicles remaining within ('synaptosome ghosts'). These synaptosome ghosts

## EXPLANATION OF PLATES 1 AND 2

PLATE 1. Unless otherwise stated, all electron-micrographs shown in Plates 1–4 are of material negatively stained as described in the text. (a) Low-magnification electron-micrograph of particles of fraction D showing large numbers of synaptic vesicles about 500Å in diameter together with smaller numbers of larger microsomes 0·1–0·2 μ in diameter. (b) High-magnification electron-micrograph of same preparation as (a). (c) Portion of pellet $D_p$ obtained by centrifuging fraction D and showing hollow ($sv_1$), dense-cored ($sv_2$) and compound (csv) synaptic vesicles. (d) Synaptosome negatively stained under slightly hypo-osmotic conditions showing synaptic vesicles of the three main types [see legend to (c)] *in situ*. A portion of axon (a) remains attached, but this synaptosome does not contain a mitochondrion.

PLATE 2. (a) Fraction E showing large numbers of microsomes, a few scattered synaptic vesicles and a portion of a myelin fragment (my). (b) Fraction F showing membrane fragments including non-vesicular fragments (psm?) that could be detached post-synaptic thickenings. (c) Fraction G showing larger oval membrane fragments (g) believed to represent synaptosome ghosts. (d) Fraction H showing partially disrupted synaptosomes (ds) and small mitochondria (m) often surrounded by small vesicles and membrane fragments.

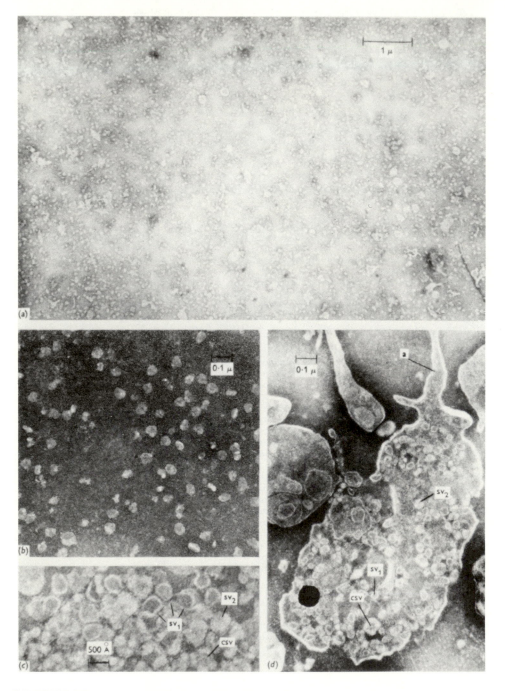

V. P. WHITTAKER, I. A. MICHAELSON AND R. J. A. KIRKLAND

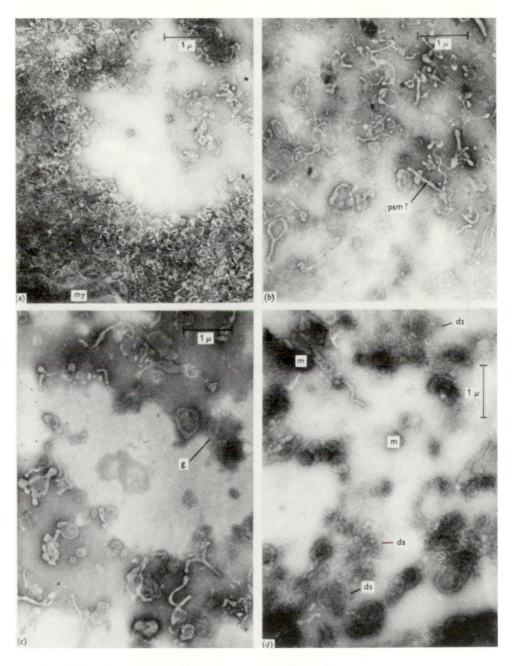

P. WHITTAKER, I. A. MICHAELSON AND R. J. A. KIRKLAND

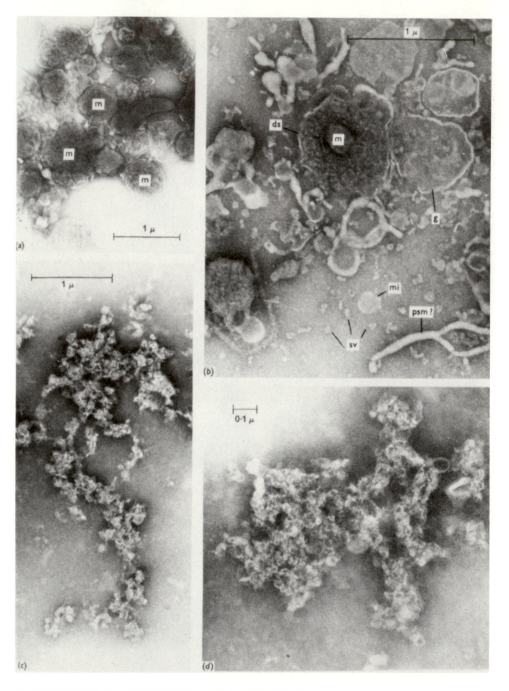

V. P. WHITTAKER, I. A. MICHAELSON AND R. J. A. KIRKLAND

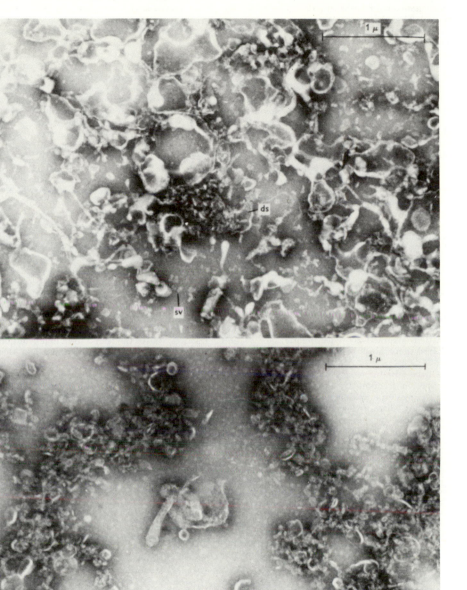

V. P. WHITTAKER, I. A. MICHAELSON AND R. J. A. KIRKLAND

were more abundant in fraction $G$ than in fraction $F$. Thick non-vesicular membranes were also common, resembling post-synaptic membranes. These were more plentiful in fraction $F$ than in fraction $G$.

Fraction $H$ (Plate 2$d$) contained a confused mass of membranes of greatly different sizes, resembling the parent fraction $W_s$, and is believed to represent incompletely disrupted synaptosomes. It is difficult to convey an adequate impression of this fraction in a single electron-micrograph. Frequently, small mitochondria of a size similar to those seen within synaptosomes could be seen surrounded by vesicular masses resembling synaptic vesicles and disrupted external membranes. It is known from previous work (summarized by Whittaker, 1963$a$) that the synaptic vesicles of ruptured endings behave as though they are embedded in a sticky cytoplasm. The equilibrium densities of the $G$ and $H$ fractions correspond to that of intact synaptosomes (Gray & Whittaker, 1960, 1962; Michaelson & Whittaker, 1962; Johnson & Whittaker, 1962, 1963).

Fraction $I$ (Plate 3$a$) consisted almost entirely of small mitochondria with the characteristic fine structure (Whittaker, 1963$a$) of swollen mitochondria. It also contained unpenetrated structures tentatively identified with the highly osmiophilic shrunken synaptosomes seen in intact preparations exposed to hyperosmotic sucrose and referred to as 'black bodies' by Gray & Whittaker (1962).

All the structures visible in fractions $O–I$ could be seen in fraction $W_s$. Occasionally, drifts of isolated synaptic vesicles could be seen, but incompletely disrupted synaptosomes (Plate 3$b$), microsomes, synaptosome ghosts, mitochondria

---

### EXPLANATION OF PLATES 3 AND 4

PLATE 3. ($a$) Fraction $I$ consisting mainly of swollen mitochondria (m). ($b$) Fraction $W_s$ showing partly damaged synaptosome (ds) containing a mitochondrion (m) and synaptic vesicles, synaptosome ghosts (g), isolated synaptic vesicles (sv), microsomes (mi) and non-vesicular membrane fragments (psm?). ($c$) Appearance of fraction $D$ after brief exposure to acid (pH 4 for 1–2 min. at 0°). The synaptic vesicles have clumped and partially fused. ($d$) Same preparations as in ($c$) at higher magnification.

PLATE 4. ($a$) Electron-micrograph of $M_2$ preparation of De Robertis et al. (1963$a$) showing isolated synaptic vesicles (sv) mixed with damaged synaptosomes (ds) and membrane fragments of varied shape and size. ($b$) The same preparation as in ($a$), negatively stained by suspending an osmic acid-treated pellet in ammonium acetate and diluting with sodium phosphotungstate as described by De Robertis et al. (1963$a$). The large membrane fragments and damaged synaptosomes of ($a$) are absent.

and non-vesicular membrane fragments were all visible in adjacent areas.

Fraction $W_p$ contained mainly large mitochondria and myelin fragments; however, considerable numbers of partially damaged synaptosomes were also present. Its morphology was consistent with the relatively high proportion of the mitochondrial marker, succinate dehydrogenase, and relatively low proportions of other components sedimenting in this fraction (Table 2).

*Activity of fractions.* The lactate-dehydrogenase, succinate-dehydrogenase, choline-acetyltransferase, cholinesterase and acetylcholine activities of the various fractions are presented in Tables 2 and 3. The rather large standard deviations in Table 2 were due to the difficulty experienced in duplicating conditions exactly each time. One source of variation was the difference in the weights of tissue processed, but the main variation was probably due to the difficulty of cutting the tubes in exactly the same way each time. Nevertheless the general pattern of distribution in each experiment was the same.

The most noteworthy finding was that acetylcholine (Table 2, l. 5) was bimodally distributed in the density gradient, the fractions with the highest activities being the synaptic-vesicle fraction, $D$, and the fraction containing incompletely disrupted synaptosomes, $H$. The acetylcholine in these fractions was in the bound form and could be sedimented with the particles contained in them by high-speed centrifuging. Further details of the properties of the acetylcholine of the $D$ fraction are given below.

Lactate dehydrogenase (Table 2, l. 1) was recovered mainly in fraction $O$, with some activity in fraction $D$ and little or none in the other fractions. This distribution was similar to that found for the potassium of the fraction (Table 2, l. 7) and for the soluble protein bovine serum albumin after a dummy run in which 28·5 mg. of albumin in 5 ml. of water was placed on top of a density gradient, centrifuged and sampled in the same way as in a normal experiment (Table 2, l. 8). This showed that soluble components do not diffuse throughout the whole gradient in 2 hr. Fraction $O$ thus contains most of the soluble cytoplasmic constituents of the synaptosome, and lactate dehydrogenase and potassium behave as one would expect of soluble cytoplasmic markers.

Succinate dehydrogenase (Table 2, l. 2) was recovered mainly in fractions $I$ and $H$, as would be expected of a mitochondrial marker. Almost half the original activity of fraction $W$ had already been removed in fraction $W_p$ by the initial low-speed centrifuging.

Cholinesterase, shown to be a microsomal marker by Toschi & Hanzon (1959) and Aldridge &

**Table 2. Distribution of enzymes, acetylcholine, nitrogen and potassium in fractions prepared from water-treated $P_2$ fractions of guinea-pig brain by density-gradient separation**

For nomenclature of the fractions see the text and Fig. 1. Values are mean values ± S.D.; numbers in parentheses indicate the numbers of experiments averaged when this differs from that given in column 3.

| Component | Unit | No. of experiments | $W$ (units/g.) | Percentage distribution | | Recovery (% of $W$) | Percentage distribution | | | | | | | Recovery (% of $W_s$) |
|---|---|---|---|---|---|---|---|---|---|---|---|---|---|---|
| | | | | In $W_p$ | In $W_s$ | | In $O$ | In $D$ | In $E$ | In $F$ | In $G$ | In $H$ | In $I$ | |
| Lactate dehydrogenase | $\Delta E_{390}$/min. | 3 | 13·4±4·1 | 9±4 | 91±4 | 123±42 | 74±18 | 16±14 | 3±3 | 1±1 | 0 | 2±2 | 3±3 | 71±17 |
| Succinate dehydrogenase | μmoles/hr. | 3 | 193·0±70 (2) | 45±10 | 55±10 | 80±2 (2) | 5±5 | 5±5 | 4±4 | 5±4 | 6±2 | 22±5 | 52±20 | 66±16 |
| Cholinesterase | μmoles/hr. | 4 | 63·0±29 | 17±8 | 83±9 | 91±11 | 5±2 | 9±3 | 20±7 | 27±5 | 21±6 | 10±4 | 8±7 | 88±22 |
| Choline acetyltransferase | μmoles/hr. | 3 | 0·46±0·07 | 9±4 | 91±4 | 116±16 | 73±6 | 8±1 | 2±1 | 5±3 | 5±1 | 4±2 | 3±1 | 83±37 |
| Acetylcholine | μm-moles | 4 | 2·70±0·39 | 24±10 | 76±10 | 100±68 | 2±2 | 30±8 | 8±5 | 5±5 | 11±5 | 35±11 | 9±6 | 81±19 |
| Nitrogen | mg. | 11 | 3·24±1·8 | 28±6 | 72±6 | 99±15 | 28±6 | 12±2 | 8±1 | 12±3 | 12±2 | 15±4 | 13±5 | 84±7 |
| Potassium | μg. | 1 | 305 | 13 | 87 | 98 | 75 | 14 | 4 | 5 | 2 | 0 | 0 | 100 |
| Bovine serum albumin* (5·7 mg./ml.) | — | 1 | — | — | — | — | 76 | 24 | 0 | 0 | 0 | 0 | 0 | 111 |

\* Dummy run.

Johnson (1959), was rather diffusely distributed throughout the density gradient but was mainly present in fractions $E$, $F$ and $G$, all rich in small membrane fragments. The highest relative specific activity was associated with the predominantly microsomal fraction $E$ (Table 3, 1. 3).

In the primary fractions of brain homogenates, the distribution of choline acetyltransferase closely parallels that of acetylcholine (Hebb & Whittaker, 1958). After water-treatment, choline acetyltransferase behaves like lactate dehydrogenase, potassium and bovine serum albumin, being recovered mainly in fraction $O$. As with these other components, the concentration in fraction $D$ is consistent with diffusion from fraction $O$. High-speed centrifuging (100000$g$ for 60 min.) or fraction $D$ gave a pellet, $D_p$, and a slightly opalescent supernatant, $D_s$; 87 % of the recovered choline acetyltransferase remained in fraction $D_s$ whereas 80 % of the recovered acetylcholine was sedimented in fraction $D_p$. Thus choline acetyltransferase, unlike acetylcholine, is not a constituent of the synaptic vesicles but is localized in the soluble cytoplasm of the synaptosome.

As seen in Table 3, the separation of fraction $W_p$ from fraction $W_s$ in the initial low-speed run produced an enrichment with respect to fraction $W$ in fraction $W_s$ of all the activities except that of succinate dehydrogenase. The enrichment was greatest, as would be expected, with the soluble cytoplasmic constituents, lactate dehydrogenase, potassium and choline acetyltransferase, which had been largely (87–95 %) released by the water-treatment, less with the microsomal cholinesterase and least with acetylcholine, nearly a quarter of which remained sequestered within the damaged synaptosomes sedimenting in fraction $W_p$. Nearly half the succinate dehydrogenase was carried down with fraction $W_p$, which is consistent with the high mitochondrial content of this fraction.

The other results in Table 3 serve to show that, in general, the fractions with the highest activities are also the fractions with the highest relative specific activities.

*Effect of inhibiting cholinesterase.* When eserine sulphate (0·2 %) was present in the water in which the $P_2$ pellet was suspended, the free acetylcholine released was not destroyed and was recovered, as one would expect, mainly in the $O$ and $D$ fractions with smaller amounts in other fractions.

*Preparation of vesicles from fraction B.* When fraction $B$, consisting almost entirely of synaptosomes, was suspended in water and fractionated on the density gradient, fractions similar to those described above were obtained. The exposure of the synaptosomes to hyperosmotic sucrose during their isolation from the $P_2$ fraction did not prevent vesicles from being released.

Table 3. *Relative specific activities of density-gradient fractions prepared from water-treated $P_2$ fractions from guinea-pig brain*

For nomenclature of the fractions see the text and Fig. 1. The relative specific activity is (percentage of total recovered activity)/(percentage of total recovered nitrogen). Fractions $W_s$ and $W_p$ are referred to fraction $W$ taken as unity, and fractions $O-I$ to fraction $W_s$ taken as unity. Values are obtained from the mean values in Table 2.

| Activity | | | | Relative specific activity | | | | | |
|---|---|---|---|---|---|---|---|---|---|
| | In $W_p$ | In $W_s$ | In $O$ | In $D$ | In $E$ | In $F$ | In $G$ | In $H$ | In $I$ |
| Lactate dehydrogenase | 0·32 | 1·26 | 2·64 | 1·33 | 0·37 | 0·08 | 0 | 0·13 | 0·23 |
| Succinate dehydrogenase | 1·61 | 0·76 | 0·18 | 0·42 | 0·50 | 0·42 | 0·50 | 1·47 | 3·77 |
| Cholinesterase | 0·61 | 1·15 | 0·18 | 0·75 | 2·50 | 2·25 | 1·75 | 0·67 | 0·61 |
| Choline acetyltransferase | 0·32 | 1·26 | 2·61 | 0·67 | 0·25 | 0·42 | 0·42 | 0·27 | 0·23 |
| Acetylcholine | 0·86 | 1·06 | 0·07 | 2·50 | 1·00 | 0·42 | 0·92 | 2·33 | 0·69 |
| Potassium | 0·46 | 1·21 | 2·68 | 1·17 | 0·50 | 0·42 | 0·17 | 0 | 0 |

### Fractionation of frozen-and-thawed and untreated preparations

For comparison with the experiments described in the preceding section, washed $P_2$ fractions were divided and one half frozen-and-thawed ten times. The frozen-and-thawed and untreated preparations were then placed on to the usual density gradients and separated as described above.

The appearance of the tubes after the centrifuging was essentially the same for both preparations but different from those in which water-treated material had been fractionated. The $D$ band was no longer visible, the $E$ band was faint and the $H$ band was intensified. Most of the lactate dehydrogenase, choline acetyltransferase, acetylcholine and nitrogen were recovered in the $H$ band; however, with the frozen-and-thawed preparations significant amounts of lactate dehydrogenase (23 %) and choline acetyltransferase (20 %) were recovered in the region 0–0·4 M-sucrose corresponding to the $O$ and $D$ bands of the water-treated preparations. These results are consistent with previous conclusions (Johnson & Whittaker, 1962, 1963) that freezing-and-thawing, though disrupting a certain proportion of synaptosomes, does not release intact synaptic vesicles.

### Properties of the acetylcholine of the synaptic-vesicle fraction

*Evidence for the association of acetylcholine and vesicles.* The acetylcholine of the $D$ fraction was in a particulate bound state as evinced by the following observations: (1) It was immune from the action of cholinesterase, until released by any of the methods mentioned below. If the method of release did not simultaneously destroy the cholinesterase present in the preparation, the prior addition of a cholinesterase inhibitor was essential to stabilize the released acetylcholine. (2) On diluting fraction $D$ with an equal volume of water and centrifuging at 100000g for 1 hr. most of the acetylcholine was sedimented along with most of the synaptic vesicles. Examination of the supernatant in the electron microscope showed that a few synaptic vesicles had not been sedimented. (3) The acetylcholine in the $D$ fraction was inactive on the leech preparation unless first released by an appropriate disruptive technique.

It was decided to compare the stability of the bound acetylcholine in the isolated synaptic vesicles of the $D$ fraction with that of synaptosomes (Whittaker, 1959). This study is not yet complete but the following preliminary observations have been made.

*Spontaneous release.* The vesicles appeared to be stable for a period of at least 2–3 hr. after preparation at 0°. On incubation at 20° about 60 % of the bound acetylcholine was released after 20 min. and 100 % after 60 min. At 35°, release was still more rapid, 60 % having been released after 5 min. and 100 % after 30 min.

*Effect of osmotic strength of suspension medium.* Synaptic vesicles, in contrast with synaptosomes, do not appear to be osmotically sensitive. This is indicated by their method of preparation and by an experiment in which there was no increase in the rate of spontaneous release from the $D$ fraction (sucrose concn. approx. 0·4 M) when this was diluted with an equal volume of water.

*Effect of acid.* Brief (1–2 min.) exposure at 0° to acid conditions (pH 4·0) released all the bound acetylcholine of the fraction. This release was accompanied by a remarkable change in the morphology of the vesicles (Plates 3c and 3d). They clumped together and apparently began to fuse. These experiments showed that it is not necessary to heat the $D$ fraction at 100° for 10 min. to release all the bound acetylcholine, as was in fact done as a routine.

### Are the particles of fraction D an artifact?

A problem that must be seriously considered is the possibility that the synaptic vesicles of fraction $D$ are simply lipoprotein micelles that have arisen as the result of the degradation of lipoprotein membranes by water-treatment and mechanical disruption during preparation. The presence of bound acetylcholine might then be accounted for by the uptake by the lipoprotein micelles of small amounts of acetylcholine released from storage sites during manipulation.

It may be difficult to disprove such a proposition until analyses on the lipid composition of the isolated vesicles are complete. Nevertheless, two types of experiments have been carried out in an attempt to test it.

*Attempted preparation of 'synaptic vesicles' from liver.* A liver-mitochondrial fraction was suspended in water and submitted to density-gradient fractionation by exactly the same procedure as was used for preparing fraction D from brain. The density gradient, illustrated diagrammatically in Fig. 2, had a very different appearance from that shown in Fig. 1. At the top was a thin layer of fat. The regions corresponding to most of fraction O and the whole of fractions D and E were clear and lemon-yellow in colour; in the electron microscope they were found to be free from organized membranous structures. Particulate material corresponding to fractions F, G, H and I was present, but only the pellet (corresponding to fraction I) contained much material. This consisted of badly damaged mitochondria often with disintegrating matrices. Swollen mitochondria also accounted for most of the layer corresponding to fraction H. The mitochondria were more damaged than in brain which is in accordance with the known greater fragility of liver mitochondria. The regions equiva-

lent to fractions F and G appeared to consist mainly of mitochondria fragments, but there were also occasional larger granular bodies which might have been lysosomes. Other work has shown that liver mitochondria are much more readily disrupted in water than brain mitochondria. It seems clear that particles like the isolated synaptic vesicles of the D fraction from brain do not arise spontaneously from lipoprotein membranes generally.

*Effect of emulsified lecithin.* Acetylcholine (5 $\mu$m-moles/ml.) and lecithin (2 $\mu$moles/ml.) were shaken together in aqueous solution and the ensuing emulsion tested on the frog rectus-abdominis-muscle preparation. No evidence of binding was obtained. The micelles formed by lecithin under these conditions vary greatly in size and are readily distinguishable from the isolated synaptic vesicles in negative staining (Dr A. D. Bangham, personal communication).

### Do synaptic vesicles contain choline acetyltransferase ?

Our findings, reported above, show that the isolated vesicles of fraction D contain acetylcholine but not choline acetyltransferase. The choline acetyltransferase of fraction D is considered to originate by diffusion from fraction O.

These results are at variance with those published by De Robertis *et al.* (1963a). In their procedure, a crude mitochondrial fraction from rat brain (corresponding to our $P_2$ fraction) is suspended in water, coarse particulate material is removed at $11500g$ for 20 min. (fraction $M_1$ corresponding to our fraction $W_p$) and the supernatant (corresponding to our $W_s$ preparation) is centrifuged at $100000g$ for 30 min. to give a pellet, $M_2$, and a supernatant, $M_3$. Fraction $M_2$ contains cholinesterase, choline acetyltransferase and acetylcholine, and is stated to consist of free synaptic vesicles mixed with some 'curved membranes'. Their published electron micrographs support this statement.

Thinking that relatively small differences of procedure might account for the divergence in the two sets of results, we have attempted to repeat experiments of De Robertis and co-workers as closely as their published account allows. Since, in their latest paper (De Robertis *et al.* 1963a) though not in their previous ones (De Robertis *et al.* 1962, 1963b), they stress the importance of the presence of a low concentration of $Ca^{2+}$ ions, sucrose solutions were deionized before use by passage through a mono-bed resin (Amberlite MB-1) to remove traces of $Ca^{2+}$ and other ions, and calcium chloride was added to give a final concentration of $10 \mu M$. The water used for resuspending the $P_2$ fraction also contained this concentration of calcium chloride.

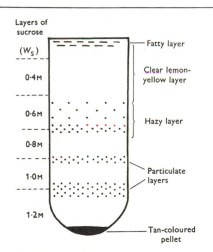

Layers of sucrose

$(W_S)$ — Fatty layer

0·4M — Clear lemon-yellow layer

0·6M — Hazy layer

0·8M

1·0M — Particulate layers

1·2M

Tan-coloured pellet

Fig. 2. Diagram showing the appearance of the density gradient when an experiment similar to that shown in Fig. 1 was performed with guinea-pig liver.

Table 4. *Comparison of distribution of activity in fractions of water-treated* $P_2$ *fractions of guinea-pig brain by using different procedures*

For nomenclature of the fractions see the text. (a) Results of De Robertis *et al.* (1963a); (b) this paper.

| | In $M_1$ | | In $M_2$ | | In $M_3$ | | Percentage recovery | | In $W_p$ (b) | In $W_s$ (b) | Percentage recovery |
|---|---|---|---|---|---|---|---|---|---|---|---|
| | (a) | (b) | (a) | (b) | (a) | (b) | (a) | (b) | | | |
| Choline acetyltransferase | 33 | 0 | 52 | 2 | 15 | 98 | 63 | 103 | 9 | 91 | 116 |
| Acetylcholine | 35 | 21 | 37 | 27 | 28 | 52 | 100 | 61 | 24 | 74 | 100 |

Our results (Table 4) were similar to those obtained with our $W_p$ and $W_s$ fractions prepared in the absence of $Ca^{2+}$ ions, on the assumption that fraction $W_s$ is equivalent to fraction $M_2$ plus fraction $M_3$. Electron microscopy, by our usual technique (Plate 4a), confirmed this. Fraction $M_2$ was extremely heterogeneous, containing disrupted synaptosomes, membrane fragments, clumps of synaptic vesicles and detached vesicles. Fraction $M_3$ was similar to fraction $M_2$ except that it was much more dilute, microsomes and synaptic vesicles predominated and there were fewer larger membrane fragments present.

Electron microscopy was also carried out on fraction $M_2$ by using the negative-staining technique of De Robertis and co-workers. The $M_2$ fraction was resuspended and treated with 2% (w/v) osmium tetroxide in 0·32M-sucrose and the osmic acid-treated particles were centrifuged to form a pellet. This pellet was resuspended in ammonium acetate and diluted 1:5 with 2% (w/v) phosphotungstic acid neutralized to pH 6·7. Droplets were applied to grids in the usual way.

The electron-micrographs showed an astonishing difference (Plate 4b) from those prepared by our usual method. The partially disrupted synaptosomes had disappeared, leaving clumps of synaptic vesicles and membrane fragments, selected areas of which resembled the electron-micrographs published by De Robertis and co-workers. It is evident that the resuspension of the osmic acid-treated particulate material of fraction $M_2$ had led to extensive disruption of the more organized structures, as indeed was predicted (see Discussion in Whittaker, 1963b) from the work of Gray & Whittaker (1960, 1962) and Horne & Whittaker (1962). These workers found that osmic acid-treated synaptosomes are extremely fragile and disintegrate on resuspension liberating vesicles stained with osmic acid. It is this property which accounts for the appearance of the previous electron-micrographs of the B fraction (Whittaker, 1959) in which resuspension techniques had been used and in which 60% of the particles were within the size range of synaptic vesicles.

We believe, therefore, that De Robertis and co-

workers may have seriously underestimated the degree of organization of their $M_2$ fraction and are mistaken in thinking that it is a reasonably homogeneous preparation of isolated synaptic vesicles. We do not attach great significance to the fact that in our hands this fraction contained a considerably lower proportion of the total choline acetyltransferase than they found, as this could be accounted for by a higher proportion of undamaged synaptosomes in their preparation. However, it is surprising that the percentage of acetylcholine which they recovered in fraction $M_2$ is not also proportionately higher. This might be explained by assuming that the less-stable synaptosomes had already been broken during their initial homogenization. Vesicles released at this stage, because of their tendency to stick together (Whittaker, 1963a), might well be recovered in fraction $M$ and subsequently in fractions $M_2$ and $M_3$, but choline acetyltransferase released from these broken synaptosomes would be recovered in fraction $S_2$ and so would not be included in their results.

## DISCUSSION

The results given in the present paper show that it is now possible to resolve fractions containing isolated nerve endings into a number of subfractions which represent its main structural features: synaptic vesicles, soluble cytoplasm, mitochondria and post-synaptic membrane. Of these, the last-named fraction is less well characterized than the others. In addition, fractions containing partially ruptured endings and microsomes are obtained. The microsomes probably represent contamination of the original preparation augmented by membrane fragments formed from larger structures during disruption. The markers lactate dehydrogenase and potassium (soluble cytoplasm) and succinate dehydrogenase (mitochondria) have assisted the characterization of the fractions.

The results clearly indicate the separate localization within the synaptic region of the three components (acetylcholine, choline acetyltransferase and cholinesterase) of the acetylcholine system. The transmitter itself appears to have a multiple localization within the neurone. When brain tissue is homogenized in sucrose containing eserine, a portion (20–30 %) of the total acetylcholine of the tissue is recovered in the soluble supernatant fraction ($S_3$). The remainder, representing bound acetylcholine, is recovered, under our conditions of homogenization, in a fraction identified as largely consisting of pinched-off nerve endings. To emphasize the relatively homogeneous nature of this fraction, and the similarity in physical properties of the isolated nerve endings to subcellular organelles, we have proposed the term 'synaptosomes' for the nerve-ending particles.

Disruption of the synaptosomes by exposure to hypo-osmotic media and other relatively mild conditions has led to the recognition of two kinds of bound acetylcholine, the 'labile' and 'stable' fractions (Whittaker, 1959). There are thus in all three states in which acetylcholine is present in nervous tissue: (a) that which is released on initial homogenization in iso-osmotic media; (b) the labile bound fraction of synaptosomes; (c) the stable bound fraction of synaptosomes.

It is well known that choline acetyltransferase is distributed throughout the length of cholinergic neurones. It seems reasonable to assume that a low steady-state concentration of acetylcholine exists in the cytoplasm of these neurones which represents the balances of synthesis and destruction by intracellular cholinesterase or spontaneous hydrolysis or both. This acetylcholine may give rise to the free acetylcholine of the $S_3$ fraction. The 'labile' bound acetylcholine released by hypo-osmotic treatment may represent the fraction of this free cytoplasmic acetylcholine sequestered within the synaptosomes. The 'stable' bound acetylcholine may represent acetylcholine bound to synaptic vesicles or contained within them, providing a device for raising the effective steady-state acetylcholine concentration at the cholinergic terminal. It is likely, however, that, even if these different acetylcholine 'compartments' exist, shifts from one 'compartment' to another may occur during the formation and subsequent disruption of the synaptosomes.

Although acetylcholine is stored, at any rate in part, in the synaptic vesicles, its synthesis in the cholinergic nerve ending appears to take place in the cytoplasm. In our experiments choline acetyltransferase is localized in the soluble cytoplasm; L. A. Mounter & V. P. Whittaker (unpublished work) also found a cytoplasmic localization for acetate–coenzyme A ligase (adenosine monophosphate) (acetylthiokinase), which provides the acetyl-coenzyme A for the acetylation of choline.

The yield of isolated synaptic vesicles cannot at present be estimated with any certainty but is probably low. About 10 % of the acetylcholine originally present in the $P_2$ fraction is eventually recovered in the $D$ band. If it is assumed that all the acetylcholine was originally present in the vesicles and that no gains or losses occurred subsequent to water-treatment, the yield would also be about 10 %. If the vesicles were not the sole 'compartment' or acetylcholine were lost from them during isolation, or both, the yield might be considerably higher. Work is continuing in an attempt to raise the yield.

## SUMMARY

1. A density-gradient procedure has been devised for fractionating pinched-off nerve endings ('synaptosomes') after disruption by suspension in water.

2. Seven fractions are obtained. These consist of soluble cytoplasmic components, synaptic vesicles, microsomes, larger membrane fragments, partially disrupted synaptosomes and mitochondria.

3. The various fractions have been characterized morphologically and biochemically. Lactate dehydrogenase (known to be a soluble-cytoplasmic marker), potassium and choline acetyltransferase were recovered mainly in the soluble-cytoplasmic fraction; succinate dehydrogenase in the mitochondrial fraction; and cholinesterase in the microsome and large-membrane fractions. Bound acetylcholine was distributed bimodally, part being recovered in the synaptic-vesicle fraction and part in the fraction containing incompletely disrupted synaptosomes.

4. The isolated synaptic vesicles had a mean diameter of $469 \pm 110 \text{Å}$, close to values reported in the literature for synaptic vesicles in whole-tissue preparations.

5. The acetylcholine in the vesicle fraction was in the bound form, but was readily released on incubation or acid treatment. The specific activity of this fraction was higher than that of preparations of intact synaptosomes.

6. The 'compartmentalization' of acetylcholine, choline acetyltransferase and cholinesterase in the cholinergic synapse is discussed in the light of these findings.

This work was supported in part by Research Grant no. B–3928 from the National Institute of Neurological Diseases and Blindness of the National Institute of Health, U.S. Public Health Service. The electron microscope was provided by the Wellcome Trust. We are most grateful to Mr G. H. C. Dowe and Mr N. Fincham for their skilled technical assistance and to Miss J. van Asch for her photographic work. Dr A. D. Bangham kindly suggested the lecithin experiment and provided the lecithin. Dr M. W. Smith kindly performed the potassium determinations. I.A.M. is a Postdoctoral Fellow of the National Heart Institute of the U.S. Public Health Service.

### REFERENCES

Aldridge, W. N. & Johnson, M. K. (1959). *Biochem. J.* **73**, 270.

Ammon, R. (1933). *Pflüg. Arch. ges. Physiol.* **233**, 486.

Andersson-Cedergren, E. (1959). *J. Ultrastruct. Res.* suppl. 1.

Berry, J. F. & Whittaker, V. P. (1959). *Biochem. J.* **73**, 447.

Carlsson, A., Falck, B. & Hillarp, N.-Å. (1962). *Acta physiol. scand.* **56** (suppl.), 196.

Chruściel, T. (1960). *Ciba Found. Symp.: Adrenergic Mechanisms*, p. 539. Ed. by Vane, J. R., Wolstenholme, G. W. E. & O'Connor, M. London: J. and A. Churchill Ltd.

del Castillo, J. & Katz, B. (1955). *J. Physiol.* **128**, 396.

del Castillo, J. & Katz, B. (1956). *Progr. Biophys. biophys. Chem.* **6**, 121.

De Robertis, E. (1958). *Exp. Cell Res.* suppl. 5, 347.

De Robertis, E., Arnaiz, G. R. de L. & de Iraldi, A. P. (1962). *Nature, Lond.*, **194**, 794.

De Robertis, E., Arnaiz, J. R. de L., Salganicoff, L., de Iraldi, A. P. & Zieher, L. (1963*a*). *J. Neurochem.* **10**, 225.

De Robertis, E. D. P. & Bennett, H. S. (1955). *J. biochem. biophys. Cytol.* **1**, 47.

De Robertis, E., Salganicoff, L., Zieher, L. M. & Arnaiz, G. R. de L. (1963*b*). *Science*, **140**, 300.

Fatt, P. & Katz, B. (1952). *J. Physiol.* **117**, 109.

Gaddum, J. H. (1961). *Proc. 1st int. Pharmacol. Meet., Stockholm*, vol. 8, p. 1. Ed. by Paton, W. D. M. & Lindgren, P. London: Pergamon Press Ltd.

Gray, E. G. & Whittaker, V. P. (1960). *J. Physiol.* **163**, 35 P.

Gray, E. G. & Whittaker, V. P. (1962). *J. Anat., Lond.*, **96**, 79.

Hebb, C. O. & Smallman, B. N. (1956). *J. Physiol.* **134**, 385.

Hebb, C. O. & Whittaker, V. P. (1958). *J. Physiol.* **142**, 187.

Horne, R. W. & Whittaker, V. P. (1962). *Z. Zellforsch.* **58**, 1.

Johnson, M. K. (1960). *Biochem. J.* **77**, 610.

Johnson, M. K. & Whittaker, V. P. (1962). *Acta neurol. scand.* **38** (suppl. 1), 60.

Johnson, M. K. & Whittaker, V. P. (1963). *Biochem. J.* **88**, 404.

Michaelson, I. A. & Whittaker, V. P. (1962). *Biochem. Pharmacol.* **11**, 505.

Michaelson, I. A. & Whittaker, V. P. (1963). *Biochem. Pharmacol.* **12**, 203.

Morán, H. F. (1957). In *Metabolism of the Nervous System*, p. 1. Ed. by Richter, D. London: Pergamon Press Ltd.

Palay, S. L. & Palade, G. E. (1954). *Anat. Rec.* **118**, 336.

Robertson, J. D. (1956). *J. biophys. biochem. Cytol.* **2**, 381.

Sjöstrand, F. S. (1953). *J. appl. Physics*, **214**, 1422.

Szèrb, J. C. (1962). *J. Physiol.* **158**, 8 P.

Toschi, G. & Hanzon, V. (1959). *Exp. Cell Res.* **16**, 256.

Whittaker, V. P. (1959). *Biochem. J.* **72**, 694.

Whittaker, V. P. (1960). *Regional Neurochemistry: The Regional Chemistry, Physiology and Pharmacology of the Central Nervous System: Proc. 4th int. Neurochem. Symp., Varenna*, p. 259. Ed. by Kety, S. S. & Elkes, J. London: Pergamon Press Ltd.

Whittaker, V. P. (1961). *Proc. 1st int. Pharmacol. Meet., Stockholm*, vol. 8, p. 61. Ed. by Lowry, O. H. & Lindgren, P. London: Pergamon Press Ltd.

Whittaker, V. P. (1963*a*). *Symp. biochem. Soc.* **23**, 109.

Whittaker, V. P. (1963*b*). In *Int. Symp. Problems of the Brain, Galesburg., Ill.* Amsterdam: Elsevier (in the Press).

Whittaker, V. P. & Gray, E. G. (1962). *Brit. med. Bull.* **18**, 223.

Whittaker, V. P., Michaelson, I. A. & Kirkland, R. J. (1963). *Biochem. Pharmacol.* **12**, 300.

# Chapter 3

# CATECHOLAMINES

The pathway of catecholamine metabolism seems almost baroque when compared with the relatively simple enzymic pathways of metabolism of ACh and GABA. No fewer than six enzymes are involved, along with their required cofactors and metals, and the various biochemical interconversions occur in three or more different subcellular compartments. At least three intermediates in the metabolic pathway are physiologically important compounds: dopamine, norepinephrine, and epinephrine. The first two serve as neurotransmitters in different neurons, and the last serves as a circulating hormone as well as a suspected transmitter. In what follows, we attempt to summarize this broad and complex field by focusing on two general topics: the enzymes of catecholamine synthesis and metabolism, and the storage and regulation of synthesis of catecholamines.

In mammals, norepinephrine is found in both the peripheral and central nervous systems. In the periphery, postganglionic sympathetic neurons secrete norepinephrine as their transmitter. Studies of norepinephrine synthesis and storage usually are carried out with sympathetically innervated tissues such as heart, spleen, and vas deferens. The adrenal medulla also contains norepinephrine, but most of the catecholamine in this tissue is epinephrine, the N-methyl derivative of norepinephrine. Although this book emphasizes chemical events that take place at synapses, much of the work presented in this chapter involves the chromaffin cells from the adrenal medulla. Investigators often compare adrenal medullary cells to peripheral sympathetic neurons on grounds that both derive from ectodermal neural crest, receive synaptic input from cholinergic neurons whose cell bodies lie in the CNS, and secrete catecholamines in response to neural stimulation. For both biochemical and physiological studies, the adrenal medulla often has been the system of choice, mainly because it yields large amounts of relatively homogeneous tissue. The cellular components of catecholamine synthesis and storage that are best characterized have been isolated from the adrenal medulla, although postganglionic sympathetic neurons invariably contain corresponding components.

## The Enzymes of Catecholamine Synthesis and Metabolism

In 1939, H. Blaschko delivered an important communication at a meeting of the British Physiological Society (abstract reprinted here). Out of the confusing array of phenolamines and catecholamines that had been characterized at the time, Blaschko accounted for epinephrine biosynthesis with an orderly series of reactions, which he felt satisfied the chemical interrelationships among these compounds. Rarely does the original version of a proposed pathway of metabolism survive the passage of time as this one has. Since its proposal, the scheme has been confirmed through isolation and characterization of the enzymes responsible for all the steps, and the pathway as now understood is as follows:

1)  tyrosine + $O_2$ $\xrightarrow[\text{hydroxylase}]{\text{tyrosine}}$ DOPA + $H_2O$

2)  DOPA $\xrightarrow[\text{decarboxylase}]{\text{DOPA}}$ dopamine + $CO_2$

3)  dopamine + $O_2$ $\xrightarrow[\beta\text{-hydroxylase}]{\text{dopamine}}$ norepinephrine + $H_2O$

4)  norepinephrine + S-adenosylmethionine $\xrightarrow{\begin{array}{c}\text{phenylethanolamine}\\\text{N-methyl transferase}\end{array}}$

    epinephrine + S-adenosyl homoserine

The first step is hydroxylation of L-tyrosine, producing 3,4-dihydroxyphenylalanine (DOPA) in a reaction that requires molecular oxygen and a tetrahydropteridine cofactor (tetrahydrobiopterin in the adrenal medulla) (Nagatsu, Levitt, and Udenfriend, 1964; Shiman, Akino, and Kaufman, 1971). Purified tyrosine hydroxylase from the adrenal medulla is stereospecific for L-tyrosine, although L-phenylalanine can serve almost as well as tyrosine as a substrate for DOPA production. A variety of catecholamines, including dopamine and norepinephrine, inhibit the enzyme. Norepinephrine inhibits tyrosine

118

hydroxylase by competing with the tetrahydropteridine cofactor. Catecholamine inhibition may be important for physiological regulation of catecholamine accumulation (see below).

The second biosynthetic enzyme, DOPA decarboxylase, converts DOPA to dopamine in a reaction requiring pyridoxal phosphate. In neurons that accumulate dopamine, this is the last synthetic step. A single enzyme, purified to homogeneity from hog kidney, catalyzes decarboxylation of 5-hydroxytryptophan, phenylalanine, tyrosine, tryptophan, and histidine (Christenson, Dairman, and Udenfriend, 1970). While the low substrate specificity of this enzyme suggests that all aromatic amines may be formed by a single decarboxylase, recent experiments indicate that in brain, different enzymes decarboxylate 5-hydroxytryptophan and DOPA (Sims, Davis, and Bloom, 1973).

The conversion of dopamine to norepinephrine (step three), catalyzed by dopamine β-hydroxylase, requires molecular oxygen, ascorbate, and enzyme-bound copper. S. Friedman and S. Kaufman (1965), in an elegant study, analyzed the properties of purified dopamine β-hydroxylase and proposed a detailed mechanism for its action. The enzyme has a relatively low substrate specificity that allows hydroxylation of a variety of phenylethylamines besides dopamine.

In the adrenal medulla and in neurons that secrete epinephrine, a final enzyme, phenylethanolamine-N-methyl transferase, catalyzes the transfer of a methyl group from S-adenosylmethionine to norepinephrine to form epinephrine (Axelrod, 1962).

Thus the pathway of catecholamine synthesis comprises three enzymes in postganglionic sympathetic neurons, and four in the adrenal medulla. Much speculation and confusion exist in the literature regarding the possible intracellular compartmentalization and transport (see Chapter 8) of these enzymes. Cell fractionation studies have suggested that tyrosine hydroxylase, DOPA decarboxylase, and phenylethanolamine-N-methyl transferase are in the soluble cytoplasmic fraction (Laduron and Belpaire, 1968); dopamine β-hydroxylase is invariably found associated with particles. These findings suggest that tyrosine is converted to dopamine in the neuronal soluble cytoplasm, and that dopamine then enters granules where it is transformed to norepinephrine. In adrenal medullary cells, norepinephrine presumably leaves the granules, is converted to epinephrine in the soluble cytoplasm, and then re-enters the granules for storage and secretion.

Further metabolism of the catecholamines involves the enzymes monoamine oxidase (MAO) and catechol-O-methyl transferase (COMT). Both enzymes are present in many tissues. MAO is a flavoprotein that is specifically associated with the mitochondrial outer membrane (Schnaitman, Erwin, and Greenawalt, 1967) and catalyzes the oxidative deamination of diverse physiological amines to the corresponding aldehydes. These in turn are reduced to alcohols or further oxidized to carboxylic acids by other tissue enzymes. COMT catalyzes transfer of the methyl group from S-adenosylmethionine preferentially to the hydroxyl group at ring position three of catechols (Axelrod and Tomchick, 1958). Both COMT and MAO are relatively nonspecific enzymes, and products of one reaction often can serve as substrates for the other. Accordingly a complex mixture of compounds is the end product of catecholamine metabolism. As we shall see in Chapter 6, it is not these enzymic modifications of catecholamines, but cellular uptake that is important for termination of the action of catecholamine transmitters. Inhibitors of either COMT or MAO fail to potentiate the effects of injected or physiologically released catecholamines.

### The Storage and Regulation of Synthesis of Catecholamines

Cells that contain catecholamines also contain dense-cored granules in their cytoplasm. These organelles can be easily demonstrated by electron microscopy of tissue treated with osmium tetroxide, and can be isolated from tissue homogenates by differential and density gradient centrifugation. Granular fractions from the adrenal medulla have been characterized far better than those isolated from sympathetic nerves or their terminals (for review see Smith and Winkler, 1972; Geffen and Livett, 1971). The adrenal granules are large (1000 to 4000 Å) and contain epinephrine, ATP, and a group of soluble proteins called chromogranins. Epinephrine and ATP are present in a molar ratio of four to one, suggesting that ATP may be a counter-ion for the catecholamine. The chromogranins comprise at least eight different soluble proteins, one of which, chromogranin A, predominates (see paper by Schneider, *et al.*, 1967, in Chapter 5). The functions of these proteins are unknown. Only two enzymic activities have been found in the granules: a membrane-bound ATPase and dopamine β-hydroxylase.

Sympathetic neurons possess several different populations of particles. L. Geffen and A. Ostberg (1969) reported that cell bodies and axons contain only a few dense-cored vesicles with an average diameter of 787 Å. In nerve terminals, these relatively large vesicles occasionally can be seen, but most of the vesicles, both with and without dense cores, have an average diameter of 443 Å. Centrifugation of homogenates of sympathetic nerve trunks of sympathetically innervated tissues yields two different fractions that presumably correspond to the large and small dense-cored vesicles (Roth, Stjarne, Bloom, and Giarman, 1968).

Each of the identified components of adrenal medullary granules (ATP, chromogranin A, and dopamine β-hydroxylase) has been found in crude vesicle preparations from noradrenergic nerves. De Potter, Smith, and De Shaepdryver (1970, reprinted here) showed that the subcellular distribution of these substances accords with their suggested association with vesicles. A more detailed examination of the biochemical properties of vesicles, important both for our understanding of norepinephrine synthesis and its control and for elucidation of the mechanism of transmitter release, awaits their further purification.

After nerve terminals release norepinephrine, at least three processes can replenish it: axonal transport of transmitter into the endings, uptake of released or exogenous transmitter, and local synthesis. Of these processes *de novo* synthesis of norepinephrine in nerve terminals is probably the most important. N. Weiner and M. Rabadjija (1969, reprinted here) demonstrated norepinephrine production from exogenous radioactive tyrosine in the vas deferens. When radioactive DOPA replaced tyrosine as precursor, there was considerably more incorporation of radioactivity into norepinephrine. Neural stimulation increased the rate of norepinephrine synthesis from tyrosine, but did not further increase norepinephrine formation from exogenous DOPA. These observations suggest that neural stimulation accelerates tyrosine hydroxylation and support the idea that this enzymic step is rate-limiting in the formation of norepinephrine. The data do not rule out the possibility that neural stimulation accelerates a rate-limiting tyrosine uptake process.

The results of Weiner and Rabadjija could be explained by a mechanism involving product inhibition of the enzyme tyrosine hydroxylase. As mentioned above, norepinephrine and dopamine inhibit partially purified tyrosine hydroxylase (Nagatsu, *et al.,* 1964). Accordingly, a pool of catecholamine in the soluble cytoplasm, in equilibrium with vesicular catecholamines, might regulate the soluble tyrosine hydroxylase. Release of catecholamines from stimulated nerve terminals, presumably emptying vesicles, could be followed by uptake of cytoplasmic catecholamines into empty vesicles. This could deplete the regulatory pool and thereby increase tyrosine hydroxylase activity. A critical test of this hypothesis has not so far been devised.

Another explanation of the increased rate of tyrosine hydroxylation with electrical stimulation could be an increase in the formation of the enzyme tyrosine hydroxylase itself. Weiner and Rabadjija did not find an increase in tyrosine hydroxylase activity in tissue homogenates after nerve stimulation. It was later found that cycloheximide, an inhibitor of protein synthesis, did not prevent the increased norepinephrine synthesis in intact tissue (Thoa, Johnson, Kopin, and Weiner, 1971). But a number of experiments in the last few years have shown that prolonged activation of sympathetic neurons or of the adrenal medulla, over periods of days rather than hours, can change the levels of several enzymes involved in catecholamine biosynthesis. For instance, chronic exposure of animals to stressful situations, such as cold or overcrowded conditions, or use of drugs that block sympathetic transmission or destroy sympathetic terminals, causes increases in tyrosine hydroxylase and dopamine $\beta$-hydroxylase activities both in the adrenal medulla and in sympathetic neurons. Reserpine, which depletes tissues of catecholamines, causes similar effects (Thoenen, Mueller, and Axelrod, 1969; Molinoff, Brimijoin, Weinshilboum, and Axelrod, 1970; Henderson, Iversen, and Black, 1973). Aromatic amino acid decarboxylase and monoamine oxidase activities do not change. These increases in enzymic activities in postganglionic sympathetic neurons can be prevented by surgical transection of the preganglionic axons, suggesting that the enzymic activities change because of increased stimulation of the postganglionic neurons via the preganglionic cells rather than because of direct effects on postganglionic cells. Other studies suggest that the normal biochemical maturation of sympathetic ganglia also requires presynaptic input. In the second week after birth, tyrosine hydroxylase activity in mouse sympathetic ganglia undergoes a dramatic increase; this increase does not occur if the preganglionic axons are severed shortly after birth (Black, Hendry, and Iversen, 1972).

A final interesting link between transmitter release and norepinephrine synthesis is illustrated in the paper by I. Kopin, G. Breese, K. Krauss, and V. Weise (1968, reprinted here). Their experiments on the spleen showed that newly synthesized norepinephrine is preferentially released. Transmitter secretion therefore must occur from a small pool, which is only part of the total tissue transmitter and which contains the newly synthesized norepinephrine. Whether this pool corresponds to norepinephrine in large or small vesicles, in vesicles close to the membrane, or in some other compartment, remains to be demonstrated.

Thus what emerges from the studies described in this chapter is a comprehensive view of the events that take place in catecholamine-secreting cells. Combination of pharmacological and biochemical methods has allowed an elegant dissection of events taking place in sympathetic neurons. This chapter also illustrates some of the difficulties encountered in investigations of transmitter synthesis and storage in intact tissues. For example, the neural elements to be studied often make up only a minute part of a tissue sample and resist isolation because of their intimate and tortuous association with non-neural components. Such contamination of neurons by other cell types might be circumvented in future work through the use of recently developed monolayer cultures of sympathetic ganglion cells (see Chapter 10).

## READING LIST

*Reprinted Papers*

1. Blaschko, H. (1939). The specific action of L-DOPA decarboxylase. *J. Physiol.* 96: 50p–51p.
2. Kopin, I.J., G.R. Breese, K.R. Krauss, and V.K. Weise (1968). Selective release of newly synthesized norepinephrine from the cat spleen during sympathetic nerve stimulation. *J. Pharmacol. Exp. Therap.* 161: 271–278.
3. Weiner, N. and M. Rabadjija (1968). The effect of nerve stimulation on the synthesis and metabolism of norepinephrine in the isolated guinea-pig hypogastric nerve–vas deferens preparation. *J. Pharmacol. Exp. Therap.* 160: 61–71.
4. De Potter, W.P., A.D. Smith, and A.F. De Schaepdryver (1970). Subcellular fractionation of splenic nerve: ATP, chromogranin A and dopamine $\beta$-hydroxylase in noradrenergic vesicles. *Tissue and Cell* 2: 529–546.

*Other Selected Papers*

5. Axelrod, J. and R. Tomchick (1958). Enzymatic O-methylation of epinephrine and other catechols. *J. Biol. Chem.* 233: 702–705.
6. Axelrod, J. (1962). Purification and properties of phenylethanolamine-N-methyl transferase. *J. Biol. Chem.* 237: 1657–1660.
7. Nagatsu, T., M. Levitt, and S. Udenfriend (1964). Tyrosine hydroxylase. The initial step in norepinephrine biosynthesis. *J. Biol. Chem.* 239: 2910–2917.
8. Friedman, S. and S. Kaufman (1965). 3,4-Dihydroxyphenylethylamine $\beta$-hydroxylase. Physical properties, copper content and role of copper in the catalytic activity. *J. Biol. Chem.* 240: 4763–4773.
9. Schnaitman, C., V.G. Erwin, and J.W. Greenawalt (1967). The

submitochondrial localization of monoamine oxidase. An enzymatic marker for the outer membrane of rat liver mitochondria. *J. Cell Biol.* 32: 719–735.

10. Smith, W.J. and N. Kirshner (1967). A specific soluble protein from the catecholamine storage vesicles of bovine adrenal medulla. I. Purification and chemical characterization. *Mol. Pharmacol.* 3: 52–62.

11. Laduron, P. and F. Belpaire (1968). Tissue fractionation and catecholamines. II. Intracellular distribution patterns of tyrosine hydroxylase, DOPA decarboxylase, dopamine β-hydroxylase, phenylethanolamine N-methyl transferase, and monoamine oxidase in adrenal medulla. *Biochem. Pharmacol.* 17: 1127–1140.

12. Roth, R.H., L. Stjarne, F.E. Bloom, and N.J. Giarman (1968). Light and heavy norepinephrine storage particles in the rat heart and in bovine splenic nerve. *J. Pharmacol. Exp. Therap.* 162: 203–212.

13. Chubb, I.W., B.N. Preston, and L. Austin (1969). Partial characterization of a naturally occurring inhibitor of dopamine β-hydroxylase. *Biochem. J.* 111: 243–244.

14. Geffen, L.B. and A. Ostberg (1969). Distribution of granular vesicles in normal and constricted sympathetic neurones. *J. Physiol.* 204: 583–592.

15. Thoenen, H., R.A. Mueller, and J. Axelrod (1969). Trans-synaptic induction of adrenal tyrosine hydroxylase. *J. Pharmacol. Exp. Therap.* 169: 249–254.

16. Christenson, J.G., W. Dairman, and S. Udenfriend (1970). Preparation and properties of a homogeneous aromatic L-amino acid decarboxylase from hog kidney. *Arch. Biochem. Biophys.* 141: 356–367.

17. Molinoff, P.B., S. Brimijoin, R. Weinshilboum, and J. Axelrod (1970). Neurally mediated increase in dopamine β-hydroxylase activity. *Proc. Nat. Acad. Sci.* 66: 453–458.

18. Geffen, L.B. and B.G. Livett (1971). Synaptic vesicles in sympathetic neurons. *Physiol. Rev.* 51: 98–157.

19. Shiman, R., M. Akino and S. Kaufman (1971). Solubilization and partial purification of tyrosine hydroxylase from bovine adrenal medulla. *J. Biol. Chem.* 246: 1330–1340.

20. Thoa, N.B., D.G. Johnson, I.J. Kopin, and N. Weiner (1971). Acceleration of catecholamine formation in the guinea-pig vas deferens after hypogastric nerve stimulation: Roles of tyrosine hydroxylase and new protein synthesis. *J. Pharmacol. Exp. Therap.* 178: 442–449.

21. Black, I.B., I.A. Hendry, and L.L. Iversen (1972). Effects of surgical decentralization and nerve growth factor on the maturation of adrenergic neurons in a mouse sympathetic ganglion. *J. Neurochem.* 19: 1367–1377.

22. Smith, A.D. and H. Winkler (1972). "Fundamental mechanisms in the release of catecholamines," in O. Eichler, A. Farah, H. Herken, A.D. Welch (Eds.), *Handbook of Experimental Pharmacology. New Series. Vol. 33,* pp. 538–617. Berlin: Springer Verlag.

23. Sims, K.L., G.A. Davis, and F.E. Bloom (1973). Activities of 3,4 dihydroxy-L-phenylalanine and 5-hydroxy-L-tryptophan decarboxylases in rat brain: Assay characteristics and distribution. *J. Neurochem.* 20: 449–464.

*Short Recent Review*

24. *The British Medical Bulletin,* Vol. 29 No. 2 (May 1973), *Catecholamines,* Ed. L.L. Iversen.

## The specific action of *l*-dopa decarboxylase. By HERMANN
BLASCHKO. (*From the Physiological Laboratory, Cambridge*)

In a paper by Holtz, Heise & Lüdtke [1938] on enzymic decarboxylation of *l*-(3:4)-dihydroxyphenylalanine (*l*-dopa) to the corresponding amine, oxytyramine, the question is discussed whether this reaction might be part of a general *l*-amino-acid deaminase, according to the scheme:

$$(1)\quad R\mathrm{CHNH_2.COOH} \xrightarrow{\text{decarboxylase}} R\mathrm{CH_2NH_2} + \mathrm{CO_2}.$$

$$(2)\quad R\mathrm{CH_2NH_2} + \mathrm{H_2O} + \mathrm{O_2} \xrightarrow{\text{amine oxidase}} R\mathrm{CHO} + \mathrm{NH_3} + \mathrm{H_2O_2}.$$

Our experiments are not in favour of this suggestion, since only *l*-dopa was decarboxylated by the enzyme. We used preparations from guinea-pigs' liver and kidney which contain the decarboxylase. None of the following amino-acids formed $CO_2$ in the presence of the enzyme: *d*-dopa, *dl*-N-methyl-dopa, *l*-tyrosine, *dl*-N-methyl-tyrosine, *l*-phenylalanine, *l*- and *d*-histidine.

This remarkable substrate specificity confines the scheme given above to *l*-dopa. It is likely that the enzyme does not only act in the breakdown of *l*-tyrosine via *l*-dopa, but also in the formation of *l*-adrenaline from tyrosine. Four changes are necessary for this transformation:

(*a*) Introduction of a phenolic OH group,
(*b*) Introduction of an OH group in the side chain,
(*c*) N-methylation,
(*d*) Decarboxylation.

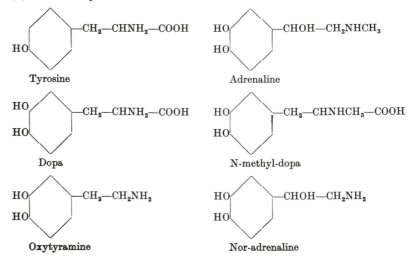

Reprinted from *The Journal of Physiology* 96: 50p–51p (1939) by permission of the publisher.

126

If the decarboxylation is brought about by this enzyme then our results establish the sequence of some of these changes. The fact that neither tyrosine nor N-methyl-dopa are decarboxylated shows that decarboxylation follows the introduction of the phenolic OH group but precedes N-methylation. Independent support for the first conclusion is given by clinical observations in tyrosinosis where tyrosine given in the diet is partly excreted as *l*-dopa [Medes, 1932]. The second conclusion is supported by the observation that in perfused adrenals no adrenaline is formed from N-methyl-dopa [Heard & Raper, 1933]. The stage at which the OH group is introduced in the side chain is at present unknown.

Our results are of interest with regard to the nature of the substance released after stimulation of the hepatic sympathetic nerves (Cannon's sympathin E). Since N-methyl-dopa is not decarboxylated by the enzyme the first step in the formation of sympathomimetic amines in the organism must lead to a non-N-methylated amine, like oxytyramine or nor-adrenaline. In 1910 Barger & Dale concluded that "of the catechol bases those with a methyl-amino-group, including adrenine, reproduce inhibitor sympathomimetic effects more powerfully than motor effects: the opposite is true of the primary bases of the same series". Nor-adrenaline has already been suggested as a possible candidate for sympathin E [Bacq, 1934, Stehle & Ellsworth, 1937] because its pressor effect, like that of sympathin E, is not reversed by ergotoxine. We find that the less active oxytyramine resembles nor-adrenaline in this respect.

The author wishes to thank Prof. C. R. Harington for a number of substances. Work was carried out with a grant from the Ella Sachs Plotz Foundation.

## REFERENCES

Bacq, Z. M. [1934]. *Ann. Physiol. Physicochim. biol.* **10**, 467.
Barger, G. & Dale, H. H. [1910]. *J. Physiol.* **41**, 19.
Heard, R. D. H. & Raper, H. S. [1933]. *Biochem. J.* **27**, 36.
Holtz, P., Heise, R. & Lüdtke, K. [1938]. *Arch. exp. Path. Pharmak.* **191**, 87.
Medes, G. [1932]. *Biochem. J.* **26**, 917.
Stehle, R. L. & Ellsworth, H. C. [1937]. *J. Pharmacol.* **59**, 114.

# SELECTIVE RELEASE OF NEWLY SYNTHESIZED NOREPINEPHRINE FROM THE CAT SPLEEN DURING SYMPATHETIC NERVE STIMULATION

IRWIN J. KOPIN, GEORGE R. BREESE, KENNETH R. KRAUSS
AND VIRGINIA K. WEISE

*Laboratory of Clinical Science, National Institute of Mental Health, Bethesda, Maryland*

Accepted for publication February 22, 1968

## ABSTRACT

KOPIN, IRWIN J., GEORGE R. BREESE, KENNETH R. KRAUSS AND VIRGINIA K. WEISE: Selective release of newly synthesized norepinephrine from the cat spleen during sympathetic nerve stimulation. J. Pharmacol. Exp. Therap. **161**: 271–278, 1968. During perfusion with tyrosine-$C^{14}$-containing solution, norepinephrine-$C^{14}$ is synthesized in the cat spleen. Rapid nerve stimulation results in release of norepinephrine-$C^{14}$ having a greater specific activity than that found in the spleen, indicating that the newly synthesized norepinephrine is selectively released. When spleens from cats which had been treated with norepinephrine-$H^3$ were perfused, the specific activity of norepinephrine released initially was similar to that in the spleen. After a period of continuous nerve stimulation, however, when the immediately available stores were depleted, the specific activity fell to about one-third that found in the spleen. If the perfusing solution contained $\alpha$-methyltyrosine, an inhibitor of norepinephrine synthesis, initial release was not altered. At later times, however, only about one-third as much norepinephrine was released and the specific activity of the released catecholamine was similar to that in the spleen. These results suggest that, during continued rapid stimulation, mobilization of stored norepinephrine does not play as great a role in maintenance of transmitter release as does new synthesis.

Stimulation of the splenic nerve results in release of norepinephrine from the spleen into the perfusing fluids (Brown and Gillespie, 1957). Administered norepinephrine-$H^3$, which is taken up by sympathetic nerves, can also be released (Hertting and Axelrod, 1961). With continued rapid stimulation there is a marked decrease in the rate of transmitter release, although splenic stores are not comparably depleted (Davies, 1963; Dearnaley and Geffen, 1966). This decline is reversible if there is a sufficient interval between periods of stimulation.

Blakeley and Brown (1966) showed that, when reuptake of norepinephrine is prevented, transmitter release from adrenergic nerves in the spleen during repeated stimulation is maintained at a diminished rate. The norepinephrine content of the spleen is only partly depleted, the stores presumably being replenished by synthesis. When norepinephrine synthesis is inhibited by pretreatment with $\alpha$-methyltyrosine during the 28-hr period prior to

Received for publication December 15, 1967.

perfusion of the spleen, the amount of norepinephrine released by nerve stimulation and the vascular responses are decreased (Thoenen et al., 1966). These observations suggest that, during continued nerve stimulation, both synthesis and mobilization of stored norepinephrine can contribute to the support of transmitter release.

The recent observation that the rate of norepinephrine synthesis, as calculated from conversion of tyrosine-$C^{14}$ to norepinephrine-$C^{14}$, exceeds calculated rates of norepinephrine turnover (Sedvall et al., 1968) suggested that newly synthesized norepinephrine may enter a small, preferentially released store of the catecholamine. These observations led us to investigate the fate of newly synthesized norepinephrine in the perfused cat spleen and to study the relative roles of mobilization and synthesis of norepinephrine in maintaining its release during maximal stimulation-induced transmitter liberation.

METHODS. The isolated spleens of cats (males, 2.0–2.8 kg) were perfused at a constant rate

(7.5 ml/min) with Krebs-Ringer bicarbonate solution (Umbreit *et al.*, 1957) saturated with 95% oxygen–5% carbon dioxide and containing 1 g of glucose per liter and $5 \times 10^{-5}$ M tyrosine or α-methyltyrosine for 20 to 30 min before the beginning of collections of the effluent perfusate. Splenic arterial perfusion pressure was monitored with a Statham P-23 AC transducer; the splenic nerve was prepared for stimulation as previously described (Fischer *et al.*, 1965). In some experiments, the cats were given 200 μc of DL-norepinephrine-7-H³ (specific activity 200 mc/mg; New England Nuclear Corporation, Boston, Mass.) i.v. 16 to 20 hr before the experiment. In other experiments, L-tyrosine-UL-C¹⁴ (400 mc/mmol, New England Nuclear Corporation) was infused at a constant rate (20 μc/min) into the perfusing solution (which contained tyrosine, $5 \times 10^{-5}$ M) during the indicated intervals.

The effluent perfusate from the splenic vein was collected during 2-min intervals and immediately cooled and mixed with 0.5 ml of 60% perchloric acid. Immediately after each experiment, the spleens were homogenized in 5 volumes of 0.4 N perchloric acid. The homogenates and effluent perfusates were stored at −20°C until the following day.

After thawing and centrifugation the clear supernatant was adjusted to pH 6.5 with sodium hydroxide. The amines were adsorbed on Dowex-50 (K⁺), and norepinephrine was eluted with 1 N HCl, as previously described (Musacchio *et al.*, 1966). The catecholamine in the eluate was then adsorbed on alumina by the method of Anton and Sayre (1962). The alumina, suspended in the solution, was poured onto a column containing 400 mg of alumina and the norepinephrine was eluted with 6 ml of 0.2 N acetic acid. Aliquots of the eluate were assayed for H³ or C¹⁴ with a liquid scintillation spectrometer and for norepinephrine by the fluorimetric method of Häggendal (1963). When tyrosine-C¹⁴ was carried through this procedure, less than 0.0001% of the C¹⁴ was recovered in the alumina eluate.

In the experiments in which tyrosine-C¹⁴ was used, the specific activity of the amino acid was calculated from the tyrosine levels (Wong *et al.*, 1964) and C¹⁴ content in the perfusate.

RESULTS. *Effect of continuous nerve stimulation on the specific activity of norepinephrine-C¹⁴ released during perfusion with tyrosine-C¹⁴.* When tyrosine-C¹⁴ was infused, the specific activity of the amino acid in the effluent perfusate rapidly reached a steady level (fig. 1). After infusion of the labeled amino acid

was stopped, its specific activity rapidly declined. During continuous splenic nerve stimulation, initially there was a marked increase in norepinephrine release. During this initial interval the specific activity in the perfusate was similar to that in the spleen at the end of the experiment and probably exceeded that in the spleen at the time of stimulation (table 1).

The amount of norepinephrine released in the next two intervals of continuous stimulation declined, but the amount of norepinephrine-C¹⁴ increased (fig. 1). The specific activity of released norepinephrine progressively increased and greatly exceeded that found in the spleen at the end of the experiment (table 1). In those experiments in which the perfusion was continued after tyrosine-C¹⁴ infusion was stopped and stimulation resumed after the specific activity of the tyrosine in the perfusate had reached low levels, there was again a marked increase in norepinephrine release. With continued stimulation, the rate of release diminished. This time, however, there was a more rapid fall in labeled than in unlabeled norepinephrine, so that the specific activity decreased (fig. 1). This decrease in specific activity was seen in all those experiments in which perfusion was continued and there was a second period of stimulation. The specific activity of the norepinephrine released during the second 2 min of the second stimulation was 60 ± 9% (S.E.M.) of that in the first 2 min.

The total amount of norepinephrine-C¹⁴ released during the second stimulation interval was less than 5% of that found in the spleen at the end of the experiment. The mean specific activity of norepinephrine-C¹⁴ found in these spleens (0.23 ± 0.03 μc/μmol) did not differ significantly from that found in the spleens in which the experiment had terminated immediately after the tyrosine-C¹⁴ infusion (0.17 ± 0.03 μc/μmol).

*Effect of α-methyltyrosine on release of norepinephrine from cat spleen.* In those spleens perfused with a solution containing tyrosine, stimulation of the splenic nerve (30 impulses/ sec) resulted in an initial outpouring of norepinephrine into the perfusing solution. This was followed by a decline in the rate of catecholamine release until, after about 6 min,

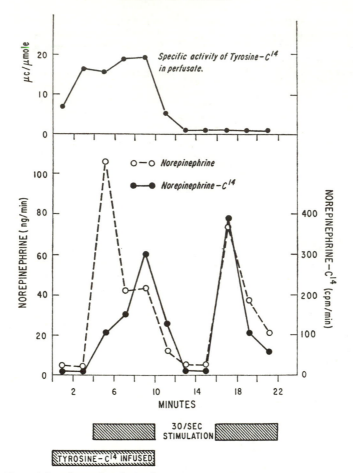

FIG. 1. Specific activity of tyrosine-C[14] in the perfusion fluid of an isolated spleen and the effect of nerve stimulation on the release of norepinephrine and norepinephrine-C[14]. Results are typical of three spleens in which there was a second stimulation period, as well as three in which the experiment was concluded after the first stimulation period.

a steady rate of efflux, at levels of 10 to 20% the initial rate, was reached (fig. 2).

In spleens perfused with a solution containing α-methyltyrosine, initial release was not significantly diminished, but there was a marked decrease in the amount of norepinephrine released in the intervals after the first 2 min (fig. 2; table 2). During the steady state reached, spleens perfused with a solution containing α-methyltyrosine released only about one-third as much norepinephrine as those perfused with a tyrosine-containing solution (table 2).

*Effect of α-methyltyrosine on the specific*

*activity of splenic and released norepinephrine-*H[3]. The cats had been given norepinephrine-H[3] 16 to 20 hr before perfusion of their spleens. There was no significant difference in the norepinephrine or norepinephrine-H[3] content of the two groups of spleens (table 4). The specific activity of the norepinephrine-H[3] which was spontaneously released from the spleens both before and after (tables 2 and 3) the stimulation interval was considerably higher than that in the spleens, perhaps as a result of washout of nonspecifically bound extraneuronal norepinephrine-H[3] having a high specific activity. Therefore, base-line levels of both radioactive and unlabeled norepinephrine had to be subtracted when the specific activity of released norepinephrine was calculated. During the first 2 min of stimulation, the specific activity of norepinephrine released was similar to that found in the spleens at the end of the experiments (102 ± 10% for tyrosine-per-

### TABLE 1

*Specific activity of norepinephrine-$C^{14}$ released by nerve stimulation or retained in the cat spleen during perfusion with tyrosine-$C^{14}$*

| Interval of Stimulation | Specific Activity of Norepinephrine-$C^{14}$ | |
| --- | --- | --- |
| | Released | Retained |
| | *$\mu c/\mu mol$* | |
| 0–2 min | 0.188 ± 0.012 | 0.199 ± 0.033 |
| 2–4 min | 0.723 ± 0.167 | |
| 4–6 min | 1.62 ± 0.47 | |

Results are the mean values ± S.E.M. from 6 experiments. Specific activity of norepinephrine in the spleen was determined at the end of the experiment. The levels of norepinephrine and norepinephrine-$C^{14}$ in the perfusate are similar to those shown in figure 1.

fused spleens and 106 ± 6% for $\alpha$-methyl-tyrosine-perfused spleens).

During the interval 6 to 16 min after initiation of continuous stimulation, there was no significant difference between the amount of norepinephrine-$H^3$ released from the spleens perfused with solutions containing tyrosine or $\alpha$-methyltyrosine (table 3). The specific activity of norepinephrine-$H^3$ released from the spleens by stimulation (table 4) was calculated from the decrements in labeled (table 3) and unlabeled norepinephrine (table 2) found in the perfusates. The decrements were estimated for each spleen by subtracting the levels found in the perfusates 2 to 4 min after stimulation from those found during the last 10 min of stimulation (tables 2 and 3). The specific activity of norepinephrine-$H^3$ released from spleens perfused with $\alpha$-methyltyrosine was similar to that found in these spleens (table 4). Because more unlabeled norepinephrine was released, the specific activity of norepinephrine-$H^3$ released from spleens perfused with a tyrosine-containing solution was only about two-fifths that of splenic norepinephrine-$H^3$ (table 4).

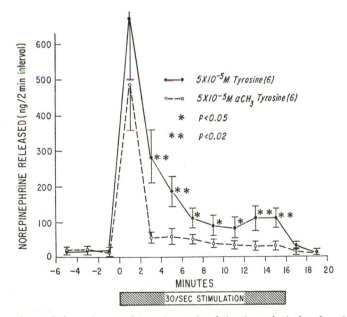

FIG. 2. Effect of $\alpha$-methyltyrosine on release of norepinephrine from the isolated perfused cat spleen during continued rapid nerve stimulation. Each point is the mean (±S.E.M.) of the results from perfusion of six spleens.

*Effect of α-methyltyrosine on the splenic perfusion pressure during continuous sympathetic nerve stimulation.* The vascular resistance in spleens perfused with the tyrosine-containing fluid rose rapidly and then gradually declined during continued nerve stimulation (fig. 3). When nerve stimulation was terminated, there was usually a distinct, although small, decrease in perfusion pressure (four of six spleens). In spleens perfused with the α-methyltyrosine-containing solution, there was also an initial increase in vascular resistance, but the decline in resistance was more rapid, and usually no fall in perfusion pressure was evident when stimulation ceased (fig. 3).

DISCUSSION. Sympathetic nerve stimulation accelerates norepinephrine synthesis in the rat heart (Gordon *et al.*, 1966) and salivary gland (Sedvall and Kopin, 1967), and in guinea-pig vas deferens (Alousi and Weiner, 1966; Roth *et al.*, 1966). In the cat spleen, norepinephrine-$C^{14}$ formed from tyrosine-$C^{14}$ is released during nerve stimulation (fig. 1; table 1). Since the specific activity of norepinephrine-$C^{14}$ released by stimulation during infusion of tyrosine-$C^{14}$ is greater than that found in the spleen (table 1), the newly synthesized catecholamine must be selectively released. This is not due to the existence of an inert or remote (not exposed to the tyrosine-$C^{14}$) store of the catecholamine in the spleen since there is a subsequent decrease in specific activity of the released catecholamine when only unlabeled tyrosine is present in the perfusate (fig. 1).

The specific activity of norepinephrine-$C^{14}$ released during stimulation is far less than

TABLE 2

*Effect of α-methyltyrosine on the stimulation-induced release of norepinephrine from the perfused cat spleen*

| Perfusion | During Continuous Stimulation | 2–4 min Post-stimulation | Stimulation-Induced Release |
|---|---|---|---|
| | *μμmol/min* | | |
| Tyrosine | 268 ± 70 | 36.2 ± 6.5 | 232 ± 65 |
| α-Methyltyrosine | 113 ± 28 | 38.4 ± 17.0 | 74.6 ± 17.8 |

Spleens from 12 cats were perfused with a solution containing 5 × 10⁻⁵ M tyrosine (six spleens) or α-methyltyrosine (six spleens). Results are the mean rates of release of norepinephrine (±S.E.M.) into the perfusate during an interval 6 to 16 min after onset of splenic nerve stimulation at 30 impulses/sec or during the indicated poststimulation interval.

TABLE 3

*Effect of α-methyltyrosine on the stimulation-induced release of norepinephrine-$H^3$ from the perfused cat spleen*

| | During Continuous Stimulation | 2–4 min Post-stimulation | Stimulation-Induced Release |
|---|---|---|---|
| | *mμc/min* | | |
| Tyrosine | 7.20 ± 1.40 | 4.01 ± 0.35 | 3.19 ± 0.95 |
| α-Methyltyrosine | 6.01 ± 0.75 | 4.60 ± 0.40 | 2.61 ± 0.65 |

Results are the radioactivity found to accompany the norepinephrine values presented in table 2 and are the mean values (±S.E.M.) for groups of six spleens. The stimulation-induced release was calculated individually for each spleen by subtracting the norepinephrine-$H^3$ released in the poststimulation interval from that of the mean release during the last 10 min of continuous stimulation. The mean of these values ± S.E.M. is shown, and the decrements are significant (P < .02).

TABLE 4

*Effect of α-methyltyrosine on specific activity of splenic and nerve stimulation-induced norepinephrine-$H^3$ in the perfused cat spleen*

| Amino Acid Perfused | Splenic Content | | Specific Activity | |
|---|---|---|---|---|
| | NE | NE-$H^3$ | Splenic NE-$H^3$ | Released NE-$H^3$ |
| | *mμmole* | *mμc* | *mμc/mμmol* | *mμc/mμmol* |
| Tyrosine | 37.3 ± 4.33 | 1100 ± 250 | 29.5 ± 8.9 | 13.7 |
| α-Methyl-tyrosine | 50.4 ± 6.27 | 1600 ± 290 | 31.7 ± 6.1 | 34.9 |

The norepinephrine (NE) and norepinephrine-$H^3$ (NE-$H^3$) contents of the spleens were determined as described in METHODS. The specific activities of norepinephrine-$H^3$ in the spleens were calculated individually for each spleen from its content of endogenous and labeled catecholamine and not from the ratio of the mean levels in the spleens shown in the table. These results are the mean values (±S.E.M.) for two groups of six spleens each. The specific activities of the released norepinephrine-$H^3$ were calculated from the data given in tables 2 and 3.

that of tyrosine-$C^{14}$ in the perfusate. During conversion of tyrosine-UL-$C^{14}$ to norepinephrine-$C^{14}$, only one-ninth of the $C^{14}$ is lost (the carboxyl group of tyrosine), which cannot account for the discrepancy in specific activities. During the 4 min of tyrosine-$C^{14}$ infusion before nerve stimulation, its specific activity in the perfusate attains a constant level, but there is no assurance that the intraneuronal tyrosine has also reached this level. Indeed, it is unlikely that the tyrosine in the sympathetic neuron has equilibrated with that in the perfusate. Because the specific activity of the intraneuronal tyrosine is

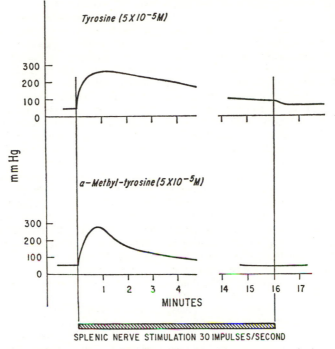

Fig. 3. Effect of α-methyltyrosine on the splenic arterial perfusion pressure during continuous nerve stimulation. Results are typical of those seen in six spleens in each group.

unknown, the proportion of released norepinephrine derived from new synthesis cannot be assessed in this experiment.

The relative proportion of newly synthesized norepinephrine in the spleen vs. that in the perfusate can be estimated by comparing the specific activities of released and retained norepinephrine (table 1). These results indicate that released norepinephrine contains a much greater proportion of the newly synthesized norepinephrine than does that retained in the spleen. Released norepinephrine, however, represents only a minute fraction (2%) of the total norepinephrine content of the spleen, and, although its specific activity is higher than that remaining in the spleen, most of the radioactive norepinephrine-C[14] formed in this short interval was found in the spleen.

At rates of stimulation as rapid as 30 impulses/sec (Brown and Gillespie, 1957) or during rapid perfusion (Hertting and Schiefthaler, 1963), reuptake of released norepinephrine is minimized. Under more physiologic conditions, a large portion of released norepinephrine is taken up by the sympathetic nerve endings and rebound in the storage vesicles (Blakely et al., 1964; Hertting and Axelrod, 1961). Part of the released amine, however, reaches the circulation or is enzymatically inactivated by catechol-O-methyl tranferase (COMT) or monoamine oxidase (MAO). To maintain a constant tissue level, this portion would have to be replaced by newly synthesized norepinephrine.

Studies of turnover reflect the rate of replacement of norepinephrine stores. Estimates of synthesis rates based on turnover are lower than estimates made using the rate of tyrosine-C[14] conversion to norepinephrine-C[14] (Sedvall et al., 1968). The discrepancy is readily explained by postulating the presence of a small, relatively rapidly utilized pool of norepinephrine. This is consistent with previous concepts that there is more than one pool of norepinephrine in sympathetic nerve endings (e.g., Trendelenburg, 1961; Kopin, 1964). Our finding of selective release of newly synthesized norepinephrine provides additional evidence for such a pool.

The amount of norepinephrine released during the first 2 min of nerve stimulation is not significantly diminished by α-methyltyrosine (fig. 1), and the specific activity of the released norepinephrine is similar to that found in the spleens. These findings suggest that newly synthesized norepinephrine is not a major source of the norepinephrine released at this time. With continued stimulation, exhaustion of this immediately available norepinephrine occurs and the situation changes.

During constant, rapid stimulation, the rate of transmitter release diminishes to a lower, steady level which is 10 to 20% of the initial rate of catecholamine release (Dearnaley and Geffen, 1966; Davies, 1963; present study, figs. 2 and 3). There are parallel changes in vascular resistance. Inhibition of norepinephrine formation by blockade of tyrosine hydroxylase with α-methyltyrosine (Spector, 1966) diminishes stimulation-induced release of norepinephrine (Thoenen et al., 1966; present study, fig. 2). The steady, low level of norepinephrine release found after 6 min of rapid splenic nerve stimulation is considerably lower during perfusion with α-methyltyrosine (fig. 2). During constant nerve stimulation, the vascular resistance diminishes more rapidly, and to lower levels, in spleens perfused with the tyrosine hydroxylase inhibitor (Thoenen et al., 1966; present study, fig. 3). These results suggest that new synthesis plays a more important role in maintenance of norepinephrine release during constant rapid nerve stimulation than does mobilization of stored norepinephrine.

A quantitative estimate of the relative amount of released transmitter which is derived from newly synthesized norepinephrine can be made by examining the effects of inhibition of synthesis. When α-methyltyrosine is perfused, there is a decrease in the amount of norepinephrine released by splenic nerve stimulation to levels of about one-third of those found in spleens perfused with physiologic levels of tyrosine (table 2). Release of norepinephrine-$H^3$ does not appear to be altered (table 3) so that the specific activity of the norepinephrine released from the α-methyltyrosine-perfused spleens is about 3 times that released from the tyrosine-perfused spleens (table 4). The specific activity of norepineph-

rine-$H^3$ released from spleens in which norepinephrine synthesis was inhibited is similar to that found in the spleens (table 4).

These results suggest that, under the conditions of rapid, continued stimulation, only one-third of the released norepinephrine is derived from tissue stores; the remainder is newly synthesized. The observations that inhibition of norepinephrine synthesis with α-methyltyrosine can diminish adrenergic neuronal function even when norepinephrine stores are not completely depleted (Spector, 1966; Thoenen et al., 1966) is consistent with the view that newly synthesized norepinephrine plays a significant role in maintaining transmitter release. The relative importance of new synthesis in maintaining transmitter release may vary with the interval and the rate of stimulation (unpublished observations) as well as with the organ or species examined.

These results may be explained if sites from which norepinephrine is released during nerve stimulation are replenished by both mobilization and new synthesis. It appears likely that vesicles nearest the nerve terminal release the catecholamine and are responsible for the accelerated synthesis accompanying nerve stimulation (Alousi and Weiner, 1966; Roth et al., 1966; Gordon et al., 1966; Sedvall and Kopin, 1967). Stimulation does not accelerate norepinephrine synthesis in the splenic nerve axon (Roth et al., 1967). It has been suggested that levels of intraneuronal cytoplasmic catecholamines may control the rate of tyrosine conversion to norepinephrine (Alousi and Weiner, 1966). When vesicles near the site of release are emptied, cytoplasmic norepinephrine and dopamine are taken up. This lowers the levels of cytoplasmic catecholamines and accelerates conversion of tyrosine to dopa. The latter reaction is believed to be rate-limiting in norepinephrine biosynthesis since trace amounts of dopa-$H^3$ are converted to norepinephrine-$H^3$ at the same rate, regardless of the levels of nerve activity (Gordon et al., 1966; Sedvall and Kopin, 1967).

If dopa-$C^{14}$ is supplied in excess, however, nerve stimulation enhances formation of norepinephrine-$C^{14}$ (Austin et al., 1967). This apparent discrepancy may be a result of excessive dopamine formation. The dopa-$C^{14}$ is readily converted to large amounts of dopamine-$C^{14}$, and conversion to norepinephrine-$C^{14}$ becomes

134

rate-limiting. Nerve stimulation results in release of norepinephrine stores and makes available empty binding sites. More dopamine-$C^{14}$ can then be taken up and converted to norepinephrine-$C^{14}$.

When excess dopamine is not present, uptake of dopamine and norepinephrine by the emptied vesicles diminishes cytoplasmic catecholamine levels and tyrosine hydroxylation is accelerated. Since empty vesicles take up cytoplasmic norepinephrine, it is likely that remote "full" storage vesicles release norepinephrine into the cytoplasm and thereby participate in transmitter replenishment by mobilization. These vesicles also take up dopamine and convert it to norepinephrine; therefore, synthesis is accelerated in vesicles remote from the site of release, but not to the same extent as in regions of the site of transmitter release.

## REFERENCES

ALOUSI, A. AND WEINER, N.: The regulation of norepinephrine synthesis in sympathetic nerves: Effect of nerve stimulation, cocaine and catecholamine-releasing agents. Proc. Nat. Acad. Sci. USA **56:** 1491–1496, 1966.

ANTON, A. H. AND SAYRE, E. D.: A study of the factors affecting the alumina oxide–trihydroxyindole procedure for the analysis of catecholamines. J. Pharmacol. Exp. Therap. **138:** 360–375, 1962.

AUSTIN, L., LIVITT, B. G. AND CHUBB I. W.: Increased synthesis and release of noradrenalin and dopamine during nerve stimulation. Life Sci. **6:** 97–104, 1967.

BLAKELEY, A. G. H. AND BROWN, G. L.: Release and turnover of the adrenergic transmitter. In Mechanisms of Release of Biogenic Amines, ed. by U. S. von Euler and B. Uvnäs, pp. 185–188, Pergamon Press, Oxford, 1966.

BLAKELEY, A. G. H., BROWN, G. L. AND GEFFEN, L. B.: Uptake and release of noradrenaline by sympathetic nerves of the transmitter they liberate. J. Physiol. (London) **173:** 22–23, 1964.

BROWN, G. L. AND GILLESPIE, J. S.: The output of sympathetic transmitter from the spleen of the cat. J. Physiol. (London) **138:** 181–192, 1957.

DAVIES, B. N.: Effect of prolonged activity on the release of the chemical transmitter at postganglionic sympathetic nerve endings. J. Physiol. (London) **167:** 52P, 1963.

DEARNALEY, D. P. AND GEFFEN, L. B.: Effect of nerve stimulation on the noradrenalin content

of the spleen. Proc. Roy. Soc. Med. **B183:** 303–313, 1966.

FISCHER, J. E., HORST, W. D. AND KOPIN, I. J.: β-Hydroxylated sympathomimetic amines as false neurochemical transmitters. Brit. J. Pharmacol. Chemotherap. **24:** 477–482, 1965.

GORDON, R., REID, J. V. O., SJOERDSMA, A. AND UDENFRIEND, S.: Increased synthesis of norepinephrine in the cat heart on electrical stimulation of the stellate ganglion. Mol. Pharmacol. **2:** 606–613, 1966.

HÄGGENDAL, J.: An improved method for fluorimetric determination of small amounts of adrenalin and noradrenalin in plasma and tissues. Acta Physiol. Scand. **57:** 242–254, 1963.

HERTTING, G. AND AXELROD, J.: Fate of tritiated norepinephrine at the sympathetic nerve endings. Nature (London) **192:** 172–173, 1961.

HERTTING, G. AND SCHIEFTHALER, T.: Beziehung zwischen Durchflußgröße und Noradrenalinfreisetzung bei Nervenreizung der isoliert durchströmten Katzenmilz. Arch. Exp. Pathol. Pharmakol. **246:** 13–14, 1963.

KOPIN, I. J.: Storage and metabolism of catecholamines: The role of monoamine oxidase. Pharmacol. Rev. **16:** 179–192, 1964.

MUSACCHIO, J. M., FISCHER, J. E. AND KOPIN, I. J.: Subcellular distribution and release by sympathetic nerve stimulation of dopamine and α-methyldopamine. J. Pharmacol. Exp. Therap. **152:** 51–55, 1966.

ROTH, R. H., STJARNE, L. AND EULER, U. S. VON: Acceleration of noradrenaline biosynthesis by nerve stimulation. Life Sci. **5:** 1071–1075, 1966.

ROTH, R. H., STJARNE, L. AND EULER, U. S. VON: Factors influencing the rate of norepinephrine biosynthesis in nerve tissue. J. Pharmacol. Exp. Therap. **158:** 373–377, 1967.

SEDVALL, G. C. AND KOPIN, I. J.: Acceleration of norepinephrine synthesis in the rat submaxillary gland in vivo during sympathetic nerve stimulation. Life Sci. **6:** 45–52, 1967.

SEDVALL, G. C., WEISE, V. K. AND KOPIN, I. J.: The rate of norepinephrine synthesis measured in vivo during short intervals; influence of adrenergic nerve impulse activity. J. Pharmacol. Exp. Therap. **159:** 274–282, 1968.

SPECTOR, S.: Inhibition of endogenous catecholamine biosynthesis. Pharmacol. Rev. **18:** 599–610, 1966.

THOENEN, H., HAEFELY, W., GEY, K. F. AND HUERLIMANN, A.: The effect of α-methyl-tyrosine on peripheral sympathetic transmission. Life Sci. **5:** 723–730, 1966.

TRENDELENBURG, U.: Modification of the effect of tyramine by various agents and procedures. J. Pharmacol. Exp. Therap. **134:** 8–17, 1961.

UMBREIT, W. W., BURRIS, R. H. AND STOUFFER, J. F.: In Manometric Techniques, p. 149, Burgess Publishing Co., Minneapolis, 1957.

WONG, P. K. W.; O'FLYNN, M. E. AND INOUYE, T.: Micromethods for measuring phenylalanine and tyrosine in serum. Clin. Chem. **10:** 1098–1104, 1964.

# THE EFFECT OF NERVE STIMULATION ON THE SYNTHESIS AND METABOLISM OF NOREPINEPHRINE IN THE ISOLATED GUINEA-PIG HYPOGASTRIC NERVE-VAS DEFERENS PREPARATION[1]

NORMAN WEINER[2] AND MIRJANA RABADJIJA[3]

*Department of Pharmacology, Harvard Medical School, and Neuropharmacology Laboratory, Massachusetts Mental Health Center, Boston, Massachusetts*

Accepted for publication November 6, 1967

ABSTRACT

WEINER, NORMAN AND MIRJANA RABADJIJA: The effect of nerve stimulation on the synthesis and metabolism of norepinephrine in the isolated guinea-pig hypogastric nerve-vas deferens preparation. J. Pharmacol. Exp. Therap. **160**: 61–71, 1968. Electrical nerve stimulation of the isolated hypogastric nerve-vas deferens preparation of the guinea-pig is associated with increased formation of $H^3$-norepinephrine from $H^3$-tyrosine. The effect is similar in the presence or absence of pargyline, a monoamine oxidase inhibitor. In contrast, nerve stimulation is not associated with a significant increase in the synthesis of $H^3$-norepinephrine from $H^3$-dihydroxyphenylalanine. The uptake of $H^3$-tyrosine and its incorporation into tissue protein is not affected by nerve stimulation. The tissue content of norepinephrine and the metabolism of exogenous labeled norepinephrine are identical in stimulated and control preparations. Norepinephrine inhibits the synthesis of $H^3$-norepinephrine from $H^3$-tyrosine and blocks the accelerated synthesis of norepinephrine which is ordinarily seen during nerve stimulation. Pargyline slightly potentiates this inhibitory effect of norepinephrine. The results indicate that a relatively small pool of intraneuronal norepinephrine which is able to interact with tyrosine hydroxylase inhibits this enzyme and thus regulates its own synthesis by a feedback inhibition mechanism. It is proposed that nerve stimulation leads to a reduction in the concentration of that norepinephrine which can interact with the tyrosine hydroxylase. This results in activation of the normally inhibited enzyme and consequent acceleration of norepinephrine synthesis.

The association of increased activity of the sympathetic nervous system and accelerated synthesis of norepinephrine has been observed in the heart and brain (Oliverio and Stjärne, 1965; Gordon *et al.*, 1966a,b) and the submaxillary gland (Sedvall and Kopin, 1967) of the intact animal. The accelerated synthesis appears to be the consequence of an increased rate of conversion of tyrosine to dihydroxyphenylalanine (dopa) (Gordon *et al.*, 1966a; Sedvall and Kopin, 1967). The hydroxylation of tyrosine has been proposed as the rate-limiting step in the biosynthesis of norepinephrine (Levitt *et al.*, 1965).

Accelerated catecholamine formation which is associated with increased sympathetic nervous activity has also been demonstrated in the isolated adrenal gland (Holland and Schümann, 1956; Butterworth and Mann, 1957; Bygdeman and von Euler, 1958) and in the isolated guinea-pig hypogastric nerve-vas deferens preparation (Weiner and Alousi, 1966; Roth *et al.*, 1966). Since catecholamine-releasing agents and norepinephrine itself inhibit the synthesis of $H^3$-norepinephrine from $H^3$-tyrosine in the vas deferens preparation and inhibit the increased synthesis of norepinephrine associated with nerve stimulation, it has been proposed that free intraneuronal norepinephrine may inhibit its own synthesis by negative feedback inhibition of tyrosine hydroxylase (Alousi and Weiner, 1966). A similar negative feedback mechanism for the regulation of norepinephrine synthesis had been

Received for publication July 14, 1967.
[1] This work was supported by U.S. Public Health Service Grants NB 02947, NB 04663 NB 05723.
[2] Present address: Department of Pharmacology, University of Colorado Medical Center, Denver, Colo.
[3] Present address: Department of Pharmacology, University of Zagreb, Zagreb, Yugoslavia.

136

suggested earlier on the basis that catechols and catecholamines inhibit purified beef adrenal tyrosine hydroxylase, presumably by competitively antagonizing the binding of the pteridine cofactor to the apoenzyme (Nagatsu *et al.*, 1964; Udenfriend *et al.*, 1965; Ikeda *et al.*, 1966). The present report is an attempt to define further the mechanism of increased norepinephrine synthesis associated with nerve stimulation in the isolated hypogastric nerve-vas deferens preparation of the guinea-pig.

METHODS. Male guinea-pigs, weighing between 400 and 700 g, were employed in all experiments. The animals were killed with a blow on the head, and the vasa deferentia with attached hypogastric nerves were dissected out according to the procedure of Huković (1961). Each organ was placed in a separate 10-ml organ bath in a solution consisting of 133 mM NaCl, 4.7 mM KCl, 16.3 mM NaHCO₃, 1.4 mM NaH₂PO₄, 2.5 mM CaCl₂, 0.1 mM MgCl₂, 0.01 mM Na₂ EDTA and 7.8 mM glucose (Gillespie, 1962). The salt solution was gassed with 95% O₂–5% CO₂ for

at least 1 hr prior to use and throughout the experiment. All experiments were performed at 37°C.

The hypogastric nerve of each preparation was placed between two platinum loop electrodes After 10 min, each nerve was stimulated for 5 sec at 25 pulses/sec employing a pulse intensity of 5 V and a pulse duration of 5 msec. If either preparation failed to respond to this test stimulus, both preparations were discarded. After the test responses, one preparation was randomly chosen to be the stimulated preparation. The hypogastric nerve of the second preparation was withdrawn from the electrodes, leaving the silk thread to which it was attached lying across the pair of electrodes (fig. 1). Throughout the experiment, both organ baths were subjected to identical electric current from the electrodes although only one preparation was stimulated. Labeled precursor was added to each bath and the stimulation was performed for 5 sec/min for 1 hr. Stimulation was performed with a Tektronix stimulator and the pulses were monitored on a Tektronix oscilloscope. The responses of the tissue were recorded on a smoked paper kymograph.

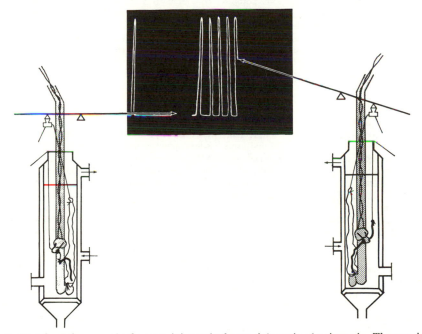

FIG. 1. Sketch of the organ baths containing paired vasa deferentia of guinea pig. The vas deferens in the bath on the right is stimulated for 1 hr. The control vas deferens (left) is stimulated only once prior to the addition of radioactive precursor. After this single stimulation, the nerve is removed from its position between the platinum electrodes and this preparation is sham-stimulated subsequently. For details, see METHODS.

At the end of the stimulation period, the tissues were removed from the bath, blotted dry, weighed, homogenized in 1 N HCl and centrifuged at 4°C. The protein precipitate was washed twice with 1 N HCl, and the supernatants were combined. The medium was similarly acid-precipitated with one-sixth of a volume of 6 N HCl. Acid extracts were stored in the cold until analysis.

In those experiments in which tyrosine was estimated, the tissue and bath proteins were removed with 10% trichloracetic acid (TCA). Tissue protein precipitates were washed twice with 5% TCA and, after centrifugation, the supernatants were combined. Tyrosine values were somewhat higher if HCl was used as protein precipitant, presumably because some bound tyrosine is liberated by this strong mineral acid.

*Norepinephrine assay.* An aliquot of the tissue sample was assayed for norepinephrine by the trihydroxyindole fluorimetric procedure (Weiner *et al.*, 1962).

*Assay of H³-dopamine and H³-norepinephrine.* To aliquots of acid extracts of both tissue and medium, 200 μg of dopamine and 200 μg of norepinephrine were added. Dopamine and norepinephrine in the tissue extracts were separated from each other and from the small amount of precursor present by ion exchange chromatography on a Dowex 50-Na⁺-X8 column, 0.5 by 3.5 cm, by a modification of the method Häggendal (1963). On this column, catecholamines are quantitatively retained while the amino acid precursors pass through in the effluent. After thorough washing of the column, norepinephrine is eluted with six 4-ml aliquots of 1 N HCl and dopamine is subsequently eluted with three 4-ml aliquots of 2 N HCl. Recoveries of norepinephrine and dopamine were determined either by measuring the optical density of the eluates at 280 mμ or by colorimetric assay of aliquots of the eluates (Barness *et al.*, 1963). The eluates were subsequently dried in a vacuum desiccator over NaOH and H₂SO₄. The dried material was dissolved in 1.5 ml of H₂O and 14 ml of dioxane scintillation fluid containing 6% naphthalene, 0.6% 2,5-diphenyloxazole (PPO) and 0.005% 2-p-phenylenebis(5-phenyloxazole) (POPOP). The samples were counted in a Nuclear-Chicago liquid scintillation counter. Counts were corrected for efficiency using the external standard technique. Results are generally expressed as millimicromoles of product formed per micromole of norepinephrine and are corrected for incomplete recovery (average norepinephrine recovery = 92%; average dopamine recovery = 83%) (Rutledge and Weiner, 1967).

The medium was assayed in a similar fashion for H³-norepinephrine and H³-dopamine. In most experiments, tyrosine was first separated from the catecholamines by adsorption of the latter compounds on alumina and elution of these substances with 0.2 N acetic acid. The catecholamines in the eluate were then separated on Dowex 50-Na⁺. If the preliminary alumina separation was omitted, some contamination of the dopamine fraction with H³-tyrosine was obtained. After the separation on alumina, very little H³-norepinephrine and virtually no H³-dopamine were demonstrable in the acid extracts of the medium.

*Separation and assay of tyrosine.* TCA extracts of medium and tissue were separately neutralized to pH 6.5 and each was passed through a Dowex 50-Na⁺-X8 column, 0.5 by 3.5 cm, which retains the amines but does not retain tyrosine. The column was washed with 0.1% Na₂EDTA (ethylenediamine tetraacetic acid) and the effluent and wash were combined. The pH of the solution was adjusted to 2.0 with HCl and passed through Dowex 50-H⁺, 0.8 by 10 cm, on which tyrosine is retained. After washing the column with 5 ml of 0.1% Na₂EDTA and 30 ml of H₂O, tyrosine was eluted with 10 ml of 1 N NH₄OH. Tyrosine in the effluent was assayed fluorimetrically (Waalkes and Udenfriend, 1957) and an aliquot was counted by liquid scintillation spectrometry using dioxane scintillation fluid as described.

*Assay of norepinephrine metabolites.* Either C¹⁴- or H³-norepinephrine was incubated with the vasa deferentia in the manner described and HCl extracts of the tissues were prepared. Carrier 3,4-dihydroxyphenylglycol (DOPEG), 3-methoxy-4-hydroxyphenylglycol (MOPEG), 3,4-dihydroxymandelic acid (DOMA) and vanilmandelic acid (VMA), 500 μg each, were added to the acid extracts. The acid extracts were divided into two fractions and one fraction was heated at pH 1.5 at 95°C under nitrogen for 30 min to hydrolyze any conjugated metabolites. The extracts were adjusted to pH 6.5 and passed over a Dowex 50-H⁺ column, 0.8 by 10 cm, to remove norepinephrine and amine metabolites. The column was washed with 10 ml of H₂O. The combined effluent and wash was extracted three times with two volumes of ethyl acetate each time. Most of the neutral metabolites were extracted in this fashion, along with a small amount of the acid metabolites. The aqueous phase was acidified to pH 1.5 and the acid metabolites were extracted with 2 volumes of ethyl acetate three times. The extracts were reduced to a small volume in a rotary evaporator under vacuum and the contents were transferred to small tubes and further evaporated *in vacuo* to a volume of approximately 0.1 ml. The entire sample was spotted on Whatman silica gel impregnated paper and chromatographed in toluene–acetic acid–ethyl acetate–$H_2O$ (16:8:4:1) for at least 20 hr. After drying, the spots were located under ultraviolet light, cut out and extracted with 0.2 N acetic acid. An aliquot was assayed by the phenol colorimetric reaction in order to determine recovery (Barness *et al.*, 1963). A second aliquot was counted by liquid scintillation spectrometry in dioxane scintillation fluid. All results are corrected for quenching and recovery. Mean recoveries ± S.E. for the four metabolites were: DOMA, 49.5% ± 1.2; DOPEG, 27.1% ± 1.0; VMA, 75.2% ± 2.0; and MOPEG, 65.1% ± 2.0.

*Incorporation of tyrosine into protein.* Protein precipitates were freed of non-protein material by successive treatment in the following solutions, followed by centrifugation at 800 × $g$ for 10 min at 4°C and discarding of the supernatant each time: 5% TCA; 5% TCA plus heating at 90°C for 30 min; 95% ethanol and heating at 65°C for 20 min; 95% ethanol–ether (3:1) and heating at 65°C for 30 min; 95% ethanol–ether (3:1) and heating at 65°C for 10 min; ether. Each protein precipitate was dried, weighed, transferred to a counting vial and dissolved in 1 ml of 1 M hyamine in methanol by heating at 60°C overnight. To each vial was added 14 ml of scintillation fluid consisting of 0.4% PPO and 0.05% dimethyl POPOP dissolved in toluene. The samples were counted by liquid scintillation spectrometry. Results were corrected for quenching by the external standard technique. Specific activity was calculated by dividing the micromicromoles of tyrosine incorporated into protein by the weight of the protein in milligrams.

The substances used in this study were: L-tyrosine, L-3,4-dihydroxyphenylalanine (dopa), 3,4-dihydroxyphenylethylamine HCl (dopamine), DL-arterenol HCl (norepinephrine), DL-3,4-dihydroxymandelic acid (DOMA), 3-methoxy-4-hydroxymandelic acid (VMA), 3,4-dihydroxyphenylglycol (DOPEG), 3-methoxy-4-hydroxyphenylglycol piperazine salt (MOPEG), 3,5-$H^3$-L-tyrosine, L-3(3,4-dihydroxyphenyl) alanine (ring-2,5,6-T) (dopa), DL-norepinephrine (carbinol-$C^{14}$) DL-bitartrate, DL-norepinephrine-7-$H^3$, 3-iodotyrosine and pargyline HCl (Eutonyl, kindly supplied by Abbott Laboratories, Chicago).

3,5-$H^3$-L-tyrosine was purified prior to use by twice passing a solution of the radioactive substance, adjusted to pH 8.4, through an alumina column, 0.8 by 4 cm, followed by adsorption of the alumina effluent (adjusted to pH 2) on Dowex 50-$H^+$ and elution with 1 N $NH_4OH$. The $NH_4OH$ was removed by distillation *in vacuo*, and the $H^3$-tyrosine was dissolved in 0.01 N HCl. Labeled dopa and norepinephrine were purified by adsorption on and elution from alumina. The purified substances were checked for purity by paper chromatography (1-butanol–acetic acid–$H_2O$, 12:3:5) and radiochromatogram scanning and each was found to exhibit only one peak whose $R_f$ was identical to that of standard material.

Statistical calculations were performed according to Snedecor (1956). The results are generally expressed as the mean ± S.E.

RESULTS. *The effect of nerve stimulation on norepinephrine formation.* Nerve stimulation is associated with a significantly increased rate of synthesis of norepinephrine from tyrosine (table 1). The increase is quite variable from preparation to preparation. In a few experiments, no increase in synthesis was observed. The reasons for the variations among preparations in the effects obtained are unknown. The increased norepinephrine synthesis associated with nerve stimulation is independent of the extracellular tyrosine concentration (table 1). At all levels of tyrosine concentration examined, the percent increase in synthesis associated with nerve stimulation was similar. As the extracellular tyrosine concentration is increased from 1 × $10^{-6}$ M to 5.5 × $10^{-5}$ M, increased amounts of norepinephrine are formed. The increased norepinephrine synthesis with increased tyrosine in the medium is similar to that reported by Levitt *et al.* (1965) for the guinea-pig perfused heart. A Lineweaver-Burk plot of the results yields a Michaelis constant ($K_m$) for tyrosine of approximately 2 × $10^{-5}$ M, identical to the results of Levitt *et al.* The $K_m$ in the stimulated preparations is not different from that seen with the controls.

Inhibition of monoamine oxidase with 1.6 × $10^{-4}$ M pargyline does not significantly alter either the rate of norepinephrine synthesis or the effect seen with nerve stimulation (table 1). The concentration of pargyline is sufficient to block monoamine oxidase at least 90% (table 4).

The synthesis of norepinephrine from dopa is much greater than that seen when $H^3$-tyrosine is used as labeled precursor. In this instance, however, nerve stimulation is no longer

TABLE 1

*Formation of norepinephrine and dopamine from tyrosine in the vas deferens-hypogastric nerve preparation of guinea-pig*

| Tyrosine Concentration | $N^a$ | Stimu-lation | Norepinephrine Tissue | Dopamine Tissue | Norepinephrine Bath | Effect of Stimulation on Norepinephrine Formation (Increase above Control) |
|---|---|---|---|---|---|---|
| *M* | | | *mμmol amine formed/μmol endogenous norepinephrine* | | | % |
| $1 \times 10^{-6}$ | 6 | 0 | $2.13 \pm 0.30^b$ | $0.17 \pm 0.03$ | $0.34 \pm 0.14$ | |
| | | + | $3.55 \pm 0.41$ | $0.17 \pm 0.03$ | $0.30 \pm 0.07$ | $+65.5 \pm 22.6^c$ |
| $5.5 \times 10^{-6}$ | 11 | 0 | $8.08 \pm 0.74$ | $0.64 \pm 0.17$ | $0.27 \pm 0.03$ | |
| | | + | $11.46 \pm 1.25$ | $0.57 \pm 0.03$ | $0.37 \pm 0.07$ | $+44.3 \pm 12.2^d$ |
| $5.5 \times 10^{-5}$ | 8 | 0 | $28.53 \pm 2.70$ | $1.69 \pm 0.40$ | $0.81 \pm 0.47$ | |
| | | + | $41.24 \pm 5.74$ | $2.54 \pm 0.64$ | $1.28 \pm 0.85$ | $+48.1 \pm 19.4^c$ |
| $5.5 \times 10^{-6} + \text{pargyline}^e$ | 13 | 0 | $9.26 \pm 1.22$ | $0.47 \pm 0.07$ | $0.47 \pm 0.07$ | |
| | | + | $12.4 \pm 1.15$ | $0.64 \pm 0.07$ | $0.47 \pm 0.07$ | $+45.3 \pm 16.1^c$ |
| $5.5 \times 10^{-5} + \text{pargyline}$ | 4 | 0 | $19.06 \pm 4.16$ | $1.79 \pm 0.37$ | $0.47 \pm 0.50$ | |
| | | + | $39.7 \pm 6.42$ | $3.04 \pm 0.64$ | $1.32 \pm 0.68$ | $+126.1 \pm 38.2^c$ |

[a] Number of experiments.
[b] Results are expressed as mean $\pm$ S.E.
[c] P < .05.
[d] P < .01.
[e] Pargyline concentration, $1.6 \times 10^{-4}$ M.

TABLE 2

*Formation of catecholamines from dopa in the hypogastric nerve-vas deferens preparation*

| Dopa Concentration | $N^a$ | Stimu-lation | Norepinephrine Tissue | Dopamine Tissue | Norepinephrine Bath | Dopamine Bath | Effect of Stimulation on Norepinephrine Formation (Increase above Control) |
|---|---|---|---|---|---|---|---|
| *M* | | | *mμmol amine formed/μmol endogenous norepinephrine* | | | | % |
| $1 \times 10^{-6}$ | 4 | 0 | $6.81 \pm 0.56^b$ | $0.17 \pm 0.05$ | $1.18 \pm 0.34$ | $0.35 \pm 0.08$ | |
| | | + | $6.69 \pm 0.61$ | $0.12 \pm 0.02$ | $0.95 \pm 0.37$ | $0.25 \pm 0.08$ | $-2.8 \pm 5.1$ |
| $1 \times 10^{-6} + \text{pargyline}^c$ | 4 | 0 | $11.23 \pm 0.88$ | $0.41 \pm 0.03$ | $1.49 \pm 0.47$ | $0.54 \pm 0.12$ | |
| | | + | $11.51 \pm 1.76$ | $0.37 \pm 0.10$ | $1.69 \pm 0.54$ | $0.52 \pm 0.07$ | $+8.9 \pm 19.1$ |
| $2.5 \times 10^{-5} + \text{pargyline}$ | 5 | 0 | $152.9 \pm 21.1$ | $14.5 \pm 3.0$ | $7.6 \pm 1.0$ | $9.3 \pm 1.0$ | |
| | | + | $182.5 \pm 26.5$ | $14.2 \pm 3.7$ | $8.1 \pm 1.7$ | $9.3 \pm 1.5$ | $+25.2 \pm 13.3$ |

[a] Number of experiments.
[b] Results are expressed as mean $\pm$ S.E.
[c] Pargyline concentration, $1.6 \times 10^{-4}$ M.

associated with an increase in the rate of norepinephrine formation. In the presence of pargyline, a significantly greater production of catecholamines from dopa is obtained (table 2). Even when monoamine oxidase is inhibited, the formation of norepinephrine from dopa is not significantly altered by nerve stimulation.

The norepinephrine contents and the weights of the stimulated organs were not significantly different from the corresponding values in the contralateral control preparations (table 3).

*The effect of nerve stimulation on the metabolism of norepinephrine.* $C^{14}$-norepinephrine, $1.2 \times 10^{-5}$ M, was incubated with the vasa deferentia and the effect of nerve simulation on the metabolism of norepinephrine was examined. The major deaminated metabolic products of norepinephrine in the guinea-pig vas deferens are the glycols, notably DOPEG (table 4). Less than 20% of the acid and neutral metabolites are present in the O-methylated form when $1.2 \times 10^{-5}$ M norepinephrine is employed. However, when a much lower

TABLE 3

*Tissue weight and norepinephrine content of guinea-pig vas deferens*

| Group[a] | $N^b$ | Tissue Weight | | Norepinephrine Content | |
|---|---|---|---|---|---|
| | | Control | Stimulated | Control | Stimulated |
| | | *mg* | | *μg* | |
| H$^3$-tyrosine, $5.5 \times 10^{-6}$ M | 11 | $183 \pm 14^c$ | $188 \pm 10$ | $1.04 \pm 0.13$ | $1.06 \pm 0.08$ |
| + Pargyline[d] | 13 | $203 \pm 10$ | $193 \pm 11$ | $1.03 \pm 0.07$ | $1.00 \pm 0.08$ |
| + Pargyline + norepinephrine[e] | 7 | $171 \pm 5$ | $185 \pm 6$ | $1.13 \pm 0.12$ | $1.17 \pm 0.09$ |
| H$^3$-dopa, $2.5 \times 10^{-5}$ M, + pargyline | 5 | $179 \pm 12$ | $185 \pm 12$ | $0.98 \pm 0.07$ | $0.98 \pm 0.09$ |

[a] Groups refer to the appropriate experimental groups in tables 1, 2 and 5.
[b] Number of experiments.
[c] Results are expressed as mean ± S.E.
[d] Pargyline, $1.6 \times 10^{-4}$ M.
[e] Norepinephrine, $6 \times 10^{-6}$ M.

TABLE 4

*The metabolism of norepinephrine[a] in isolated vas deferens-hypogastric nerve preparation*

| Metabolite[b] | Acid Hydrolysis[c] | Effect of Nerve Stimulation | | | |
|---|---|---|---|---|---|
| | | Control | Stimulated | Control + pargyline[d] | Stimulated + pargyline |
| | | *μμmol metabolite formed/g tissue* | | | |
| DOMA | 0 | $2610 \pm 123^e$ | $2515 \pm 145^e$ | 150 (129, 171)[f] | 86 (61, 112)[f] |
| | + | $2451 \pm 135$ | $2452 \pm 133$ | 158 (89, 228) | 148 (73, 224) |
| VMA | 0 | $565 \pm 72$ | $569 \pm 60$ | 78 (89, 67) | 54 (61, 47) |
| | + | $582 \pm 84$ | $538 \pm 44$ | 80 (83, 76) | 63 (61, 65) |
| DOPEG | 0 | $4371 \pm 232$ | $4347 \pm 328$ | 230 (278, 181) | 146 (179, 112) |
| | + | $4520 \pm 319$ | $4477 \pm 314$ | 298 (264, 333) | 176 (240, 112) |
| MOPEG | 0 | $1334 \pm 89$ | $1225 \pm 36$ | 108 (139, 76) | 66 (86, 47) |
| | + | $1386 \pm 72$ | $1300 \pm 40$ | 108 (122, 95) | 75 (102, 47) |

[a] C$^{14}$-norepinephrine concentration, $1.2 \times 10^{-5}$ M.
[b] DOMA, 3,4-dihydroxymandelic acid; VMA, vanilmandelic acid; DOPEG, 3,4-dihydroxyphenylglycol; MOPEG, 3-methoxy-4-hydroxyphenylglycol.
[c] Acid hydrolysis = heating at 95°C for 30 min at pH 1.5.
[d] Pargyline, $1.6 \times 10^{-4}$ M.
[e] Values are means ± S.E. of six determinations.
[f] Values are means with individual values given in parentheses.

concentration of norepinephrine is employed (H$^3$-norepinephrine, $2.5 \times 10^{-7}$ M), a greater proportion of the acid and neutral metabolites is acted upon by catechol-O-methyl transferase. No conjugated catecholamine metabolites were demonstrable.

*The effect of norepinephrine on catecholamine synthesis from tyrosine.* When the vasa deferentia are incubated with $6 \times 10^{-6}$ M norepinephrine, synthesis of H$^3$-norepinephrine from tyrosine is reduced to approximately 30% of that seen in the absence of norepinephrine. There is no significant increase in the amount of H$^3$-catecholamines present in the medium (table 5). In confirmation of previous results, nerve stimulation is no longer associated with increased norepinephrine synthesis (Alousi and Weiner, 1966). In the presence of $1.6 \times 10^{-4}$ M pargyline, norepinephrine synthesis is inhibited by norepinephrine to an even greater degree. Synthesis in the presence of pargyline plus norepinephrine is ap-

TABLE 5

*Effect of norepinephrine on catecholamine synthesis from tyrosine[a] in the vas deferens-hypogastric nerve preparation of guinea-pig*

| Group | $N^b$ | Stimula-tion | Norepinephrine Tissue | Norepinephrine Bath | Dopamine Tissue | Effect of Stimulation on Norepinephrine Formation (Increase above Control) |
|---|---|---|---|---|---|---|
| | | | *μμmol amine formed/organ* | | | % |
| Control | 3 | 0 | $45.8 \pm 8.1^c$ | $1.8 \pm 0.6$ | $2.6 \pm 0.4$ | |
| | | + | $55.8 \pm 5.4$ | $2.2 \pm 0.8$ | $3.6 \pm 0.4$ | $+36.2 \pm 9.8^d$ |
| Norepinephrine[e] | 3 | 0 | $19.2 \pm 3.6$ | $1.8 \pm 0.8$ | $1.8 \pm 0.2$ | |
| | | + | $17.0 \pm 3.0$ | $1.6 \pm 0.6$ | $2.0 \pm 0.2$ | $+4.2 \pm 18.7$ |
| Pargyline[f] | 7 | 0 | $49.6 \pm 7.0$ | $2.4 \pm 0.4$ | $2.4 \pm 0.2$ | |
| | | + | $66.4 \pm 4.6$ | $2.6 \pm 0.2$ | $2.8 \pm 0.2$ | $+45.6 \pm 15.3^d$ |
| Pargyline + norepineph-rine | 7 | 0 | $9.6 \pm 1.0$ | $2.2 \pm 0.2$ | $1.4 \pm 0.4$ | |
| | | + | $12.8 \pm 1.8$ | $2.6 \pm 0.4$ | $1.6 \pm 0.4$ | $+32.9 \pm 15.4$ |

[a] Tyrosine concentration, $5.5 \times 10^{-6}$ M (20 μc).
[b] Number of experiments.
[c] Results are expressed as mean ± S.E.
[d] P < .05.
[e] Norepinephrine concentration, $6 \times 10^{-6}$ M.
[f] Pargyline concentration, $1.6 \times 10^{-4}$ M.

TABLE 6

*Effect of 3-iodotyrosine[a] on catecholamine formation from tyrosine in the isolated vas deferens-hypogastric nerve preparation of guinea-pig*

| Tyrosine Concentration | Stimula-tion | Norepinephrine Tissue | Dopamine Tissue | Norepinephrine Bath |
|---|---|---|---|---|
| *M* | | *mμmol catecholamine formed/μmol norepinephrine* | | |
| $5.5 \times 10^{-6}$ + pargyline[b] | 0 | $0.30 \ (0.37, 0.24)^c$ | $0.15 \ (0.14, 0.17)$ | $0.51 \ (0.44, 0.57)$ |
| | + | $0.37 \ (0.44, 0.30)$ | $0.10 \ (0.10, 0.10)$ | $0.46 \ (0.51, 0.41)$ |
| $5.5 \times 10^{-5}$ | 0 | $5.63 \ (4.87, 6.39)$ | $1.44 \ (1.76, 1.12)$ | $0.64 \ (1.01, 0.27)$ |
| | + | $5.46 \ (6.35, 4.56)$ | $1.00 \ (1.45, 0.54)$ | $0.66 \ (1.05, 0.27)$ |
| $5.5 \times 10^{-5}$ + pargyline | 0 | $4.41 \ (2.87, 5.95)$ | $0.85 \ (1.08, 0.61)$ | $0.44 \ (0.64, 0.24)$ |
| | + | $6.51 \ (5.17, 7.84)$ | $1.81 \ (2.64, 0.98)$ | $0.76 \ (1.25, 0.27)$ |

[a] 3-Iodotyrosine concentration, $1 \times 10^{-4}$ M.
[b] Pargyline concentration, $1.6 \times 10^{-4}$ M.
[c] The means of 2 experiments are presented, with individual values in parentheses.

proximately 20% of that seen with pargyline alone. Nerve stimulation is associated with a slight, although insignificant, increase in the formation of $H^3$-norepinephrine from $H^3$-tyrosine, when both exogenous norepinephrine and monoamine oxidase inhibitor are in the bath.

*The effect of 3-iodotyrosine on the formation of norepinephrine from tyrosine.* 3-Iodotyrosine, $10^{-4}$ M, markedly inhibits the synthesis of catecholamines from tyrosine. The inhibitory effect of 3-iodotyrosine is greater when $5.5 \times 10^{-6}$ M tyrosine is employed

than when $5.5 \times 10^{-5}$ M tyrosine is present in the medium, suggesting that the inhibition by 3-iodotyrosine is competitive with tyrosine (table 6) (Udenfriend *et al.*, 1965).

*The uptake of tyrosine by the isolated vas deferens preparation.* Vasa deferentia were set up in organ baths as described and incubated for 1 hr in the presence of 25 μc of $H^3$-tyrosine and different amounts of unlabeled tyrosine. After the incubation, tissue and bath tyrosine were isolated and separately assayed and counted, and the specific activities of the tyrosine in tissue and bath were determined. Both the radioisotopic assay and the fluorimetric assay indicate that relatively little of the added tyrosine is taken up by the tissue during a 1-hr incubation period, amounting to 1 to 2% of that added (table 7). It is clear that added tyrosine does not completely equilibrate with endogenous tyrosine in this preparation during a 1-hr period, since the specific activity of added tyrosine exceeds that of endogenous tyrosine by 50-fold at $1 \times 10^{-6}$ M added tyrosine and by 3-fold at $5.5 \times 10^{-5}$ M exogenous amino acid. Tissue equilibration is probably less than the results in table 7 indicate, since a small amount of medium was doubtless assayed with the tissue. The uptake of tyrosine and the failure to approach equilibrium were similar in both stimulated and control preparations.

*The incorporation of tyrosine into tissue*

protein. In order to determine whether nerve stimulation results in a general increase in tyrosine metabolism in the tissue, incorporation of $H^3$-tyrosine into norepinephrine and into protein was assessed in stimulated and unstimulated vasa deferentia. Tyrosine is incorporated into the tissue protein of this organ at a rate which is 10 to 20 times greater than the rate of formation of norepinephrine from tyrosine. The increase in formation of norepinephrine and the incorporation of tyrosine into protein are proportional when the medium tyrosine concentration is increased 10-fold. However, in contrast to the formation of norepinephrine from tyrosine, incorporation of tyrosine into protein is unaffected by stimulation of the hypogastric nerve (table 8).

DISCUSSION. The present results confirm the

TABLE 7

*Uptake of $H^3$-tyrosine in guinea-pig vas deferens preparation*

| Tyrosine Added to Bath | $N^a$ | Tyrosine Content[b] | | Tyrosine | | Specific Activity | | Added Tyrosine Taken up by Tissue[c] |
|---|---|---|---|---|---|---|---|---|
| | | Tissue | Bath | Tissue | Bath | Tissue | Bath | |
| | | μg | | μc | | μc/μg | | μg |
| $1.0 \times 10^{-6}$ M[d] (1.8 μg) | 4 | 1.8 ± 0.13 | 3.1 ± 0.52 | 0.32 ± 0.06 | 24.8 ± 0.74 | 0.17 ± 0.024 | 8.6 ± 0.96 | 0.023 ± 0.004 |
| $5.5 \times 10^{-5}$ M[d] (101.8 μg) | 4 | 3.8 ± 0.16 | 92.4 ± 6.9 | 0.32 ± 0.05 | 19.8 ± 0.74 | 0.084 ± 0.015 | 0.22 ± 0.015 | 1.30 ± 0.20 |
| $5.5 \times 10^{-5}$ M[e] (11.8 μg) | 4 | 1.5 ± 0.17 | 12.7 ± 0.30 | | | | | |

[a] Number of experiments.
[b] Total tyrosine in tissue or bath determined fluorimetrically. The tyrosine content of guinea-pig vas deferens-hypogastric nerve preparations which were not incubated was 2.81 ± 0.24 μg (14.4 ± 1.0 μg/g tissue) ($N = 6$).
[c] Determined by dividing the microcuries of tyrosine in the tissue by the specific activity of the added tyrosine.
[d] To obtain the concentrations shown, 25 μc were diluted with unlabeled tyrosine.
[e] No added radioactive tyrosine.

TABLE 8

*The incorporation of $H^3$-tyrosine into protein in the guinea-pig vas deferens-hypogastric nerve preparation*

| Tyrosine Concentration | $N^a$ | Effect of Nerve Stimulation | | | |
|---|---|---|---|---|---|
| | | Incorporation of tyrosine into protein | | Norepinephrine synthesis | |
| | | Control | Stimulated | Control | Stimulated |
| | | μμmol tyrosine/mg protein | | mμmol/μmol norepinephrine | |
| $5.5 \times 10^{-6}$ M | 9 | 40.4 ± 4.5 | 40.1 ± 6.6 | 6.8 ± 0.7 | 8.2 ± 1.1 |
| $5.5 \times 10^{-5}$ M | 3 | 102.0 ± 17.5 | 117.9 ± 28.6 | 19.2 ± 2.5 | 34.0 ± 6.4 |
| Effect of nerve stimulation (% increase over control) | 12 | +4.7 ± 9.5 | | +35.7 ± 11.9[b] | |

[a] Number of experiments.
[b] P <.05.

earlier observations (Roth *et al.*, 1966; Alousi and Weiner, 1966) that nerve stimulation *in vitro* is associated with an accelerated formation of norepinephrine from tyrosine. Since nerve stimulation results in accelerated synthesis of norepinephrine from tyrosine, but is without significant effect on the synthesis of norepinephrine from dopa, the increased synthesis must be due either to an alteration in the metabolism of tyrosine or to an effect on the hydroxylation of tyrosine to dopa. It appears that overall tyrosine metabolism is not profoundly affected by nerve stimulation, since this procedure is without effect on the incorporation of tyrosine into tissue protein. Thus the altered rate of transformation of tyrosine to dopa and ultimately to norepinephrine which is associated with nerve stimulation appears to be a relatively selective effect on tyrosine metabolism.

The absence of an effect of nerve stimulation on protein synthesis also indicates that the uptake of tyrosine into the cells of the vas deferens is not altered. Conceivably, either the uptake of tyrosine or the overall metabolism of tyrosine might be selectively altered in the nervous tissue of the organ, and this effect might be masked by the quantitatively greater uptake and utilization of tyrosine in the muscle cells. However, it is believed that tyrosine and other aromatic amino acids are taken up into cells by an identical energy-dependent process (Guroff *et al.*, 1961). Since the synthesis of norepinephrine from dopa is not significantly affected by nerve stimulation, it would appear that aromatic amino acid uptake is not altered by nerve stimulation.

After incubation of exogenous tyrosine with the isolated vas deferens preparation for 1 hr, the complete equilibration of this tyrosine pool with endogenous tissue tyrosine is not achieved. The incomplete equilibration of exogenous and endogenous tyrosine has also been noted in the isolated, perfused guinea-pig heart (Spector *et al.*, 1963). It is not certain whether this is also true in the nerve endings. If equilibrium is not achieved in the nerve endings, the synthesis of norepinephrine from tyrosine may be greater than that which can be calculated from the formation of $H^3$-norepinephrine from labeled amino acid precursor. The specific activity of tyrosine in the tissue

and in the bath of the stimulated preparations is not different from analogous values in the control preparations, providing further evidence that nerve stimulation is not associated with an altered rate of uptake or equilibration of tyrosine in the system. Thus, although the rate of synthesis of $H^3$-norepinephrine from $H^3$-tyrosine in the isolated preparations may yield a low estimate of the true rate of norepinephrine synthesis, the increase in synthesis associated with nerve stimulation appears real and does not seem to be the result of altered rates of uptake or equilibration of exogenous tyrosine with the endogenous pool.

Evidence is also presented which indicates that the effect of nerve stimulation on the formation of norepinephrine from tyrosine is not the result of altered norepinephrine metabolism. The metabolism of exogenous norepinephrine in control and stimulated vas deferens preparations is virtually identical. Furthermore, marked inhibition of the oxidative deamination of norepinephrine does not significantly affect the increased synthesis associated with nerve stimulation. Finally, since the synthesis of norepinephrine from dopa is unaffected by nerve stimulation, it is hardly likely that the effect of nerve stimulation on the formation of $H^3$-norepinephrine from $H^3$-tyrosine is the result of some effect on an event beyond the formation of dopa.

It would thus appear that the effect of nerve stimulation is directly on the hydroxylation of tyrosine to dopa, the step which is presumed to be the rate-limiting reaction in the formation of norepinephrine (Nagatsu *et al.*, 1964). The observation that an increase in the concentration of exogenous norepinephrine is associated with a marked reduction in the synthesis of norepinephrine from tyrosine suggests that norepinephrine may regulate its own synthesis by feedback inhibition. If a monoamine oxidase inhibitor is also employed, the inhibitory effect of norepinephrine on its own synthesis is even more profound. This suggests that the action of norepinephrine is directly on synthesis and is not due to the releasing effect of this amine, with a consequent increase in the metabolism of the liberated norepinephrine stores. Norepinephrine is also able to inhibit the increase in the formation of norepinephrine from tyrosine which is ordinarily associated with nerve stimulation.

The present results suggest that tyrosine hydroxylase is normally inhibited by tissue norepinephrine, and that nerve stimulation leads to the release of tissue norepinephrine, activation of tyrosine hydroxylase and consequent accelerated synthesis of norepinephrine. Since the concentrations of norepinephrine in control preparations and in stimulated preparations are not significantly different, it is unlikely that total tissue norepinephrine is critical to this aspect of the regulation of norepinephrine synthesis. It seems more feasible that a small pool of intraneuronal norepinephrine which is able to interact with tyrosine hydroxylase is shifted either extraneuronally or into a noninteracting site during nerve stimulation. Udenfriend *et al.* (1965) have shown that catechols, including norepinephrine, inhibit tyrosine hydroxylase and that the inhibition appears to be competitive with the pteridine co-factor which is required for enzymatic activity. Ordinarily, the reduced co-factor apparently combines with the oxidized enzyme and reduces the enzyme to the active form for binding with oxygen and tyrosine prior to the catalytic formation of dopa. Norepinephrine and other catechols presumably compete with the reduced pteridine co-factor for the oxidized enzyme and thus prevent the succeeding catalytic reaction (Ikeda *et al.*, 1966). Stimulation in some way may reduce the intraneuronal norepinephrine concentration at the enzyme site. This would facilitate the binding of reduced pteridine with the enzyme and subsequent enzyme activation. Studies are in progress to evaluate this hypothesis.

Inhibition of monoamine oxidase would be expected to result in the preservation of free intraneuronal norepinephrine, and thus, according to the above hypothesis, might lead to an inhibition of norepinephrine synthesis. However, in the present results, addition of pargyline to the organ bath does not significantly affect the rate of formation of norepinephrine from tyrosine. This result is in agreement with the work of Levitt *et al.* (1965) on the isolated perfused guinea-pig heart. It might be argued that norepinephrine synthesis is actually inhibited by an amount which is equal to that amount of newly formed norepinephrine which otherwise would be degraded by monoamine oxidase. In favor of this hypothesis is the observation that, when dopa is used as precursor, formation of norepinephrine is approximately doubled in the presence of pargyline. This would suggest that pargyline inhibits the hydroxylation of tyrosine by approximately 50%. A reduction in the synthesis of norepinephrine by pargyline of this degree is consistent with the reported effect of monoamine oxidase inhibitors on norepinephrine turnover (Neff and Costa, 1966). The definitive evaluation of the effect of pargyline on norepinephrine synthesis must await the quantitative assessment of the formation of both norepinephrine and norepinephrine metabolites from tyrosine under experimental conditions similar to those in which net norepinephrine synthesis is evaluated.

ACKNOWLEDGMENT. The excellent technical assistance of Miss Sandra K. Svihovec is gratefully acknowledged.

## REFERENCES

ALOUSI, A. AND WEINER, N.: The regulation of norepinephrine synthesis in sympathetic nerves: Effect of nerve stimulation, cocaine and catecholamine-releasing agents. Proc. Nat. Acad. Sci. USA **56:** 1491–1496, 1966.

BARNESS, L. A., MELLMEAN, W. J., TEDESCO, T., YOUNG, D. G. AND NOCHO, R.: A quantitative method of determining urinary phenols. Clin. Chem. **9:** 600–607, 1963.

BUTTERWORTH, K. R. AND MANN, M.: The release of adrenaline and noradrenaline from the adrenal glands of the cat by acetylcholine. Brit. J. Pharmacol. Chemotherap. **12:** 422–426, 1957.

BYGDEMAN, S. AND EULER, U. S, VON: Resynthesis of catechol hormones in the cat's adrenal medulla. Acta Physiol. Scand. **44:** 375–383, 1958.

GILLESPIE, J. S.: Spontaneous mechanical and electrical activity of stretched and unstretched intestinal smooth muscle cells and their response to sympathetic nerve stimulation. J. Physiol. (London) **162:** 54–75, 1962.

GORDON, R., REID, J. V. O., SJOERDSMA, A. AND UDENFRIEND, S.: Increased synthesis of norepinephrine in the rat heart on electrical stimulation of the stellate ganglion. Mol. Pharmacol. **2:** 610–613, 1966a.

GORDON, R., SPECTOR, S., SJOERDSMA, A. AND UDENFRIEND, S.: Increased synthesis of norepinephrine and epinephrine in the intact rat during exercise and exposure to cold. J. Pharmacol. Exp. Therap. **153:** 440–447, 1966b.

GUROFF, G., KING, W. AND UDENFRIEND, S.: The uptake of tyrosine by rat brain *in vitro.* J. Biol. Chem. **236:** 1773–1777, 1961.

HÄGGENDAL, J.: An improved method for fluorimetric determination of small amounts of adrenaline and noradrenaline in plasma and tissues. Acta Physiol. Scand. **59:** 242–254, 1963.

HOLLAND, W. C. AND SCHÜMANN, H. V.: Formation

of catecholamines during splanchnic stimulation of the adrenal gland of the cat. Brit. J. Pharmacol. Chemotherap. **11**: 449–453, 1956.

HUKOVIĆ, S.: Responses of the isolated sympathetic nerve-ductus deferens preparation of the guinea pig. Brit. J. Pharmacol. Chemotherap. **16**: 188–194, 1961.

IKEDA, M., FAHIEN, L. A. AND UDENFRIEND, S.: A kinetic study of bovine adrenal tyrosine hydroxylase. J. Biol. Chem. **241**: 4452–4456, 1966.

LEVITT, M., SPECTOR, S., SJOERDSMA, A. AND UDENFRIEND, S.: Elucidation of the rate-limiting step in norepinephrine biosynthesis in the perfused guinea-pig heart. J. Pharmacol. Exp. Therap. **148**: 1–8, 1965.

NAGATSU, T., LEVITT, M. AND UDENFRIEND, S.: Tyrosine hydroxylase: The initial step in norepinephrine biosynthesis. J. Biol. Chem. **239**: 2910–2917, 1964.

NEFF, N. H. AND COSTA, E.: The influence of monoamine oxidase inhibition on catecholamine synthesis. Life Sci. **5**: 951–959, 1966.

OLIVERIO, A. AND STJÄRNE, L.: Acceleration of noradrenaline turnover in the mouse heart by cold exposure. Life Sci. **4**: 2339–2343, 1965.

ROTH, R. H., STJÄRNE, L. AND EULER, U. S. VON: Acceleration of noradrenaline biosynthesis by nerve stimulation. Life Sci. **5**: 1071–1075, 1966.

RUTLEDGE, C. O. AND WEINER, N.: The effect of reserpine upon the synthesis of norepinephrine in the isolated rabbit heart. J. Pharmacol. Exp. Therap. **157**: 290–302, 1967.

SEDVALL, G. C. AND KOPIN, I. J.: Acceleration of norepinephrine synthesis in the rat submaxillary gland *in vivo* during sympathetic nerve stimulation. Life Sci. **6**: 45–51, 1967.

SNEDECOR, C. W.: Statistical Methods, Iowa State University Press, Ames, 1956.

SPECTOR, S., SJOERDSMA, A., ZALTZMAN-NIRENBERG, P., LEVITT, M. AND UDENFRIEND, S.: Norepinephrine synthesis from tyrosine-C¹⁴ in isolated perfused guinea pig heart. Science (Washington) **139**: 1299–1301, 1963.

UDENFRIEND, S., ZALTZMAN-NIRENBERG, P. AND NAGATSU, T.: Inhibitors of purified beef adrenal tyrosine hydroxylase. Biochem. Pharmacol. **14**: 837–845, 1965.

WAALKES, T. P. AND UDENFRIEND, S.: A fluorometric method for the estimation of tyrosine in plasma and tissues. J. Lab. Clin. Med. **50**: 733–736, 1957.

WEINER, N. AND ALOUSI, A.: Influence of nerve stimulation on rate of synthesis of norepinephrine (NE). Federation Proc. **25**: 259, 1966.

WEINER, N., DRASKÓCZY, P. R. AND BURACK, W. R.: The ability of tyramine to liberate catecholamines *in vivo*. J. Pharmacol. Exp. Therap. **137**: 47–55, 1962.

W. P. DE POTTER,* A. D. SMITH† and
A. F. DE SCHAEPDRYVER*

# SUBCELLULAR FRACTIONATION OF SPLENIC NERVE: ATP, CHROMOGRANIN A AND DOPAMINE β-HYDROXYLASE IN NORADRENERGIC VESICLES

ABSTRACT. The subcellular particles in axons of the splenic nerve have been studied by centifrugation techniques. By differential centifrugation, five different types of particle could be distinguished and partly separated: noradrenaline-containing particles (noradrenergic vesicles), large and small lysosomes, mitochondria, and microsomal particles. In density gradient centrifugation, only one type of noradrenergic vesicle could be demonstrated.

The noradrenergic vesicles and the mitochondria contain ATP. Two proteins (chromogranin A and dopamine β-hydroxylase) are present in the noradrenergic vesicles.

## Introduction

SINCE the discovery by von Euler and Hillarp (1956) that noradrenaline is present in a particulate fraction of bovine splenic nerve, there have been many studies on the properties of this particulate fraction (see reviews by Stjärne, 1966a; Potter, 1966, and Potter, 1967). However, there is still relatively little information about the chemical composition of the noradrenaline-containing particles (noradrenergic vesicles) compared with what is known about the composition of other catecholamine-containing particles, such as adrenal chromaffin granules (see review by Smith, 1968).

Two approaches can be used to determine the composition of a subcellular particle: first, the distribution of a substance between different subcellular fractions of the tissue can be compared with that of a known constituent of the particle. Second, if the particle in question can be obtained free from significant contamination with other particles then its chemical composition can be determined directly, as was done by Hillarp (1959) for adrenal chromaffin granules. In practice, both these approaches have to be applied and both require a detailed knowledge of the distribution of all the different types of subcellular particle between the fractions obtained by centrifugation.

This paper compares the distribution of noradrenaline between fractions obtained by differential and density gradient centrifugation of homogenates of bovine splenic nerve, with the distribution of marker enzymes for mitochondria, lysosomes and microsomes. The subcellular distribution of the enzymes involved in the biosynthesis of noradrenaline and the distribution of the acidic protein chromogranin A will also be described. Some

* Heymans Institute of Pharmacology, University of Ghent, 9000 Ghent, Belgium.
† Department of Pharmacology, University of Ox ord, Oxford OX1 3QT, England.

Received 9 June 1970.

Reprinted from *Tissue and Cell* 2: 529–546 (1970) by permission of the publisher, Longman Group Ltd.

147

of these results have been communicated to the Belgian Physiological Society (Smith, De Potter and De Schaepdryver, 1969).

## Methods

*Tissue fractionation*

Bovine splenic nerves were obtained from the slaughterhouse within 30 min. of the death of the animals and were immediately placed on ice. The nerves were dissected free from contaminating tissue, desheathed, and washed with ice-cold 0·25 M sucrose. The tissue was chopped finely with a knife, suspended in 5 volumes of 0·25 M sucrose, and homogenised in a Potter-Elvehjem homogenizer (Braun, Melsungen, Germany; Kontes, Vineland, New Jersey, U.S.A.) using a Teflon pestle (clearance Braun: 0·12 mm, Kontes: 0·08 mm). The homogenization was continued until the pestle had been passed up and down twice (Braun) or five times (Kontes). The homogenate was filtered through a single layer of surgical gauze and the filtrate was then passed through four layers of gauze.

The subsequent differential centrifugation, in which five successive sediments and a final supernatant were obtained, was carried out with the A40 rotor of the Spinco model L ultracentrifuge at 2°C. The filtrate was centrifuged at 10,000 r.p.m. (6,596 g, $r_{av}$) for 8 min. to obtain sediment 1; the supernatant was centrifuged at 17,500 r.p.m. (20,203 g) for 15 min to obtain a sediment. The latter sediment was resuspended gently by hand in 10 ml 0·25 M sucrose with an homogenizer. The suspension was re-centrifuged at 17,500 r.p.m. for 15 min. to yield sediment 2 and a supernatant which was combined with the previous supernatant. The combined supernatants were centrifuged at 17,500 r.p.m. (20,203 g) for 30 min. to give sediment 3; the supernatant was centrifuged at 30,000 r.p.m. (59,364 g) for 22 min. to give sediment 4. The supernatant was centrifuged at 30,000 r.p.m. for 35 min. to give sediment 5 and the final supernatant.

For density gradient centrifugation, a sediment corresponding to the particulate fractions 2 to 5 was resuspended in 0·25 M sucrose (0·2 ml per g of original tissue) and 0·2 ml was applied to each density gradient. Linear density gradients (prepared with a mixing chamber) ranging from 0·3 M to 1·7 M-sucrose, were used. The bottom of each tube contained 0·5 ml of 2·0 M sucrose. The tubes containing the density gradients were centrifuged for 150 min. in the SW 39 head of the Spinco ultracentrifuge at 39,000 r.p.m. (125,000 g). After centrifugation, the tubes were punctured at the bottom and fractions of 23 drops were collected for analysis. Densities of the fractions were determined by the method of Hvidt, Johansen, Linderstrøm-Lang and Vaslow (1954) using a gradient of o–dichlorobenzene and petroleum ether (b.p. 60°–80°).

*Analysis of subcellular fractions*

For the assay of protein and noradrenaline, the fractions were mixed with cold perchloric acid to give a final concentration of 0·4 N. The resulting precipitate was analysed for protein by the method of Lowry, Rosebrough, Far and Randall (1951) using bovine serum albumin as a standard. The supernatants were neutralised and subjected to column chromatography to separate noradrenaline (Bertler, Carlsson and Rosengren, 1958; Sharman, Vanov and Vogt, 1962) which was estimated by the method of Laverty and Taylor (1968). ATP was measured in the neutralized supernatants after precipitation of the protein, by the method of Stanley and Williams (1969).

Lipids were extracted from the fractions with chloroform/methanol according to Folch, Lees and Sloane-Stanley (1957), using the KCl solution for washing. Lipid-phosphorus (Bartlett, 1959) and total cholesterol (Zlatkis, Zak and Boyle, 1953) were determined on aliquots of the chloroform phase.

Enzyme activities in the fractions were determined by the following methods: cytochrome oxidase (Appelmans, Wattiaux and de Duve, 1955); succinate-tetrazolium reductase (Pennington, 1961; Porteous and Clark, 1965); glucose-6-phosphatase (de Duve, Pressman, Gianetto, Wattiaux and

Appelmans, 1955); tyrosine hydroxylase (Nagatsu, Levitt and Udenfriend, 1964); dopa decarboxylase (Laduron and Belpaire, 1968); monoamine oxidase (Wurtman and Axelrod, 1963). The following enzymes were assayed in solutions containing Triton X-100 (0·02% W/V): alkaline and acid phenyl-phosphatase (Kind and King, 1954); β-gluc-uronidase (Gianetto and de Duve, 1955); acid ribonuclease (Smith and Winkler, 1966); β-gly-cerophosphatase (Berthet and de Duve, 1951).

Dopamine β-hydroxylase activity was estimated by measuring the conversion of [³H] tyramine to [³H] octopamine (Friedman and Kaufman, 1965; Viveros, Arqueros and Kirshner, 1968). The incubation mixture (1 ml) contained 2 μC of [³H] tyramine (0·0038 mM), ATP (5 mM), sodium fumarate (20 mM), tranylcypromine sulphate (0·5 mM), catalase (115 units/ml), ascorbic acid (1 mM), Triton X-100 (0·02% W/V), p-hydroxymercuri-benzoate (0.1 mM) and potassium phosphate buffer, pH 6·0 (100 mM). The mixture was incubated for 20 min at 25° and the reaction was stopped by addition of 1 ml of cold perchloric acid (0·8 N). The [³H]-octopamine in the supernatant was determined by periodate extraction according to the method of Friedman and Kaufman (1965).

For each of the above enzymes, incubation conditions were chosen so that the amount of substrate broken down was proportional to the amount of added enzyme. This is particularly important in the assays in which radioactively-labelled substrates were used, i.e. dopamine-β-hydroxylase, tyrosine hydroxylase, dopa-decarboxylase and mono-amine oxidase, since the substrate concentrations are below those required to saturate the enzymes. Except for cytochrome oxidase and dopamine β-hydroxylase, one unit of enzymic activity refers to the decomposition of 1 μmole of substrate per hr (see de Duve et al., 1955). One unit of cytochrome oxidase activity is defined (Cooperstein and Lazarow, 1951) as the amount of enzyme causing the decadic logarithm of the concentration of reduced cytochrome C to decrease by one unit/min/100 ml of incubation mixture. One

unit of dopamine β-hydroxylase activity refers to the formation one pmole of [³H] octopamine from [³H] tyramine during 20 min at 25°.

Immunochemical procedures were used to estimate material reacting with rabbit anti-serum to bovine adrenal chromogranin A. The chromogranin A was purified by the method of Smith and Winkler (1967) and only the fractions corresponding to the upper third of peak 2 were used to prepare anti-serum (Schneider, Smith and Winkler, 1967). The antisera were examined by immuno-electrophoresis using standard conditions (Grabar and Williams, 1955) and give a single precipitation line with chromogranin A. However, when the antisera were tested against the soluble lysate of bovine adrenal chromaffin granules a major precipitation line in the position of chromogranin A was formed, together with a minor line due to another faster moving chromogranin, and a very faint slow moving line due to dopamine β-hydroxylase (see Sage, Smith and Kirshner, 1967). The latter line was not present in antisera that had been incubated with dopa-mine β-hydroxylase purified by procedure of Goldstein, Lauber and McKereghan (1965) from the soluble lysate of bovine adrenal chromaffin granules. This treated antiserum (diluted 1:150) was used for the assay of chromogranin A by complement fixation as described by Schneider et al. (1967). The results will be expressed in terms of the amount of purified chromogranin A required to fix the same amount of complement.

*Lysis of particles by osmotic shock*

A particulate fraction corresponding to the sum of fractions 2, 3, 4 and 5 described above was suspended in Na, K phosphate buffer (0·005 M, pH 7·0) and left for 1 h at 0°C. An equal volume of 0·2 M KCl was added, and the suspension was then centrifuged for 90 min at 37,500 r.p.m. (92,739 g) in the A40 rotor of the Spinco ultracentrifuge. Samples of the pellet and supernatant were analysed for noradrenaline, chromogranin A and for dopamine β-hydroxylase activity as described above.

149

## Materials

U-[³H] tyramine, 2-[¹⁴C] tryptamine and 2-[¹⁴C]-dopa were purchased from NEN Chemicals, Boston, Mass. Tranylcypromine sulphate was given by Smith, Kline & French Ltd. The following substances were obtained from Sigma Chemicals, London: ATP (disodium), catalase (crystalline), 2-p-(iodophenyl) - 3 - (p - nitrophenyl) - 5 -phenyltetrazolium chloride, D-glucose 6-phosphate, phenophthalein mono- β -glucuronic acid, yeast ribonucleic acid and firefly lanterns. Disodium β-glycerophosphate and disodium phenylphosphate were purchased from Merck & Co., Darmstadt, Germany. Oxoid complement fixation test diluent tablets (BR 16) were used in the immunochemical experiments.

## Results

Homogenates of bovine splenic nerve contain several enzymes which have been shown in other tissues to be characteristic of different types of cell particle. The specific activities of these enzymes are given in Table 1. In addition to typical mitochondrial enzymes (cytochrome oxidase, succinate-tetrazolium reductase and monoamine oxidase) several hydrolases were present. It was found that some of the hydrolases were optimally active at low pH: ribonuclease (pH 5·4), β-glucuronidase (pH 5·0), phenylphosphatase (pH 5·0) and β-glycerophosphatase (pH 5·0). In other tissues such acid hydrolases are localized in lysosomes. An alkaline phosphatase was also present in splenic nerve, as indicated by second pH optima for phenylphosphatase (pH 9·8) and β-glycerosphosphatase (pH 9·0): in some tissues this enzyme is found in microsomal elements which may have been derived from the cell membrane (see Reid, 1967). Glucose-6-phosphatase, an enzyme characteristic of endoplasmic reticulum (Reid, 1967) was present. It had a pH optimum at 6·5.

Three enzymes concerned in the biosynthesis of noradrenaline from tyrosine, i.e. tyrosine hydroxylase, dopa decarboxylase

and dopamine β-hydroxylase are present, and each has a high specific activity in homogenates of splenic nerve. The specific activities given for these enzymes were measured at substrate concentrations of 0·1 mM, 0·93 mM and 0·0038 mM respectively and so do not necessarily represent the maximum rates since the concentration of substrate necessary to saturate each enzyme was not determined.

## Differential centrifugation of homogenates

The distribution of noradrenaline between five particulate fractions and the final supernatant was compared with that of two classes of enzyme: first, enzymes which, as described above, are believed to be characteristic of certain subcellular particles and, second, enzymes involved in the biosynthesis of noradrenaline. The results are given in Table 1 in terms of the proportion of the total enzymic activity found in each fraction and in Fig. 1 the results are plotted in the manner introduced by de Duve et al. (1955). The latter method compares the relative specific activity of the enzymes with the percentage distribution of protein.

It can be seen from Table 1 that some enzymes (cytochrome oxidase, succinate-tetrazolium reductase, monoamine oxidase and dopamine β-hydroxylase) were largely recovered in particulate fractions. In contrast, nearly 90% of the protein and all of the tyrosine hydroxylase and dopa decarboxylase activities were found in the final supernatant. In between these extremes lie the other enzymes, together with noradrenaline, ATP and chromogranin A, which were partly particle-bound and partly soluble.

Between 28% and 53% of the activities of the acid hydrolases were present in particles, which are likely to be lysosomes. Some of the activities of the acid hydrolases in the final supernatant may have been released from damaged lysosomes during homogenisation and centrifugation. Nearly 60% of the glucose-6-phosphatase activity was particulate, and most of this was present in small particles.

The advantage of plotting the results by

the method of de Duve *et al.* (1955), as shown in Fig. 1, is that it makes it possible to distinguish several different types of particle. Five different distribution patterns were obtained, and these are listed below in order of decreasing sedimentation rate of the particle-bound components:

(i) acid $\beta$-glucuronidase and acid ribonuclease;

(ii) cytochrome oxidase and succinate-tetrazolium reductase;

(iii) noradrenaline and dopamine $\beta$-hydroxylase;

(iv) acid phenylphosphatase and acid $\beta$-glycerophosphatase;

(v) alkaline phosphatase and glucose-6-phosphatase.

Monoamine oxidase had a distribution similar to that of mitochondria (type ii), but some of the enzymic activity sedimented more slowly and was recovered in sediments 3 to 5. The distribution of ATP was intermediate between type (ii) and type (iii) and the distribution of the lipids was similar to that of type (v).

*Distribution of chromogranin A and dopamine $\beta$-hydroxylase after differential centrifugation*

As shown above, the distributions of particulate dopamine $\beta$-hydroxylase and noradrenaline were very similar. Further evidence that noradrenaline and dopamine $\beta$-hydroxylase are present in the same particle is given in Fig. 2. In these experiments the amount of material reacting with antiserum to chromagranin A was also determined in each fraction. The histograms on the left of Fig. 2 are the results obtained when the centrifugation procedure of Schümann, Schmidt and Philippu (1966) was followed: in these experiments 19% of the noradrenaline was recovered in the second sediment and only 12% was in sediment 3. However, when the second sediment was resuspended and re-centrifuged the distribution of noradrenaline changed so that 9% was recovered in sediment 2 whereas the proportion in sediment 3 increased to 24·5%. This is shown on the right of Fig. 2. There is a parallel shift in

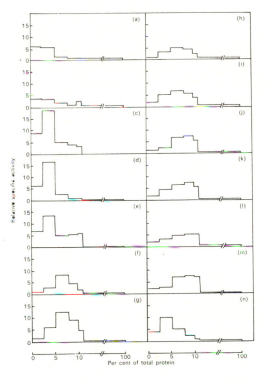

Fig. 1. Distribution of mitochondria, lysosomes, noradrenergic vesicles and microsomal elements between fractions obtained by differential centrifugation of bovine splenic nerve homogenates. The abscissa gives the proportion of the total protein in each fraction, beginning with the low speed sediment on the left; the ordinate gives the relative specific activity of each substance, which is the proportion of the constituent in a fraction divided by the proportion of the total protein in the fraction. The distributions are the means from several different experiments and the number of experiments is given in Table 1. (a) $\beta$-glucuronidase, (b) acid ribonuclease, (c) cytochrome oxidase, (d) succinate–tetrazolium reductase, (e) monoamine oxidase, (f) noradrenaline, (g) dopamine $\beta$-hydroxylase, (h) acid phenylphosphatase, (i) acid $\beta$-glycerophosphatase, (j) alkaline phosphatase, (k) glucose-6-phosphatase, (l) lipid-phosphorus, (m) cholesterol, (n) ATP.

the distributions of noradrenaline, of dopamine $\beta$-hydroxylase activity and of chromogranin A, but no corresponding change in the distribution of cytochrome oxidase.

*Composition of a particulate fraction rich in noradrenaline*

Although the particulate fraction (sediment 3) containing the highest concentration of noradrenaline is by no means free from other cell particles, it seemed of interest to determine the composition of this fraction. The results are given in Table 2, together with the composition of highly purified bovine adrenal chromaffin granules taken from the literature.

Experiments were carried out, as described in Methods, to determine the proportions of noradrenaline, dopamine $\beta$-hydroxylase and chromogranin A which become soluble when the particles are exposed to hypo-osmotic shock. When sediment 3 was exposed to hypo-osmotic shock 76% of the noradrenaline, 65% of the chromogranin A and 18% of the dopamine $\beta$-hydroxylase activity were released into the supernatant. The proportion of dopamine $\beta$-hydroxylase that was released into the supernatant was only 9% when the combined sediments 2 to 5 were exposed to hypo-osmotic shock. This is very similar to the proportion (8%) found by Hörtnagl, Hörtnagl and Winkler (1969) upon lysis of a fraction obtained by gradient centrifugation of a microsomal sediment from splenic nerve.

*Density gradient centrifugation*

The results of the differential centrifugation experiments indicated that homogenates of splenic nerve contain several different populations of particles which differ in their sedimentation properties in isotonic sucrose. Sucrose density gradient centrifugation was carried out to see whether these particles could also be distinguished on the basis of their equilibrium densities.

A fraction containing all the cell particles apart from those present in the first sediment was subjected to centrifugation over a linear gradient (0·3 M to 1·7 M-sucrose) and the results are given in Fig. 3. It is possible to distinguish five different distribution patterns. These are, in order of decreasing density of the particle-bound components:

  (a) $\beta$-glucuronidase;
  (b) cytochrome oxidase;
  (c) noradrenaline;
  (d) acid phenylphosphatase;
  (e) alkaline phosphatase and (not shown) glucose-6-phosphatase.

The distribution of monoamine oxidase was similar to, but not identical with, that of cytochrome oxidase: some of the monoamine oxidase was recovered in a region of lower density. The proportion of monoamine oxidase in less dense particles was found to depend upon the severity of homogenization. When the pestle was passed up and down only twice (as in the experiment in Fig. 3b) only a small part of the enzymic activity was found in particles less dense than mitochondria. However, when the pestle was passed up and down 5 or more times (as in the experiment in Fig. 3j) a distinct peak of monoamine oxidase activity appeared in particles present in the density range 1·09–1·11.

The noradrenaline-containing particles were only slightly less dense than the mitochondria, and were recovered in the density range 1·15 to 1·17. Some of the noradrenaline remained at the top of the gradient in a particle-free layer. The particles containing dopamine $\beta$-hydroxylase had a distribution close to that of the noradrenaline-containing particles, but a proportion of the enzymic activity was recovered in regions of lower density.

In these experiments no evidence was found for a population of noradrenaline-containing particles equilibrating at a low density, such has been found in sympathetically innervated tissues, e.g. rat heart (Potter and Axelrod, 1963; Roth *et al.*, 1968), rat vas deferens (Potter and Axelrod, 1963; Austin, Chubb and Livett, 1967) and dog spleen (De Potter, 1968). The finding of only one population of noradrenergic vesicles in splenic nerve homogenates confirms the work of Roth *et al.* (1968).

Table 1. *Distribution of constituents of bovine splenic nerve among fractions obtained by differential centrifugation of homogenates*

| Constituent | No. of experiments | Absolute value in total homogenate | Fraction 1 | Fraction 2 | Fraction 3 | Fraction 4 | Fraction 5 | Fraction 6 | Recovery |
|---|---|---|---|---|---|---|---|---|---|
| Protein | 8 | 12·57±2·15 | 2·51±0·63 | 2·82±1·01 | 2·76±0·83 | 2·02±0·66 | 1·06±0·36 | 88·72±3·18 | 91·5±10·2 |
| Cytochrome oxidase | 7 | 0·089±0·014 | 21·87±4·9 | 52·60±6·7 | 14·04±3·15 | 7·87±2·11 | 3·52±1·86 | 0 | 27·7±5·2 |
| Succinate dehydrogenase | 5 | 1·58±0·34 | 16·00±4·74 | 46·22±4·74 | 7·20±2·05 | 2·08±0·6 | 1·10±0·35 | 27·28±8·04 | 71·0±13·5 |
| Monoamine oxidase | 8 | 0·064±0·024 | 17·61±3·84 | 38·28±5·89 | 14·42±2·01 | 11·56±1·97 | 6·30±1·27 | 11·76±3·92 | 60·8±6·0 |
| Acid phenylphosphatase | 7 | 12·6±5·8 | 2·30±0·37 | 9·30±3·2 | 14·07±4·17 | 9·14±2·41 | 2·71±0·67 | 61·91±10·29 | 73·1±8·8 |
| Acid β-glycerophosphatase | 5 | 0·420±0·168 | 5·42±0·67 | 13·94±2·67 | 17·98±2·05 | 11·36±2·63 | 3·98±0·46 | 47·24±6·39 | 61·2±8·0 |
| β-glucuronidase | 7 | 0·354±0·066 | 15·17±2·22 | 15·22±3·57 | 4·31±1·12 | 1·85±0·57 | 0·84±0·17 | 62·52±4·92 | 80·5±7·4 |
| Acid ribonuclease | 4 | 7·2±2·4 | 8·97±2·67 | 9·47±4·07 | 4·70±1·14 | 2·25±0·58 | 2·40±0·27 | 72·10±7·02 | 110·6±21·8 |
| Alkaline phosphatase | 7 | 9·6±2·8 | 3·50±0·69 | 7·24±1·94 | 18·57±3·67 | 14·82±2·93 | 6·00±1·72 | 49·85±7·38 | 66·8±16·5 |
| Glucose-6-phosphatase | 4 | 1·56±0·14 | 4·60±0·55 | 12·72±1·02 | 18·47±0·98 | 15·12±0·47 | 6·42±1·66 | 42·62±2·9 | 78·0±6·1 |
| Phospholipid | 2 | 3·83±0·57 | 5·05±2·54 | 9·05±2·14 | 13·25±0·55 | 10·65±1·24 | 5·50±1·00 | 56·30±0·2 | 76·5±10·4 |
| Cholesterol | 2 | 0·83±0·29 | 5·4 | 6·95 | 19·75 | 15·2 | 7·5 | 45·3 | 71·5 |
| Dopa decarboxylase | 2 | 3·55±0·15 | 0 | 0 | 0 | 0 | 0 | 100 | 83·0±3·0 |
| Tyrosine hydroxylase | 2 | 0·205±0·045 | 0 | 0 | 0 | 0 | 0 | 100 | 76·0±5·0 |
| Dopamine β-hydroxylase | 6 | 4030±5·73 | 3·63±1·46 | 17·01±3·32 | 34·13±6·8 | 17·33±3·5 | 5·06±1·58 | 22·66±8·15 | 69·7±3·1 |
| Noradrenaline | 5 | 13·7±3·5 | 2·44±0·62 | 7·84±4·78 | 22·66±4·78 | 9·06±3·16 | 1·88±0·67 | 56·12±5·5 | 87·0±10·9 |
| ATP | 4 | 2·87±0·351 | 10·2±2·01 | 28·7±3·8 | 14·3±2·3 | 5·0±0·74 | 1·3±0·65 | 40·7±3·88 | 91·6±10·4 |
| Chromogranin A | 3 | 3·53±1·4 | 1·45 | 11·6 | 23·2 | 14·6 | 2·9 | 46·5 | 86·1±9·2 |

The concentration of each constituent in the filtered homogenate is expressed per g wet weight of original tissue: the enzymic activities are given in enzyme units, protein in mg, noradrenaline and ATP in nmoles, phospholipid and cholesterol in μmoles, and chromogranin A in μg. The results are means ± S.D. The proportion of each constituent found in a fraction is given as a percentage of the total recovered; the actual recoveries are given in the last column. Fractions 1–5 were the sediments obtained by centrifugation, and fraction 6 is the final supernatant (see Methods).

Table 2. *Composition of fraction 3 obtained by differential centrifugation of splenic nerve homogenates*

| Constituent | Units | Fraction 3 from bovine splenic nerve | Chromaffin granules from bovine adrenal medulla |
|---|---|---|---|
| Catecholamine | nmole | 1 | 1 |
| ATP | nmole | 0·132 | 0·22 |
| Dopamine β-hydroxylase | unit | 443 | 7·25 |
| Chromogranin A | μg | 0·26 | 0·10 |
| Protein | μg | 110·0 | 0·29 |
| Lipid-phosphorus | nmole | 161·0 | 0·18 |
| Cholesterol | nmole | 52·0 | 0·10 |

The composition of each particle is expressed per nmole of catecholamine.

The data for adrenal chromaffin granules were calculated from data given in the review by Smith (1968), with the exception of the activity of dopamine β-hydroxylase which was determined with the same incubation mixture (substrate [$^3$H] tyramine at 3·8 μM) as used for the splenic nerve (see Methods).

## Discussion

### Different types of subcellular particle in splenic nerve

The proportion of the total protein of the homogenate which is recovered in particles is very low (11·3%) compared with that found in other tissues such as rat liver (62·5%; de Duve et al., 1955), dog spleen (43%; De Potter, 1968) and bovine adrenal medulla (59%; see Smith, 1968). This may be a reflection of the relative paucity of particles in the axoplasm of splenic nerve, as seen in the electron microscope (Elfvin, 1958).

From the results of differential centrifugation experiments it can be concluded that homogenates of splenic nerve contain at least five different populations of particles which are, in order of decreasing sedimentation rate: large lysosomes (containing β-glucuronidase and acid ribonuclease); mitochondria; noradrenergic vesicles; small lysosomes (containing acid phosphatase); and microsomal elements (containing glucose-6-phosphatase and alkaline phosphatase).

Although defined by their biochemical composition, the above particles differ in some respects from similar particles in other tissues. The mitochondria sediment much more slowly than do those from other tissues: most of the mitochondria from rat liver are sedimented after centrifugation for 33,000 g-min (de Duve et al., 1955) whereas only a small proportion of the mitochondria from splenic nerve were sedimented at 53,000 g-min (sediment 1). Centrifugation for 302,000 g-min was required to sediment the bulk of the mitochondria of the splenic nerve. Similarly, the noradrenergic vesicles sediment more slowly, requiring 600,000 g-min, than do the chromaffin granules of adrenal medulla, which require 242,000 g-min (Smith and Winkler, 1966). The small size of both the mitochondria and the noradrenergic vesicles is consistent with electron microscopic studies of splenic nerve (Elfvin, 1958; Geffen and Ostberg, 1969) which show small mitochondria and small membrane-limited vesicles (diameter 500–800 Å); the latter are believed to contain the catecholamines.

The finding of two populations of lysosomes, one sedimenting at about the same rate as in other tissues and the other sedimenting much less rapidly, cannot yet be correlated with ultrastructural studies. However, it is of interest that Gordon, Bensch,

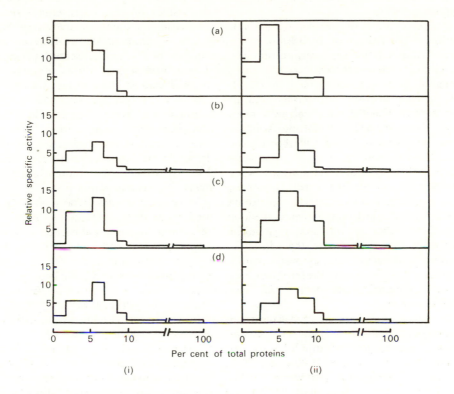

Fig. 2. Effect of resuspending sediment 2 on the distribution of mitochondria and noradrenergic vesicles. (i) Homogenates of splenic nerve fractionated by the method of Schümann *et al.* (1966). (ii) Homogenates of splenic nerve fractionated as described in Methods: sediment 2 was resuspended and re-sedimented. (a) cytochrome oxidase, (b) noradrenaline, (c) dopamine β-hydroxylase, (d) chromogranin A.

155

Deanin and Gordon (1968) reported that nerve terminals contain small-acid phosphatase-containing particles which may be a type of lysosome.

Further evidence for the occurrence of five different populations of particles was obtained by density gradient centrifugation. The results of these experiments confirm those recently reported by Hörtnagl et al. (1969), who concluded from their density gradient experiments that the noradrenergic vesicles could be distinguished from mitochondria, from lysosomes containing acid ribonuclease, and from microsomal elements containing glucose-6-phosphatase. The present work further shows that the small lysosomes, which contain acid phosphatase, can also be distinguished from the noradrenergic vesicles by their behaviour in density gradient centrifugation. Furthermore, the acid phosphatase-containing particles were readily distinguished from the denser lysosomes which contained acid ribonuclease and $\beta$-glucuronidase.

Several workers have found that the noradrenergic vesicles of splenic nerve equilibrate in density gradients in a layer initially containing 1·2 M sucrose (Roth et al., 1968; Burger, Philippu and Schümann, 1969; Hörtnagl et al., 1969) and the present experiments confirm these observations. The noradrenergic vesicles had an equilibrium density of 1·16 which corresponds to a sucrose molarity of 1·2.

In our gradient experiments, in which the lowest concentration of sucrose was 0·3 M, no evidence was found for a second population of noradrenergic vesicles equilibrating at a lower density.

*Possible constituents of noradrenergic vesicles*

By means of differential centrifugation alone or by density gradient centrifugation alone, as shown in the present work, or by a combination of both methods as shown by Hörtnagl et al. (1969) it is possible to distinguish noradrenergic vesicles from four other types of subcellular particle. However, these experiments also show that even the fractions richest in noradrenaline are by no means free from serious contamination by other cell particles. It is, therefore, not possible to form any conclusions about the composition of the noradrenergic vesicle by an analysis of only that fraction which is richest in noradrenaline. However, constituents of the noradrenergic vesicles can still be identified, if these substances are mainly located in the vesicles, by a comparison of the subcellular distribution of the substance with that of noradrenaline. We shall now discuss the evidence from the present experiments for the localisation in noradrenergic vesicles of monoamine oxidase, ATP, the enzymes of noradrenaline biosynthesis, and chromogranin A.

*Monoamine oxidase.* The possibility has been raised that monoamine oxidase might be present in the noradrenergic vesicles of splenic nerve (Roth and Stjärne, 1966; Stjärne, 1966b) and in the vesicles of other sympathetic nerves (Champlain, Axelrod, Krakoff and Müller, 1968; Champlain, Müller and Axelrod, 1969).

In the present experiments, the major part of the monoamine oxidase activity had a distribution close to that of the mitochondrial enzymes succinate-tetrazolium reductase and cytochrome oxidase, which is in agreement with the finding of Hörtnagl et al. (1969). However, both Stjärne, Roth and Giarman (1968) and Hörtnagl et al. (1969) found monoamine oxidase activity in a microsomal fraction. Our differential centrifugation experiments confirm that some monoamine oxidase is in smaller particles, and the gradient experiments show that a proportion of the enzyme is in particles which are not as dense as mitochondria.

The finding that the proportion of these less dense monoamine oxidase-containing particles increases when the tissue is homogenized more strongly is noteworthy. First, it probably accounts for the finding of Hörtnägl et al. (1969) that a large part of the microsomal monoamine oxidase in their experiments remained just below the top of the density gradient (0·8 M sucrose, corresponding to a density of 1·105) since their homogenization conditions (Kontes homogenizer,

156

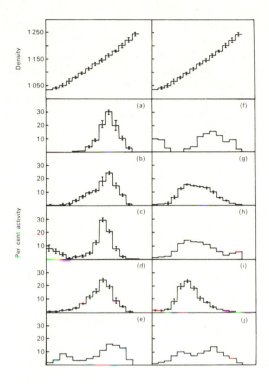

Fig. 3. Sucrose density gradient centrifugation of particles from bovine splenic nerve. A particulate fraction equivalent to fractions 2 to 5 (see Methods) was suspended in 0·25 M sucrose and centrifuged on a linear gradient (0·3 to 1·7 M sucrose). The abscissa is divided into the number of fractions with the top of the gradient at the left. The ordinate is the percent of the total activity recovered in each fraction. At the top of each set of histograms, the density of each fraction is given at 20°C. Vertical bars on the columns of the histograms give the standard deviation, and the number of experiments is given in parenthesis: (a) cytochrome oxidase (3), (b) monoamine oxidase: normal homogenisation (4), (c) noradrenaline (3), (d) dopamine β-hydroxylase (5), (e) β-glucuronidase (1), (f) acid ribonuclease (1), (g) acid phenyl-phosphatase (3), (h) β-glycerophosphatase (1), (i) alkaline phosphatase (4), (j) monoamine oxidase : prolonged homogenisation (2).

ten times up and down) were stronger than in the present work. Second, it raises the question of the origin of the less dense mono-amine oxidase-containing particles. Two possibilities have to be considered (see also Hörtnagl et al., 1969): this part of the monoamine oxidase may either be a component of cellular membranes which give rise to small particles of a lower density than mitochondria, or it may be derived artefactually from the mitochondria by fragmentation of the outer membrane (see also Stjärne et al., 1968; Jarrot and Iversen, 1968). In other tissues, the mitochondrial monoamine oxidase is localized in the outer membrane which is less dense than the intact mitochondrion (Schnaitman, Erwin and Greenwalt, 1967). The second possibility is supported by the decrease in the amount of monoamine oxidase in the mitochondrial layer of the gradient after strong homogenisation of the tissue (see Fig. 3).

It is concluded that the monoamine oxidase of splenic nerve is predominantly located in mitochondria and, in agreement with Hörtnagl et al. (1969), that the noradrenergic vesicles contain little, if any, monoamine oxidase.

*Adenosinetriphosphate.* Particulate fractions from bovine splenic nerve have been found to contain ATP (Schümann, 1958; Euler, Lishajko and Stjärne, 1963; Stjärne, 1964; Stjärne and Lishajko, 1966; Banks, Helle and Mayor, 1969) and the molar ratio of noradrenaline to ATP found by these workers ranged from 3·0 to 5·2. Stjärne (1964) and Stjärne and Lishajko (1966) pointed out that the fractions analysed were unlikely to be free of contamination by other cell particles and that these particles might also contain ATP. The present work shows that ATP has a distribution in differential centrifugation consistent with its presence in both mitochondria and noradrenergic vesicles. Since the fractions analysed by the authors quoted above contained mitochondria, their values for the molar ratio of noradrenaline to ATP do not represent the molar ratio actually present in noradrenergic vesicles.

The molar ratio of noradrenaline to ATP

in the combined fractions 2, 3 and 4, approximately equivalent to the sediment obtained by Stjärne and Lishajko (1966), was 2·9, which is similar to the ratio (range 3·0–3·8) found by these workers. However, when the contribution of the ATP present in mitochondria which contaminate fractions 3 and 4 is allowed for, it can be calculated that the molar ratio of noradrenaline to ATP in the noradrenergic vesicles is in the range 7·5–12.

These findings are of interest for two reasons. First, they could account for the differences observed by Euler et al. (1963), Stjärne (1964) and Stjärne and Lishajko (1966) between the rate of loss of ATP from 'nerve vesicles' compared with that from chromaffin granules. These authors found that whereas there was a parallel release of catecholamines and ATP from chromaffin granules incubated *in vitro*, the rate of loss of ATP from a particulate fraction of splenic nerve was much less than that of noradrenaline. This apparent difference between the two types of particle is now readily explained by the fact that the bulk of the ATP in the particulate fraction of splenic nerve was not present in noradrenergic vesicles.

The second point of interest, revealing a genuine difference between the above two types of particle, is the molar ratio of catecholamine to ATP which is about twice as high in nerve vesicles as it is in adrenal chromaffin granules. A similar relative lack of ATP has been found in chromaffin granules from some, but not all, phaeochromocytomas and this raised the question whether ATP is the only factor involved in the binding of the catecholamines (see Winkler and Smith, 1968). It is possible that the relative lack of ATP in the noradrenergic vesicles of splenic nerve is one of the causes of the rapid loss of noradrenaline from isolated vesicles compared with the slower loss of catecholamines from adrenal chromaffin granules incubated at 37°C (Stjärne, 1964).

*Enzymes of noradrenaline biosynthesis.* It has recently been suggested that, in sympathetic nerves, all the enzymes involved in the conversion of tyrosine to noradrenaline might be present within the same subcellular particle (Udenfriend, 1966, 1968). However, studies by Stjärne and Lishajko (1967) and Stjärne, Roth and Lishajko (1967) on fractions of bovine splenic nerve demonstrated that the conversion of tyrosine to dopa was exclusively a property of the particle-free supernatant, that the enzyme converting dopa to dopamine was also mainly located in the supernatant, but that the conversion of dopamine to noradrenaline only took place in a particulate fraction. The present experiments confirm that tyrosine hydroxylase activity and dopa decarboxylase activity are localized in the supernatant fraction, and they show that dopamine β-hydroxylase is a constituent of the noradrenergic vesicles. The distribution of dopamine β-hydroxylase and that of noradrenaline are very similar in two types of differential centrifugation and in density gradient centrifugation. Hörtnagl et al. (1969) also found a close similarity between the distribution of dopamine β-hydroxylase and noradrenaline in their two types of density gradient, and concluded that this enzyme is present in the noradrenergic vesicles.

The present work reveals slight differences between the subcellular distribution of dopamine β-hydroxylase and that of noradrenaline. The greatest difference is in the proportion of each recovered in the final supernatant: this can in part be explained by the finding that only 18% of the dopamine β-hydroxylase activity of the vesicles becomes soluble after osmotic shock, whereas 76% of the noradrenaline is solubilized by this procedure. During homogenization and centrifugation it is likely that a considerable proportion of the vesicles become damaged, and lose their soluble contents. This would leave behind an insoluble residue (including the vesicle-membrane) containing dopamine β-hydroxylase. It is suggested that these empty membranes account for the slight differences in the distributions of particulate noradrenaline and dopamine β-hydroxylase which were found in both differential and gradient centrifugation.

If the distribution of alkaline phosphatase and glucose-6-phosphatase is taken as a marker for that of microsomes derived from the endoplasmic reticulum, then it can be concluded from the gradient experiments that dopamine β-hydroxylase is not a constituent of these membranes, in agreement with Hörtnagl et al. (1969).

It is concluded that the major subcellular location of dopamine-β-hydroxylase is the noradrenergic vesicle, but that a small proportion may normally be present in the soluble cytoplasm.

*Chromogranin A.* The soluble proteins of adrenal chromaffin granules have been called 'chromogranins' (Blaschko, Comline, Schneider, Silver and Smith, 1967) and the major component of these proteins was called chromogranin A (Schneider et al., 1967). Using rabbit antisera to whole adrenal chromaffin granules, Hopwood (1968) found evidence for the presence of antigenic material of a similar nature in sympathetic nerves. This was not surprising since both tissues contain the enzyme dopamine β-hydroxylase, which is strongly antigenic (Sage et al., 1967). However, Hopwood (1968) also found, by an immunohistochemical method, evidence for antigenic material in bovine sympathetic nerves reacting with antisera to purified bovine adrenal chromogranin A. Further immunohistochemical studies by Geffen, Livett and Rush (1969) independently demonstrated that sheep sympathetic nerves reacted with antisera to two purified sheep adrenal chromogranins, one of which was dopamine β-hydroxylase, the other being the main component of the chromogranins. Geffen et al. (1969) found that both antigens accumulated proximal to the ligature in constricted sympathetic nerves at about the same rate as did noradrenaline. These findings raise the question whether the proteins are present in the noradrenergic vesicles and indirect evidence in favour of this was obtained by Banks, Helle and Mayor (1969) who found a chromogranin-like protein in a particulate fraction of bovine splenic nerve.

By using rabbit antisera to purified chromogranin A, we have been able to demonstrate that the antigenic material in bovine splenic nerve has a subcellular distribution in two types of differential centrifugation almost identical with that of noradrenaline: the chromogranin is, therefore, a constituent of the noradrenergic vesicles. The antigen in the vesicles was largely solublized upon osmotic shock just as is chromogranin A in adrenal chromaffin granules (Winkler, Hörtnagl, Hörtnagl and Smith, 1970). When the amount of antigenic material in the vesicles is expressed in terms of immunochemically equivalent amounts of chromogranin A, a ratio of chromogranin A ($\mu$g) to noradrenaline (nmoles) of 0·26 is found. This is of the same order of magnitude as the ratio of chromogranin A to catecholamines in bovine adrenal chromaffin granules: values of 0·14 (Kirshner, Sage and Smith, 1967) and of 0·10 (Schneider *et al.*, 1967) have been reported. This finding, as well as providing further biochemical evidence for the similarity of sympathetic nerve and adrenal medulla, raises again the question, what is the function of this acidic protein in catecholamine-containing particles?

*The storage of catecholamines in splenic nerve*

The biochemical approach to the subcellular composition of the splenic nerve as illustrated by the present work and that of Hörtnagl *et al.* (1969) can be compared with similar studies on chromaffin tissue (see review by Smith, 1968). In both tissues the catecholamines are stored in a highly specific type of cell particle which can be distinguished from other cell particles by its mass and density. The noradrenergic vesicles of splenic nerve are smaller and less dense than the chromaffin granules of adrenal medulla and yet both particles have the following constituents in common: catecholamine, ATP, dopamine $\beta$-hydroxylase and chromogranin A. By comparing the amount of each constituent with the amount of catecholamine present (see Table 2) it can be concluded that the noradrenergic vesicles are relatively deficient in ATP, but contain about twice as much chromogranin A and 60 times as much dopamine $\beta$-hydroxylase activity as adrenal chromaffin granules.

The possibility of identifying additional components of the noradrenergic vesicle depends upon whether these components are unique, or nearly so, to the vesicle. Components, such as phospholipids or cholesterol, which are also present in the other cell particles, cannot be studied until methods are available to purify the vesicles. An indication of the amount of purification required can be obtained by assuming that the ratio of total protein to catecholamine in the vesicles may be similar to that in chromaffin granules; in the latter particle this ratio is 0·29 $\mu$g protein per nmole catecholamine. In sediment 3, obtained by differential centrifugation of splenic nerve, this ratio was 110 $\mu$g/nmole, which is of the same order of magnitude as the ratios of 345 and 206 found for fractions from density gradients by Hörtnagl *et al.* (1969) and Burger, Philippu and Schümann (1969), respectively.

The present work has shown that two specific proteins are present in the noradrenergic vesicle, and that a proportion of each protein becomes soluble upon lysis of the vesicles. The occurrence of both these proteins, as well as noradrenaline, in the final supernatant of the homogenate can be accounted for in two ways. Either the proteins and noradrenaline exist both in particles and in the soluble axoplasm, or they are normally confined to the vesicles but are released from them during homogenization and centrifugation. The proportion of the total dopamine $\beta$-hydroxylase activity recovered in the final supernatant (23%) is greater than the value of 14% which can be predicted from the lysis of 56% of the noradrenergic vesicles during homogenization. It is possible, therefore, that a small proportion (about 10%) of the dopamine $\beta$-hydroxylase is localised in the soluble axoplasm. By using similar arguments, Viveros *et al.* (1968) came to the same conclusion for the adrenal medulla. However, the distribution of chromogranin A among fractions of the adrenal medulla is consistent with the localisation of all of it within chromaffin granules (Kirshner, Sage and Smith, 1967). The present work suggests that the chromogranin of splenic nerve is present only in the noradrenergic vesicles because the amount of chromogranin A found in the final supernatant is close to that which would be released upon lysis of vesicles during homogenization.

It can be concluded that, in both the adrenal medulla and splenic nerve, the catecholamines are stored in a highly specific type of cell particle. The question as to whether there are also similarities between the mode of release of catecholamines from these two tissues is examined in the next paper.

## Summary

1. Homogenates of bovine splenic nerve were fractionated by differential and sucrose density gradient centrifugation.
2. By differential centrifugation, five different types of particle could be distinguished and partly separated; these were, in order of decreasing sedimentation rate: large lysosomes, mitochondria, noradrenergic vesicles, small lysosomes, and microsomal elements.
3. Density gradient centrifugation of the combined particulate fractions confirmed the distinction between the five types of particle. The noradrenergic vesicles equilibrated in the gradient at the density of 1·2 M sucrose. No evidence for the presence of a less dense population of noradrenergic vesicles was obtained.
4. From their distribution among fractions obtained by differential centrifugation, it was concluded that tyrosine hydroxylase and dopa decarboxylase are not present in particles; that dopamine $\beta$-hydroxylase and chromogranin A are present in noradrenergic vesicles; that ATP is present in both mitochondria and noradrenergic vesicles; and that monoamine oxidase is present mainly in mitochondria. Confirmation that dopamine $\beta$-hydroxylase is present in noradrenergic vesicles was obtained by density gradient centrifugation.
5. The composition of the particulate fraction richest in noradrenaline was compared with that of bovine adrenal chromaffin granules: the noradrenergic vesicles are relatively rich in dopamine $\beta$-hydroxylase, contain twice as much chromagranin A, and half as much ATP per mole of catecholamine. The protein, phospholipid and cholesterol content of the fraction was very much higher than that of chromaffin granules due to contamination with other cell particles.

## Acknowledgements

This work was supported by grants from the Fund for Collective Fundamental Research, Belgium and the Medical Research Council, London. The excellent technical assistance of Miss M. Vanneste, Mrs B. Baeden and Miss H. Geffens is gratefully acknowledged. A. D. Smith is a Royal Society Stothert Research Fellow.

## References

APPLEMANS, F., WATTIAUX, R. and DE DUVE, C. 1955. Tissue fractionation studies. 5. The association of acid phosphatase with a special class of cytoplasmic granules. *Biochem. J.*, **59**, 438–445.

AUSTIN, L., CHUBB, I. W. and LIVETT, B. G. 1967. The subcellular localization of catecholamines in nerve terminals in smooth muscle tissue. *J. Neurochem.*, **14**, 473–478.

BANKS, P., HELLE, K. B. and MAYOR, D. 1969. Evidence for the presence of a chromogranin-like protein in bovine splenic nerve granules. *Molec. Pharmac.*, **5**, 210–212.

BARTLETT, G. R. 1959. Phosphorus assay in column chromatography. *J. Biol. Chem.*, **234**, 466–468.

BERTHET, J. and DE DUVE, C. 1951. Tissue fractionation studies. The existence of a mitochondria-linked, enzymically inactive form of acid phosphatase in rat-liver tissue. *Biochem. J.*, **50**, 174–181.

BERTLER, A., CARLSSON, A. and ROSENGREN, E. 1958. A method for the fluorimetric determination of adrenaline and noradrenaline in tissues. *Acta Physiol. scand.*, **44**, 273–292.

BLASCHKO, H., COMLINE, R. S., SCHNEIDER, F. H., SILVER, M. and SMITH, A. D. 1967. Secretion of a chromaffin granule protein, chromogranin, from the adrenal gland after splanchnic stimulation. *Nature, Lond.*, **215**, 58–59.

Burger, A., Philippu, A. and Schümann, H. J. 1969. ATP-Spaltung und Aminaufnahme dürch Milznervengranula. *Arch. exp. Path. Pharmak.*, **262**, 208–220.

Champlain, J. de, Axelrod, J., Krakoff, L. R. and Müller, R. A. 1968. Microsomal localization of monoamine oxidase in the heart and salivary gland. *Fedn. Proc.*, **27**, 399.

Champlain, J. de, Müller, R. A. and Axelrod, J. 1969. Subcellular localization of monoamine oxidase in rat tissues. *J. Pharmac. exp. Ther.*, **166**, 339–345.

Cooperstein, S. J. and Lazarow, A. 1951. A microspectrometric method for the determination of cytochrome oxidase. *J. biol. Chem.*, **189**, 665–670.

de Duve, C., Pressman, B. C., Gianetto, R., Wattiaux, R. and Appelmans, F. 1955. Tissue fractionation studies 6. Intracellular distribution patterns of enzymes in rat liver tissue. *Biochem. J.*, **60**, 604–617.

de Potter, W. P. 1968. Doctoral Thesis, University of Ghent, Belgium.

Elfvin, L.-G. 1958. The ultrastructure of unmyelinated fibers in the splenic nerve of the cat. *J. Ultrastruct. Res.*, **1**, 428–454.

Euler, U. S. von and Hillarp, N.-Å. 1956. Evidence for the presence of noradrenaline in submicroscopic structures of adrenergic axons. *Nature, Lond.*, **177**, 44–45.

Euler, U. S. von, Lishajko, F. and Stjärne, L. 1963. Catecholamines and ATP in isolated adrenergic nerve granules. *Acta physiol. scand.*, **59**, 495–496.

Folch, J., Lees, M. and Sloane-Stanley, G. H. 1957. A simple method for the isolation and purification of total lipides from animal tissues. *J. biol. Chem.*, **266**, 497–509.

Friedman, S. and Kaufman, S. 1965. 3,4-dihydroxyphenylethylamine $\beta$-hydroxylase: Physical properties, copper content, and role of copper in the catalytic activity. *J. biol. Chem.*, **240**, 4763–4773.

Gabar, P. and Williams, C. A. 1955. Méthode immunoélectrophorétique d'analyse de mélange de substances antigéniques. *Biochim. biophys. Acta*, **17**, 67–74.

Geffen, L. B., Livett, B. G. and Rush, R. A. 1969. Immunohistochemical localization of protein components of catecholamine storage vesicles, *J. Physiol.*, **204**, 593–605.

Geffen, L. B. and Ostberg, A. 1969. Distribution of granular vesicles in normal and constricted sympathetic neurones. *J. Physiol.*, **204**, 583–592.

Gianetto, R. and de Duve, C. 1955. Tissue fractionation studies. 4. Comparative study of the binding of acid phosphatase, $\beta$-glucuronidase and cathepsin by rat liver particles. *Biochem. J.*, **59**, 433–438.

Goldstein, M., Lauber, E. and McKereghan, M. R. 1965. Studies on the purification and characterisation of 3,4-dihydroxyphenylethanolamine-$\beta$-hydroxylase. *J. biol. Chem.*, **240**, 2066–2072.

Gordon, M. K., Bensch, K. G., Deanin, G. G. and Gordon, M. W. 1968. Histochemical and biochemical study of synaptic lysosomes. *Nature, Lond.*, **217**, 523–527.

Hillarp, N.-Å. 1959. Further observations on the state of the catecholamines stored in the adrenal medullary granules. *Acta physiol. scand.*, **47**, 271–279.

Hopwood, D. 1968. An immunhistochemical study of the adrenal medulla of the ox. A comparison of antibodies against whole ox chromaffin granules and ox chromogranin A. *Histochemie*, **13**, 323–330.

Hörtnagl, H., Hörtnagl, H. and Winkler, H. 1969. Bovine splenic nerve: characterization of noradrenaline-containing vesicles and other cell organelles by density gradient centrifugation. *J. Physiol.*, **205**, 103–114.

Hvidt, A., Johansen, G., Linderström-Lang, K. and Vaslow, F. 1954. Exchange of deuterium and [$^{18}$O] between water and other substances. 1. Methods. *C.r. Trav. Lab. Carlsberg*, **29**, 129–157.

Jarrot, B. and Iversen, L. L. 1968. Subcellular distribution of monoamine oxidase activity in rat liver and vas deferens. *Biochem. Pharmac.*, **17**, 1619–1625.

Kind, P. R. N. and King, E. J. 1954. Estimation of plasma phosphatase by determination of hydrolysed phenol with amino-antipyrine. *J. clin. Path.*, **7**, 322–326.

Kirshner, H., Sage, H. J. and Smith, W. J. 1967. Mechanism of secretion from the adrenal medulla. 2. Release of catecholamines and storage vesicle protein in response to chemical stimulation. *Molec. Pharmac.*, **3**, 254–265.

Laduron, P. and Belpaire, F. 1968. A rapid assay and partial purification of dopa decarboxylase. *Analyt. Biochem.*, **26**, 210–218.

Laverty, R. and Taylor, K. M. 1968. The fluorimetric assay of catecholamines and related compounds. *Analyt. Biochem.*, **22**, 269–279.

Lowry, O. H. and Rosenbrough, N. J., Farr, A. L. and Randall, R. J. 1951. Protein measurement with the Folin phenol reagent. *J. biol. Chem.*, **193**, 265–275.

NAGATSU, T., LEVITT, M. and UDENFRIEND, S. 1964. A rapid and simple radioassay for tyrosine hydroxylase activity. *Analyt. Biochem.*, **9**, 122–126.

PENNINGTON, R. J. 1961. Biochemistry of dystrophic muscle. Mitochondrial succinate-tetrazolium reductase and adenosinetriphosphatase. *Biochem. J.*, **80**, 649–654.

PORTEOUS, J. W. and CLARK, B. 1965. The isolation and characterisation of subcellular components of the epithelial cells of rabbit small intestine. *Biochem. J.*, **96**, 159–171.

POTTER, L. T. 1966. Storage of norepinephrine in sympathetic nerves. *Pharmac. Rev.*, **18**, 439–451.

POTTER, L. T. 1967. Role of intraneuronal vesicles in the synthesis, storage, and release of noradrenaline. *Circulation Res.*, **21**, (Suppl. 3), 13–24.

POTTER, L. T. and AXELROD, J. 1963. Subcellular localization of catecholamines in tissues of the rat. *J. Pharmac. exp. Ther.*, **142**, 291–298.

REID, E. 1967. Membrane systems. *Enzyme Cytology*, (ed. Roodyn, D. B.), pp. 321–406. London, Academic Press.

ROTH, R. H. and STJÄRNE, L. 1966. Monoamine oxidase activity in bovine splenic nerve granule preparation. *Acta Phys. scand.*, **68**, 342–346.

ROTH, R. H., STJÄRNE, L., BLOOM, F. E. and GIARMAN, N. J. 1968. Light and heavy norephinephrine storage particles in the rat heart and in bovine splenic nerve. *J. Pharmac. exp. Ther.*, **162**, 203–212.

SAGE, H. J., SMITH, W. J. and KIRSHNER, N. 1967. Mechanism of secretion from the adrenal medulla. 1. A microquantitative immunologic assay for bovine adrenal catecholamine storage vesicle protein and its application to studies of the secretory process. *Molec. Pharmac.*, **3**, 81–89.

SCHNAITMAN, C. A., ERWIN, V. G. and GREENWALT, J. W. 1967. The submitochondrial localization of monoamine oxidase. An enzymatic marker for the outer memebrane of rat liver mitochondria. *J. Cell Biol.*, **32**, 719–735.

SCHNEIDER, F. H., SMITH, A. D. and WINKLER, H. 1967. Secretion from the adrenal medulla: biochemical evidence for exocytosis. *Br. J. Pharmac. Chemother.*, **31**, 94–104.

SCHÜMANN, H. J. 1958. Über den Noradrenalin- und ATP-Gehalt sympatischer Nerven. *Arch. exp. Path. Pharmak.*, **233**, 296–300.

SCHÜMANN, H. J., SCHMIDT, K. and PHILIPPU, A. 1966. Storage of norepinephrine in sympathetic ganglia. *Life Sci.*, Oxford, **5**, 1809–1815.

SHARMAN, D. F., VANOV, S. and VOGT, M. 1962. Noradrenaline content in the heart and spleen of the mouse under normal conditions and after administration of some drugs. *Brit. J. Pharmac.*, **19**, 527–533.

SMITH, A. D. 1968. Biochemistry of adrenal chromaffin granules. In: *The Interaction of Drugs and Subcellular Components in Animal Cells*, pp. 239–292. Ed. Campbell, P. N., London, Churchill Ltd.

SMITH, A. D., DE POTTER, W. P. and DE SCHAEPDRYVER, A. F. 1969. Subcellular fractionation of bovine splenic nerves. *Arch. int. Pharmacodyn. Ther.*, **179**, 495–496.

SMITH, A. D. and WINKLER, H. 1966. The localization of lysosomal enzymes in chromaffin tissue. *J. Physiol.*, **183**, 179–188.

SMITH, A. D. and WINKLER, H. 1967. Purification and properties of an acid protein from chromaffin granules of bovine adrenal medulla. *Biochem. J.*, **103**, 483–492.

STANLEY, P. E. and WILLIAMS, S. G. 1969. Use of the liquid scintillation spectrometer for determining adenosine triphosphate by the luciferase enzyme. *Analyt. Biochem.*, **29**, 381–392.

STJÄRNE, L. 1964. Studies of catecholamine uptake storage and release mechanisms. *Acta physiol. scand.*, **62**, Suppl. 228, pp. 1–60.

STJÄRNE, L. 1966a. Storage particles in adrenergic tissues. *Pharmac. Rev.*, **18**, 425–432.

STJÄRNE, L. 1966b. Studies of noradrenaline biosynthesis in nerve tissue. *Acta physiol. scand.*, **67**, 441–454.

STJÄRNE, L. and LISHAJKO, F. 1966. Comparison of spontaneous loss of catecholamines and ATP *in vitro* from isolated bovine adrenomedullary, vesicular gland, vas deferens and splenic nerve granules. *J. Neurochem.*, **13**, 1213–1216.

STJÄRNE, L. and LISHAJKO, F. 1967. Localization of different steps in noradrenaline synthesis to different fractions of a bovine splenic nerve homogenate. *Biochem. Pharmac.*, **16**, 1719–1728.

STJÄRNE, L., ROTH, R. H. and LISHAJKO, F. 1967. Noradrenaline formation from dopamine in isolated subcellular particles from bovine splenic nerve. *Biochem. Pharmac.*, **16**, 1729–1739.

STJÄRNE, L., ROTH, R. H. and GIARMAN, N. J. 1968. Microsomal monoamine oxidase in sympathetically innervated tissue. *Biochem. Pharmac.*, **17**, 2008–2012.

UDENFRIEND, S. 1966. Tyrosine hydroxylase. *Pharmac. Rev.*, **18**, 43–51.

UNDERFRIEND, S. 1968. Physiological regulation of noradrenaline biosynthesis. *Adrenergic neurotransmission*, pp. 3–11. Ed. Wolstenholme, G. E. W. and O'Connor, M. London: Churchill.

VIVEROS, O. H., ARQUEROS, L. and KIRSHNER, N. 1968. Release of catecholamines and dopamine-$\beta$-oxidase from the adrenal medulla. *Life Sci.*, Oxford, **7**, 609–618.

WINKLER, H., HÖRTNAGL, H., HÖRTNAGL, H. and SMITH, A. D. 1970. Membranes of the adrenal medulla. Behaviour of insoluble proteins of chromaffin granules on gel electrophoresis. *Biochem. J.*, **118**, 303–310.

WINKLER, H. and SMITH, A. D. 1968. Catecholamines in phaeochromocytoma. Normal storage but abnormal release? *Lancet* (*i*), 793–795.

WURTMAN, R. J. and AXELROD, J. 1963. A sensitive and specific assay for the estimation of monoamine oxidase. *Biochem. Pharmac.*, **12**, 1439–1441.

ZLATKIS, A., ZAK, B. and BOYLE, A. J. 1953. A new method for the direct determination of serum cholesterol. *J. Lab. clin. Med.*, **41**, 486–492.

*Chapter 4*

# GAMMA-AMINOBUTYRIC ACID

Acetylcholine and catecholamines were well recognized as physiologically important compounds some forty years before their synthesis
and degradation in nervous tissue were significantly understood. In
contrast, about twenty years ago, biochemists isolated gamma-aminobutyric acid (GABA) and its biosynthetic enzyme, demonstrated
that they are exclusively located in brain tissue (Awapara, Landua,
Fuerst, and Seale, 1950; Roberts and Frankel, 1950; Wingo and
Awapara, 1950), and quickly and completely elucidated the metabolic
pathway, without shedding light on the physiological role played by
GABA. When GABA was found to support respiration in brain slices
as well as does glucose or glutamic acid, much attention focused on
the possibility that the GABA metabolic pathway functions solely for
energy production in brain (McKhann, Albers, Sokoloff, Mickelsen,
and Tower, 1960). The first clue of a more important physiological
role for GABA came some years later when it was identified as the
major inhibitory compound in a mammalian central nervous system
(CNS) extract that could block firing of a crustacean stretch receptor
neuron (see Chapter 1). Since that time GABA has been firmly established as an inhibitory neuromuscular transmitter in Crustacea. It
almost certainly functions as a transmitter in the mammalian CNS
as well (see Chapter 9). In this chapter we focus on the synthesis and
degradation of GABA in crustacean nervous tissue, where the physiological role of GABA is well defined.

The metabolic pathway for GABA is the same in both mammalian
and crustacean tissues. The enzyme L-glutamic acid decarboxylase
forms GABA from glutamic acid and requires pyridoxal phosphate as
a cofactor (Susz, Haber, and Roberts, 1966; Molinoff and Kravitz,
1968). GABA is an effective inhibitor of lobster glutamic decarboxylase. The mammalian enzyme, which has recently been highly purified

165

(Wu, Matsuda, and Roberts, 1973), is not inhibited by GABA, but elevated levels of chloride ion decrease activity.

GABA breakdown takes place in two steps. In the first, the amino group of GABA is transferred to $\alpha$-ketoglutarate to form glutamate and succinic semialdehyde. This is a reversible reaction catalyzed by GABA-glutamic transaminase, for which pyridoxal phosphate again serves as the cofactor (Bessman, Rossen, and Layne, 1953; Hall and Kravitz, 1967a). In the second step, the enzyme succinic semialdehyde dehydrogenase converts succinic semialdehyde to succinate. In this nearly irreversible oxidation, the electron acceptor is nicotinamide adenine dinucleotide ($NAD^+$) (Albers and Koval, 1961; Hall and Kravitz, 1967b).

$$\text{L-glutamate} \xrightarrow{\overset{\text{Glutamic acid}}{\text{decarboxylase}}} \text{GABA} + CO_2$$

$$\text{GABA} + \alpha\text{-ketoglutarate} \underset{\overset{\text{GABA-glutamic acid}}{\text{transaminase}}}{\rightleftharpoons} \text{succinic semialdehyde} + \text{L-glutamate}$$

$$\text{Succinic semialdehyde} + NAD^+ + H_2O \underset{\overset{\text{Succinic semialdehyde}}{\text{dehydrogenase}}}{\rightleftharpoons} \text{succinate} + NADH + H^+$$

$$\text{Sum: } \alpha\text{-ketoglutarate} + NAD^+ + H_2O \longrightarrow \text{Succinate} + NADH + H^+ + CO_2$$

The net effect of these three reactions is the oxidative decarboxylation of $\alpha$-ketoglutarate to succinate. Accordingly, the pathway has been called the "GABA shunt," as it provides an alternative to the $\alpha$-ketoglutarate oxidase portion of the tricarboxylic acid cycle. High activities of the GABA shunt enzymes in the mammalian CNS, coupled with active uptake of GABA (see Chapter 6), account for the efficient use of GABA as an energy source by brain slices.

The papers reprinted in this chapter deal with the identification of neurons containing GABA and the accumulation of GABA by these cells in the lobster nervous system. The investigations provide valuable information on the cellular neurochemistry of GABA and illustrate the general usefulness of invertebrate preparations for neurochemical studies. In the lobster nervous system, single, large, physiologically identified neurons can be located and isolated repeatedly by dissection from a series of animals. Thus, detailed chemical analyses can be performed on the contents of specific neurons, and functionally different neurons can be compared.

The studies under consideration began in the early 1960s, when there was still considerable doubt about the presence of GABA in crustacean tissues, despite earlier experiments that had shown that GABA could mimic the effects of inhibitory nerve stimulation. The paper by E. Kravitz, S. Kuffler, and D. Potter (1963, reprinted here) was the third in a series of papers establishing that GABA is present in lobster nervous tissue and demonstrating that GABA possesses the highest physiological specific activity of ten inhibitory compounds extracted from the tissues. The reprinted paper reports analyses at the level of single axons. The distribution of inhibitory compounds was examined in specific inhibitory and excitatory axons innervating lobster walking leg muscles. Of the inhibitory compounds, only GABA is highly concentrated in inhibitory axons. The levels of all the other inhibitory substances and of glutamate, the only excitatory compound found, are similar in the two types of axons. In a subsequent investigation, E. Kravitz and D. Potter (1965) showed that the GABA concentration in inhibitory axons is about one hundred millimolar, while in excitatory axons it is less than one millimolar.

Z. Hall, M.D. Bownds, and E. Kravitz (1970, reprinted here) attempted to understand this difference in GABA concentration by measuring enzymic activities and substrate levels of the GABA pathway in single axons. Glutamate, $\alpha$-ketoglutarate, and GABA-glutamic transaminase are present in equivalent amounts in excitatory and inhibitory axons, but glutamic decarboxylase is found only in inhibitory axons. From quantitative measurements of enzymic activities in neuronal extracts, these investigators calculated that inhibitory axons could synthesize GABA faster than they could degrade it, thereby providing a potential mechanism for GABA accumulation. Moreover, the normal GABA concentration (one hundred millimolar) in inhibitory axonal homogenates inhibits glutamic decarboxylase enough to reduce the synthetic activity to the level of the degradative activity, suggesting that GABA inhibition of glutamic decarboxylase may regulate the rate of GABA synthesis.

In order to analyze further the contents of inhibitory and excitatory neurons, M. Otsuka, E. Kravitz, and D. Potter (1967, reprinted here) demonstrated that functionally identified cell bodies can be reproducibly located in abdominal ganglia of the lobster ventral nerve cord. The somata of efferent inhibitory neurons contain a high level of GABA (about one-fourth that found in axons), while excitatory cell bodies have little or no GABA. As in axons, glutamate is equally concentrated in cell bodies of the two types of neurons. Thus in the lobster nervous system, high levels of GABA exist throughout inhibitory neurons and not just in terminals. This contrasts with the situation in certain neurons using other transmitters. For example, in mammalian sympathetic neurons, norepinephrine achieves high concentrations only in terminals.

It is disappointing that although lobster inhibitory neurons contain extraordinarily high levels of GABA, we do not know whether these cells have a special mechanism for GABA storage. As with mammalian cholinergic or noradrenergic terminals, electron micrographs of lobster inhibitory terminals show numerous vesicles. Moreover, miniature endplate potentials observed at these synapses give evidence of quantal release of GABA and thereby implicate vesicles in inhibitory synaptic function (see Chapter 5). Yet to date no one has convincingly demonstrated a bound or particulate form of GABA in either lobster or mammalian nervous tissue. It is not clear if technical difficulties alone can account for this failure to find GABA associated with vesicles, but until the problem of GABA storage is resolved it remains a challenge to the generality of our notions about the mechanisms of transmitter storage and release.

## READING LIST

*Reprinted Papers*

1. Kravitz, E.A., S.W. Kuffler, and D.D. Potter (1963). Gamma-aminobutyric acid and other blocking compounds in Crustacea. III. Their relative concentrations in separated motor and inhibitory axons. *J. Neurophysiol.* 26: 739–751.
2. Otsuka, M., E.A. Kravitz, and D.D. Potter (1967). Physiological and chemical architecture of a lobster ganglion with particular reference to gamma-aminobutyrate and glutamate. *J. Neurophysiol.* 30: 725–752.
3. Hall, Z.W., M.D. Bownds, and E.A. Kravitz (1970). The metabolism of gamma-aminobutyric acid in the lobster nervous system—Enzymes in single excitatory and inhibitory axons. *J. Cell Biol.* 46: 290–299.

*Other Selected Papers*

4. Awapara, J., A.J. Landua, R. Fuerst, and B. Seale (1950). Free γ-aminobutyric acid in brain. *J. Biol. Chem.* 187: 35–39.
5. Roberts, E. and S. Frankel (1950). γ-Aminobutyric acid in brain: its formation from glutamic acid. *J. Biol. Chem.* 187: 55–63.

6. Wingo, W.J. and J. Awapara (1950). Decarboxylation of L-glutamic acid by brain. *J. Biol. Chem.* 187: 267–271.

7. Bessman, S.P., J. Rossen, and E.C. Layne (1953). γ-Aminobutyric acid-glutamic acid transamination in brain. *J. Biol. Chem.* 201: 385–391.

8. McKhann, G.M., R.W. Albers, L. Sokoloff, O. Mickelsen, and D.B. Tower (1960). "The quantitative significance of the gamma-aminobutyric acid pathway in cerebral oxidative metabolism," in E. Roberts (Ed.), *Inhibition in the Nervous System and Gamma-Aminobutyric Acid,* pp. 169–181, New York: Pergamon Press.

9. Albers, R.W. and G.J. Koval (1961). Succinic semialdehyde dehydrogenase: Purification and properties of the enzyme from monkey brain. *Biochim. Biophys. Acta* 52: 29–35.

10. Kravitz, E.A. and D.D. Potter (1965). A further study of the distribution of gamma-aminobutyric acid between excitatory and inhibitory axons of the lobster. *J. Neurochem.* 12: 323–328.

11. Susz, J.P., B. Haber, and E. Roberts (1966). Purification and some properties of mouse brain L-glutamic decarboxylase. *Biochem.* 5: 2870–2877.

12. Hall, Z.W. and E.A. Kravitz (1967a). The metabolism of γ-aminobutyric acid (GABA) in the lobster nervous system. I. GABA-glutamate transaminase. *J. Neurochem.* 14: 45–54.

13. Hall, Z.W. and E.A. Kravitz (1967b). The metabolism of γ-aminobutyric acid (GABA) in the lobster nervous system. II. Succinic semialdehyde dehydrogenase. *J. Neurochem.* 14: 55–61.

14. Molinoff, P.B. and E.A. Kravitz (1968). The metabolism of γ-aminobutyric acid (GABA) in the lobster nervous system— Glutamic decarboxylase. *J. Neurochem.* 15: 391–409.

15. Wu, J., T. Matsuda, and E. Roberts (1973). Purification and characterization of glutamate decarboxylase from mouse brain. *J. Biol. Chem.* 248: 3029–3034.

16. Schousboe, A., J.-Y. Wu, and E. Roberts (1973). Purification and characterization of the 4-aminobutyrate — 2-ketoglutarate transaminase from mouse brain. *Biochem.* 12: 2868–2873.

# GAMMA-AMINOBUTYRIC ACID AND OTHER BLOCKING COMPOUNDS IN CRUSTACEA

## III. THEIR RELATIVE CONCENTRATIONS IN SEPARATED MOTOR AND INHIBITORY AXONS[1]

E. A. KRAVITZ,[2] S. W. KUFFLER, AND D. D. POTTER

*Neurophysiology Laboratory, Department of Pharmacology, Harvard Medical School, Boston, Massachusetts*

(Received for publication February 1, 1963)

### INTRODUCTION

IN THE TWO PRECEDING PAPERS it was reported that gamma-aminobutyric acid (GABA) was the most active of ten blocking substances extracted from the nervous systems of lobsters and crabs. The concentrations of GABA in several peripheral nerves were measured and found to be highest in a nerve that contained only one motor and one inhibitory axon. It was natural to wonder if GABA was specifically concentrated in the inhibitory axon. In the present study, therefore, we have isolated individual axons and found, within the limits of sensitivity of our enzymic assay, that motor fibers contained no GABA while inhibitory neurons contained surprisingly high concentrations. Other blocking compounds were also extracted from separated motor and inhibitory axons, but in contrast to GABA, these are present in both neuron types, as is the precursor of GABA, glutamic acid.

The current studies strongly suggest that GABA has a specific physiological role confined to inhibitory neurons.

#### METHODS

Two types of experiments were performed. The first was to compare enzymically the GABA contents of isolated motor and inhibitory axons and the second was to compare chromatographically the concentrations of other blocking compounds.

*Isolation of single motor and inhibitory axons.* Long stretches of isolated fibers were most easily obtained from a small nerve bundle in the meropodite (Fig. 1A in ref. 18). This bundle contains two prominent axons, one motor and one inhibitory, running side by side unbranched for 90–110 mm. (in 8- to 12-lb. lobsters) with a group of smaller sensory fibers. The motor fiber innervates the stretcher of the carpopodite and the opener (abductor) of the dactyl in the walking leg. The inhibitory axon also innervates the stretcher of the carpopodite but beyond that muscle it separates from the motor axon to supply the closer (adductor) of the dactyl (28). The axons are of similar and uniform diameter (50–60 $\mu$) during their course in the meropodite. The tissue around them and the accompanying smaller nerve fibers were removed and the two axons separated and identified by electrical stimulation through fluid electrodes, noting excitation or inhibition of the innervated

---

[1] This research was supported by Public Health Service Grants NB-02253-04, NB-03813-02, and NB-K3-7833.

[2] Special Research Fellow of the National Institute of Neurological Diseases and Blindness.

muscles (8). During dissection and separation most of the adhering connective tissue was removed (Fig. 1). Each dissection took about 3 hours and was performed at 6–12° C. in un-buffered saline containing (mM/liter) NaCl 462; KCl 15.6; and CaCl₂ 25.9. Several lengths, each up to 120 mm., of the two fiber types were pooled to obtain sufficient material for the analyses (Table 1). Our emphasis lies in comparing the relative amounts of certain materials contained in fibers of similar diameter and of similar length. As far as possible the handling and chemical treatment of fibers were identical.

For GABA assay, the separated fibers were homogenized in ice-cold 5% trichloroacetic acid or 0.5 M acetic acid and assayed as described below. For blocking compounds other than GABA the axons were homogenized in 0.5 M acetic acid, and after centrifugation the supernatant fluid was applied to a continuous flow electrophoresis apparatus as described in the preceding paper (18). The resulting physiologically active regions, B₁, B₂, and B₃ (18) were fractionated further by ascending paper chromatography in the solvent butanol-acetic acid-water (60-15-25). Region E was chromatographed in the solvent ethanol-acetic acid-water (160-15-25) at 4° and two strips, one containing betaine, the other aspartic acid plus glutamine, were eluted, the first for physiological assay, the second for further fractionation (paper chromatography in butanol-acetic acid-water, and phenol-water (70-30): for further details on the methods, see first paper, 7).

GABA assays were also done on the pairs of motor and inhibitory fibers which inner-vate the opener muscle of the dactyl of the walking leg of lobsters (Fig. 1B, ref. 18). No other fibers are known to accompany these two axons in their course over the inner surface of the muscle. The axons were separated for a few millimeters and then stimulated with a fluid electrode. In some experiments recordings were made from a muscle fiber with an intracellular electrode to observe the resulting excitatory or inhibitory junctional poten-tials. In other experiments the excitatory nerve alone was identified simply by observing muscular contractions. The two fibers were then pulled apart with whatever connective tissue adhered to them, extracted, and treated in the same way as the fibers from the mer-opodite. There were a number of uncertainties in these dissections. There was a possibility of false identification through escape of the stimulus from the fluid electrode to the fiber lying nearby. Furthermore, when many short lengths of axon had to be pooled for the spectrophotometric enzymic assay (Table 2, exp. 1–4), the chances were increased that seg-ments of inhibitory axon were mistakenly placed in the excitatory pool. Moreover, branches of the two fibers sometimes ran in the main connective tissue sheath for a distance (Fig. 2, ref. 18), and there was a chance that they did not separate properly with the parent stems. Separation was also more difficult than in the meropodite due to the relatively small size and tapering diameters towards the periphery; the range of diameters of isolated fibers in various sizes of lobsters was 40–15 μ. The method was improved by increasing the sensi-tivity of the enzymic assay until single axon segments of 30–40 mm. could be used. But, in contrast to the meropodite dissection, the possibility of contamination of one fiber with fragments of the other remained.

*Enzyme assays for GABA.* When sufficient material was available, assays were per-formed spectrophotometrically as described in the preceding paper (18). If less than 10⁻⁹ moles of GABA was expected, a fluorimetric procedure was used. The enzyme preparation was the same as that in the spectrophotometric method, but the reduced nicotinamide adenine dinucleotide phosphate (NADPH) was measured by chemical conversion to its oxidized form (NADP) which was measured fluorometrically. The techniques were based on the procedures of Lowry and co-workers (22, 23) and were similar to the GABA assay described by Hirsch and Robins (17). Assay tubes contained enzyme, NADP ($9 \times 10^{-4}$ μmoles), β-mercaptoethanol (0.09 μmole), α-ketoglutarate ($9 \times 10^{-3}$ μmoles), tris buffer, pH 7.9 (1.8 μmoles), and experimental samples in 12-μl. volumes. Zero-time controls (to which α-ketoglutarate had not been added) were run with experimental samples to establish tissue blank levels of fluorescence, and five GABA standards (within the range $2.5 \times 10^{-11}$ moles to $1.25 \times 10^{-10}$ moles) were run with each assay. Incubations were for 45 min. at room temperature except for zero-time controls. The reactions were ended, and excess NADP destroyed, by pipetting 10 μl. of the samples into 50 μl. of 0.25 M Na₃PO₄:0.35 M K₂HPO₄ buffer, and heating at 60° for 15 min. One hundred microliters of 10 N NaOH containing 0.03% H₂O₂ was added and the tubes were heated at 60° for 10 min. Finally, 1 ml. of water was added and the fluorescence measured in a Farrand fluorometer, model A, with a Corning 5860 primary filter (365 mμ) and a Baird-Atomic B-1 type interference filter (460 mμ peak transmission) as the secondary filter.

## RESULTS

*GABA content of motor and inhibitory fibers.* The results of the analyses of isolated axons from the meropodite region are presented in Table 1. The total material was over 5 m. of axon length. In each case we have compared the GABA content of paired inhibitory and excitatory neurons; these were of similar diameter and were treated in the same way.

No GABA was found in the meropodite excitatory axons; if it was present at all, it was in amounts too small to be detected by the enzymic assay.

Table 1. *GABA content of isolated motor (M) and inhibitory (I) axons from the meropodite*

| Nerve | Length, mm. | Separation Technique* | GABA, $\mu g/100$ mm. | Total GABA | | |
|---|---|---|---|---|---|---|
| | | | | Moles | Threshold,[†] moles | $I/M_T$[‡] |
| M-I | 200 | Columns | 1.2 | $2.35 \times 10^{-8}$ | | |
| I | 370 | Columns | 1.0 | $3.61 \times 10^{-8}$ | | 90 |
| M | 350 | | 0 | 0 | $4 \times 10^{-10}$ | |
| I | 500 | Columns | 2.4 | $1.2 \times 10^{-7}$ | | 300 |
| M | 500 | | 0 | 0 | $4 \times 10^{-10}$ | |
| I | 500 | Electrophoresis | 1.1 | $5.3 \times 10^{-8}$ | | 130 |
| M | 500 | | 0 | 0 | $4 \times 10^{-10}$ | |
| I | 1,085 | Electrophoresis | 1.25 | $1.32 \times 10^{-7}$ | | 1,200 |
| M | 1,085 | | 0 | 0 | $1.1 \times 10^{-10}$ | |

* Separation techniques: columns refers to the Dowex-50-H$^+$ techniques described in preceding paper (18); electrophoresis means crude extracts were separated by electrophoresis and GABA regions were pooled and assayed for GABA. † The minimum amounts of GABA which could be detected were $10^{-10}$ moles spectrophotometrically and $8 \times 10^{-12}$ moles fluorimetrically. The threshold values in the table are higher than this because only part of the sample was used for the assay. ‡ No GABA was detected in the M fiber. This calculation uses the threshold value for GABA ($M_T$) and represents a minimum ratio of GABA contents.

Therefore, no reliable value can be given to the ratio of GABA concentrations in the two types of fibers. However, it was possible to calculate how much GABA could have been present in the motor fibers and yet have remained undetected by the assay ("Threshold" in Table 1); this amount was dependent on the sensitivity of the assay and the quantity of material used. The threshold value was then compared to the measured GABA content of the corresponding inhibitory fiber to give the minimum value of the ratio of GABA concentrations in the two types of fibers ($I/M_T$ of Table 1). In our most striking experiment, in which the sensitivity of the assay was highest, if GABA was present at all in the motor axons it could not have been more than 1 part in 1,200 of that in the inhibitory fibers. In the other tests, smaller amounts of tissue were used, the assay was less sensitive and therefore the $I/M_T$ values were lower.

In one experiment of this series we also assayed combined motor and inhibitory fibers (no. 1). These contained 1.2 $\mu$g. of GABA/100 mm., an amount per unit length similar to the average of inhibitory axons alone.

The GABA contents of isolated axons from the surface of the opener muscle were compared in seven of the eight experiments of Table 2. Assays in the first four experiments were done spectrophotometrically and to obtain

Table 2. *GABA content of isolated M and I axons from the opener muscle surface*

| Nerve | Length, mm. | Separation Technique* | GABA, $\mu$g/100 mm. | Total GABA | | | |
| --- | --- | --- | --- | --- | --- | --- | --- |
| | | | | Moles | I/M | Threshold,† moles | I/M$_T$‡ |
| M-I | 320 | Columns | 0.11 | $3.4 \times 10^{-9}$ | | | |
| I | 350 | Columns | 0.14 | $4.6 \times 10^{-9}$ | 11.5 | | |
| M | 340 | | 0.012 | $4 \times 10^{-10}$ | | | |
| I | 1,010 | Columns | 0.19 | $1.91 \times 10^{-8}$ | 9.9 | | |
| M | 1,010 | | 0.02 | $1.96 \times 10^{-9}$ | | | |
| I | 300 | Columns | 0.37 | $1.07 \times 10^{-8}$ | | | |
| M | 275 | | 0 | 0 | | $10^{-9}$ | |
| Connective tissue | § | Columns | 0 | 0 | | $10^{-9}$ | 10 |
| I | 30 | No separation | 0.16 | $4.8 \times 10^{-10}$ | | | 24 |
| M | 30 | | 0 | 0 | | $2 \times 10^{-11}$ | |
| I | 36 | No separation | 0.14 | $4.8 \times 10^{-10}$ | | | 24 |
| M | 36 | | 0 | 0 | | $2 \times 10^{-10}$ | |
| I | 30 | No separation | 0.15 | $4.3 \times 10^{-10}$ | 6.2 | | |
| M | 30 | | 0.023 | $6.9 \times 10^{-11}$ | | | |
| I | 27 | No separation | 0.13 | $3.3 \times 10^{-10}$ | 4.8 | | |
| M | 27 | | 0.026 | $6.9 \times 10^{-11}$ | | | |

* No separation, GABA assays were performed directly on crude extracts; columns refers to the Dowex-50-H$^+$ techniques described in preceding paper (18).  † See Table 1 for explanation of threshold.  ‡ See Table 1 for explanation of I/M$_T$.  § The volume of this tissue was greater than that of the axons.

sufficient material many short fiber segments (8–20 mm. each from 2-lb. lobsters) were pooled. In the last four experiments with single pieces of individual axons from large lobsters, the fluorometric assay was used. In three cases no GABA was found in motor fibers and the I/M$_T$ values were 10 and 24. On the other hand, traces of GABA were found in four experiments, including two (no. 7 and no. 8) in which single fibers were assayed. In experiment no. 4 the connective tissue that was removed from the axons was also analyzed but no GABA could be detected. It should also be noted that while the GABA content of the inhibitory axon of the opener was only 0.1–0.2 µg/ 100 mm. length, approximately one-tenth that of the meropodite axons, the fiber diameter was smaller; in addition, as mentioned earlier (METHODS), a different inhibitory neuron was involved while the motor axon to the opener was the same as the one analyzed in the meropodite.

The results on the opener fibers raise the unexpected possibility that while GABA is absent in a motor axon along its course, it appears toward the periphery of the same cell. However, such a change in the chemistry of a motor axon in respect to GABA should not be considered seriously on the basis of our results because the experimental conditions were not satisfactory.

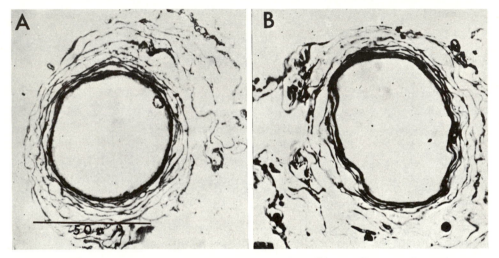

FIG. 1. Cross sections of isolated motor (A) and inhibitory (B) axons from the meropodite of the walking leg of a large (10 lb.) lobster. The axons were fixed in Millonig's solution after isolation, embedded in Araldite and stained with toluidine blue. In this sample the motor axon is somewhat better cleaned of connective tissue. The scale is the same for the two fibers. Note that diameter of the motor axon is greater in the meropodite than in its peripheral portion (Fig. 2, ref. 18). The sections were kindly provided by Dr. W. Fahrenbach.

There was a good chance of contamination of the excitatory axons by sections of the inhibitory axons, as already discussed (METHODS). It is hoped that with improved techniques of separation and even more sensitive assay methods the opener nerves may be studied more profitably.

One should note that the isolated fibers we analyzed were still a complex tissue because the dissections left varying amounts of connective tissue and the Schwann cell layer around the neuron membrane as indicated in the histological section of isolated axons in Fig. 1. It seems quite unlikely that connective tissue around motor fibers is different from that surrounding inhibitory axons. As far as Schwann cells are concerned there is no evidence at present that their chemical composition differs around various axon types. We therefore attribute the differences in GABA content to the axoplasm. From the data of Table 1 one obtains a GABA content of about 0.5 g. of GABA/ 100 g. of wet wt. of inhibitory axon. The following figures were used for this calculation: average fiber diameter 60 $\mu$; GABA content 1.4 $\mu$g/100 mm.; density of axoplasm, 1.0.

*Distribution of other blocking compounds in motor and inhibitory fibers.* We did not have specific sensitive enzymic assays for the blocking compounds other than GABA (18). Therefore the relative amounts of these compounds were estimated by comparing the density of Ninhydrin-stained spots on paper chromatograms, or, in the case of betaine, by elution from the paper chromatograms and bio-assay. While these techniques are not quantitative, they easily detected marked differences between motor and inhibitory fibers. The results of an experiment with 1,085 mm. of each type of axon are presented in Figs. 2 and 3. The Ninhydrin-stained spots in the principal physiologically active regions ($B_1$, $B_3$, E) are shown for inhibitory (I) and motor (M) fibers along with standard compounds run for comparison. The greatest difference between the two types of fibers occurs in the region $B_1$ to which GABA runs. There is no GABA spot in the motor axon chromatogram. The absence of GABA was confirmed by fluorometric assay of one-tenth of each $B_1$ fraction set aside at the time the remainder was chromatographed (see last experiment, Table 1). A spot-absorbing ultraviolet light was present in the GABA regions of I as well as M fibers (lightly outlined) but the material was physiologically inactive. $\beta$-Alanine occurred in both fibers, but in greater concentration in inhibitory than in motor axons (dotted circle). Since there was far less $\beta$-alanine than GABA and it is only about 1/50 as active as GABA in our physiological assay, this unequal distribution has not been studied further. There is a prominent spot high on the chromatogram ($R_F$ = 0.7) in the inhibitory fiber only. We believe this compound to be the cyclic amide (lactam) of GABA, for it has the $R_F$ value and staining characteristics (yellow, slowly turning blue) reported for GABA lactam (27). Presumably it was formed during spotting for chromatography. If this is the case, it is not surprising that we found it only in the inhibitor. The experiment illustrated in Fig. 2 was the only one in which we have seen this fast-moving spot, a fact which strengthens our suspicion that it was an artifact. One of the lower spots in region $B_1$ is the blocking substance "unknown A" (18), a very weakly active guanido compound which is present equally in the two fibers.

The blocking region, $B_3$, was subdivided; the bulk of the taurine was in one fraction, (on right in Fig. 2) the remaining taurine and homarine in the other (left). These blocking compounds were present in about equal concentration in the two types of fibers. The position and relative amounts of homarine on the chromatogram were determined with ultraviolet light (254 m$\mu$). The excitatory regions, E, of M and I fibers were not spotted on the same chromatogram, but streaked along the base lines of two chromatograms for 25 cm. Narrow side strips of these chromatograms were stained with Ninhydrin and are shown in Fig. 3. Glutamate was present in both fibers but more prominent in the motor axon. Aspartate and glutamine (no standard

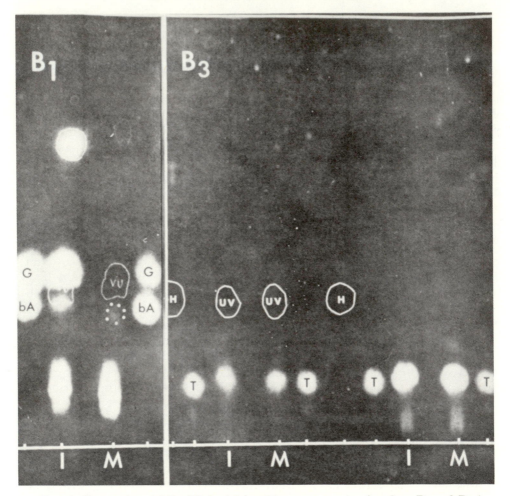

FIG. 2. Comparison of the Ninhydrin-positive components of regions $B_1$ and $B_3$ (see also Fig. 3, ref. 18) from electrophoretic fractionation of isolated inhibitory (I) and motor (M) axons; ascending paper chromatography in butanol-acetic acid-water (60-15-25). Standard components were not labeled at the base line but were marked on the spots as follows: G, GABA; bA, beta-alanine; H, homarine; T, taurine; UV, absorption of ultraviolet light. Taurine was present in both fractions of $B_3$, homarine in one (left). Areas of ultraviolet light absorption and homarine are outlined. In $B_1$, the outline of the beta-alanine spot in the motor fiber was faint and was dotted in. Solvent fronts and origins are retouched. Note that the large GABA spot appearing in the inhibitor is absent in the motor axon. Both neurons had an UV-absorbing region in GABA area (lightly outlined). The fast-moving spot in the inhibitory fibers is believed to be the cyclic amide of GABA (see text).

illustrated) run together in this solvent, but after elution from the chromatograms they were separated in another solvent and found to be uniformly distributed between the two fibers (not shown). Betaine is not revealed by Ninhydrin but was eluted from the chromatograms and bio-assayed; weak activity was found in both types of fibers. The weak blocking substance

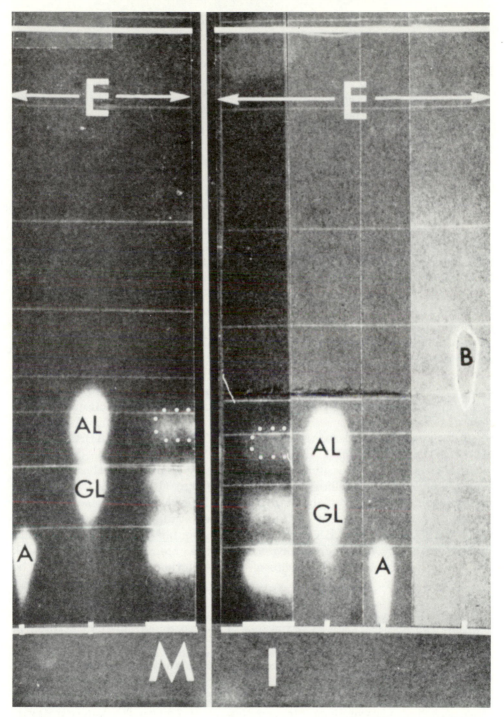

(*Legend on next page*) ⇉⟶

alanine (dotted in) may have been present in higher concentration in the motor than in the inhibitory fiber. A large part of the alanine was in region $B_2$ and is not shown. Ninhydrin-staining of the other regions of the electrophoretically separated extracts failed to reveal any other differences between motor and inhibitory axons.

Therefore, of the ten blocking compounds found in peripheral nerve (see 18) GABA may be the only one which is present exclusively in inhibitory fibers. The other nine are more or less evenly distributed between motor and inhibitory axons, with the possible exception of $\beta$-alanine, whose distribution has not been settled with the present material.

## DISCUSSION

Widespread interest in GABA was stimulated by the discovery that it occurred in the mammalian CNS in surprisingly high concentrations (for a review see ref. 2). It has been suggested that GABA functions as a key metabolic intermediate in a pathway of glutamate (or $\alpha$-ketoglutarate) metabolism, bypassing the oxidative decarboxylation of $\alpha$-ketoglutarate to succinyl coenzyme A. The sequence of enzyme reactions in this pathway is shown in Fig. 4. The enzymes catalyzing these reactions have been demonstrated in extracts prepared from brains of various species (2).

The possible reasons for GABA accumulation in cells have been extensively discussed in the literature (e.g., 17, 25). The relative rates of enzymic synthesis and destruction of GABA and factors which influence these enzymes are considered to be explanations for differences in GABA content of cells. The mechanisms of GABA accumulation are of special interest in the case of crustacean motor and inhibitory axons. At present, the distribution of glutamic decarboxylase, the enzyme which synthesizes GABA, is under study in separated axons.

Physiological interest in GABA was largely sparked by the important findings of Bazemore, Elliott, and Florey (1) that GABA was the principle compound in an extract of the mammalian CNS that blocked the discharges in crustacean stretch receptors. There followed studies by many workers on the pharmacology of GABA and of allied compounds on the vertebrate and invertebrate nervous systems (for reviews of the extensive literature see 4, 9, 14, 21). The physiological aspects of GABA action at synapses could be

---

FIG. 3. Comparison of the Ninhydrin-stained substances contained in the E region (see Fig. 3, ref. 18) from electrophoretic fractionation of isolated motor (M) and inhibitory (I) axons: two ascending paper chromatograms in ethanol-acetic acid-water (160-15-25) at 4°. Standard compounds (labeled on spots) were indicated as follows: A, aspartate; Al, alanine; Gl, glutamate; B, betaine. Faint horizontal lines mark subdivisions of paper which were eluted for physiological assay. Since tissue betaine was not stained by Ninhydrin, the horizontal strips opposite betaine standards (stained and identified with Dragendorff's reagent) were eluted for bio-asssay. The lowest horizontal strips of I and M contained both aspartate and glutamine; they were also eluted for further chromatography. Solvent fronts are indicated by white lines at top (see *Methods,* ref. 7 for details). Alanine spots were faint and were dotted in.

analyzed most thoroughly in invertebrates. In the CNS of crayfish (13) and in peripheral tissues of Crustacea such as the stretch receptor (20, 16) and the neuromuscular junction (14, 15, 19) GABA imitates the postsynaptic action of the inhibitory transmitter. Recently this analogy was extended to presynaptic inhibition in the crayfish (8) and an effect on the impulse spread in motor nerve terminals has been demonstrated (6). The results of experiments with GABA in the mammalian CNS have been less favorable for an assumption that this compound has a specific synaptic action. For instance,

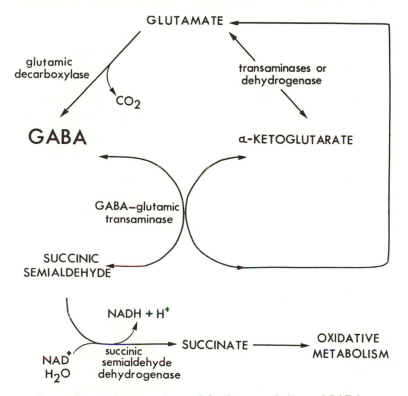

FIG. 4. Enzymic formation and further metabolism of GABA.

Curtis and his colleagues (3, 4), using electrophoretic application from micropipettes on spinal motoneurons, suggested that GABA as well as many of its analogues acted only as general depressants. In recent studies, however, the effect of GABA on the Mauthner cell, a large neuron in the goldfish medulla, was more striking and apparently more specific. Its action was similar to that of the neural transmitter substance and was confined to certain regions of the Mauthner neuron (5).

It has been proposed by many that GABA is an inhibitory transmitter. This hypothesis had the following weakness: the basic requirement that it be present in crustacean tissues, where it had been extensively studied and where its mechanism was best known, had not been met. In fact, it was emphatically stated (12) that there was no GABA in the crustacean nervous system. In the mammalian nervous system, on the other hand, where the presence of GABA had been known for a long time, the evidence was far from convincing that GABA imitated the action of the neurally released transmitter. It was natural, therefore, that in several recent symposia and reviews (e.g., 24, 10, 26, 4) the concensus developed that GABA was not a candidate for a role as an inhibitory transmitter.

Some studies that in several respects are similar to ours were made by Florey and co-workers (11, 12). From motor, sensory, and inhibitory axons they obtained extracts which they tested by physiological assay for blocking activity. It is interesting that in inhibitory neuron extracts they found strong blocking activity but none in sensory and motor fibers. One of the major discrepancies between our findings and theirs is that they could not detect any GABA. Further, their inhibitory material (11) was believed to be more active than GABA. They were led to this conclusion because, in order to explain the great activity of their extract, they would have had to assume that "up to" 3% of wet wt. of their inhibitory neurons was GABA. So far we have not been able to find substances more effective than GABA and in fact there may be no need for them to explain the calculated physiological blocking activity in extracts from crabs (11). Our measured GABA content in lobster inhibitory fibers was about 0.5% of the wet wt. GABA actually accounted for only 30–50% of the total blocking activity in our tissues, the rest being contributed largely by taurine and betaine. If these latter substances, as well as GABA, were present in Florey and Biederman's (11) extracts, much of their blocking activity would be accounted for. In view of the inherent inaccuracies in calculation of fiber weight and in the quantitation by bio-assays, and the fact that different species were used, it is uncertain whether any substantial discrepancies remain. The absence of blocking effects in their motor and sensory extracts (11) was presumably due to the small amount of tissue that was used for the assays and the admixture of excitatory substances.

The present series of studies have a direct bearing on the possible physiological role of GABA in Crustacea only. The following conclusions can be drawn: 1) GABA is a constituent of the peripheral as well as the central nervous system (7, 18). 2) GABA is present in surprisingly high concentration in isolated inhibitory axons. It makes up about 0.5% of the wet wt. along the unbranched course of this neuron. We have no way at present to determine the GABA concentration in the nerve terminal regions. 3) GABA may be confined to inhibitory neurons. On this important point the results are not complete. Principally, we know little about sensory neurons in which a small amount of GABA was found (18). Further, because of technical difficulties, we cannot exclude the presence of GABA in the peripheral portions of motor fibers.

The above conclusions indicate that GABA has a specific role linked with the function of inhibitory neurons. The crucial test that could establish it as a transmitter has not been made. It would have to be shown that it is released from the inhibitory terminals by the inhibitory nerve impulse in adequate amounts at the appropriate time during the process of transmission. In respect to the other blocking compounds all we can conclude is that their function is not uniquely related to inhibitory neurons since they are present in motor and inhibitory fibers.

As far as the vertebrate nervous system is concerned, an extension of single cell analyses, such as those of Hirsch and Robins (17), to known inhibitory and excitatory neurons would be very interesting.

## Summary

1. Two efferent axons of similar diameter, one inhibitory, the other excitatory, run side by side in the leg of the lobster (*Homarus americanus*). Long unbranched stretches of these neurons were removed and separated; the isolated axons were analyzed for their content of gamma-aminobutyric acid (GABA) and nine other synaptic blocking compounds that had been previously found in the crustacean nervous system (18). The GABA contents were compared enzymically; the contents of the other blocking substances were compared chromatographically or by physiological assay.

2. The GABA content along the course of the inhibitory axon was about 0.5% of its wet wt., while no GABA was detected in the accompanying excitatory fiber. GABA may therefore be confined to inhibitory nerves. The other blocking compounds, with the possible exception of $\beta$-alanine, were found in both neuron types. The distribution of $\beta$-alanine (a much weaker blocking substance than GABA) cannot be stated with confidence.

3. The findings indicate that GABA has a function specifically related to inhibitory neurons.

#### ACKNOWLEDGMENTS

We express our thanks to Dr. Nico van Gelder for valuable assistance in some of the experiments and Dr. W. Fahrenbach who kindly provided histological material for illustration. We also acknowledge continued technical help by R. B. Bosler and Peter Lockwood. Mrs. Marcia Feinlieb and Miss Star Martin contributed greatly in the biochemical laboratory.

## REFERENCES

1. BAZEMORE, A., ELLIOTT, K. A. C., AND FLOREY, E. Isolation of Factor I. *J. Neurochem.*, 1957, *1*: 334–339.
2. BAXTER, C. F. AND ROBERTS, E. Gamma-aminobutyric acid and cerebral metabolism. In: *The Neurochemistry of Nucleotides and Amino Acids*, edited by R. O. Brady and D. B. Tower. New York, Wiley, 1960, pp. 127–145.
3. CURTIS, D. R., PHILLIS, J. W., AND WATKINS, J. C. The depression of spinal neurones by $\gamma$-amino-n-butyric acid and $\beta$-alanine. *J. Physiol.*, 1959, *146*: 185–203.
4. CURTIS, D. R. AND WATKINS, J. C. The excitation and depression of spinal neurones by structurally related amino acids. *J. Neurochem.*, 1960, *6*: 117–141.
5. DIAMOND, J. Variation in the sensitivity to GABA of different regions of the Mauthner neurone. *Nature*. In press.
6. DUDEL, J. Effect of inhibition on the presynaptic nerve terminal in the neuromuscular junction of the crayfish. *Nature*, 1962, *193*: 587–588.
7. DUDEL, J., GRYDER, R., KAJI, A., KUFFLER, S. W., AND POTTER, D. D. Gamma-

aminobutyric acid and other blocking compounds in Crustacea. I. Central nervous system. *J. Neurophysiol.*, 1963, *26*: 721–728.

8. DUDEL, J. AND KUFFLER, S. W. Presynaptic inhibition at the crayfish neuromuscular junction. *J. Physiol.*, 1961, *155*: 543–562.

9. ELLIOTT, K. A. C. AND JASPER, H. H. Gamma-aminobutyric acid. *Physiol. Rev.*, 1959, *39*: 383–406.

10. FLOREY, E. Comparative physiology: transmitter substances. *Annu. Rev. Physiol.*, 1961, *23*: 501–528.

11. FLOREY, E. AND BIEDERMAN, M. A. Studies on the distribuiton of Factor I and acetylcholine in crustacean peripheral nerve. *J. gen. Physiol.*, 1960, *43*: 509–522.

12. FLOREY, E. AND CHAPMAN, D. D. The non-identity of the transmitter substance of crustacean inhibitory neurons and gamma-aminobutyric acid. *Comp. Biochem. Physiol.*, 1961, *3*: 92–98.

13. FURSHPAN, E. J. AND POTTER, D. D. Slow post-synaptic potentials recorded from the giant motor fibre of the crayfish. *J. Physiol.*, 1959, *145*: 326–335.

14. GRUNDFEST, H. AND REUBEN, J. P. Neuromuscular synaptic activity in lobster. In: *Nervous Inhibition*, edited by E. Florey. New York, Pergamon, 1961, pp. 92–104.

15. GRUNDFEST, H., REUBEN, J. P., AND RICKLES, W. H., JR. The electrophysiology and pharmacology of lobster neuromuscular synapses. *J. gen. Physiol.*, 1959, *42*: 1301–1323.

16. HAGIWARA, S., KUSANO, K., AND SAITO, S. Membrane changes in crayfish stretch receptor neuron during synaptic inhibition and under action of gamma-aminobutyric acid. *J. Neurophysiol.*, 1960, *23*: 505–515.

17. HIRSCH, H. E. AND ROBINS, E. Distribution of $\gamma$-aminobutyric acid in the layers of the cerebral and cerebellar cortex. Implications for its physiological role. *J. Neurochem.*, 1962, *9*: 63–70.

18. KRAVITZ, E. A., KUFFLER, S. W., POTTER, D. D., AND VAN GELDER, N. M. Gamma-aminobutyric acid and other blocking compounds in Crustacea. II. Peripheral nervous system. *J. Neurophysiol.*, 1963, *26*: 729–738.

19. KUFFLER, S. W. Excitation and inhibition in single nerve cells. *Harvey Lectures*. New York, Academic, 1960, pp. 176–218.

20. KUFFLER, S. W. AND EDWARDS, C. Mechanism of gamma-aminobutyric acid (GABA) action and its relation to synaptic inhibition. *J. Neurophysiol.*, 1958, *21*: 589–610.

21. LISSAK, E., ENDRÖCZI, E., AND VINCZE, E. Further observations concerning the inhibitory substance extracted from brain. In: *Nervous Inhibition*, edited by E. Florey. New York, Pergamon, 1961, pp. 369–375.

22. LOWRY, O. H., ROBERTS, N. R., AND KAPPHAHN, J. L. The fluorometric measurement of pyridine nucleotides. *J. Biol. Chem.*, 1957, *224*: 1047–1064.

23. LOWRY, O. H., ROBERTS, N. R., SCHULZ, D. W., CLOW, J. E., AND CLARK, J. R. Quantitative histochemistry of retina. II. Enzymes of glucose metabolism. *J. Biol. Chem.*, 1961, *236*: 2813–2820.

24. McLENNAN, H. Inhibitory transmitters—A review. In: *Nervous Inhibition*, edited by E. Florey. New York, Pergamon 1961, pp. 350–368.

25. ROBERTS, E. Free amino acids of nervous tissue: some aspects of metabolism of gamma-aminobutyric acid. In: *Inhibition in the Nervous System and Gamma-aminobutyric Acid*, edited by E. Roberts. New York, Pergamon, 1960, pp. 144–158.

26. ROBERTS, E. (ed.). *Inhibition in the Nervous System and Gamma-aminobutyric Acid*. New York, Pergamon, 1960, 591 pp.

27. VAN DER HORST, C. J. G. Artifacts of ornithine and $\alpha$-$\gamma$-diaminobutyric acid found during chromatographic investigation of Rumen liquid. *Nature*, 1962, *196*: 147–148.

28. WIERSMA, C. A. G. AND RIPLEY, S. H. Innervation patterns of crustacean limbs. *Physiol. Comparata et Oecol.*, 1952, *2*: 391–405.

# PHYSIOLOGICAL AND CHEMICAL ARCHITECTURE OF A LOBSTER GANGLION WITH PARTICULAR REFERENCE TO GAMMA-AMINOBUTYRATE AND GLUTAMATE[1]

M. OTSUKA,[2] E. A. KRAVITZ, AND D. D. POTTER

*Department of Neurobiology, Harvard Medical School, Boston, Massachusetts*

(Received for publication November 18, 1966)

THERE IS LITTLE DOUBT that gamma-aminobutyric acid (GABA) is the inhibitory transmitter compound at the lobster neuromuscular junction (see 20). Special interest, therefore, is attached to the chemistry of this compound. GABA is about 100 times more concentrated in inhibitory than in excitatory axons; the concentration is about 0.1 M in inhibitory fibers if GABA is freely dissolved in the axoplasm (13, 15). The origin of the GABA difference appears to lie in an asymmetric distribution of the enzyme that synthesizes GABA from glutamate, glutamic decarboxylase, the pathway for subsequent degradation being about equally active in the two types of axons (14). The mechanisms regulating the levels of the enzymes, on the other hand, are unknown; it is possible that differential enzyme synthesis or destruction accounts for the decarboxylase difference. Since the neuronal cell body is presumably the site of enzyme synthesis, the aim of the present work was to develop methods for finding and isolating the cell bodies of efferent excitatory and inhibitory neurons within the lobster central nervous system. As a first step toward understanding enzyme regulation in the GABA pathway, the contents of the substrates, GABA and glutamate, were measured. During the course of this work observations were made on the physiological organization of a ganglion, and these are also presented.

The present study, like earlier ones on peripheral axons, was aided by the favorable anatomy of the lobster. The total number of efferent neurons is small, usually between two and six per muscle, at least one of which is inhibitory (cf. 12, 31); this eases the problem of locating any particular cell body. Like the axons, the cell bodies are large enough to be isolated with hand-held instruments. In contrast to the cell bodies of most vertebrate neurons, they are apparently free of synapses (1); thus interpretation of the chemical analysis is simplified. Finally, the ganglia, like the peripheral nerves, show a striking constancy of organization; many of the efferent cell bodies can be recognized by their size and position alone.

A brief abstract of this work has been published (21).

---

[1] This work was supported by Public Health Service Grants 5 K3 NB 7833-05, 6 K3 HD 5899-01A1, NB 02253-06, and NB 02253-07.

[2] Rockefeller Foundation Fellow. Present address: Dept. of Pharmacology, Faculty of Medicine, Tokyo Medical and Dental University, Tokyo, Japan.

Reprinted from the *Journal of Neurophysiology* 30: 725–752 (1967) by permission of The American Physiological Society.

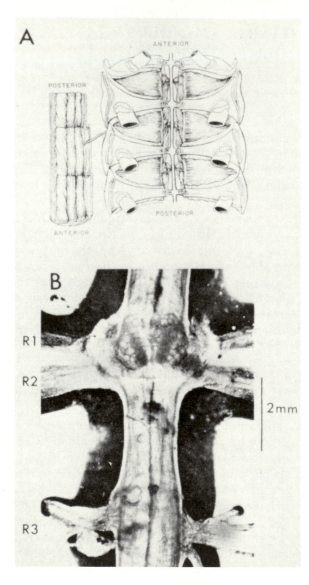

FIG. 1. *A:* an abdominal segment of the lobster, viewed from the ventral side. The ganglionic chain was exposed by removing ribs and skin in the midline. Flexor muscles were divided at the midline. At the left, the extensor muscles are attached to the preparation by the nerve supply of one segment (the main branch of the second root). *B:* ventral surface of the nerve cord, showing the second abdominal ganglion. The cell bodies were exposed by removing the connective tissue sheath and perineural tissue. The cell bodies are shown at higher magnification in Fig. 3. R1, R2, and R3; first, second, and third ganglionic roots.

## METHODS

*Animals.* Lobsters (*Homarus americanus*) were obtained from local dealers and kept in moist seaweed in a cold room at 3 C, sometimes for several days. They weighed 0.5–1.5 kg.

*Preparation.* A portion of the abdomen containing the first through the fourth ganglia was isolated (Fig. 1*A*). If the extensor muscles (cf. Fig. 12*B*) were used, the main branch of the second ganglionic root was exposed by removing the overlying shell, skin, and muscle. The extensor muscles were isolated, remaining connected to the rest of the abdomen by the nerve bundle. The nerve is sufficiently long to permit the extensor muscles to be placed with their deep face exposed when the rest of the abdomen is placed ventral side up (Fig. 1*A*).

If the extensor muscles were not needed, they were cut away with the shell to which they are attached. Further dissection was done in oxygenated physiological solution (hereafter called saline, see below for composition), with the temperature maintained between 7 and 14 C by thermoelectric cooling units upon which the chamber rested. The ventral surface of the ganglionic chain was exposed by removing midline portions of the overlying ribs, the joint membranes, and the underlying pigmented skin (Fig. 1*A*). To permit transmitted light to reach the ganglia, the flexor musculature dorsal to the ganglionic chain was divided in the midline, care being taken to minimize damage to the third roots. The only

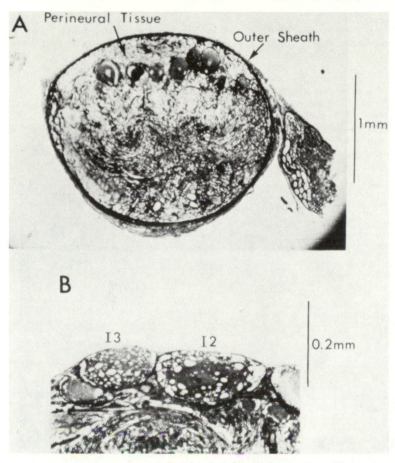

FIG. 2. *A*: transverse section of the third abdominal ganglion. The ventral surface, on which the cell bodies lie, is uppermost. The main mass of the ganglion consists of neuropil in which synapses are found. The ganglion was stained with toluidine blue. *B*: transverse section of a second abdominal ganglion in which the cell bodies were exposed before fixation. The highly vacuolated cytoplasm is characteristic of I2 and I3.

structure joining the two sides was now the ganglionic chain with its roots. The two halves were fixed with forceps or pins so that slight tension was placed on the roots, holding the ganglia taut (see Fig. 1, *A* and *B*). Light was reflected obliquely from below to give a dark-field effect.

To expose the cell bodies, the outer connective tissue sheath (Fig. 2*A*) was cut along a lateral margin, reflected to one side, and removed. The mass of soft perineural tissue (Fig. 2*A*) was washed away with a gentle stream of saline from a fine-tipped pipette (see Fig. 2*B*). The washing process was stopped as soon as the cells were clearly recognized. Under the dissecting microscope the ganglion now had the appearance shown in Figs. 1*B* and 3.

Cold, oxygenated saline was usually directed into the neighborhood of the ganglion throughout the experiment. An outlet attached to a suction line maintained a fluid level barely covering the tissues. In some experiments the bath was oxygenated directly without perfusion.

The methods for identifying the cell bodies of efferent excitatory and inhibitory neurons are described in RESULTS section.

*Isolation and transfer procedures.* Two procedures for isolating the cells were used. In method 1, the cell bodies were isolated by free-hand dissection using forceps under a dissecting microscope at a magnification of 40 ×. The sharpened points of stainless forceps were polished with rouge to reduce the tendency of the isolated cells to stick to the forceps. The cell body was first separated from its neighbors by softening and separating the surrounding tissue with a fine stream of saline or with forceps. When the cell body had been freed, the axon was grasped with forceps as far from the cell body as possible and severed (Fig. 4A). Remaining tissue was removed from the isolated cell as thoroughly as possible to reduce the chance of contamination by small cell bodies that lie beneath the large cells (Fig. 2). A histological section of such an isolated cell body is shown in Fig. 4C; some contaminating tissue remains, but most of the sample consists of the nerve cell body.

**Anterior**

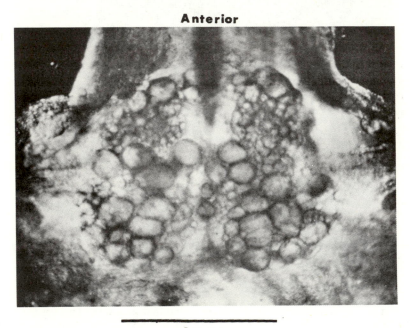

**1 mm**

FIG. 3. The third abdominal ganglion, showing the appearance of the living cell bodies under the dissecting microscope. This is the same ganglion as Fig. 14B.

Resting potentials of isolated cells were usually between 15 and 40 mv, with none higher than 45 mv; in most cases, the resting potential was not measured.

The isolated cell was then drawn into a pipette with a constricted neck (Fig. 4B) and transferred to a 0.2-ml conical tube with about 1 μl of saline. Two microliters of 0.2 N HCl were added to extract GABA and glutamate and to denature enzymes. The sample was then stored at −20 C until analyzed. Isolation and extraction usually took less than 4 min.

Method 2 for isolating the cell bodies resulted in more consistent chemical measurements. The whole ganglion was quickly removed and placed in isopentane kept near its freezing point with liquid nitrogen. The preparation was dried in vacuo (about 20 μ Hg) for a week at −30 C. The dry ganglion was placed in xylene to make it more transparent. The desired cells were removed with forceps and transferred and extracted as above. Xylene was chosen as a clearing agent because GABA and glutamate are virtually insoluble in it. In one series of experiments, cells were physiologically identified before the ganglia were frozen; neighboring cells were stained by dye injection (see below) so that the identified cells could be recognized in the dried ganglia. In another series of experiments (reported

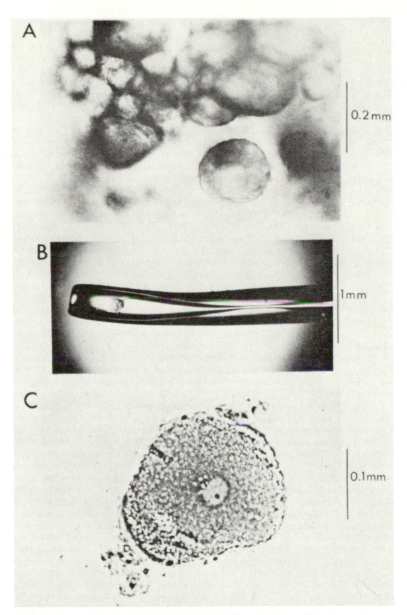

FIG. 4. Isolation and transfer of single cell bodies. *A*: the cell body at the lower right was separated from its neighbors by free-hand dissection. Its axon was severed, and the cell lies free on the ganglion. *B*: the cell body has been drawn into a transfer pipette. The constricted neck of the pipette prevents the cell from being lost, and by slowing fluid movement improves control. *C*: section of an isolated cell body, which was fixed in 1% OsO₄, embedded in Epon and stained with toluidine blue. Adhering tissue is present at the upper right and lower left.

in the bottom two columns of Table 3) an attempt was made to minimize disturbance to the ganglia before freezing. Instead of isolating a segment of the abdomen in the usual way, the brain was crushed and the whole animal immobilized. The second abdominal ganglion was exposed and the connective tissue sheath and perineural tissue over the ventral surface removed. Circulating blood was cleared from the ganglion during this operation with a jet of cooled, oxygenated saline. The ganglion was removed and frozen, the operation taking about 10 min in all. Less than 1 min elapsed from cutting the roots and connectives to immersing in the isopentane. The cell bodies were presumably frozen instantly since they were directly exposed to the freezing solution (cf. Fig. 2B). The cells were identified in the dried ganglion by visual inspection.

*GABA and glutamate assays.* The microtubes containing the cell bodies were lyophilized. GABA was assayed by a modification of the method of Jakoby and Scott (7). The details of this assay have already been published (15). With large inhibitory cell bodies the sample could be divided, so that a control tube containing aminooxyacetic acid could be run to give tissue blank levels of fluorescence.

Glutamate was determined by dividing the sample in half and treating one portion with a bacterial decarboxylase which converts glutamate to GABA. Both portions were then assayed for GABA; the difference between them represents the glutamate in the sample. Glutamine will also react in this assay but independent checks have demonstrated that glutamine levels are low in these cells. The details of the glutamate assay were as follows: The lyophilized sample was dissolved in 5 $\mu$l of pyridine-hydrochloride buffer, pH 4.6 adjusted to 0.1 M chloride with NaCl (25). Samples of 2 $\mu$l were transferred to two 0.1-ml test tubes. Two microliters of decarboxylase were added to the first tube (containing sufficient enzyme to convert all the glutamate present to GABA within 15 min) and 2 $\mu$l of heated decarboxylase to the second tube. The tubes were capped with parafilm and incubated for 15 min at room temperature. They were heated at 95 C for 1 min, 1 $\mu$l of 1 M Tris, pH 7.9 was added and a standard GABA assay was run, as previously described. The bacterial decarboxylase was prepared from dried *Escherichia coli* cells purchased from Worthington Biochemical Corp. The enzyme was extracted by homogenization in a French pressure cell, precipitation of contaminating proteins at pH 4.6, fractionation with solid $(NH_4)_2SO_4$ (0–60% saturation) and dialysis against 1,000 volumes of 0.01 M potassium phosphate, pH 6.5. This purification procedure is a modification of the method of Shukuya and Schwert (25).

*Estimation of cell body volume.* Only rough measurements of cell volume could be made on the living cell with the dissecting microscope. It was found that the manipulation required to measure the diameter of living cells under the compound microscope (cell transfers, temperature changes, etc.) resulted in reduced GABA contents. The method used, therefore, was to derive an average volume for each cell type by reconstruction from serial sections of fixed, plastic-embedded ganglia. These ganglia were from lobsters of the same size and condition as those used for chemical analyses. In two ganglia, certain cells were physiologically identified in the usual way and their positions in the ganglion sketched. The ganglia were then fixed in ice-cold acrolein-glutaraldehyde fixative modified after Sandborn et al. (23) and postfixed in phosphate-buffered OsO₄. The ganglia were dehydrated in methanol, stained with toluidine blue, and embedded in Epon 9. They were serially sectioned with a steel knife (J. Alvarez and E. J. Furshpan, unpublished data) at 4 $\mu$. Shrinkage of the ganglia during these procedures was found to be negligible. The cells could be easily identified by comparing a reconstructed ventral view from the serial sections with the sketch of the living ganglion. The volume of a cell was derived by tracing each section at known magnification on paper, weighing the tracings to determine their area, and multiplying the area by the known thickness of the sections. It was found that the large inhibitory cells could be confidently identified on histological grounds alone; they contained a higher proportion of large vacuoles (5–50 $\mu$ in diameter; see Fig. 2B) than neighboring excitatory cells. Moreover, certain excitatory cells could be identified from their positions in the ganglion. The second abdominal ganglia from five other animals were fixed without physiological manipulation. They were treated as described above, except that they were sectioned at 11 or 13 $\mu$. The proportion of the cell volume occupied by vacuoles was estimated in 13 cells.

*Physiological solution.* The solution had the following composition (millimoles): NaCl, 462; KCl, 15.6; CaCl₂, 25.9; MgSO₄, 8.3; Tris(hydroxymethyl)aminomethane, 10.0;

maleic acid, 10.0; NaOH, about 10 to bring the pH to 7.5. Just before using, glucose (2 mg/ml) was added. The saline was cooled and oxygenated.

*Electrodes.* Glass micropipettes were used for recording and passing current. They were filled with 3 M KCl or 2 M K- or Na-citrate and had resistances of 2–20 megohms when measured in 3 M KCl. The electrodes could be connected via a manual switch either to a high impedance preamplifier or to a pulse generator.

For marking cell bodies, organic dyes were injected electrophoretically from the microelectrodes. Electrodes with tips about 1 μ in diameter were filled with dye solutions, about one-quarter saturated, by pushing the dye down the shank with a fine glass filament (Alvarez and Furshpan, unpublished). The dyes used were fluorescein sodium, chromotrope 2R, light green S F yellowish, and fast green FCF. They are listed in order of decreasing rate of diffusion within the cells.

It was frequently necessary to stimulate a peripheral nerve in the middle of its course without disturbing its central and peripheral connections. A convenient electrode for doing this was made by enclosing a platinum wire with a flattened end in a polyethylene tube about 4 cm long (Fig. 5). The end of the polyethylene tube was sealed and a groove for supporting the nerve and confining the current was made with a hot needle. The wire

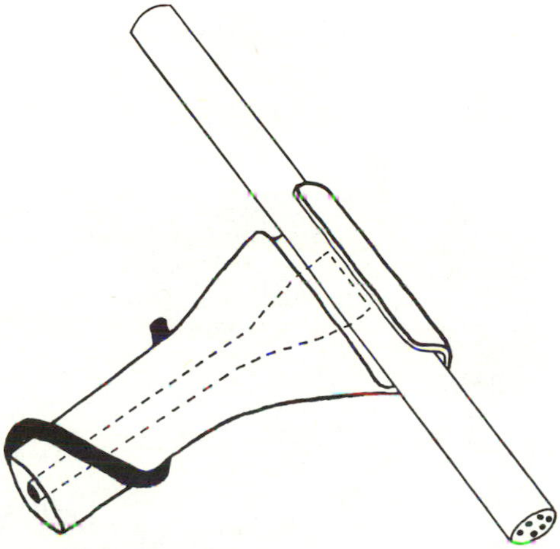

FIG. 5. Electrode used for stimulating the peripheral nerve in the middle of its course. One lead (dotted line) is surrounded by a polyethylene tube and is exposed to the bath only at the bottom of the groove in which the nerve lies. The other lead (solid black line) is wound around the polyethylene tube.

was exposed to the saline only in the groove. A second lead was wound on the outside of the tube. Stimulating voltages were as small as those used with suction electrodes. The assembly was carried on a ball-joint manipulator and could easily be bent into any position. When the nerve in the groove was stimulated, impulses spread in both centripetal and centrifugal directions at the same threshold.

## RESULTS

**PART I**

### *Physiological architecture of the ganglion*

The abdominal ganglia were used because the cell bodies lie nearly in one plane (Figs. 2A, 3), and are among the largest in the lobster nervous system, several being over 200 μ in diameter. Usually the second and third abdominal ganglia were chosen. Cells of exposed ganglia were impaled under visual control. The resting potentials recorded with our low-resistance microelectrodes were usually 40–70 mv, and with few exceptions the cell bodies showed action potentials of less than 25 mv, suggesting that the membrane of the cell body and its slender process behaved passively under our experimental conditions (cf. 26).

At the outset our problem was to find the efferent neurons among all the cells in the ganglion (Fig. 3) and to determine the function of each. Efferent excitatory cells were found relatively easily because a visible muscle contraction usually appeared when they were stimulated intracellularly with a single shock. The possibility that the cell was an interneuron could then be virtually eliminated by showing that antidromic impulses reached the cell body. The first efferent inhibitory cell body was located by trial and error, after a prolonged search. Following the demonstration that this cell was rich in GABA, chemical analysis provided a rapid means for discovering others. Our progress was entirely dependent on the fact that each cell has a characteristic size and position, so that once identified it could readily be found from animal to animal.

*Identification of efferent inhibitory cell bodies.* The first inhibitory cell body identified innervates the superficial flexor muscle illustrated in Fig. 12*B*-muscle 1. Advantage was taken of the fact that this muscle receives a spon

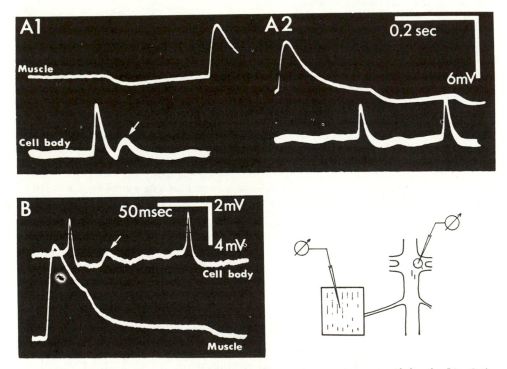

FIG. 6. Simultaneous intracellular recordings of spontaneous activity in I1 of the second ganglion and in the superficial flexor muscle innervated by this neuron. *A* and *B* are different preparations. Arrows: EPSP's. This figure illustrates the correspondence between impulses in I1 and IJP's in the opposite superficial flexor muscle. In *B*, the first IJP was superimposed on the decline of a spontaneous EJP. The time course of the action potential is shorter than in *A*; such variation was frequently seen in our preparations. In *B*, 2-mv scale refers to upper trace; 4-mv scale to lower trace.

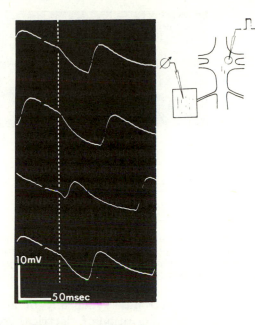

FIG. 7. Effect of stimulating I1 on the membrane potential of the superficial flexor muscle innervated by this cell. Short current pulses were delivered to I1 of the second ganglion through an intracellular electrode. The muscle received a high-frequency barrage of spontaneous EJP's upon which the evoked IJP's were superimposed at nearly constant latency (dotted line).

10mV

50msec

taneous barrage of excitatory and inhibitory impulses, as can be seen in Figs. 6 and 7 (cf. 12). The inhibitory junctional potentials (IJP's) in the muscle disappeared if the ganglion of the same segment was cut away. Thereupon, in a series of such ganglia, cell bodies were impaled systematically in search of one whose spontaneous activity was related to the IJP's in the muscle. Eventually such a cell was found on the contralateral side; this cell is shown, labeled I1, in Figs. 12A and 14. Simultaneous recordings in the cell body and the muscle are shown in Fig. 6; an action potential an the cell body invariably preceded the IJP's in the muscle by about 20 msec. The one-to-one relation between the action potential in the cell body and an IJP in the muscle demonstrated that the neuron was at least associated with the inhibitory pathway to the muscle fiber. Two further observations indicated that the neuron lay directly in the inhibitory pathway; subthreshold activity in the cell body (arrows, Fig. 6) were not followed by IJP's in the muscle, and when the cell body was stimulated with injected current, an IJP appeared in the muscle with about the same delay as with spontaneous firing (Fig. 7).

To test whether the neuron was directly connected to the muscle, the nerve leading to the muscle was stimulated in midcourse with gradually increasing intensity. At a sharply defined threshold an IJP appeared in the muscle fiber and an antidromic action potential was observed in the cell body (Fig. 8B); this observation greatly reduced the chances that we were dealing with an interneuron. The action potential in the cell body of this neuron was characteristically less than 10 mv in size; nevertheless, it could be distinguished from excitatory postsynaptic potentials (EPSP's) by its faster time course and conspicuous afterpositivity (cf. Figs. 6, 9).

When the I1 cell bodies (one on either side of the ganglion) were impaled

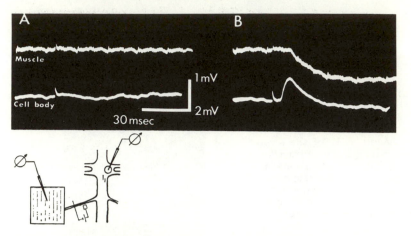

FIG. 8. Stimulation of the nerve to the superficial flexor muscle while recording intracellularly from the muscle and from the opposite I1 of the third ganglion. In *A*, the stimulus intensity was subthreshold. In *B*, activity appeared in the muscle fiber and neuron at the same stimulus strength. 1-mv scale refers to upper trace.

with microelectrodes, synchrony of action potentials was often observed (Fig. 9*A*; see description of electrical coupling, below). The procedures discussed above would, therefore, not have distinguished which of the two cells was attached to a particular muscle. However, as the experiment proceeded, the action potentials did not remain synchronous, an impulse in one cell being accompanied only by an EPSP in the other (Fig. 9*A*2). An IJP in the superficial flexor muscle was invariably associated with an impulse in the

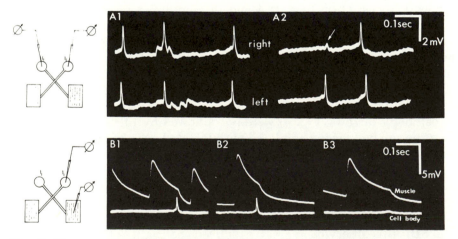

FIG. 9. The upper part of the figure shows simultaneous recording of spontaneous activity in both I1 cell bodies of the second abdominal ganglion. In *A*1, early in the experiment, action potentials in the two cells are synchronous. Later in the experiment, *A*2, the synchrony is no longer perfect. Arrow indicates an EPSP. Part *B* is from a different preparation, in the same condition as *A*2. It shows that IJP's in the superficial flexor muscle are not invariably associated with impulses in the homolateral I1. (*B*3; compare with Fig. 6.) All records are intracellular.

contralateral cell body, but this correspondence did not hold for the ipsi-lateral cell body (Fig. 9B). From this consistent finding we conclude that the axons are crossed.

The presence of bidirectional one-to-one synapses in crustacean ganglia (described below; see also 27) still leaves some doubt whether the I1's are efferent cells or interneurons. However, if they are interneurons there should be other cells in the ganglion, the true efferent neurons, with the same be-havior; thorough exploration in many preparations never revealed such cells. Moreover, the cells in question consistently have a high GABA content (PART II) not seen in excitatory neurons. From all this evidence we conclude that the I1's are the efferent inhibitory neurons innervating the superficial flexor muscles.

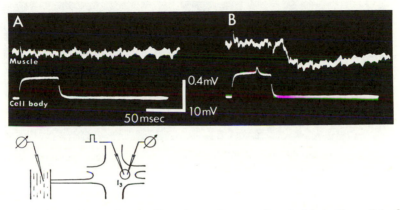

FIG. 10. Stimulating and recording electrodes were inserted into the cell body of I3, while recording from the extensor muscle it innervates, M. dorsalis prof. In A, the current pulse was just subthreshold for I3; in B just suprathreshold. An IJP appeared in the muscle at the same stimulus strength as the impulse in I3. 0.4-mv scale refers to the upper beam.

GABA analysis was then used to locate two more pairs of inhibitory cell bodies, I2's and I3's. The characteristic position of these high GABA cells is shown in Figs. 12A and 14. The physiological procedures for demonstrating an inhibitory function were similar to those just described for I1.

One-to-one correspondence between the neuronal action potential and the IJP in the muscle was established for I2 and I3 with stimulation in the cell body and in the periphery. The experiment with conduction in the orthodromic direction is illustrated for I3 in Fig. 10; at a sharply defined threshold an all-or-none action potential was produced in the cell body and an IJP in the muscle about 30 msec later.

*Identification of efferent excitatory cell bodies.* The cells that produced visible contraction in the periphery are labeled M1 through M14 in Fig. 12A. In the smaller cell bodies (M8's, M11) trains of stimuli were occasionally required to produce contraction; in the others a single suprathreshold pulse was sufficient. For six cells, M2, M5, M6, M9, M10, and M14, a one-to-one correspondence between an antidromic action potential in the cell body and an excitatory junctional potential (EJP) in the muscle leaves little doubt that the cells are connected directly to the muscles. Such an experiment is shown for M9 in Fig. 11. There is little doubt that M4 is the giant moto-neuron described by Johnson (8) and Wiersma (28) since its axon is crossed and leaves through the third root of the same segment, and since it was the only cell that regularly produced contraction in more than one flexor muscle. The other M cells are probably directly connected to muscles since a single shock or low frequency of stimulation produced EJP's in muscle fibers.

The ganglion contains a pair of interneurons that form segments of the lateral giant fiber system. These cells drive the M4 axons and other efferent axons on a one-to-one basis (32) and ought to produce a pronounced contrac-tion when stimulated, but we did not succeed in finding their cell bodies.

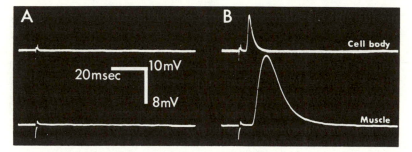

FIG. 11. Stimulation of the third root while recording intracellularly from M9 of the second ganglion and the muscle it innervates, M. obliquus ant. 4. (The experimental arrangement is thus similar to that of Fig. 8.) The stimulus strength was subthreshold in A. Activity appeared in both cell body and muscle at the same threshold (B). The 10-mv scale applies to the upper beam.

*Functional architecture of the abdominal ganglia.* There are three conspic-uous features of the ganglionic organization: *1*) Each cell has a functional partner with the same size and position on the opposite side of the ganglion; *2*) each cell lies in close association with particular other cells, forming a characteristic grouping; and *3*) the groups are quite constant in location, but within each group relative positions of cells are not necessarily constant.

The positions and certain features of the identified cells are described below. The description applies to the second and third abdominal ganglia; all but the sixth ganglion appear to be similar, but the others have not been studied in detail. No consistent differences were observed between 0.5-kg and 1.5-kg lobsters except that the cells were somewhat smaller in the former. The identified cells are shown in six representative ganglia in Figs. 12, 13, and 14, and the muscles they control are listed in Table 1. We did not at-tempt to find the entire field of innervation of any neuron. Most cells were traced to a single muscle only, but it is highly likely that the innervations of

---

domen. The numbered muscles are named in Table 1. Muscle 7 corresponds to 10; like muscle 4 it has been cut to reveal 8 and 9 more clearly. A = anterior; P = posterior; V = ventral; D = dorsal. G1 = first abdominal ganglion.

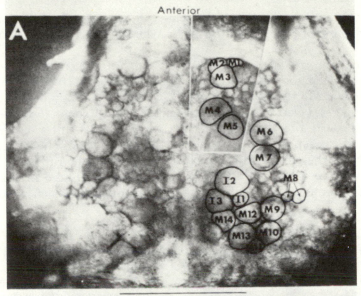

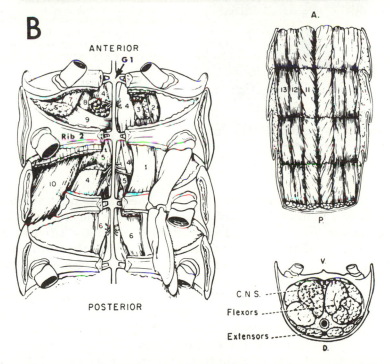

FIG. 12. Identified excitatory and inhibitory neurons of the second ganglion and the muscles they innervate. *A*: a composite physiological map derived from two ganglia from different animals. Physiologically identified cell bodies are traced with black lines. The cell bodies are named as described in the text. The peripheral field of innervation of each cell is given in Table 1. Not all of the M8 cell bodies were identified in this experiment (compare with the right side of Fig. 14*A*). *B*: drawing of the musculature of the lobster ab-

I2, I3, and M4 are broader than is indicated in Table 1. The functions of the cells are indicated in Fig. 14 and the destinations of the axons are shown with arrows.

*Anterior flexor excitatory cells, M1, M2, and M3.* These three cells lie at the anterior pole of the ganglion; their relative sizes are constant, M1 being the smallest and M3 the largest (Figs. 12, 13, and 14). They innervate flexor muscles and are labeled with an F in Fig. 14. Their axons cross the midline and leave through the third root of the ganglion just anterior. While the groups are in corresponding positions on the two sides of the ganglion, the arrangement of the cells within the cluster appears to be random (Figs. 12, 13, and 14). Since other cell bodies of similar size are found in this region, these three neurons must be physiologically identified in each preparation.

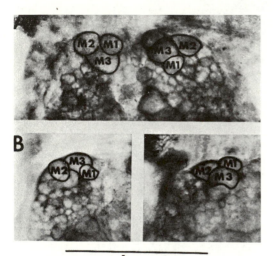

FIG. 13. Physiological maps of the anterior flexor excitatory neurons in three ganglia. In *B* and *C* the midline of the ganglion falls approximately at the right border of the photograph. This figure illustrates the variability of the relative positions of M1, M2, and M3 (compare also Fig. 12*A*) but it can be seen that the relative sizes of the cells and their position as a group are constant.

1 mm

*Medial flexor excitatory cells, M4 and M5.* These two large cell bodies are always adjacent and in the center of the ganglion near the midline, M4 being usually the larger (Fig. 12*A*). M4 lies anterior or anteromedial to M5. As indicated in Fig. 14, their axons cross and leave through the third root of the same segment. These cells are so constant in size and position that they can be recognized by visual cues alone.

*Lateral flexor excitatory cells, M6 and M7.* These are two cell bodies of about the same size, usually in contact, and, with I2, the largest in the ganglion (Fig. 12). Their axons emerge, uncrossed, through the third root of the same segment (Fig. 14, *A* and *B1*). As a pair they are conspicuous, lying over the base of the first root in relation to a cluster of small cells (M8's) and to I2; however, their relative positions are variable (Figs. 12*A*; 14, *A* and *B1*). These neurons often show a burst of action potentials, usually overshooting, after penetration with a microelectrode. It is sometimes difficult to produce contraction by intracellular stimulation of these cells.

196

*Swimmeret excitatory cells, M8's.* These are part of a compact cluster of relatively small cell bodies lying at the base of the first root and usually bordered by I2 and the lateral and posterior flexor excitatory cells. They are labeled "s" in Fig. 14, *A* and *B*1. Their axons leave uncrossed through the first root. As many as five cell bodies have been found in this group (e.g., Fig. 14*A*). They must be identified by intracellular stimulation.

*Posterior flexor excitatory cells M9, M10, and M11.* These are two cell bodies (M9, M10) of similar size and a smaller one (M11, labeled with an "f" in Fig. 14) located at the posterior-lateral part of the ganglion. All send axons through the ipsilateral third root of the same segment. Since we have not distinguished M9 and M10 functionally, we arbitrarily call the cell adjoining the small cell cluster M9. The positions of M9 and M10 are variable, and at least one of the two often needs physiological identification. They probably innervate different parts of M. obliquus ant. The small cell, M11, is usually located medial or posterior to the larger ones, but in many preparations it was difficult to find, possibly because it lies deeper. M11 can be recognized only by stimulation.

*Extensor excitatory cells M12, M13, and M14.* These three neurons lie posterior to the inhibitory group and medial to the posterior flexor excitatory cells (Figs. 12*A* and 14). Their axons run through the ipsilateral second root of the same segment (Fig. 14). Their relative positions are variable, and usually they can be recognized only by intracellular stimulation.

*Inhibitory cells I1, I2, and I3.* These cells are adjacent to each other in spite of the fact that I1 innervates a weak tonic flexor, I2 innervates the main twitch flexor and I3 extensor muscles. This is in contrast to the groups of excitatory cells which always innervate synergist muscles. The inhibitory axons decussate while the axons of neighboring excitatory cells do not (Fig. 14). Therefore, inhibitory cells are not associated with excitatory cells which innervate the same muscles (Fig. 17), nor is there a consistent relation between inhibitory and excitatory cells which innervate synergistic or antagonistic muscles (Fig. 12, Fig. 14). For these reasons, I1, I2, and I3 appear to form a natural group.

I2 is the largest cell in the ganglion. I3 lies posterior or posteromedial to I2. I1 is usually in contact with I2, but its position is variable. I2 and I3 could be located with reasonable confidence by visual inspection, but I1 required physiological identification. I1 and I2 send their axons through the third root, I3 through the second. Confirmation of the identity of I2 and I3 was easy since no other large cells near I2 and I3 send their axons to the contralateral roots. When the superficial or main branch of the third root was stimulated with low intensity, the only large cell in the posterior and contralateral half of the ganglion responding with an antidromic action potential was I2. Similarly, on stimulation of the second root, I3 was the only large cell responding with antidromic action potentials. It is likely that I2 corresponds to the common flexor inhibitor described in the crayfish abdomen by Kennedy and Takeda (11), since it sends branches into all major subdivisions of the third root.

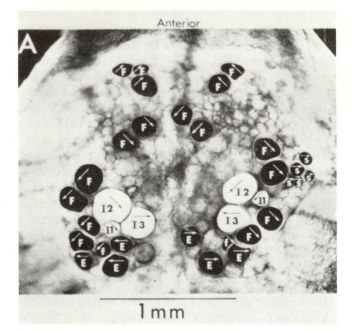

Fig. 14A. (*See opposite page.*)

*General remarks.* We have seen no exception to the observations by Wiersma (29) that efferent axons to the swimmeret, extensor, and flexor muscles run through the first, second, and third roots, respectively. In Fig. 14, *A* and *B*, it can be seen that the excitatory cell bodies in the anterior part of the ganglion send axons to the opposite side, while the posterior groups of excitatory cells give rise to uncrossed axons. The three pairs of identified inhibitory axons on each side are crossed. About 80% of the large cells in the ganglion have been identified: this constitutes about 10% of the total cell population (30).

*Electrical coupling between cell bodies.* Electrical synapses were sought between pairs of inhibitory cells by the methods used in earlier studies (e.g., 5, 27); the membrane potential of one cell was altered by passing hyperpolarizing pulses while recording from both cells. The potential changes in pairs of I1's and pairs of I2's had the characteristics of passive spread of current, and hyperpolarizations spread equally well in either direction. These results show that these cells are linked to each other by electrical synapses. We have no convincing demonstration of electrical coupling between I3's.

The attenuation of the potential spreading from one I2 cell body to the other was usually about 60:1. In the case of I1's, the attenuation was about 50:1. Evidence from histology and from experiments with injections of dyes that diffuse rapidly within the cells indicates that the axons of the inhibitory neurons decussate near the dorsal surface of the ganglion. If this is the place

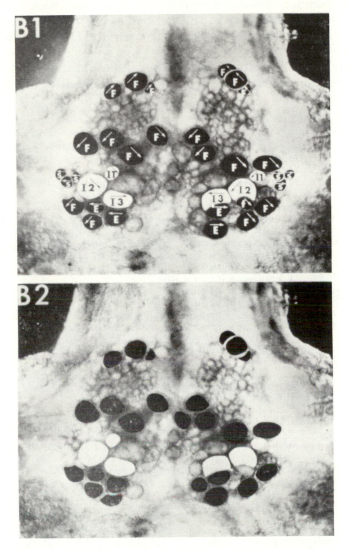

FIG. 14. Physiological and chemical maps of two ganglia. Part *A* shows the second ganglion of a 1.5-kg lobster, and *B* the third ganglion of a 0.5-kg lobster. In *A* and *B*1, physiologically identified inhibitors have been marked with white and excitors with black. *B*2 is a chemical map of the same ganglion as *B*1; cells containing more than $2 \times 10^{-11}$ moles of GABA were marked white; others containing no detectable GABA were marked black. F = excitatory cells innervating flexor muscles; f = excitatory cells innervating the superficial flexor muscles (i.e., M11). E = excitatory cells of the extensor musculature. s = excitatory cells of the swimmeret muscles (i.e., M8). I1, I2, and I3 = inhibitory cell bodies. Arrows indicate whether the axons are crossed or uncrossed; a diagonal arrow indicates that the axon leaves through the third root. All but the most anterior cells send axons through roots of the same ganglion. Not all cells were identified in both ganglia, e.g., the swimmeret neurons on the left side of photograph *A*. This figure may be compared with Fig. 12*A*.

of electrical coupling, it is not surprising that the interaction appears to be weak when recorded far away in the cell bodies on the ventral surface. As was mentioned above, the spontaneous activity of the I1's was often synchronous (Fig. 9A).

The experiment illustrated in Fig. 15 suggests that this synchrony is not produced by common interneurons, but is achieved directly. When one of the

*Table 1. Cells of the second abdominal ganglion and the muscles they control\**

Axons crossed, emerging through 3rd root of 1st ganglion
M1     M. obliquus posterior 2 (3), medial part
M2     M. obliquus anterior 2 (2)
M3     M. transversus abdominis 2, ventral part (9)

Axons crossed, emerging through 2nd root of 2nd ganglion
I3     M. dorsalis profundus, lateral part (13)

Axons crossed, emerging through 3rd root of 2nd ganglion
M4     M. obliquus posterior 3 (5), lateral part
         M. obliquus anterior 2, caudal part (10)
         M. obliquus anterior 4 (6)
         M. transversus abdominis 3, dorsal part †
M5     M. obliquus anterior 3 (4)
I1     M. ventralis superficialis abdominis 2, 3 (1)
I2     M. obliquus anterior 2, caudal part (10)

Axons uncrossed, emerging through 1st root of 2nd ganglion
M8     M. remotor II pedis spuris (swimmeret muscle)

Axons uncrossed, emerging through 2nd root of 2nd ganglion
M12   M. dorsalis profundus, medial part (11)
M13   M. dorsalis profundus, middle part (12)
M14   M. dorsalis profundus, lateral part (13)

Axons uncrossed, emerging through 3rd root of 2nd ganglion
M6     M. transversus abdominis 3, dorsal part †
M7     M. obliquus anterior 2, caudal part (10)
M9     M. obliquus anterior 4(6)
M10   M. obliquus anterior 4 (6)
M11   M. ventralis superficialis abdominis 2, 3 (1), lateral part

\* Positions of the cells and muscles are shown in Fig. 12. Numbers in parentheses refer to the labels on the muscles in Fig. 12B. The nomenclature is that of Schmidt (24).      † Muscle corresponding to 8 in segment posterior to second rib.

I1's was internally stimulated, the muscle innervated by the other consistently showed IJP's. It is probable that the electrical synapse is the mechanism for coupling the activities of the two inhibitory neurons.

Weak electrical interaction was also observed between neighboring large excitatory cells within the anterior, medial, and lateral flexor groups. This coupling persisted after the cell bodies were separated by removing the tissue between them, demonstrating that the site of the current spread is not at the cell body.

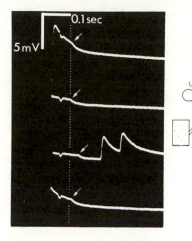

FIG. 15. Effect of stimulating homolateral I1 of the third ganglion on the membrane potential of the superficial flexor muscle 3, 4. Short current pulses were delivered to I1 cell body through an intracellular electrode. Note that latency is variable from stimulation to stimulation. Arrow indicates the onset of the IJP.

PART II

### Chemical architecture of the ganglion

*GABA content of excitatory and inhibitory cell bodies.* A correlation between GABA content and physiological function was established in experiments in which many cells were removed by free-hand dissection from living ganglia, following physiological identification. The results of such assays are shown in Table 2. Individual values are given to illustrate the variability of the results.

GABA analyses were made on 36 excitatory cell bodies. In 32, no GABA was detected (less than $10^{-11}$ moles per cell). Four of the cells appeared to contain $1–1.7 \times 10^{-11}$ moles, but this is below the limit of accurate measure-

*Table 2. GABA contents of excitatory and inhibitory cell bodies from fresh ganglia*

| Cell Type | GABA, $10^{-11}$ moles | Average, $10^{-11}$ moles |
|---|---|---|
| Excitors | | |
| Anterior flexor | 0, 0;  0, 0, 0;  0, 0, 0;  0, 1.0;  0 | |
| Medial flexor | 0, 1.7;  0, 0;  0, 0 | |
| Lateral flexor | 1.3, 0;  1.1, 0;  0, 0;  0 | |
| Posterior flexor | 0;  0, 0;  0, 0;  0 | |
| Extensor | 0;  0;  0, 0;  0 | |
| Inhibitors | | |
| I1 | 2.1, 3.5, 2.6 | 2.7 |
| I2 | 7.2, 12.5, 5.1, 7.1, 10.0, 6.3, 7.1, 7.3, 7.8, 7.3, 7.9, 7.3, 8.0, 9.0 | 7.9 |
| I3 | 6.9, 2.6, 1.9, 6.8, 2.7, 5.7 | 4.4 |

Both 0.5- and 1.5-kg lobsters were used. The limit of accurate measurement of GABA was $2 \times 10^{-11}$ moles. Semicolons separate values obtained from cells on opposite sides of the same ganglion or from different ganglia.

ment ($2 \times 10^{-11}$ moles). In these cases the possibility of contamination of samples with small inhibitory cell bodies must be considered.

In an attempt to determine more accurately the GABA content within excitatory cell bodies, two samples containing six and eight cells were analyzed. The GABA contents of these samples were less than $1.3 \times 10^{-11}$ moles, again below the limit of accurate measurement; the average GABA content per cell was therefore less than $2 \times 10^{-12}$ moles. The conclusion was that GABA if present in excitatory cell bodies is in amounts too small to be reliably measured by our methods.

This stands in sharp contrast to the results with physiologically identified inhibitory cells from fresh ganglia (Table 2); in all but one of the 23 cells more than $2 \times 10^{-11}$ moles of GABA was present. The differences in average GABA content are due mainly to differences in cell volume. I1 is small and difficult to isolate with hand-held instruments; therefore few analyses were performed on this cell.

Figure 14B illustrates the correlation between inhibitory function and a high GABA content, and excitatory function and a low GABA content. All the marked cells in Fig. 14B1 were physiologically identified and then the ganglion was photographed. Cells with more than $2 \times 10^{-11}$ moles of GABA are presented in white in Fig. 14B2; those without detectable GABA in black. Twenty-three of the cells were assayed for GABA including many of the identified cells. The GABA contents of eight identified cells were assumed from the data of Table 2, and these cells have been marked black or white accordingly.

While the procedures described above established a clear difference between excitatory and inhibitory cells, within each type of inhibitory cell there was considerable variation in the GABA content. This could be due to 1) differences in cell volume from animal to animal (see below), 2) leakage or changed GABA metabolism during the impalement and stimulation required for physiological identification, and 3) damage during isolation of the living cell with forceps. The results of three experiments designed to test these points are shown in Table 3. In the first experiment the inhibitory cells were identified by visual inspection alone and were removed quickly from the living ganglia with forceps; there were no failures to detect GABA and the average GABA contents were somewhat higher than those reported in Table 2. In the second experiment the cells were physiologically identified, but they were removed after the ganglia had been freeze-dried, as described in METH-ODS. Again, the GABA contents were higher, especially in the I3's. Finally, the two lower columns of Table 3 show the results obtained when ganglia were rapidly removed from the whole animal and frozen, as described in METHODS. These cells were visually identified. The average GABA contents were highest of all. These values are the most reliable because there was the least chance for damage to the cells, and because it is unlikely that the GABA contents were affected significantly by altered metabolism, assuming that the enzyme activities in the cell bodies are similar to the optimal ac-

Table 3. *GABA contents of excitatory and inhibitory cell bodies isolated in several ways* *

| | GABA Content, $10^{-11}$ moles† | Average, $10^{-11}$ moles† |
|---|---|---|
| Visually identified inhibitors from fresh ganglia | | |
| I2 | 8.3, 11.4, 6.5, 8.6 | 8.7 |
| I3 | 5.0, 5.7, 5.2, 7.8, 4.1, 4.5 | 5.4 |
| Physiologically identified inhibitors from dried ganglia | | |
| I2 | 7.6, 9.0, 8.4 | 8.3 |
| I3 | 6.6, 8.4, 6.0, 5.0 | 6.5 |
| Visually identified inhibitors from dried ganglia | | |
| I2 | 11.0, 6.5, 9.7, 9.8 | 9.2 |
| I3 | 6.1, 7.5, 5.9, 7.8 | 6.8 |
| Visually identified excitors from dried ganglia | | |
| M4 and M5 | 4 cells pooled | 0.5 |
| M6 and M7 | 0, 0.5, 0, 0, 1.3 | |
| M9 and M10 | 0, 0 | |
| M1 and M2 | 2 cells pooled | 0.5 |

\* For the methods of identifying and isolating the cells, see text of PART II. Data from 0.5-kg lobsters only.      † The limit of accurate measurement was $2 \times 10^{-11}$ moles.

tivities measured in peripheral axons (14). (These ganglia were immersed in circulating blood, and the neurons were intact, until less than 1 min before freezing. In 1 min, a volume of homogenized axoplasm equal to the I2 cell body (see Table 5) is able to synthesize or degrade only about 0.3% of the amount of GABA in the I2 cell body.) It should be noted that the highest GABA contents per cell found with the various isolation procedures were similar (Tables 2 and 3); we conclude that the major causes of variation in the results were damage during isolation and differences in cell volume from ganglion to ganglion (see below).

*Glutamate content of excitatory and inhibitory cell bodies.* Glutamate analyses were performed on I2, I3, M6, and M7 cell bodies (Table 4). The limit of accurate measurement in all cases was $4 \times 10^{-11}$ moles. In contrast to

Table 4. *Glutamate contents of excitatory and inhibitory cell bodies from fresh ganglia* *

| Cell | Glutamate, $10^{-11}$ moles | Average, $10^{-11}$ moles |
|---|---|---|
| I2 | 15.0, 8.2, 5.9, 13.0, 11.0, 6.8, 14.0, 16.5, 11.4, 5.2, 9.9, 6.5 | 10.3 |
| I3 | 8.6, 15.0, 7.2, 9.5, 7.8 | 9.6 |
| M (6 or 7) | 9.6, 6.5, 12.7, 6.5, 7.3 | 8.5 |

\* Data are from 0.5-kg lobsters only.

*Table 5. Volumes of cell bodies of efferent neurons**

| Cell | Total Volume, $10^{-9}$ liter | Cytoplasm, $10^{-9}$ liter† | Average, $10^{-9}$ liter‡ |
|---|---|---|---|
| I2 | 6.74-6.48<br>7.2-7.0<br>8.42-8.07<br>6.65-6.25<br>8.93-6.79<br>5.3§-4.9§ | 3.34-3.42<br>3.85<br>3.57<br>3.4<br>4.51-4.63 | Total volume: 6.89<br>Cytoplasm:     3.75 |
| I3 | 3.64-3.5<br>4.97-4.95<br>5.4 -5.4<br>4.21<br>6.29-6.73<br>3.4§-3.3§ | 2.24<br>2.32<br>3.32<br>2.5<br>4.4-4.5 | Total volume: 4.67<br>Cytoplasm:     2.97 |
| M6 and M7 | 4.16-4.23-3.79-3.81<br>4.95-4.4 -5.13<br>6.05-4.14 | | Total volume: 4.64 |
| M4 | 3.81<br>5.32<br>4.47<br>4.38 | | Total volume: 4.49 |
| M5 | 3.32<br>3.75<br>5.33<br>3.05 | | Total volume: 3.86 |

* All cells are from second abdominal ganglia of 0.5-kg lobsters treated as described in METHODS. Measurements (§) were on physiologically identified cells; all others were visually identified. Hyphens separate measurements on the same ganglion.     † This represents the total volume of the cell body less the volume of cytoplasmic vacuoles (cf. Fig. 2B). ‡ When two values were available for a ganglion, they were averaged and the mean used in computing the value in this column.

the result with GABA, excitatory and inhibitory cells contained similar amounts of glutamate. This is similar to the findings in isolated axons (14). It provides an internal control for the GABA analyses, demonstrating that the excitatory cells were not selectively damaged by the isolation procedures.

Glutamate is a fairly uniform constituent of tissues, and the uncertainty introduced by contamination with glia and connective tissue is greater than with the GABA analyses. An isolated cell with a small amount of adhering tissue is shown in section in Fig. 4C. This qualification must be borne in mind in considering the results obtained with these methods.

*Concentration of GABA and glutamate in excitatory and inhibitory cell bodies.* Our calculations of the concentrations of these substances depend on volume measurements made from sections of fixed ganglia (see METHODS). These volumes are given in Table 5. Values obtained from cells of the same ganglion are separated by hyphens; such pairs of cells generally had similar volumes. A conspicuous feature of the cell bodies was vacuoles of an uncertain nature (Fig. 2*B*). In I2 and I3 these vacuoles consistently formed a large portion of the cell body, about 40%. Usually less than 15% of the cytoplasm of M6, and M7, and other excitatory cells was composed of the vacuoles. This difference between the large excitatory and inhibitory cells was so pronounced that it could be used to locate I2 and I3 rapidly in the sections. In I3 cells an independent measure of the vacuoles was available; this was subtracted from the total volume to give the "cytoplasmic volume." The nucleus was found to comprise about 1% of the total, but the contributions of mitochondria, endoplasmic reticulum, and other cellular components are not yet known.

In Table 6 the concentrations of GABA and glutamate are shown, computed both for total volume and cytoplasmic volume, using the average

*Table 6. GABA and glutamate concentrations in excitatory and inhibitory cell bodies\**

| Cell | GABA, $10^{-3}$ moles/liter[1] | | Glutamate, $10^{-3}$ moles/liter | |
|------|-------------------|-----------|-------------------|-----------|
| | Total cell volume | Cytoplasm | Total cell volume | Cytoplasm |
| I2 | 13.4 | 24.5 | 14.9 | 27.5 |
| I3 | 14.6 | 22.9 | 20.6 | 32.3 |
| M (6 or 7) | | | 18.3 | |
| M (4 or 5) | (1.2) | | | |

\* These values were obtained by dividing the average GABA and glutamate contents (Table 3, bottom categories and Table 4) by the average volumes (Table 5). It should be noted that the concentration of GABA in M (4 and 5) is uncertain because the GABA content is below the limit of accurate measurement.

GABA contents shown in the lower columns of Table 3 and glutamate contents shown in Table 4.

## Discussion

*Architecture of the abdominal ganglia.* A high degree of constancy in the size, position, and connections of individual neurons appears to be general in invertebrate nervous systems (e.g., 1). Indeed, from available physiological and anatomical information there is no reason to doubt that this is also true of chordate nervous systems. This constancy was essential to the present study, as it was in studies on other forms (e.g., 4, 9, 10, 19).

With regard to the way cells are arranged in the ganglion, it is found that neurons controlling certain muscles do not lie together, or even at corresponding points in successive ganglia. For example, at least seven excitatory cells innervate M. obliquus ant. 3 (Fig. 16); these lie in four cell groups in three ganglia, both sides being represented.

Figure 17 illustrates that the identified inhibitory cells are not found adjacent to the excitatory cells with which their axons run in the periphery. (It should be noted that the course of axons through the ganglion is not known in detail; Figs. 16 and 17 are diagrammatic in this regard.) That cells lying at widely separate points may send axons to the same target is familiar

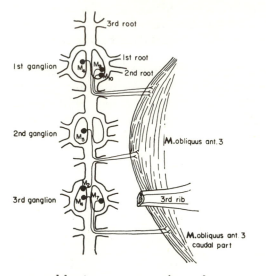

FIG. 16. Excitatory innervation of M. obliquus ant. 3. For description, see text.

in neuroanatomy; an example from primates is the convergence of spinal interneurons and cortical cells on spinal motoneurons. In such instances the converging neurons have different inputs. Kennedy and Takeda (12) have demonstrated that axons innervating the superficial flexor muscle of the crayfish abdomen subserve different reflexes, and it is reasonable to suppose that the same is true of the cells illustrated in Figs. 16 and 17.

Similarly, we may suppose that the excitatory cells are grouped according to their reflex connections. In some cases adjacent excitatory cells send axons to the same muscle (e.g., M8's; M9 and M10), in other cases synergistic muscles are innervated (e.g., M1-M3; M4 and M5; M6 and M7). One is reminded that in the mammalian spinal cord, motoneurons innervating the same muscle are clustered and may also be closely associated with motoneurons innervating synergistic muscles (e.g., 22).

The invariable clustering of the inhibitory cells I1, I2, and I3 is more surprising. These cells innervate muscles of different or contrary function

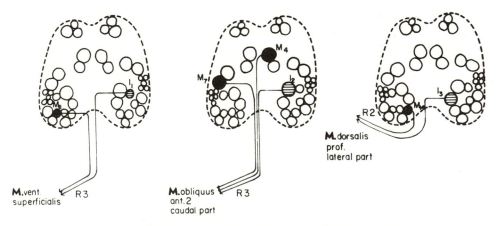

FIG. 17. Locations of excitatory and inhibitory cell bodies innervating three muscles. For description, see text. R2 and R3 indicate that the axons lie in the second and third ganglionic roots, respectively.

and doubtless receive quite different inputs. It is possible that they do have certain connections in common or that they interact in a way that we did not detect; still another possibility is that I1, I2, and I3 have a common embryological origin. Perhaps cells destined to have inhibitory chemistry differentiate at special points in the developing ganglia and then acquire distinct and appropriate incoming and outgoing connections. In this regard it may be noted that another pair of high-GABA cells of unknown function lie in the midline in the immediate vicinity of this cluster.

It must be borne in mind that so far only three inhibitory neurons have been identified; of course, clustering of synergistic inhibitory neurons may also occur in the lobster CNS. The present point is simply that in this instance neurons of antagonistic function are consistently found together.

The grouping of neurons with common transmitter chemistry is familiar in the mammalian nervous system. Motoneurons are clustered, as are cell bodies of preganglionic neurons of the autonomic nervous system. In the cerebellum it has been reported that the layers of cells are discrete with respect to function, e.g., granule cells being excitatory and Purkinje cells inhibitory (3, 6).

Another point of interest concerns the constant relative sizes of the cell bodies. Almost certainly this is related to the number of muscle fibers innervated, as in the case of mammalian motoneurons (18). The largest cell body is I2 which innervates the massive caudal part of the anterior oblique muscle, and doubtless other flexor bundles as well. In contrast, one of the smallest of the identified cells, I1, innervates only the thin superficial flexor muscle. The smallest excitatory neurons we identified innervate the diminutive swimmeret muscles.

The possible role of electrical coupling in coordinating the activities of cells on the two sides of the ganglion was discussed above. We find that neurons with chemical inhibitory synapses in muscle also form excitatory synapses in the CNS that are electrical. Thus a cell can be excitatory and inhibitory without the need for a second transmitter compound or an altered postsynaptic chemistry. Another case of a neuron that forms both excitatory and inhibitory contacts has recently been reported in the snail *Aplysia* by Kandel et al. (9). In this case, a single transmitter, acetylcholine, and two different postsynaptic chemistries are apparently involved.

*GABA and glutamate in the cell bodies of efferent neurons.* Our long-term interest in the cell bodies is to discover the mechanism of regulation of the enzymes of the GABA pathway in excitatory and inhibitory neurons. As yet we have no information about the enzymes; the present paper provides information only about the substrates, GABA and glutamate.

There is no doubt that the GABA content of inhibitory cell bodies is considerably higher than that of excitatory cell bodies and that glutamate is present in about equal amounts in the two types of cells. We have confidence in the values for GABA contents of inhibitory cells because similar high values were obtained with several methods of identification and isolation

(Tables 2 and 3). The glutamate contents are more tentative because of inevitable contamination with small amounts of other tissues.

Our calculations of concentration within the cells are less certain for several reasons. First, we do not know how these amino acids are distributed in the cytoplasm. Since there is no evidence in lobsters that either the substrates or enzymes are bound to cellular constituents in axons or cell bodies (cf. 14), it would be reasonable to assign GABA and glutamate contents to cytoplasm exclusive of organelles. Light microscopy provides a rough estimate of the volume occupied by vacuoles and nucleus (Table 5), but the volumes of mitochondria and other formed elements are not yet known. In view of these uncertainties, the only safe conclusion is that the concentrations calculated from total cell volumes represent lower limits.

Another uncertainty regarding GABA and glutamate concentrations arises from the fact that we could not measure the volumes of the cells that were chemically analyzed. By dividing average substrate contents by average volumes we may be obscuring differences from animal to animal. It would be interesting to know why the volumes of I2 and I3 vary over about a twofold range (Table 5).

It is unlikely that there are great differences in GABA concentration between cell bodies and axons of inhibitory neurons. The average concentrations of GABA in the abdominal cell bodies (Table 6) are about one-seventh (total volume) or one-fourth (cytoplasmic volume) those previously found in inhibitory axons of the walking legs (15). Since we have not measured substrate contents in two parts of the same neuron, however, this comparison between cell body and axon is tentative. If the concentration of GABA in excitatory cell bodies is similar to that in limb axons ($10^{-3}$ M or less), it is not surprising that the amounts we observed were below the limit of accurate measurement; a cell body with a volume of $4.5 \times 10^{-9}$ liter would contain $4.5 \times 10^{-12}$ moles or less (cf. Table 3).

The rather high concentrations of the physiologically active compounds glutamate and GABA throughout the lobster neurons may be compared with the distribution of acetylcholine and catecholamines in mammalian nerve cells. By histochemical means it has been demonstrated that catecholamines are found throughout the cells (2), but the concentration gradient from cell body to nerve terminal is reported to be steep (1:100 to 1:1000). Acetylcholine is found in axons (17) at a considerable distance from the terminals, but the concentration in axoplasm is not known. The relatively high concentration of GABA and catecholamines in cell bodies permits a conclusion about transmitter chemistry from analyses of this part of the cell. It is not yet known whether this is also true of cholinergic neurons.

So far, in the lobster nervous system a high content of GABA has labeled a cell as inhibitory. If this is true in other nervous systems it could be valuable in mapping certain inhibitory pathways. Recent work on the cerebellum has indicated that Purkinje cells are inhibitory. The layer in which they lie contains considerably more GABA than other cerebellar layers (16). Analyses of single cells could show whether GABA is an index of inhibitory function in the mammalian CNS. Neither acetylcholine nor noradrenaline analyses can be used in this way to indicate neuronal function.

## SUMMARY

1. The physiological organization of lobster ganglia has been correlated with certain chemical properties of excitatory and inhibitory neurons. Methods were developed for physiologically identifying and then isolating the cell bodies of efferent neurons. Gamma-aminobutyric acid (GABA) and glutamate contents of the cell bodies were assayed by enzymic methods.

2. The physiological functions of 21 pairs of neurons were determined. The cell bodies occur in clusters which are constant in location and composition. Adjoining excitatory cells innervate the same or synergistic muscles. In contrast, the identified inhibitory cells are grouped together although they innervate muscles with different or opposing action. Certain cell bodies are so constant in size and position that they can be recognized with confidence by visual inspection alone.

3. In conformity with previous studies on axons, GABA analysis revealed two populations of cell bodies; inhibitory cells with a high GABA content (the lower limit being about 0.014 M) and excitatory cells with a low GABA content (below the limit of accurate measurement with our assay). Glutamate is about equally concentrated in the two types of cell bodies.

#### ACKNOWLEDGMENTS

We gratefully acknowledge the histological assistance of Mrs. Florence Foster and Miss Karen Fischer. Robert Bosler gave us unfailing assistance throughout the work. We received much helpful advice from Professors Kuffler, Furshpan, Hubel, and Wiesel.

## REFERENCES

1. BULLOCK, T. H. AND HORRIDGE, G. A. *Structure and Function in the Nervous Systems of Invertebrates.* San Francisco: Freeman, vols. I and II, 1965.
2. DAHLSTRÖM, A., FUXE, K., AND HILLARP, N.-Å. Site of action of reserpine. *Acta Pharmacol. Toxicol.* 22: 277–292, 1965.
3. ECCLES, J. C., LLINÁS, R., AND SASAKI, K. Intracellularly recorded responses of the cerebellar Purkinje cells. *Exptl. Brain Res.* 1: 161–183, 1966.
4. FURSHPAN, E. J. AND FURUKAWA, T. Intracellular and extracellular responses of the several regions of the Mauthner cell of the goldfish. *J. Neurophysiol.* 25: 732–771, 1962.
5. FURSHPAN, E. J. AND POTTER, D. D. Transmission at the giant motor synapses of the crayfish. *J. Physiol., London,* 145: 289–325, 1959.
6. ITO, M. The origin of cerebellar inhibition on Deiters' and intracellebellar nuclei. In: *Studies in Physiology,* edited by D. R. Curtis and A. K. McIntyre, Berlin: Springer, 1965, p. 100–106.
7. JAKOBY, W. B. AND SCOTT, E. M. Aldehyde oxidation. III. Succinic semialdehyde dehydrogenase. *J. Biol. Chem.* 234: 937–940, 1959.
8. JOHNSON, G. E. Giant nerve fibers in crustaceans with special reference to *Cambarus* and *Palaemonetes. J. Comp. Neurol.* 36: 323–373, 1924.
9. KANDEL, E. R., FRAZIER, W. T., AND COGGESHALL, R. E. Opposite synaptic actions mediated by different branches of an identifiable interneuron in *Aplysia. Science* 155: 346–349, 1967.
10. KANDEL, E. R. AND TAUC, L. Heterosynaptic facilitation in neurones of the abdominal ganglion of *Aplysia depilans. J. Physiol., London* 181: 1–27, 1965.
11. KENNEDY, D. AND TAKEDA, K. Reflex control of abdominal flexor muscles in the crayfish. I. The twitch system. *J. Exptl. Biol.* 43: 211–227, 1965.

12. KENNEDY, D. AND TAKEDA, K.   Reflex control of abdominal flexor muscles in the crayfish. II. The tonic system. *J. Exptl. Biol.* 43: 229–246, 1965.
13. KRAVITZ, E. A., KUFFLER, S. W., AND POTTER, D. D.   Gamma-aminobutyric acid and other blocking compounds in Crustacea. III. Their relative concentrations in separated motor and inhibitory axons. *J. Neurophysiol.* 26: 739–751, 1963.
14. KRAVITZ, E. A., MOLINOFF, P. B., AND HALL, Z. W.   A comparison of the enzymes and substrates of gamma-aminobutyric acid metabolism in lobster excitatory and inhibitory axons. *Proc. Natl. Acad. Sci. U. S.* 54: 778–782, 1965.
15. KRAVITZ, E. A. AND POTTER, D. D.   A further study of the distribution of $\gamma$-aminobutyric acid between excitatory and inhibitory axons of the lobster. *J. Neurochem.* 12: 323–328, 1965.
16. KURIYAMA, K., HABER, B., SISKEN, B., AND ROBERTS, E.   The $\gamma$-aminobutyric acid system in rabbit cerebellum. *Proc. Natl. Acad. Sci. U.S.* 55: 846–852, 1966.
17. LOEWI, O. AND HELLAUER, H.   Über das Acetylcholin in peripheren Nerven. *Arch. Ges. Physiol.* 240: 760–775, 1938.
18. McPHEDRAN, A. M., WUERKER, R. B., AND HENNEMAN, E.   Properties of motor units in a homogeneous red muscle (soleus) of the cat. *J. Neurophysiol.* 28: 71–84, 1965.
19. NICHOLLS, J. G. AND KUFFLER, S. W.   Extracellular space as a pathway for exchange between blood and neurons in the central nervous system of the leech: ionic composition of glial cells and neurons. *J. Neurophysiol.* 27: 645–671, 1964.
20. OTSUKA, M., IVERSEN, L. L., HALL, Z. W., AND KRAVITZ, E. A.   Release of gamma-aminobutyric acid from inhibitory nerves of lobster. *Proc. Natl. Acad. Sci. U. S.* 56: 1110–1115, 1966.
21. OTSUKA, M., KRAVITZ, E. A., AND POTTER, D. D.   The $\gamma$-aminobutyric acid (GABA) content of cell bodies of excitatory and inhibitory neurons of the lobster. *Federation Proc.* 24: 399, 1965.
22. ROMANES, G. J.   The motor pools of the spinal cord. In: *Progress in Brain Research: Organization of the Spinal Cord*, edited by J. C. Eccles and J. P. Schadé. Amsterdam: Elsevier, 1964, vol. 11, p. 93–119.
23. SANDBORN, E., KOEN, P. F., McNABB, J. D., AND MOORE, G.   Cytoplasmic microtubules in mammalian cells. *J. Ultrastruct. Res.* 11: 123–138, 1964.
24. SCHMIDT, W.   Die Muskulatur von *Astacus fluviatilis* (*Potamobius astacus L.*) Ein Beitrag zur Morphologie der Decapoden. *Z. Wiss. Zool.* 113: 165–251, 1915.
25. SHUKUYA, R. AND SCHWERT, G. W.   Glutamic acid decarboxylase. I. Isolation procedures and properties of the enzyme. *J. Biol. Chem.* 235: 1649–1661, 1957.
26. TAKEDA, K. AND KENNEDY, D.   Soma potentials and modes of activation of crayfish motoneurons. *J. Cell. Comp. Physiol.* 64: 165–182, 1964.
27. WATANABE, A. AND GRUNDFEST, H.   Impulse propagation at the septal and commissural junctions of crayfish lateral giant axons. *J. Gen. Physiol.* 45: 267–308, 1961.
28. WIERSMA, C. A. G.   Giant nerve fiber system of the crayfish. A contribution to comparative physiology of synapse. *J. Neurophysiol.* 10: 23–38, 1947.
29. WIERSMA, C. A. G.   On the motor nerve supply of some segmented muscles of the crayfish. *Arch. Neerl. Sci.* 28: 413–422, 1947.
30. WIERSMA, C. A. G.   On the number of nerve cells in a crustacean central nervous system. *Acta Physiol. Pharmacol. Neerl.* 6: 135–142, 1957.
31. WIERSMA, C. A. G. AND RIPLEY, S. H.   Innervation patterns of crustacean limbs. *Physiol. Comparata et Oecol.* 2: 391–405, 1952.
32. WIERSMA, C. A. G. AND SCHALLEK, W.   Potentials from motor roots of the crustacean central nervous system. *J. Neurophysiol.* 10: 323–329, 1947.

# THE METABOLISM OF GAMMA AMINOBUTYRIC
# ACID IN THE LOBSTER NERVOUS SYSTEM

## Enzymes in Single
## Excitatory and Inhibitory Axons

Z. W. HALL, M. D. BOWNDS, and E. A. KRAVITZ

From the Department of Neurobiology, Harvard Medical School, Boston, Massachusetts 02115.
Dr. Bownds' present address is the Laboratory of Molecular Biology, University of Wisconsin,
Madison, Wisconsin 53706

ABSTRACT

$\gamma$-aminobutyric acid (GABA) is the inhibitory transmitter compound at the lobster neuromuscular junction. This paper presents a comparison of the enzymes of GABA metabolism
in single identified inhibitory and excitatory axons from lobster walking legs. Inhibitory
axons contain more than 100 times as much glutamic decarboxylase activity as do excitatory
axons. GABA–glutamic transaminase is found in both excitatory and inhibitory axons,
but about 50% more enzyme is present in inhibitory axons. The kinetic and electrophoretic
behavior of the transaminase activity in excitatory and inhibitory axons is similar. Succinic
semialdehyde dehydrogenase is found in both axon types, as is an unknown enzyme which
converts a contaminant in radioactive glutamic acid to GABA. In lobster inhibitory neurons,
therefore, the ability to accumulate GABA ultimately rests on the ability of the neuron to
accumulate the enzyme glutamic decarboxylase.

## INTRODUCTION

There is considerable heterogeneity among nerve
cells, which can be recognized in several ways.
The most obvious is the variation in geometrical
shape. Neurons can also differ in the chemical
transmitter compound which they secrete. There
are more subtle differences which are shown up
by the ability of neurons to recognize and contact
other cells specifically. This heterogeneity will
depend upon protein differences between the
individual cells. To deduce the type of information
specified in determining neuronal function it
therefore seems desirable to search for and catalog
specific protein differences between neurons.

The lobster nervous system is a useful preparation to begin studies in this direction. Biochemical
analyses can be performed on single large nerve
cells which can be recognized, physiologically
identified, and readily isolated. Moreover, cells
serving precisely the same function can be isolated
repeatedly from different animals.

Our studies have been concerned with the
biochemistry of transmitter compounds. Lobster
exoskeletal muscles are innervated by both
excitatory (E)[1] and inhibitory (I) axons. $\gamma$-amino-

---

[1] *Abbreviations used in this paper:* CNS, central nervous
system; DPN, diphosphopyridine nucleotide; E, excitatory axons; GABA, $\gamma$-aminobutyric acid; I, inhibitory axons; NAD, nicotinamide adenine dinucleotide;
TCA, trichloroacetic acid.

Reprinted from *The Journal of Cell Biology* 46: 290–299 (1970) by permission of the
publisher.

butyric acid (GABA) is the transmitter compound released by inhibitory nerves (1) and the leading candidate for the excitatory transmitter substance is glutamate (2, 3). We previously reported that I axons contain about 0.1 M GABA, while E axons contain less than 1% as much, and that the glutamic decarboxylase activity is about 10 times higher in I-axon extracts (4). Other components of the pathway of GABA metabolism (Fig. 1), α-ketoglutarate, glutamate, and GABA–glutamic transaminase, show little or no difference in extracts of E- and I-axons.

This study presents further data on enzymes isolated from single axons and will begin a comparison of the properties of enzymes in functionally different axons.

## MATERIALS AND METHODS

### Tissues

Live lobsters (*Homarus americanus*) weighing 0.5–2.5 kg were obtained from a local dealer and stored in a cold room at 4°C or in a circulating sea-water tank at 12°C until used. Dissections from the meropodite segment of the walking legs of lobsters were carried out as described previously (5) to obtain 5–6-cm lengths of the I- and E-axons (Fig. 2), which respectively innervate the closer and opener muscles of the dactyl. Occasionally, other identified axons were used (6). Axons were 40–50 μ in diameter and were surrounded by a glial sheath about 1 μ in thickness and a variable small amount of connective tissue. Contaminating tissues represented less than 10% of the total volume of each axon. The approximate volume of axoplasm per cm of axon was 0.01 μl.

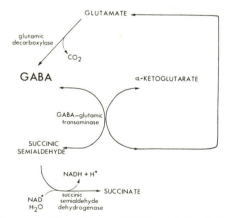

FIGURE 1  The pathway of GABA metabolism in the lobster nervous system.

### Enzyme Preparations and Assays

After dissection, single axons were picked up on the tip of a ground-glass microhomogenizer plunger, rinsed gently in isotonic KCl, or lobster physiological salt solution (6) for enzyme assays, or water (for gel electrophoresis), and then homogenized in 5 μl of buffer (see below) in microhomogenizer tubes. The homogenizers were contructed by cutting off the top half of a conical 0.1 ml test tube (Misco Scientific Corp., Berkeley, Calif.) and grinding the inside of the bottom half with an approximately fitting glass-rod in a graded series of abrasives until the rod fit snugly into the tube.

For the decarboxylase assay, axons were homogenized in 5 μl of 0.1 M potassium phosphate (pH 7.2–7.4), 0.025–0.032 M β-mercaptoethanol and 0.1 mM pyridoxal phosphate (I axon), or in the same medium with 0.003 M GABA (E axon), except where noted in the text. The volume of fluid in the microhomogenizer tubes was measured by weighing the tubes. Suitable dilutions were made and samples were removed for assay. Reactions were started by adding 2 μl of substrate (0.25–0.5 μmoles of glutamate-U-$^{14}$C, approximate specific activity; 30 mCi/mmole) to 3 μl of enzyme. For $^{14}CO_2$ collection, reactions were carried out at 25°C in closed tubes and experiments were ended at appropriate times by injection of 50 μl of 5% trichloroacetic acid (TCA). The $^{14}CO_2$ evolved was collected overnight in 50 μl of Hyamine hydroxide (1 M solution in methanol) in a 0.2 ml test tube suspended above the reaction mixture. The Hyamine solution was transferred to a toluene scintillation fluid and the radioactivity measured in a liquid scintillation spectrometer (see reference 7). In certain experiments acidic amino acids were removed from reaction mixtures with ion-exchange columns. In these cases, the reaction was stopped by transferring the incubation mixtures to small (0.5 × 5 cm) Dowex 1–acetate (AG-1-x2, 100–200 mesh, Bio-Rad Laboratories, Richmond, Calif.) ion-exchange columns. Reaction products were eluted with 5 ml of $H_2O$, taken to dryness in a Rotary Evapo-Mix (Buchler Instruments, Inc., Fort Lee, N.J.) and a portion counted. The remainder was chromatographed by ascending paper-chromatography at room temperature to identify the compounds formed. The solvents used were: phenol:water, 160 gm:40 ml (solvent 1) and butanol:acetic acid:water, 12:3:5 (solvent 2) using water-washed Whatman No. 1 paper. Strips from chromatograms were scanned for radioactivity in a Savant strip counter (Savant Instruments, Inc., Hicksville, N.Y.). Since no radioactive basic amino acids were detected, this fraction is subsequently called *neutral amino acids*.

For the transaminase assay, axons were homogenized in 5 μl of 0.4 M glycylglycine buffer, pH 8.5, 30 mM β-mercaptoethanol, and 2 mM pyridoxal phosphate. After homogenization, the volume was meas-

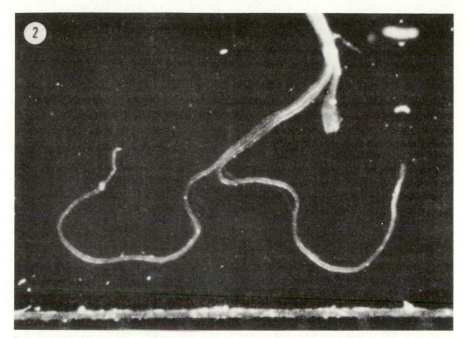

FIGURE 2 Single axons dissected from the meropodite segment of the walking leg of the lobster, as viewed through a dissecting microscope. The ruler divisions are 1 mm and individual axons are 40–50 $\mu$ in diameter. Axons are identified by stimulation. A knot is tied in one axon (the E in this case) to facilitate identification in case of axon damage during the dissection. About 5–6 cm lengths of axon are routinely obtained (see reference 5 and Methods for details).

ured as above, a suitable dilution was made, and samples were placed in 0.2 ml test tubes for assay. Substrates and cofactors were added so that final incubation concentrations were 2 mM $\alpha$-ketoglutarate, 3 mM diphosphopyridine nucleotide (DPN), 1 mM succinate, and 3 mM GABA-U-$^{14}$C (20–140 mCi/mmole). The final incubation volume was 20 $\mu$l. After 1–3 hr at 25°C, 5 $\mu$l of 40% trichloroacetic acid was added and the incubation mixture applied to a 0.5 × 5 cm column of Dowex 50–H$^+$ (Dowex 50-W-x2, 100–200 mesh, J. T. Baker Chemical Co., Phillipsburg, N.J.). The column was washed with 5 ml of water and the radioactivity of a portion of the fluid passing through the column was measured. The remainder was freeze-dried and the products were separated by either paper chromatography or high voltage electrophoresis. The paper chromatographic solvent used was $n$-butanol:acetic acid:pyridine:water, 120:20:-25:35 (solvent 3). High-voltage electrophoreses were performed at pH 6.4 in pyridine:acetic acid:water (10:0.8:90) at 50 V/cm as described by Naughton and Hagopian (15).

*Gel Electrophoresis*

Separations of proteins from single-axon homogenates were carried out by electrophoresis in 1 mm-diameter columns of polyacrylamide gel. A single buffer system was used, Tris-glycine (pH 9.3). Gel solutions and buffers were prepared as described by Matson (8). Unpolymerized gel solution was drawn into capillary tubes 30 mm long (made from 100 $\mu$l Drummond microcaps, Drummond Scientific Co., Inc., Plymouth, Mich.). The tubes were placed upright in soft paraffin as a support and 5 $\mu$l of gel solution removed and replaced with 5 $\mu$l of water. After polymerization of the gel (30 min), the water was removed and the tubes placed in an electrophoresis apparatus at 4°C. Unreacted persulfate and other toxic by-products of the polymerization were removed by applying a potential of 10 V/cm for 1 hr. Enzyme solutions were prepared as above (in 5–10 $\mu$l of fluid, see section on enzyme preparation) in 0.02 M potassium-phosphate buffer containing 2% sucrose and centrifuged at 20,000 $g$ in a Misco microcentrifuge (Misco Corp.)

213

for 20 min to remove particulate matter. 5-μl samples were applied to the top of the pretreated gels and electrophoresis was run at 10 V/cm for 30 min, followed by approximately 30 min at 20 V/cm. Bromophenol blue was used as a marker dye to determine the end of the electrophoresis run. Gels were extruded from the glass capillaries with a metal plunger and sliced lengthwise in half. One-half was placed in 10% trichloroacetic acid to precipitate the proteins in the gel and the other half was sliced by hand into 20–25 1-mm portions. Each slice was placed into 5 μl of incubation medium and assayed as above for transaminase or, with the $^{14}CO_2$ assay, for decarboxylase. The half gel in TCA was stained with fluorescent dansyl reagent (9) to visualize the proteins present as follows: The gel was rinsed in 0.5 ml 0.1 N NaHCO₃ for 15 min and placed in a second portion (0.5 ml) of 0.1 N NaHCO₃. Dansyl chloride (0.5 ml of a 1 mg/ml solution in acetone) was added and the gel left for 3 hr at 23°C. Excess dansyl reagent was removed by rinsing overnight in 0.1 N NaHCO₃ and the protein bands were observed using an ultraviolet hand lamp (Mineralight Inc., San Gabriel, Calif., model SL 3660) and graphed by visual inspection.

## Substrates

Glutamate-U-$^{14}C$ (approximately 200 mCi/mmole) was obtained from New England Nuclear Corp., Boston, Mass. It was diluted to an appropriate specific activity and purified shortly before use. The isotope in 0.01 N HCl was taken to dryness in a Rotary Evapo-Mix, dissolved in a small volume of 1 N NH₄OH, and taken to dryness again. The residue was dissolved in water and applied to a column of Dowex 1-acetate (0.6 × 3 cm). The column was washed with water and the glutamate was eluted with about 10 ml of 1 N acetic acid. The eluate was evaporated to dryness, a small volume of 1 N formic acid was added, and the solution again evaporated to dryness. The residue was dissolved in water and applied to an 0.6 × 1.5 cm column of Dowex 50–Tris. Glutamate passed through the column with the water wash, was evaporated to dryness, and made up to a standard volume. Purified isotope was used for about a month before it was repurified. GABA-U-$^{14}C$ was prepared from glutamic acid-U-$^{14}C$, using glutamic decarboxylase partially purified from an acetone powder of *Escherichia coli* (Worthington Biochemical Corp, Freehold, N.J.) by modification of the procedure of Shukuya and Schwert (10). Glutamate-U-$^{14}C$ (0.2 mCi) was incubated with 300 μmoles of sodium acetate, pH 4.4, and 0.8 units of decarboxylase in a volume of 2.6 ml for 2 hr at 23°C. The extent of the reaction was followed by collection of $^{14}CO_2$ in Hyamine hydroxide. When the reaction was complete, the incubation mixture was applied to a 0.5 × 5 cm column of Dowex 50–H⁺.

GABA was eluted with 1 N NH₄OH, evaporated to dryness, dissolved in water, and passed over a 0.5 × 3 cm column of Dowex 1–acetate. The radioactive GABA was collected in the first 5 ml of water washed through the column.

Pyridoxal phosphate, nicotinamide adenine dinucleotide (NAD), α-ketoglutarate, and dansyl chloride were purchased from Sigma Chemical Co., St. Louis, Mo. Guinea pig succinic semialdehyde dehydrogenase was prepared by the method of Pitts, Quick, and Robins (11).

## RESULTS

### Decarboxylase in Single-Axon Extracts

We previously reported that inhibitory axon extracts could synthesize about 100 μμmoles of GABA/cm axon/hour while the value for excitatory extracts was about 9 (4). These values were determined using an assay in which we measured the production of radioactive GABA from high specific-activity glutamate-U-$^{14}C$ using an ion-exchange procedure to separate glutamate and GABA. The identification of the reaction product as GABA was verified in two ways: (a) by paper chromatography in two solvent systems (Fig. 3 illustrates a radioactive scan of a chromatogram using solvent 1); and (b) by the enzymic conversion of the product to an acidic substance (presumably succinate) upon reaction with a bacterial enzyme system containing GABA–glutamic transaminase and succinic semialdehyde dehydrogenase (12). Recently we found that a highly purified lobster glutamic-decarboxylase preparation contained a contaminating enzyme which converted a contaminant in radioactive glutamic acid to GABA without the simultaneous evolution of $^{14}CO_2$ (7). The contaminating enzyme does not require β-mercaptoethanol for activity, while the glutamic decarboxylase does.

In the present experiments, glutamic decarboxylase activity was measured by the production of $^{14}CO_2$ from glutamate-U-$^{14}C$, and we observed a serious discrepancy with the previous results. In the I-axon extracts there was a linear evolution of $^{14}CO_2$ for at least 3 hr, while there was essentially no $^{14}CO_2$ produced in E-axon extracts. The average decarboxylase activity using the $^{14}CO_2$ assay was 90 μμmoles per cm of axon per hr (six I-axons pooled; total length 40 cm), a value comparable to that previously reported with the neutral amino acid assay. In the E axon, on the

214

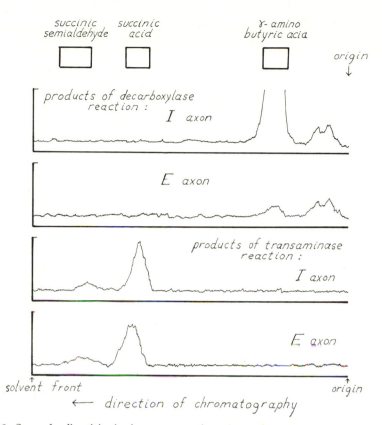

FIGURE 3 Scans of radioactivity in chromatograms of reaction products of decarboxylase and trans-aminase reactions. The double peak near the origin in decarboxylase incubations is also seen in boiled enzyme controls and is a contaminant. The principal product formed in both E- and I-axon decarboxylase incubations corresponds to GABA. There are no radioactive contaminants seen in controls of trans-aminase incubations, and the products formed correspond to succinate and succinic semialdehyde. Paper chromatography was ascending at room temperature and solvent 2 was used for decarboxylase products and solvent 3 for transaminase products. See Methods for experimental details. Full scale (indicated by bar) was 500 cpm.

other hand, there was no detectable $^{14}CO_2$ (five E axons pooled; total length 40 cm). Thus, E axons seemed to have less than 0.3% of the decarboxylase activity of I axons with the $^{14}CO_2$ assay.

To help verify this we next measured the production of $^{14}CO_2$ and radioactive neutral-amino acids in single-axon extracts in the presence and absence of $\beta$-mercaptoethanol (Table I) In order to emphasize any contribution by the radioactive substrate contaminant in this experiment, a relatively impure substrate was used. This should have the effect of drastically reducing the apparent I/E decarboxylase ratio as measured by the

production of neutral amino acids. $^{14}CO_2$ was formed in I-axon extracts and this required $\beta$-mercaptoethanol, while neutral amino acid production was reduced by about 40% in the I-axon extracts in the absence of $\beta$-mercapto-ethanol. In contrast, E-axon extracts produced a negligible amount of $^{14}CO_2$ and the amounts of neutral amino acids were the same with or without added $\beta$-mercaptoethanol. Thus the enzyme forming GABA from the contaminant in the substrate was present in both E- and I-axon extracts and accounted for the previous report of decarboxylase activity in E-axon extracts (4). In

TABLE I

*Neutral Amino Acids and $^{14}CO_2$ Production from Glutamate-U-$^{14}C$ in the Presence and Absence of β-Mercaptoethanol*

| | Neutral amino acids/4 | | | $^{14}CO_2$ | |
|---|---|---|---|---|---|
| | *dpm/hr/cm* | *Δ dpm* | *Δ μμmoles/hr/cm* | *dpm/hr/cm* | *μμmoles/hr/cm* |
| Excitor | | | | | |
| (+) β-mercaptoethanol | 13500 | 300+ | — | 35+ | — |
| (−) β-mercaptoethanol | 13200 | | | 25+ | — |
| Inhibitor | | | | | |
| (+) β-mercaptoethanol | 19500 | 8100 | 72 | 5230 | 47 |
| (−) β-mercaptoethanol | 11400 | | | 0 | — |

The experimental details were as in the methods except that axons were homogenized in buffer without β-mercaptoethanol. The substrate used was not highly purified. β-mercaptoethanol was added to specified experimental vessels to give a final concentration of 0.03 M. Since glutamate-U-$^{14}C$ was used as substrate the neutral amino acid figure (GABA) is divided by four to make it equivalent to the $CO_2$ figure. +, these values are not significant. The lower limits of detection in this experiment were about 1 μμmole/hr/ cm for the $^{14}CO_2$ assay and about 5 μμmoles/hr/cm for the neutral amino acids.

I-axon extracts, even when the correction for the contaminant-metabolizing enzyme is subtracted, we still observe a discrepancy in $^{14}CO_2$ collected and neutral amino acids produced. This discrepancy could result from some binding of $^{14}CO_2$ or from yet another source of neutral amino acid production, and could significantly affect the absolute I-axon decarboxylase values. Therefore, further experimentation is required before assigning an absolute figure to the I-axon decarboxylase level.

The absence of decarboxylase from E axons could be due to the presence of a specific decarboxylase inhibitor, to the presence of an inactivated enzyme, or to the absence of the enzyme. E- and I-axon extracts were mixed and there was no depression of the decarboxylase activity of the I-axon extracts. If an inhibitor was present, therefore, it was exactly titrated to the amount of enzyme in E axons. The failure to demonstrate decarboxylase activity after gel electrophoresis of E-axon extracts (see below) is a further argument against the existence of an enzyme inhibitor. It is possible that enzyme was present but inactive in E-axon extracts. However, agents known to increase the activity of purified lobster glutamic-decarboxylase (K+, β-mercaptoethanol, pyridoxal phosphate) did not restore E-axon activity (7).

## GABA–Glutamic Transaminase Activity in Single-Axon Homogenates

Prior to measurements of single-axon activities, homogenates of pooled E and I axons were used to show that the transaminase-reaction velocity was constant for at least 3.5 hr and was proportional to the amount of homogenate used. The pH optimum of the reaction determined with this preparation was approximately 8.0.

Assays were then carried out on single E- and I-axon extracts and paper chromatograms of the reaction products are shown in Fig. 3. Similar results were obtained upon high-voltage electrophoresis of the products. In the standard assay, with DPN present, succinate-$^{14}C$ was the principal product (61–88% in eight experiments). This suggested that succinic semialdehyde dehydrogenase activity in both E- and I-homogenates was in excess of transaminase activity. To test this, portions were assayed with and without added guinea pig kidney succinic–semialdehyde dehydrogenase. No increase in the production of radioactive acids from GABA-U-$^{14}C$ was observed with exogenous dehydrogenase. Therefore, transaminase activity in both axons is rate-limiting for the metabolism of GABA, and succinic semialdehyde dehydrogenase–activity was not studied further.

When GABA–glutamic transaminase activity was assayed in 12 pairs of I axons, an average value of 32 μμmoles/cm axon/hr was obtained. In E-axon homogenates the average value was 23 μμmoles/cm/hr. The values obtained for both kinds of axons were quite variable. Much of the variability was apparently due to differences between animals, since when pairs of axons from opposite legs of the same animal were compared

(2 and 3, 8 and 9, 11 and 12 in Table II) the values were more consistent. Transaminase activity was about 1.5 times higher in I than in E axons (Table II).

## Single-Axon Enzyme Comparisons

The presence of transaminase activity in both axons offered an opportunity to compare the kinetic properties and electrophoretic behavior of the enzyme in each homogenate, to see if the presence of different isozymes in functionally different axons could be detected.

Kinetic constants for both GABA and α-ketoglutarate at a fixed concentration of the other substrate were determined. The lobster GABA–glutamic transaminase has been previously shown (13) to have kinetic behavior consistent with a reaction mechanism in which each substrate reacts alternately with the enzyme ("ping-pong bi-bi"). Determination of true kinetic constants requires variations of both substrates. Because of limitation of material, this was not possible. The simpler procedure of varying one substrate at a fixed concentration of the other gives an apparent Michaelis constant adequate for comparison.

The determination of an apparent Km for GABA was complicated by the presence of large amounts of endogenous GABA in I-axon extracts. This difficulty was overcome by using a high concentration (40 mM) of α-ketoglutarate, which is a competitive inhibitor for GABA as well as a substrate in the reaction. The high α-ketoglutarate concentration raised the apparent Km for GABA to a value high enough to be accurately measured. Under these conditions, in two experiments the apparent Km for GABA for the enzyme in E-axon extracts was 1.8 and 1.5 mM, while in I-axon extracts, the values were 2.9 and 2.5 mM. A kinetic plot of the data from one of these experiments is shown in Fig. 4. The observed apparent Km differences between E- and I-axons were within experimental error.

For α-ketoglutarate there was considerable

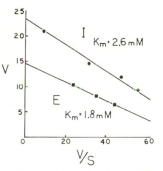

FIGURE 4 Kinetic plot of the effect of GABA concentration on transaminase activity in single E- and I-axon homogenates. The velocity (V) is expressed as moles × $10^{11}$/hr. For experimental details see text, Methods, and reference 13. The apparent Km's in the E- and I-axon homogenates are not significantly different.

### TABLE II

GABA–Glutamic Transaminase Activity in Separated E- and I-Axons

| Experiment No. | Activity | | |
|---|---|---|---|
| | E | I | I/E |
| | μμmoles/cm/hr | | |
| 1 | 15 | 25 | 1.7 |
| 2 | 11 | 19 | 1.7 |
| 3 | 12 | 18 | 1.6 |
| 4 | 23 | 28 | 1.2 |
| 5 | 29 | 32 | 1.1 |
| 6 | 35 | 43 | 1.3 |
| 7 | 26 | 40 | 1.5 |
| 8 | 23 | 33 | 1.4 |
| 9 | 24 | 32 | 1.4 |
| 10 | 27 | 41 | 1.5 |
| 11 | 22 | 33 | 1.5 |
| 12 | 24 | 37 | 1.5 |
| Average | 23 | 32 | 1.5 ± 0.1* |

Experiments 2 and 3, 8 and 9, and 11 and 12 were pairs carried out on opposite legs of the same animal. The experimental details were as in Methods.
* Standard error of the mean.

### TABLE III

Apparent Km (Km') for α-Ketoglutarate of the Transaminase in E- and I-Axons

| Experiment No. | Km' (mM) | |
|---|---|---|
| | E | I |
| 1 | 2.7 | 2.0 |
| 2 | 1.2 | 1.1 |
| 3 | 0.7 | 0.8 |

Prior to homogenization, axons were rinsed in calcium-free lobster saline in Experiment Nos. 1 and 2 and in 1 M sucrose in Experiment No. 3. The other experimental details are as in Methods.

variation of the apparent Km from experiment to experiment but E- and I-axon values in any single experiment were similar (Table III). All of the measured values exceeded the previous reported value with the partially purified lobster central nervous system (CNS) enzyme. The reasons for this discrepancy and the variation between experiments were not found, but the consistency within experiments allowed the tentative conclusion that the kinetic properties of the E- and I-enzymes were the same.

As with the partially purified enzyme, transaminase activity in both E- and I-homogenates was inhibited by high concentrations of α-ketoglutarate (Table IV).

## Polyacrylamide Gel Electrophoresis of Single-Axon Extracts

The electrophoresis of the decarboxylase and transaminase enzymes from single axons is shown in Fig. 5. Approximately 90% of the activity applied to the gel was recovered in the single bands of activity observed. The resolution of fluorescent protein bands and enzyme activities was not good enough for the identification of enzyme activities with single protein bands. However, the method was sufficient to demonstrate that the transaminase enzymes from E- and I-axons have similar mobilities, slightly higher than the mobility of the I-axon decarboxylase. There was no measurable decarboxylase activity in the E-axon extract. Glutamic decarboxylase and GABA–glutamic transaminase prepared from homogenates of the lobster central nervous system and electrophoresed on standard gels (5 mm

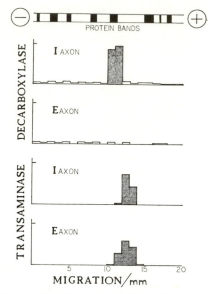

FIGURE 5  Decarboxylase and transaminase enzyme activities measured in slices of micropolyacrylamide gel columns. The experimental procedure is described in Methods. The gel pattern illustrated at the top is a typical distribution of protein bands seen on inspection after conjugation of proteins with fluorescent dansyl reagent. No significant differences were noted between E- and I-axons, and it was not possible to associate particular bands with specific enzymes. Full scale (indicated by bar) was 400 cpm.

TABLE IV

*Comparison of α-Ketoglutarate Inhibition of Transaminase Activity in E- and I-Axons*

|  | μμmoles/ hr/cm | % Inhibition |
|---|---|---|
| Excitor |  |  |
| 4 mM α-ketoglutarate | 91 |  |
| 40 mM α-ketoglutarate | 59 | 35 |
| Inhibitor |  |  |
| 4 mM α-ketoglutarate | 128 |  |
| 40 mM α-ketoglutarate | 94 | 27 |

The experimental details are as in Methods. The α-ketoglutarate concentrations used are listed in the table.

diameter) moved to the same relative positions on gels as the single-axon enzymes.

## DISCUSSION

One goal of these studies is to explain how inhibitory and excitatory nerve cells control their transmitter levels. The axon terminals of these cells, the regions directly involved in transmitter release, cannot be studied because techniques are not yet available for physically separating them from the muscle tissue they innervate. However, transmitter accumulation along the length of the nerve cells can be studied, and may provide a model for what occurs in the nerve endings.

An intensive study of the synthesis and metabolism of the inhibitory transmitter, GABA, in single lobster E- and I-axons has been carried out in this laboratory (4). The enzymes involved have been isolated and purified from the lobster nervous system and their properties studied (7, 13).

Such studies revealed, among other things, that glutamic decarboxylase is inhibited by its product, GABA. The levels of GABA, glutamate, and $\alpha$-ketoglutarate, and the activities of glutamic decarboxylase and GABA–glutamic transaminase were measured in single E- and I-axon extracts. The measurements allowed us to postulate a mechanism for the selective accumulation of GABA in I axons. The I axon can synthesize more GABA than it can destroy, and therefore GABA will accumulate. The increasing GABA concentration progressively produces a greater inhibition of the decarboxylase until synthesis is balanced by destruction. Of course, our inference of in vivo enzyme activities from in vitro measurements of optimum enzyme activities and steady-state levels of substrates is necessarily indirect. Clearly, a direct demonstration that the GABA level in I neurons is maintained by a steady-state system of the type proposed would be most desirable.

What still remains unexplained is the presence of GABA in E axons, where we are unable to demonstrate decarboxylase activity. A small, as yet undetected, amount of decarboxylase could account for the GABA found. However, it is also possible that GABA is not present in the axon at all but in the small, variable amount of connective tissue surrounding the preparations. Lobster nerve-muscle preparations contain a transport system for GABA (14). The principal site of GABA uptake has recently been found to be the connective tissue and Schwann cells which surround lobster nerve and muscle (P. Orkand, unpublished). Whether this accounts for the GABA in E-axon extracts remains an unresolved problem.

A selective comparison of the protein composition of individual, identified nerve cells can begin with the results presented in this paper. For enzymes concerned with GABA metabolism, the glutamic decarboxylase activity is found only in I-axon extracts, while transaminase, dehydrogenase, and the unknown enzyme converting glutamate contaminant to GABA are found in both axon types. As is the case with the enzymes that degrade acetylcholine and norepinephrine, therefore, the GABA–glutamic transaminase and succinic semialdehyde dehydrogenase are not confined to neurons that secrete GABA as a neurotransmitter compound. Moreover, the kinetic and electrophoretic data, although preliminary in characterizing an enzyme, suggest that the same protein catalyzes the transaminase reaction in E- and I-axons. Thus, the ability to accumulate GABA ultimately depends on the ability of I cells to accumulate the enzyme glutamic decarboxylase.

We wish to acknowledge technical assistance of Mrs. D. Dyett, Mrs. M. Kozodoy, Mr. J. Gagliardi, Mrs. T. Bolino, and Mrs. C. O'Neill.

Dr. Hall is a Medical Foundation Fellow and is supported by a grant from the Muscular Dystrophy Associations of America, Inc. and National Science Foundation Grant No. 6B 8478. Dr. Bownds was supported by a postdoctoral fellowship from NINDB, No. F2 NB 23 415 VSN. Dr. Kravitz is supported by a Career Development Award from the National Institute of Child Health and Human Development (No. K03 HD 05 899) and National Institute of Health Grants No. NB 07848 (NINDS) and NB-02253 (NINDB).

*Received for publication 22 December 1969, and in revised form 9 March 1970.*

## REFERENCES

1. Otsuka, M., L. L. Iversen, Z. W. Hall, and E. A. Kravitz. 1966. Release of gamma-aminobutyric acid from inhibitory nerves of lobster. *Proc. Nat. Acad. Sci. U.S.A.* **56**:1110.

2. Takeuchi, A., and N. Takeuchi. 1964. The effect on crayfish muscle of iontophoretically applied glutamate. *J. Physiol. (London).* **170**:296.

3. Kravitz, E. A., C. R. Slater, K. Takahashi, M. D. Bownds, and R. M. Grossfeld. 1970. Excitatory transmission in invertebrates-glutamate as a potential neuromuscular transmitter compound. *Proc. 5th Int. Meet. Neurobiol.* In press.

4. Kravitz, E. A., P. B. Molinoff, and Z. W. Hall. 1965. A comparison of the enzymes and substrates of gamma-aminobutyric acid metabolism in lobster excitatory and inhibitory axons. *Proc. Nat. Acad. Sci. U.S.A.* **54**:778.

5. Kravitz, E. A., S. W. Kuffler, and D. D. Potter. 1963. Gamma-aminobutyric acid and other blocking compounds in Crustacea. III. Their relative concentrations in separated motor and inhibitory axons. *J. Neurophysiol.* **26**:739.

6. Kravitz, E. A., and D. D. Potter. 1965. A further study of the distribution of gamma-aminobutyric acid between excitatory and inhibitory axons of the lobster. *J. Neurochem.* **12**:323.

7. MOLINOFF, P. B., and E. A. KRAVITZ. 1968. The metabolism of γ-aminobutyric acid (GABA) in the lobster nervous system-glutamic decarboxylase. *J. Neurochem.* **15**:391.

8. MATSON, C. F. 1965. Polyacrylamide gel electrophoresis—a simple system using gel columns. *Anal. Biochem.* **13**:291.

9. WEBER, G. 1952. Polarization of the fluorescence of macromolecules. 2. Fluorescent conjugates of ovalbumin and bovine serum albumin. *Biochem. J.* **51**:155.

10. SHUKUYA, R., and G. W. SCHWERT. 1960. Glutamic acid decarboxylase. I. Isolation procedures and properties of the enzyme. *J. Biol. Chem.* **235**:1649.

11. PITTS, F. N., JR., C. QUICK, and E. ROBINS. 1965. The enzymic measurement of γ-aminobutyric-α-oxoglutaric transaminase. *J. Neurochem.* **12**:93.

12. JAKOBY, W. B., and E. M. SCOTT. 1958. Aldehyde oxidation. III. Succinic semialdehyde dehydrogenase. *J. Biol. Chem.* **234**:937.

13. HALL, Z. W., and E. A. KRAVITZ. 1967. The metabolism of γ-aminobutyric acid (GABA) in the lobster nervous system-I. GABA-glutamic transaminase. *J. Neurochem.* **14**:45.

14. IVERSEN, L. L., and E. A. KRAVITZ. 1968. The metabolism of γ-aminobutyric acid (GABA) in the lobster nervous system—Uptake of GABA in nerve-muscle preparations. *J. Neurochem.* **15**:609.

15. NAUGHTON, M. A., and H. HAGOPIAN. 1962. Some applications of two-dimensional ionophoresis. *Anal Biochem.* **3**:276.

*Chapter 5*

# TRANSMITTER RELEASE

Nerve terminals spontaneously secrete small amounts of transmitter at random intervals. When an action potential invades a terminal, the rate of release increases enormously for a few milliseconds, resulting in a burst of transmitter in the synaptic cleft. A series of elegant experiments by B. Katz and R. Miledi have shown that the first step in this process is the entry of calcium into the terminals during the action potential.

Katz and Miledi performed their experiments on the frog neuro-muscular junction and on the giant synapse in the squid stellate ganglion. The squid synapse has the advantage that intracellular recordings can be made from both pre- and postsynaptic cells. Their experiments (Katz and Miledi, 1965; 1967) showed that the following series of events occurs: an action potential invades the nerve terminal; the resulting depolarization increases calcium permeability; calcium enters the terminal; and, after a variable delay, transmitter secretion occurs. Neither the sodium influx nor the potassium efflux associated with the action potential is required for normal transmitter release, nor is the action potential required; any means of depolarizing the terminals elicits secretion provided that sufficient calcium is present in the bathing fluid.

Nerve terminals appear to be specialized to allow the rapid entry of calcium. Katz and Miledi (1969, reprinted here) showed that under suitable experimental conditions the rate of calcium entry can be high enough to support a regenerative response resembling an action potential. Recently Miledi (1973) found that direct injection of calcium into the presynaptic terminal of the squid synapse causes transmitter release even in the absence of external calcium. How calcium causes release is still unknown. Transmitter secretion shows a fourth-power dependence on the external calcium concentration

(Dodge and Rahamimoff, 1967), suggesting that four calcium ions must be bound for each release event.

In 1954, J. del Castillo and B. Katz demonstrated that ACh is released from nerve endings in fixed units or "quanta" consisting of many thousands of molecules. Shortly thereafter, electron microscopy of nerve terminals showed that they contain numerous vesicles of approximately uniform size. These two observations immediately suggested the idea that the vesicles contain transmitter, and that the amount of transmitter in a single vesicle corresponds to a quantum. This hypothesis, which implies that vesicles are directly involved in the release process, has dominated research on transmitter secretion for the last twenty years. Although much indirect evidence supports the vesicle hypothesis, alternative mechanisms for transmitter release have not been excluded. For instance, vesicles may simply store transmitter that is released from the neuronal cytoplasm by selective, discrete changes in membrane permeability.

The strongest support for the role of vesicles in transmitter release from neurons actually comes from studies of catecholamine secretion in the adrenal medulla. In adrenal medullary cells, the large (*ca.* 1000 to 4000 Å) membrane-bound granules that contain most of the epinephrine and norepinephrine in the tissue also contain ATP and at least eight soluble proteins called chromogranins. Two granule proteins have been characterized: the predominant soluble protein, chromogranin A; and dopamine $\beta$-hydroxylase, which is found in the membrane of the granule and among its soluble components (see Chapter 3). The presence in granules of substances other than catecholamines provides a test of the mechanism of secretion. If the substances are released selectively and in proportion to their contents in the granules, then secretion must occur directly from the granules.

W. Douglas and A. Poisner (1966a, reprinted here) first demonstrated that granule constituents other than catecholamines are released during stimulation of the adrenal medulla. They showed that adenine nucleotides appeared along with catecholamines in fluid perfusing a stimulated gland, and that the ratio of nucleotide to amine equalled that in isolated granules (one to four). In the article reprinted here, Douglas and Poisner reported that the principal nucleotide collected was AMP, but in a companion paper (Douglas and Poisner, 1966b) they demonstrated that when extracellular hydrolysis of ATP was prevented, the predominant nucleotide was ATP.

Stimulation also causes the release of granule proteins. F. Schneider, A. Smith, and H. Winkler (1967, reprinted here) showed that the soluble proteins found in adrenal granules were recovered in the perfusates of stimulated glands. In contrast, the cytoplasmic enzyme, lactic dehydrogenase, is not released, nor are components of the granule membrane, such as phospholipid or cholesterol (Trifaro, Poisner, and Douglas, 1967). These experiments provide strong support for the proposal that secretion in the adrenal medulla occurs by a mechanism of exocytosis in which the granular membrane fuses with the cell membrane, liberating soluble granule components.

Experiments similar to these have been performed with postganglionic sympathetic neurons, but have yielded less definitive results. Vesicle fractions prepared from noradrenergic neurons contain norepinephrine, dopamine β-hydroxylase, and a protein that is immunologically similar to chromogranin A. A. Smith, et al. (1970, reprinted here), showed that splenic nerve stimulation caused release of the two proteins in addition to norepinephrine. Release required calcium, and the ratios of the proteins to catecholamine in the perfusate were approximately the same in different experiments. Comparison of these ratios with the ratios of the components in a vesicle fraction, however, revealed that the perfusate had much lower levels of both proteins than expected. One possible explanation for this discrepancy is that Smith, et al., used a vesicle fraction derived from splenic nerve axons, rather than from the terminals. Vesicles found in axons have a larger diameter than those in terminals, and may differ biochemically as well.

Weinshilboum, et al. (1971) performed an experiment similar to that of Smith, et al., but used the vas deferens and analyzed the ratio of catecholamine to dopamine β-hydroxylase in the whole postganglionic neuron. The ratio in the perfusate after nerve stimulation was close to that found in homogenates of whole tissue. While the experiments on noradrenergic neurons tend to support the idea that exocytosis is the mechanism of secretion, more definitive experiments will require further purification and characterization of the various types of vesicles in these neurons.

The mechanism of transmitter release has also been investigated by seeking ultrastructural changes in cells during secretion. If secretion occurs by exocytosis, it might be possible to observe vesicles fused with the surface membrane during secretion. Such profiles have been seen, both in the adrenal medulla and in nerve terminals, but it has been difficult to correlate them with normal secretion. Generally, stimulation of neurons at moderate frequencies for short periods of time causes little change in the number or appearance of vesicles in terminals. The paper by B. Ceccarelli, W. Hurlbut, and A. Mauro (1972, reprinted here) is one of several recent reports showing that prolonged stimulation or stimulation at high frequencies does cause depletion of vesicles.

In related experiments, several investigators have shown that nerve stimulation increases the uptake of horseradish peroxidase (a macromolecule that can be detected in the electron microscope) from the extracellular fluid into small vesicles in the terminals. This uptake could reflect the transient opening of vesicles to the external medium or represent increased endocytosis (the pinching-off of vesicles from the surface membrane into the cell interior). In studying this phenomenon, J. Heuser and T. Reese (1973) have suggested that during secretion vesicles fuse with the surface membrane and release their contents; at a later time, the extra membrane is recovered by endocytosis; the endocytotic vesicles fuse and appear as large cisternae in the terminals; and the cisternae subsequently divide to form new vesicles. The experiments on the morphology of nerve terminals during transmitter release do not establish exocytosis as the mechanism of secretion. Vesicle depletion after prolonged stimulation, for instance, could be the result of general metabolic stress. The experiments do, however, provide strong circumstantial evidence for a link between vesicles and transmitter release, and they offer a new approach to elucidation of the relation between various types of membranes in nerve terminals.

The amount of transmitter released by an action potential may be subject to physiological modification. The presynaptic inhibition studied by Dudel and Kuffler at crustacean neuromuscular junctions is one example of such a mechanism. Stimulation of the inhibitory nerve in these preparations reduces the amount of transmitter released by the motor or excitatory nerve. This effect is thought to be mediated by branches of the inhibitory nerve that terminate on the excitatory nerve endings, and can be mimicked by gamma-aminobutyric acid (GABA), the transmitter released by the inhibitory nerve. GABA, by increasing the chloride conductance of the nerve terminal membrane, decreases the depolarization in the excitatory nerve terminals produced by an action potential. The decreased depolarization probably results in reduced calcium entry, in turn causing a reduction in transmitter release.

Recent experiments suggest that the release of norepinephrine from postganglionic sympathetic neurons can also be modified. Three different effects have been described. First, $\alpha$-receptor antagonists increase the amount of norepinephrine and dopamine $\beta$-hydroxylase recovered after stimulation of sympathetic nerves. Conversely, $\alpha$-receptor agonists decrease the recovery of these substances (De Potter, et al., 1971). These results raise the possibility that released norepinephrine limits its own further secretion by interaction with $\alpha$-receptors on the nerve terminals.

Second, prostaglandins decrease the amount of norepinephrine and dopamine β-hydroxylase released per impluse. Because the formation and release of prostaglandins in the tissue is increased by sympathetic nerve stimulation, their effects on secretion may also have physiological significance (Samuelsson and Wennmalm, 1971). The effect of prostaglandins appears to be independent of that caused by α-receptor agents. Finally, ACh also depresses norepinephrine secretion, an action that can be blocked by atropine. In the heart, stimulation of parasympathetic nerves reduces the norepinephrine release caused by sympathetic nerve stimulation (Löffelholz and Muscholl, 1970).

All of these effects appear to be mediated by presynaptic receptors on sympathetic nerve terminals. The physiological function of these effects and the way in which they interact are uncertain, but the possibility that a complex control system modifies the secretion of transmitters is an intriguing one.

Future research on the mechanism of transmitter release obviously will continue to require the coordinated application of many different techniques. One important approach may be the use of natural toxins that selectively interfere with the processes of normal secretion. A number of these are now available: botulinum toxin, the β toxin in the venom of *Bungarus multicinctus,* a toxin in black widow spider venom, and a toxin in Australian tiger snake venom. As with receptors, protein toxins may be useful probes for the dissection of the molecular mechanism of transmitter release.

## READING LIST

*Reprinted Papers*

1. Douglas, W.W. and A.M. Poisner (1966a). Evidence that the secreting adrenal chromaffin cell releases catecholamines directly from ATP-rich granules. *J. Physiol.* 183: 236–248.
2. Schneider, F.H., A.D. Smith, and H. Winkler (1967). Secretion from the adrenal medulla: biochemical evidence for exocytosis. *Brit. J. Pharm. Chemotherap.* 31: 94–104.
3. Katz, B. and R. Miledi (1969). Tetrodotoxin-resistent electric activity in presynaptic terminals. *J. Physiol.* 203: 459–487.
4. Smith, A.D., W.P. De Potter, E.J. Moerman, and A.F. De Schaepdryver (1970). Release of dopamine β-hydroxylase and chromogranin A upon stimulation of the splenic nerve. *Tissue and Cell* 2: 547–568.
5. Ceccarelli, B., W.P. Hurlbut, and A. Mauro (1972). Depletion of vesicles from frog neuromuscular junctions by prolonged tetanic stimulation. *J. Cell Biol.* 54: 30–38.

*Other Selected Papers*

6. Dudel, J. and S.W. Kuffler (1961). Presynaptic inhibition at the crayfish neuromuscular junction. *J. Physiol.* 155: 543–562.
7. Katz, B. and R. Miledi (1965). The measurement of synaptic delay, and the time course of acetylcholine release at the neuromuscular junction. *Proc. Roy. Soc. B.* 161: 483–495.
8. Douglas, W.W. and A.M. Poisner (1966b). On the relation between ATP splitting and secretion in the adrenal chromaffin cell: Extrusion of ATP (unhydrolyzed) during release of catecholamines. *J. Physiol.* 183: 249–256.
9. Dodge, F.A., Jr. and R. Rahamimoff (1967). Co-operative action of calcium ions in transmitter release at the neuromuscular junction. *J. Physiol.* 193: 419–432.
10. Katz, B. and R. Miledi (1967). A study of synaptic transmission in the absence of nerve impulses. *J. Physiol.* 192: 407–436.
11. Trifaró, J.M., A.M. Poisner, and W.W. Douglas (1967). The fate of the chromaffin granule during catecholamine release from the adrenal medulla: I. Unchanged efflux of phospholipid and cholesterol. *Biochem Pharmacol.* 16: 2095–2100.
12. Löffelholz, K. and E. Muscholl (1970). Inhibition by parasympathetic nerve stimulation of the release of the adrenergic transmitter. *Naunyn-Schmiedebergs Arch. Pharmak.* 267: 181–184.
13. De Potter, W.P., I.W. Chubb, A. Put, and A.F. De Schaepdryver (1971). Facilitation of the release of noradrenaline and dopamine β-hydroxylase at low stimulation frequencies by α-blocking agents. *Arch. Int. Pharmacodyn. Ther.* 193: 191–197.
14. Samuelsson, B. and A. Wennmalm (1971). Increased nerve stimulation induced release of noradrenaline from the rabbit heart after inhibition of prostaglandin synthesis. *Acta Physiol. Scand.* 83: 163–168.
15. Weinshilboum, R.M., N.B. Thoa, D.G. Johnson, I.J. Kopin, and J. Axelrod (1971). Proportional release of norepinephrine and dopamine β-hydroxylase from sympathetic nerves. *Science* 174: 1349–1351.
16. Heuser, J.E. and T.S. Reese (1973). Evidence for recycling of synaptic vesicle membrane during transmitter release at the frog neuromuscular junction. *J. Cell. Biol.* 57: 315–344.
17. Miledi, R. (1973). Transmitter release induced by injection of calcium ions into nerve terminals. *Proc. Roy. Soc. B.* 183: 421–425.

# EVIDENCE THAT THE SECRETING ADRENAL CHROMAFFIN CELL RELEASES CATECHOLAMINES DIRECTLY FROM ATP-RICH GRANULES

By W. W. DOUGLAS and A. M. POISNER*

*From the Department of Pharmacology, Albert Einstein College of Medicine, Yeshiva University, New York 61, N.Y., U.S.A.*

(*Received 4 August* 1965)

## SUMMARY

1. Cats' adrenal glands were perfused with Locke's solution and stimulated through the splanchnic nerves or by acetylcholine.

2. In response to such stimulation there appeared in the venous effluent, in addition to catecholamines, large amounts of AMP and adenosine and smaller amounts of ATP and ADP. Like the catecholamines, these substances had their origin in the chromaffin cells as was shown by their failure to appear when the splanchnic nerves were stimulated during perfusion with drugs blocking the adrenal synapses.

3. During stimulation the ratio of catecholamines:ATP and metabolites in the venous effluent corresponded closely with the reported ratio of catecholamines:adenine nucleotides in the 'heavy' chromaffin granules.

4. Adenine nucleotide appeared in the adrenal effluent *pari passu* with catecholamines within a second or two of beginning stimulation.

5. It is concluded that the nucleotide-rich granules are the immediate source of catecholamines released from the stimulated adrenal chromaffin cell, and that the other two intracellular 'pools' that have been described, nucleotide-poor and 'free' cytoplasmic catecholamines, contribute little or not at all.

## INTRODUCTION

Although the cellular events underlying adrenal medullary secretion have long been studied they are still obscure. A principal difficulty is that several distinct 'pools' of catecholamines have been described as occurring within the adrenal chromaffin cell, and it is not known which is immediately involved when the cell is stimulated to secrete.

The cell fractionation studies carried out by Blaschko & Welch (1953), and many others since, have indicated that while the bulk of the catechol-

---

* Career Development Awardee of the U.S. Public Health Service.

Reprinted from *The Journal of Physiology* 183: 236–248 (1966) by permission of the publisher.

amine within the chromaffin cell is contained in the membrane-limited 'chromaffin granules' there is a considerable amount 'free' in the cell cytoplasm. Blaschko & Welch (1953) suggested that when the chromaffin cell was stimulated there might occur some increase in the permeability of the plasma membrane allowing the 'free' amine to escape, and that this loss might then be made up by transfer of catecholamines from the granule 'stores' to the cytoplasm. This view that 'free' cytoplasmic amine may play the central role in the acute secretory response has been advanced repeatedly since (e.g. Hillarp, 1960a; Paton, 1960; Schümann, 1961). On the other hand, it has frequently been suggested, principally on evidence obtained with light or electron microscopy, that the chromaffin granules may be more directly involved and transfer their amines, in one way or another, to the cell exterior during the secretory response (e.g. Cramer, 1928; Hillarp, Hökfelt & Nilson, 1954; De Robertis & Vas Ferreira, 1957; Wetzstein, 1957, 1961; De Robertis & Sabatini, 1960; Coupland, 1965). These granules, according to Hillarp (1960b), are of two types: the classical 'heavy' chromaffin granule in which catecholamine is stored in equivalent amounts with adenine nucleotides (principally ATP), and a less numerous 'light' chromaffin granule in which the catecholamines are held without such nucleotide. Hillarp (1960b) made a point of the fact that the latter granules released their amines most readily *in vitro*, a finding of relevance to their possible involvement in secretion in the intact cell.

Douglas, Poisner & Rubin (1965) have recently attempted to identify the 'pool' of catecholamines immediately involved in the acute secretory response by examining the effluent from perfused adrenal glands for adenine nucleotides. Their experiments revealed that whenever the adrenal gland was exposed to acetylcholine or various other medullary secreto-gogues large amounts of AMP appeared in the venous effluent along with the catecholamines; and, further, that the effluxes of AMP and catechol-amines during stimulation were highly correlated. Such evidence provides a strong indication that the 'heavy' nucleotide-rich, chromaffin granules are involved in the acute secretory process.

In the present study we have further pursued this line of experiment. We have shown first, by stimulating the medulla selectively through the splanchnic nerves, that the ATP metabolites do indeed derive from the chromaffin cells; secondly, that the molar ratio of catecholamines: ATP and metabolites in the venous effluent from secreting glands corresponds closely with that in the 'heavy' chromaffin granules; and third, that the adenine nucleotide appears *pari passu* with the catecholamine in the adrenal effluent within a second or so of beginning stimulation. From such results we conclude that the 'heavy' chromaffin granules are the principal, and possibly sole, source of catecholamines released from the adrenal medullary chromaffin cell during physiological stimulation. Brief accounts of our findings were presented by one of us at symposia last year (Douglas, 1965 a, b).

## METHODS

Cats were anaesthetized with chloralose (90 mg/kg, i.v.) following ethyl chloride and ether, and one adrenal gland, acutely denervated, was perfused in situ through the abdominal aorta with Locke's solution at 22–25° C. The procedure followed that described by Douglas & Rubin (1961) except that the venous effluent from the adrenal gland was collected with a fine polyethylene cannula tied into the adrenolumbar vein at the medial edge of the gland. The adrenolumbar vein was tied at the lateral edge of the gland, as were all small branches that entered it between the cannula and the lateral tie. In this way the cannula received effluent from the adrenal gland only. Samples of venous effluent were taken for measurement of catecholamines and ATP and its derivatives 20 min or more after beginning perfusion when the resting output of catecholamines had reached a low, stable level (Douglas & Rubin, 1961, 1963) and when the amount of blood in the effluent had fallen far below that which might interfere with the assay for adenine nucleotides (see below).

*The perfusion fluid* used was a modified Locke's solution of the following composition (mM): NaCl, 154; KCl, 5·6; CaCl, 2·2; MgCl$_2$, 1·0; Na$_2$HPO$_4$, 2·15; NaH$_2$PO$_4$, 0·85; glucose, 10. It was equilibrated with O$_2$. Perfusion could be switched at will to other reservoirs of this solution to which had been added acetylcholine (ACh) or atropine and hexamethonium (C$_6$).

*Splanchnic stimulation.* The greater and lesser splanchnic nerves on the ipsilateral side were tied together above the diaphragm and their peripheral ends were drawn into a glass pipette containing Locke's solution. The abdomen and thorax were then flooded with Locke's solution and the nerves were stimulated, when appropriate, by passing current between the inside of the pipette and the bath so formed in the manner described by Furshpan & Potter (1959). Supramaximal stimuli (about 50 V) of 0·5 msec duration were applied at a frequency of 30 shocks/sec. The duration of stimulation was always less than 40 sec in order to obtain high secretory rates.

*Analytical methods.* The catecholamines, *adrenaline* and *noradrenaline* were assayed fluorimetrically by the trihydroxyindole method as modified by Anton & Sayre (1962). *Adenosine* was determined spectrophotometrically with adenosine deaminase as described by Möllering & Bergmeyer (1963a). The method was scaled down to use 0·25 ml. sample and 0·05 ml. 0·25 M phosphate buffer. AMP was measured in one of two ways: when its concentration was low, the firefly method (see below) was used; when its concentration was high it was measured by the method of Möllering & Bergmeyer (1963b) using adenosine deaminase and alkaline phosphatase (0·25 ml. sample was used with 0·05 ml. 0·25 M triethanolamine buffer). *Hypoxanthine* was determined by the method of Jørgensen (1963) employing xanthine oxidase and uricase. The initial deproteinization and preliminary incubation with uricase were omitted. ATP was determined using a modification of the luciferase method as described by Strehler (1963) that permitted determination of ATP at concentrations in the cuvette as low as 1 p-mole/ml. ($10^{-12}$ moles/ml.). To obtain this sensitivity, the phototube filter unit of an Aminco Bowman spectrophotofluorometer was machined to hold a 1 cm diameter cuvette so that the cuvette was close to the phototube but separated from it by the shutter. A light-tight lid covering the cuvette carried a fine stainless-steel tube through which firefly extract could be injected. The output from the photomultiplier unit (set at maximum sensitivity) was further amplified by a Grass P5 amplifier whose output in turn activated a pen recorder (Texas Rectiriter). To measure ATP the procedure was as follows: 1 ml. sample, or standard, was placed in a cuvette along with 0·6 ml. glycylglycine-Mg buffer (0·025 M glycylglycine, 0·1 M-MgSO$_4$, pH 7·5) and mixed. The cuvette was then placed in the light-tight compartment and the shutter was opened. After a flat base line had been obtained on the pen recorder, 1·0 ml. of ice-cold firefly lantern extract was rapidly injected through the tube into the cuvette and the response was recorded for about 10 sec. The peak excursion of the pen was linearly related to the ATP concentration as shown in Fig. 1. *ADP* and *AMP* were also determined with this luciferase technique after first converting them to ATP by a modification of the method of Imai, Riley & Berne (1964). To measure ADP the sample was first incubated for 10 min at room temperature with pyruvic kinase (0·001 ml.) in the following incubation mixture (mM final concentration): phosphoenolpyruvate, 0·25; $MgSO_4$, 7·5; KCl, 75; glycylglycine buffer, 50; pH, 7·5. To measure AMP the sample was incubated in the same way as for ADP except that the incubation mixture contained, in addition, 0·01 ml. myokinase plus a trace of ADP (1 p-mole/ml.), and that the duration of incubation was extended to 60 min. The amounts of AMP and ADP in the samples were determined from standard curves obtained using the same incubation procedure and known amounts of these substances.

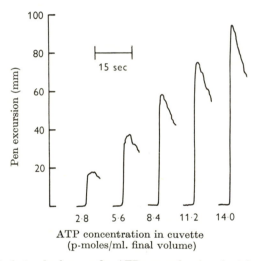

Fig. 1. A typical standard curve for ATP assay showing the ink-written records obtained from successive injections of a constant amount of firefly lantern extract into five cuvettes containing progressively greater amounts of ATP following the procedure described in the text. The rapid upward deflexion in each record coincides with the injection of firefly lantern extract. The time course of the responses can be measured from the inset calibration.

Although blood contains some adenine nucleotide (principally ATP), it was not a significant source in the present study. By the time the first samples of perfusates were collected the vasculature had been very thoroughly washed out; the perfusates were crystal clear and, after freezing and thawing to disrupt any RBC's, contained less than 1 part in 100,000 Hb when tested by the O-toluidine method as described by Watson-Williams (1955). A single estimate of the ATP content of cats' blood yielded a value of 0·2 $\mu$-moles/ml. blood, a value within the reported range (0·1–0·9 $\mu$-moles/ml.) for various mammalian species (*Handbook of Biological Data*, 1956). Cat's blood in a dilution of 1:100,000 would thus yield a concentration of ATP of 2 p-moles/ml. which is several orders below the concentration of ATP or total ATP metabolites we found in the venous effluent from stimulated adrenal glands.

*Drugs and enzymes.* The drugs used were acetylcholine chloride (ACh), hexamethonium chloride ($C_6$) and atropine sulphate. Their concentrations are expressed in terms of the salts. The following enzyme preparations were obtained from Sigma Chemical Co., St Louis, Mo.: adenosine deaminase, alkaline phosphatase, uricase, xanthine oxidase, and firefly lantern extract (FLE-250). The firefly lantern extract was made up in arsenate-$MgSO_4$ buffer (0·05 M arsenate; 0·02 M-$MgSO_4$, pH 7·4) so that 1 ml. contained the extract of 5 mg of dried firefly lanterns. Myokinase and pyruvate kinase were obtained from Boehringer, New York.

## RESULTS

### The chromaffin cells as the source of adenine nucleotide in the adrenal effluent

Stimulation of the splanchnic nerves for 10–40 sec caused AMP to appear in the adrenal venous effluent along with the catecholamines, adrenaline and noradrenaline, in each of sixteen tests on seven glands. Owing to variation among the glands and differences in the duration of stimulation the rates of catecholamine secretion ranged from 14 to 172 n-moles/min with a mean of 56·5 n-moles/min. Over this wide range the efflux of AMP paralleled that of the catecholamines and the mean molar ratio of catecholamines:AMP was 6·1 ± 0·3. This value is close to that obtained in the previous study by Douglas *et al.* (1965) using as stimuli the secretogogues acetylcholine, nicotine, excess potassium, and calcium reintroduction, where the corresponding ratio was 6·4 ± 0·6. The results obtained with splanchnic nerve stimulation are plotted in Fig. 2 where, for the purpose of comparison, they are presented along with ten values obtained in response to perfusion with Locke's solution containing acetylcholine, the chemical transmitter released by the splanchnic nerves.

Since small amounts of adenine nucleotides are released from stimulated nerves (Holton, 1959; Abood, Koketsu & Miyamoto, 1962; Kuperman, Volpert & Okamoto, 1964), some experiments were done to observe the effects of stimulating the splanchnic nerves while transmission across the adrenal synapses was interrupted by drugs. To obtain a profound block both hexamethonium ($5 \times 10^{-4}$ g/ml.) and atropine ($10^{-5}$ g/ml.) were added to the perfusion fluid since acetylcholine receptors of both 'nicotinic' and 'muscarinic' type are present in the adrenal chromaffin cell (Feldberg, Minz & Tsudzimura, 1934; Douglas & Poisner, 1965). Splanchnic stimulation during exposure to these drugs released only small amounts of catecholamines and AMP in each of six experiments. Catecholamine output ranged from 0·65 to 2·57 n-moles/min with a mean of 1·55 n-moles/min and AMP efflux was correspondingly lowered so that the mean molar ratio of catecholamines:AMP was 6·6 ± 2·0. These tests were made on the same glands that, subsequently, during perfusion with drug-free Locke's solution, yielded the much higher secretory outputs described earlier.

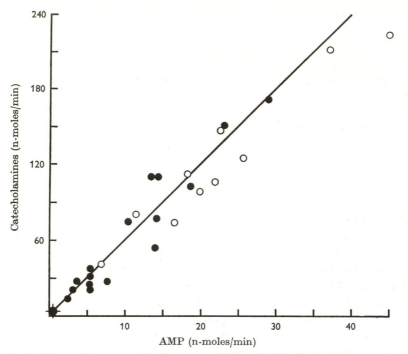

Fig. 2. Relation between catecholamine secretion and AMP efflux during splanchnic nerve stimulation and exposure to ACh. The values indicated by the closed circles were obtained in response to stimulation of both the greater and lesser splanchnic nerves: the symbols, ●, represent values obtained when nerve stimulation was performed during perfusion with Locke's solution. Six other responses to nerve stimulation obtained during perfusion with Locke's solution containing both hexamethonium ($5 \times 10^{-4}$ g/ml.) and atropine ($10^{-5}$ g/ml.) fell within the areas defined by the symbol, ◆. The open circles represent responses to perfusion with Locke's solution containing ACh ($1$–$2 \times 10^{-5}$ g/ml.). Six of these were obtained in the previous series of experiments (Douglas *et al.* 1965) and the remaining four in the present study.

### The ratio of catecholamines to total ATP metabolites

The ratio of catecholamines: AMP of about 6:1 found in the effluent escaping from the adrenal gland in the present and previous experiments falls short of the corresponding ratio of catecholamines: total adenine nucleotides in the chromaffin granules of the cat which, according to Hillarp & Thieme (1959), is 3·7:1. It therefore seemed worth while to measure the amounts of other metabolites of ATP in the adrenal effluent. In the previous experiments (Douglas *et al.* 1965), the amounts of ATP and ADP detected in addition to AMP in the effluent from adrenal glands exposed to nicotine were small and close to the limits of sensitivity of the method then used. With the much more sensitive luciferase technique adopted in the present experiments we were readily able to show that small amounts of ATP and ADP escaped along with the AMP in response to ACh or nerve stimulation. Further, since adenosine had also been found to be one of the break-down products of ATP perfused through the adrenal vasculature (W. W. Douglas, A. M. Poisner & R. P. Rubin, unpublished), this substance too was sought. It was regularly found in the venous effluent from stimulated glands in a concentration intermediate between AMP on the one hand and ATP and ADP on the other.

Six samples of venous effluent obtained from four glands stimulated with ACh or by splanchnic stimulation were analysed for ATP and all the above metabolites. Samples sufficiently rich in these substances to allow all the measurements were obtained usually by pooling the effluents escaping during several short periods of stimulation applied at intervals of about 5 min. The mean ratio of catecholamine efflux to the combined efflux of ATP and its metabolites in these samples was $4 \cdot 22 \pm 0 \cdot 07$ (Table 1). Although Stjärne (1964) and Banks (1965) have found hypoxanthine in the effluent from perfused bovine adrenal glands, we were unable to detect this compound in the venous effluents from seven cats' adrenal glands, five of which were stimulated with ACh and two through the splanchnic nerves, where the catecholamine concentration in the effluent ranged from 80 to 346 nmoles/ml. (The method used for measuring hypoxanthine was capable of detecting about 1 nmole/ml.). The different results may reflect some species variation or they may be due to the differences in experimental procedure. For example, both Stjärne and Banks perfused the adrenal glands in retrograde fashion through the adrenal vein so that the perfusion fluid, after traversing the medulla, passed through the cortex.

### Temporal relation between the efflux of AMP and that of the catecholamines

In three experiments, each conducted on a different adrenal gland, the temporal relation between the efflux of catecholamines and that of AMP was studied by measuring their concentration in successive drops escaping from the venous cannula after applying the stimulus to the splanchnic nerves. The total collection times in the three experiments ranged from 9 to 16 sec and five or six drops were obtained in these periods. As shown in Fig. 3, the first drop collected after beginning stimulation had little catecholamine or AMP, but thereafter the concentration of both substances rose together to reach a maximum in the third to fifth drop, depending on the preparation and the rate of flow. The delay in appearance of both substances was principally due to the dead space of the adrenal vein and venous cannula which was always greater than one drop. Calculation

TABLE 1. Efflux of catecholamines and of ATP and its derivatives during stimulation of perfused adrenal glands

| Stimulus | Duration of stimulus and times applied | Efflux (n-moles/min) | | | | | | Sum of ATP and derivatives | Ratio: Catecholamines / ATP and derivatives |
| | | Catechol-amines | ATP | ADP | AMP | Adenosine | | | |
|---|---|---|---|---|---|---|---|---|---|
| Splanchnic nerve stimulation (30 shocks/sec) | 10 sec × 6 | 151 | 0·72 | 0·67 | 23·1 | 9·6 | | 34·1 | 4·43 |
| | 12 sec × 4 | 177 | 1·04 | 0·42 | 29·9 | 12·6 | | 44·0 | 4·02 |
| Acetylcholine (2 × 10⁻⁵ g/ml.) | 20 sec × 6 | 77 | 0·79 | 0·14 | 16·0 | 1·49 | | 18·4 | 4·18 |
| | 20 sec × 4 | 101 | 0·73 | 0·15 | 20·0 | 3·10 | | 24·0 | 4·21 |
| | 20 sec × 4 | 212 | 0·95 | 1·58 | 37·3 | 12·6 | | 52·4 | 4·05 |
| | 25 sec × 1 | 223 | 1·64 | 0·32 | 45·0 | 3·53 | | 50·5 | 4·42 |

Each series of measurements (except the last) was made on samples obtained by pooling the effluents in several successive short periods of stimulation as indicated in the second column from the left.

showed that both catecholamines and AMP were discharged within 1 or 2 sec of beginning stimulation.

In a fourth gland exposed to ACh ($2 \times 10^{-5}$ g/ml.) for 5 min 25 sec, the mean molar ratio of catecholamines:AMP during the first 25 sec when catecholamine secretion was high (249 n-moles/min) was similar to that in the following 5 min when the rate of catecholamine secretion was much lower (57 n-moles/min): this ratio in the first period was 5·0, and in the second period 5·5.

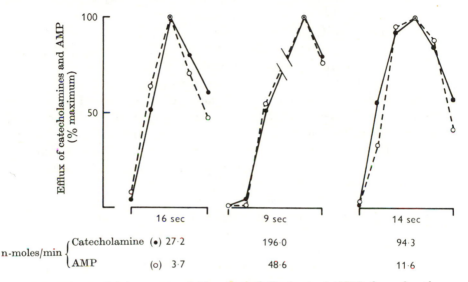

| | | 16 sec | 9 sec | 14 sec |
|---|---|---|---|---|
| n-moles/min | Catecholamine (●) | 27·2 | 196·0 | 94·3 |
| | AMP (○) | 3·7 | 48·6 | 11·6 |

Fig. 3. The parallel time courses of efflux of catecholamines and AMP in three adrenal glands stimulated for 16, 9 and 14 sec through their splanchnic nerves. Each pair of curves was constructed by measuring the catecholamines and AMP in successive drops emerging from the venous cannula after beginning stimulation and expressing the results as a percentage of the maximal value in each experiment. The figures below each graph show the absolute value of this maximum (one drop was lost in the middle experiment). See text for further details.

As shown in Fig. 3 the peak rate of secretion occurred within about 10 sec of beginning splanchnic stimulation and thereafter catecholamine output fell off sharply. A similar time course of catecholamine efflux was seen in several other experiments in which ACh was used as the stimulus. The rapid decline in secretory rate is thus not entirely due to presynaptic phenomena. Whatever its explanation, such behaviour led us to adopt very short periods of stimulation and collection in order to obtain high rates of secretion.

DISCUSSION

The AMP and related substances that appear in the venous effluent from the adrenal gland upon stimulation of the splanchnic nerves do not derive, to any significant extent, from the nerves, but must escape from the cells they innervate, the adrenal chromaffin cells. This is clearly demonstrated by the inhibitory effects of hexamethonium and atropine, substances that act post-synaptically to prevent the chromaffin cells from responding to acetylcholine, the chemical transmitter liberated by the splanchnic nerves (Marley & Paton, 1961; Douglas & Poisner, 1965).

The mean molar ratio of catecholamines:AMP in the 16 tests ($6 \cdot 1 \pm 0 \cdot 3$) was close to that ($6 \cdot 4 \pm 0 \cdot 6$) previously found by Douglas *et al.* (1965) when the adrenal gland was exposed to a variety of medullary secretogogues including acetylcholine, nicotine, excess potassium and calcium. Thus, although having access to the whole adrenal gland, cortex as well as medulla, these diverse secretogogues apparently owe all, or almost all, of their effect on nucleotide efflux to their action on chromaffin cells, as was indeed suspected in the earlier report. In addition to AMP, splanchnic stimulation (as well as the secretogogues ACh and nicotine) also released substantial amounts of adenosine and some ADP and ATP. There can now be little doubt that the release of this family of compounds is an event accompanying secretory activity in adrenal chromaffin cells.

The only source of adenine nucleotide in the chromaffin cells that is rich enough to yield such large amounts of AMP and related substances is the 'heavy', nucleotide-rich, chromaffin granules. The demonstration that the molar ratio of catecholamines:ATP and its derivatives in the adrenal venous effluent ($4 \cdot 22 \pm 0 \cdot 07$) closely approximates the corresponding ratio in 'heavy' granules, taken in conjunction with the finding that the nucleotide appears in the venous effluent as soon as the catecholamines, compels us to conclude that these granules are the principal and immediate source of catecholamines released from the adrenal chromaffin cell when it is physiologically stimulated.

Such a conclusion is counter to the view that the chromaffin granules are simply reserve stores, and that stimulation draws on the pool of the catecholamine which is 'free' in the cytoplasm. As stated in the introduction, this alternative scheme rests mainly on the finding of what appears to be a sizeable pool of extragranular catecholamines within the adrenal chromaffin cell (Hillarp, 1960*b*). But the scheme is also attractive in that it offers a simple, and seemingly plausible, explanation of the process of catecholamine release. Thus, largely on general and theoretical grounds, it has been commonly supposed that when the chromaffin cell is stimulated, either through its nerves or by acetylcholine, its membrane is depolarized and made more permeable; and such changes have been considered appropriate to allow escape of 'free' cytoplasmic catecholamine (Blaschko & Welch, 1953; Hillarp, 1960*a*; Paton, 1960; Schümann, 1961). Indeed, just this sort of release mechanism has repeatedly been suggested to obtain in sympathetic nerves, which are developmental homologues of the medullary chromaffin cells (Paton, 1960; Schümann, 1961; Euler & Lishajko, 1962). The present experiments, however, have offered no evidence of discharge of 'free' catecholamines. The catecholamines that were released were accompanied by AMP and related substances in equivalent amounts and these metabolites of ATP appeared in the adrenal effluent *pari passu* with the catecholamines within a second or two of beginning stimulation. Moreover, the ratio of ATP metabolites:catecholamines, judging by the measurements of AMP, was maintained whether stimulation lasted only a second or two or several minutes. Such results make it unlikely that any pool of 'free' catecholamines contributes significantly to the acute secretory response. This conclusion is reinforced when one considers the evidence now available concerning membrane permeability, depolarization and the release of catecholamines. Thus it has been shown that removal of calcium from the extracellular environment, a procedure well known to increase membrane permeability (Morrill, Kaback & Robbins, 1964), and one that demonstrably promotes potassium escape from the adrenal gland (W. W. Douglas, A. M. Poisner & R. P. Rubin, unpublished) does not cause the release of catecholamines: on the contrary, it depresses release well below the normal spontaneous levels. Nor can the release of catecholamines be evoked in such circumstances by the addition of acetylcholine or by raising the potassium content of the medium to high, depolarizing levels: even in combination these permeability-increasing manoeuvres fail to release catecholamines (Douglas & Rubin, 1961, 1963). Such evidence provides grounds for doubting the existence of any significant pool of 'free' catecholamines. Perhaps, arguments to the contrary notwithsanding (Hillarp, 1960*b*), the non-granular catecholamine that is found in the supernatant from homogenized chromaffin cells—and which makes up only about 10% of total amines under the best homogenization procedures currently employed—is an artifact of cell fractionation (see also Weiner, 1964).

The present results also make it unlikely that the pool of catecholamines sequestered in the 'light' (nucleotide-poor) chromaffin granules (Hillarp, 1960*b*) plays an important part in the acute secretory process, and the function of this third amine pool also remains obscure.

If, as our evidence indicates, the nucleotide-rich chromaffin granules are the source of the catecholamines released from the physiologically stimulated chromaffin cell, the question that must next be answered is this: How are these granules made to give up amines during stimulation? The discovery that release of catecholamines is accompanied by discharge of ATP metabolites in equivalent amount appears to provide a persuasive new argument for the possibility that splitting of intragranular ATP may by a key event in the catecholamine release process (Blaschko, 1959; Hillarp, 1958). This possibility is examined in the following paper (Douglas & Poisner, 1966).

It is a pleasure to acknowledge the valuable assistance provided by Miss Agatha Palazzolo and Mrs Marie Perlstein in these experiments. The work was supported by grants from the National Institutes of Health of the United States Public Health Service (B-4006 and 1-K3-GM-25, 304).

## REFERENCES

ABOOD, L. G., KOKETSU, K. & MIYAMOTO, S. (1962). Outflux of various phosphates during membrane depolarization of excitable tissues. *Am. J. Physiol.* **202**, 469–474.

ANTON, A. H. & SAYRE, D. F. (1962). A study of the factors affecting the aluminum oxide-trihydroxyindole procedure for the analysis of catecholamines. *J. Pharmac. exp. Ther.* **138**, 360–375.

BANKS, P. (1965). Quoted from BANKS, P. & BLASCHKO, H. (1965). Chromaffin tissue. *Pharmac. Rev.* (In the Press.)

BLASCHKO, H. (1959). The development of current concepts of catecholamine formation. *Pharac. Rev.* **11**, 307–316.

BLASCHKO, H. & WELCH, A. D. (1953). Localization of adrenaline in cytoplasmic particles of the bovine adrenal medulla. *Arch. exp. Path. Pharmak.* **219**, 17–22.

COUPLAND, R. E. (1965). Electron microscopic observations on the structure of the rat adrenal medulla. I. The ultrastructure and organization of chromaffin cells in the normal adrenal medulla. *J. Anat.* **99**, 231–254.

CRAMER, W. (1928). *Fever, Heat Regulation, Climate and the Thyroid-Adrenal Apparatus.* London: Longmans, Green and Co.

DE ROBERTIS, E. D. P. & SABATINI, D. D. (1960). Submicroscopic analysis of the secretory process in the adrenal medulla. *Fedn Proc.* suppl. **5**, 70–73.

DE ROBERTIS, E. D. P. & VAZ FERREIRA, A. (1957). Electron microscope study of the excretion of catechol-containing droplets in the adrenal medulla. *Expl. Cell Res.* **12**, 568–574.

DOUGLAS, W. W. (1965a). Calcium-dependent links in stimulus-secretion coupling in the adrenal medulla and neurohypophysis. In *Mechanisms of Release of Biogenic Amines*, Wenner Gren Symposium, February 1965. Oxford: Pergamon Press.

DOUGLAS, W. W. (1965b). The mechanism of release of catecholamines. In Proc. of 2nd International Catecholamine Meeting, Milan, July 1965. *Pharmac. Rev.* (In the Press.)

DOUGLAS, W. W. & POISNER, A. M. (1965). Preferential release of adrenaline from the adrenal medulla by muscarine and pilocarpine. *Nature, Lond.* (In the Press.)

DOUGLAS, W. W. & POISNER, A. M. (1966). On the relation between ATP splitting and secretion in the adrenal chromaffin cell: discharge of ATP (unhydrolysed) during release of catecholamines. *J. Physiol.* **183**, 249–256.

DOUGLAS, W. W., POISNER, A. M. & RUBIN, R. P. (1965). Efflux of adenine nucleotides from perfused adrenal glands exposed to nicotine and other chromaffin cell stimulants. *J. Physiol.* **179**, 130–137.

DOUGLAS, W. W. & RUBIN, R. P. (1961). The role of calcium in the secretory response of the adrenal medulla to acetylcholine. *J. Physiol.* **159**, 40–57.

DOUGLAS, W. W. & RUBIN. (1963). The mechanism of catecholamine release from the adrenal medulla and the role of calcium in stimulus-secretion coupling. *J. Physiol.* **167**, 288–310.

EULER, U. S. VON & LISHAJKO, F. (1962). Catecholamine release and uptake in isolated adrenergic nerve granules. *Acta physiol. scand.* **57**, 468–480.

FELDBERG, W., MINZ, B. & TSUDZIMURA, H. (1934). The mechanism of the nervous discharge of adrenaline. *J. Physiol.* **81**, 286–304.

FURSHPAN, E. J. & POTTER, D. D. (1959). Transmission at the giant motor synapses of the crayfish. *J. Physiol.* **145**, 289–325.

*Handbook of Biological Data* (1956), ed. SPECTOR, W. S. p. 53. Philadelphia: W. B. Saunders.

HILLARP, N-Å. (1958). Enzymic systems involving adenosinephosphates in the adrenaline and noradrenaline containing granules of the adrenal medulla. *Acta physiol. scand.* **42**, 144–165.

HILLARP, N-Å. (1960a). Catecholamines: mechanisms of storage and release. *Acta endocr., Copenh.*, suppl. **50**, 181–185.

HILLARP, N-Å. (1960b). Different pools of catecholamines stored in the adrenal medulla. *Acta physiol. scand.* **50**, 8–22.

HILLARP, N-Å., HÖKFELT, B. & NILSON, B. (1954). The cytology of the adrenal medullary cells with special reference to the storage and secretion of the sympathomimetic amines. *Acta anat.* **21**, 155–167.

HILLARP, N-Å. & THIEME, G. (1959). Nucleotides in the catechol amine granules of the adrenal medulla. *Acta physiol. scand.* **45**, 328–338.

HOLTON, P. (1959). The liberation of adenosine triphosphate on antidromic stimulation of sensory nerves. *J. Physiol.* **145**, 494–504.

IMAI, S., RILEY, A. L. & BERNE, R. M. (1964). Effect of ischemia on adenine nucleotides in cardiac and skeletal muscle. *Circulation Res.* **15**, 443–450.

JØRGENSEN, S. (1963). Hypoxanthine and xanthine. *Methods of Enzymatic Analysis*, ed. BERGMEYER, H.-U., pp. 495–499. New York: Academic Press.

KUPERMAN, A. S., VOLPERT, W. A. & OKAMOTO, M. (1964). Release of adenine nucleotide from nerve axons. *Nature, Lond.*, **204**, 1000–1001.

MARLEY, E. & PATON, W. D. M. (1961). The output of sympathetic amines from the cat's adrenal gland in response to splanchnic nerve activity. *J. Physiol.* **155**, 1–27.

MÖLLERING, H. & BERGMEYER, H.-U. (1963a). Adenosine. *Methods of Enzymatic Analysis*, ed. BERGMEYER, H.-U., pp. 491–494. New York: Academic Press.

MÖLLERING, H. & BERGMEYER, H.-U. (1963b). Adenosine phosphates. *Methods of Enzymatic Analysis*, ed. BERGMEYER, H.-U., pp. 578–580. New York: Academic Press.

MORRILL, G. A., KABACK, H. R. & ROBBINS, E. (1964). Effect of calcium on intracellular sodium and potassium concentrations in plant and animal cells. *Nature, Lond.*, **204**, 641–642.

PATON, W. D. M. (1960). In: *Adrenergic Mechanisms*. CIBA Foundation Symposium, p. 127. Boston: Little, Brown and Co.

SCHÜMANN, H. J. (1961). Speicherung und Freisetzung der Brenzcatechinamine. *Symp. d. Dtsch. Ges. f. Endokrinologie*, 8, 23–32.

STJÄRNE, L. (1964). Studies of catecholamine uptake storage and release mechanisms. *Acta physiol. scand.* **62**, suppl. 228, 1–97.

STREHLER, B. L. (1963). Adenosine-5′-triphosphate and creatine phosphate. Determination with luciferase. *Methods of Enzymatic Analysis*, ed. BERGMEYER, H.-U., pp. 559–572. New York: Academic Press.

WATSON-WILLIAMS, E. J. (1955). A tablet test for blood in urine. *Br. med. J.* **1**, 1511–1513.

WEINER, N. (1964). The catecholamines: biosynthesis, storage and release, metabolism, and metabolic effects. In *The Hormones*. vol. IV, ed. PINCUS, G. THIMANN, K. V. & ASTWOOD, E. B., p. 429. New York: Academic Press.

WETZSTEIN, R. (1957). Elektronenmikroskopische Untersuchungen am Nebennierenmark von Maus, Meerschweinchen und Katze. *Z. Zellforsch. mikrosk. Anat.* **46**, 517–576.

WETZSTEIN, R. (1961). Die phäochromen Granula des Nebennierenmarks im elektronenmikroskopischen Bild. *Symp. d. Dtsch. Ges. f. Endokrinologie*, 8, 33–41.

# SECRETION FROM THE ADRENAL MEDULLA:
# BIOCHEMICAL EVIDENCE FOR EXOCYTOSIS

BY

F. H. SCHNEIDER,* A. D. SMITH AND H. WINKLER †

*From the Department of Pharmacology, Oxford University*

*(Received April 25, 1967)*

Catecholamines are secreted from the adrenal gland under many physiological and experimental conditions (for a review see Coupland, 1965a). In order to explain catechol-amine secretion at a cellular level, De Robertis & Vaz Ferreira (1957) suggested that the amines of the adrenal medulla may be released from the intracellular storage granules directly into the extracellular spaces by a process which was called reverse pinocytosis. This suggestion was based on evidence obtained from electron microscopy, which has since been confirmed by Coupland (1965b). Since that time several workers have presented biochemical evidence in agreement with this hypothesis. Douglas and his co-workers (see Douglas, 1966) have shown that stimulation of the perfused cat adrenal by acetylcholine leads to the secretion of adenine nucleotides and their metabolites; the molar ratio of catecholamines to adenine derivatives in the perfusates was similar to that in chromaffin granules. Similar observations have been made using the perfused bovine adrenal gland (Banks, 1966). Furthermore, Banks & Helle (1965), using an immunochemical method, have shown that the major protein component of the chromaffin granules is also secreted upon stimulation with carbachol. This finding has been confirmed with quantitative immunochemical methods (Kirshner, Sage, Smith & Kirshner, 1966; Sage, Smith & Kirshner, 1967). The same protein was also secreted from the calf adrenal gland *in situ* upon splanchnic nerve stimulation (Blaschko, Comline, Schneider, Silver & Smith, 1967); the soluble proteins of chromaffin granules were called chromo-granins by these authors. Accordingly, we shall call the major component of these proteins " chromogranin A ".

Additional biochemical evidence in support of the idea that catecholamine release occurs by reverse pinocytosis is presented in this paper. For this type of secretion mechanism the term exocytosis has been proposed by de Duve (1963).

## METHODS

*Perfused adrenal gland*

Bovine adrenal glands, weighing between 8 and 15.5 g, were obtained approximately 20 min after the animals were killed, and kept in ice for about 30 min until perfusion was begun. The

---

\* Present address: Department of Pharmacology, University of Colorado Medical Center, Denver, Colorado, U.S.A.

† Permanent address: Pharmakologisches Institut der Universität, Innsbruck, Austria.

Reprinted from the *British Journal of Pharmacology and Chemotherapy* 31: 94–104 (1967) by permission of the publisher.

glands were perfused in a retrograde manner through the adrenal vein (Hechter, Jacobsen, Schenker, Levy, Jeanloz, Marshall & Pincus, 1953 ; Banks, 1965) with Tyrode solution (137 mM NaCl, 2.68 mM KCl, 1.80 mM $CaCl_2$, 0.28 mM $NaH_2PO_4$, 0.001 mM $MgCl_2$, 11.60 mM $NaHCO_3$ and 5.56 mM glucose) at 37°, and gassed with a mixture of 95% $O_2$ and 5% $CO_2$. Flow rates varied between 7 and 20 ml./min, with a rate of 10 to 12 ml./min in most experiments. Secretion of catecholamines was induced by injection of 15 mM-carbamoylcholine chloride (Carbachol, British Drug Houses Ltd.) into the perfusion fluid immediately before the fluid entered the gland. Carbachol was injected in volumes of 0.4 ml. or less, in a series of six separate injections, each separated by 30 sec.

*Chemical assays*

Perfusates from the glands and extracts of chromaffin granules (prepared according to Smith & Winkler, 1967a, b) were analysed for catecholamines by the colorimetric method of Euler & Hamberg (1949), using citrate-phosphate buffer (McIlvaine, 1921). In the calculation of the results, catecholamines were expressed in terms of adrenaline. Protein was precipitated by trichloroacetic acid (final concentration of 5% (W/V)), and measured by the microbiuret method (Goa, 1953).

For the analysis of lipids, the perfusates were evaporated to dryness at 37° under reduced pressure and extracted by the method of Folch, Lees & Sloane-Stanley (1957). Fatty acids were determined by the method of Sheath (1965), and cholesterol by the method of Zlatkis, Zak & Boyle (1953). Separation by thin-layer chromatography and subsequent analysis of phospholipids was carried out according to the method described by Skipski, Peterson & Barclay (1964). Lipid phosphorus was determined directly on silica scraped from the plates by the method of Bartlett (1959).

Starch gel electrophoresis (Poulik, 1957) and amino acid analysis (following hydrolysis of the protein for 17 hr at 110° in 6N HCl) were performed on perfusates and soluble lysates which had been reduced in volume by ultrafiltration (Sober, Gutter, Wyckoff & Peterson, 1956) at 4° C and dialysed for a minimum of 12 hr against tris Na-succinate buffer (I 0.015, pH 5.9).

*Immunological procedures*

Rabbit antiserum was prepared against the major soluble protein (chromogranin A) of chromaffin granules, which was purified by the method of Smith & Winkler (1967b). The animals were injected (intramuscularly) with 0.5 ml. pure protein (1.6 mg/ml.) mixed with an equal volume of Freund's complete adjuvant. Injections were repeated 7 days later with half as much material. On the 34th day after the initial injection the animals were given subcutaneous injections of a mixture of 0.5 ml. protein solution (1.6 mg/ml.) and 25 mg aluminium phosphate. Blood was collected from the marginal ear vein between 3 and 4 weeks after the final injection. Thereafter subcutaneous injections of the protein-aluminium phosphate mixture was given every 4 to 5 weeks and the rabbits were bled 2 weeks after each injection. The antiserum was stored at 4° in the presence of 0.01% merthiolate and 25% undiluted complement, and was used at dilutions of $\frac{1}{50}$–$\frac{1}{100}$ ; it was incubated for 30 min at 56° immediately before use in order to destroy complement.

A microcomplement fixation method similar to that described by Fulton & Dumbell (1949) was used to titrate the amount of antigen. The diluent was made by the alternative procedure of Kabat & Mayer (1961), and contained 0.1% gelatine. Complement fixation was carried out in Perspex agglutination trays (Prestware Ltd., London), each well of which contained complement (0.1 ml.) antigen (0.1 ml.) and antibody (0.1 ml.) or the appropriate control. Complement was used at a dilution which provided $2\frac{1}{2}$ $C'H_{50}$. The trays were incubated for $1\frac{1}{2}$ hr at 37°. One-tenth of a ml. of 2% (V/V) sheep red blood cells, sensitized with an optimum amount of haemolysin for 10 min at 37° immediately before use, was then added, and incubation continued at 37° for an additional $1\frac{1}{2}$ hr. Dilutions of antigen and antiserum were used which were free of anticomplement activity. The titre was obtained from the dilution of the antigen at which approximately 50% of the cells were haemolyzed. The amount of antigenic protein was determined by comparing the titres of the unknown with that of the standard antigen solutions. Since doubling dilutions were used, this method was accurate within the limits of 0.5 to 2 times the observed value.

*Lactate dehydrogenase activity*

This was determined by the method of, and expressed in the units of, Wróblewski & La Due (1955).

241

*Materials*

Complement (preserved guinea-pig serum), sheep red blood cells (sheep blood in alsever solution), and haemolysin (rabbit haemolytic serum) were purchased from Burroughs Wellcome & Co., London. Freund's adjuvant, complete, was purchased from Difco Laboratories, Detroit.

## RESULTS

*Catecholamine secretion*

Resting secretion of catecholamines from the adrenal gland was low, usually less than 0.1 $\mu$-mole/min. Injection of 15 mM-carbachol (2.4 ml. over a $2\frac{1}{2}$-min period) caused the secretion of large amounts of catecholamines (Fig. 1). The amount of catecholamine

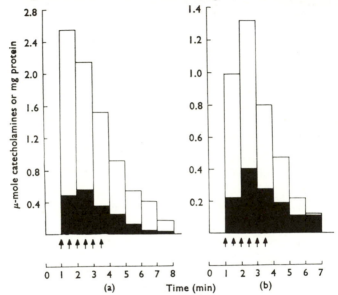

Fig. 1. Secretion of catecholamines and protein from a bovine adrenal gland during two periods of stimulation. The heights of the open columns indicate the increment of the catecholamines and those of the black columns indicate the increment of protein above control level. The arrows indicate the injection of carbamylcholine (see Methods). Experiments (a) and (b) were separated by 2 hr. The flow rate of perfusion fluid was 13 ml./min for experiment (a), and was 9 ml./min for experiment (b). Spontaneous release of catecholamines and of protein, respectively: (a) 0.02 $\mu$-mole/min and 0.43 mg/min, (b) 0.02 $\mu$-mole/min and 0.16 mg/min.

released at different flow rates was similar, although the appearance of the amines in the perfusate was slightly delayed at the lower flow rates. The amount of catecholamine secreted in each stimulation period decreased upon repeated stimulation. The flow rate decreased by up to 15% as a result of the injection of carbachol in 13 out of 14 experiments.

*Secretion of protein*

The perfusates contained considerable amounts of protein during the first 30 min of perfusion. The amount of protein decreased exponentially, and reached a fairly constant level within 40 to 60 min (Fig. 2). Due to the high protein content of the perfusate

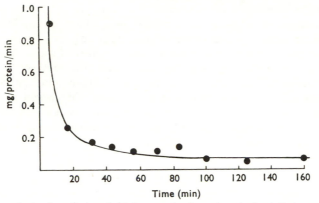

Fig. 2. Protein content of perfusion fluid from a bovine adrenal gland that was not stimulated. Protein was determined by the microbiuret method. The flow rate of perfusion fluid was approximately 14 ml./min.

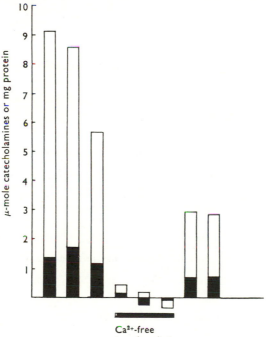

Ca²⁺-free
tyrode solution

Fig. 3. The requirement for calcium in the secretion of protein and catecholamines induced by carbamylcholine. Each column represents a 3-min stimulation period; 20 min elapsed between each stimulation period. The heights of the open columns indicate the increment of the catecholamines and those of the black columns indicate the increment of protein above control level. Ca²⁺-free perfusion fluid was used during (and for 20 min beforehand) the 4th, 5th and 6th periods of stimulation. Normal Tyrode solution was perfused for 20 min before the two final stimulation periods. Between the stimulation periods the amounts of catecholamines and protein, respectively, in the perfusate ranged from 0.2–0.3 μ-mole/min and from 0.1–0.5 mg/min.

during the early stages of perfusion, perfusates were not collected for analysis during the first hour. Stimulation of the gland with carbachol, in addition to inducing catecholamine secretion, caused an increase in the amount of protein in the perfusate, as shown in Fig. 1. The release of protein was almost simultaneous with that of catecholamines.

The dependence of several secretory processes upon the presence of calcium (see Douglas, 1966) prompted an examination of the effects of calcium depletion upon carbachol-induced secretion of protein. Figure 3 shows that protein secretion, as well as catecholamine release, was abolished when calcium was left out of the perfusion medium. When the gland was again perfused with complete Tyrode solution secretion of both protein and hormones could be induced.

*Relationship of catecholamine to protein in perfusates*

The ratio of the amount of catecholamines to that of protein secreted above the resting level was fairly constant. This ratio depended somewhat upon the length of time for which the perfusate was collected after the initial injection of carbachol, and was close to the ratio of catecholamines to total protein in the soluble lysate of chromaffin granules (see Table 1).

*Secretion of specific protein*

The complement fixation method enabled us to detect 10 ng of chromogranin A. Analysis of 4 different perfusates showed that about half of the protein secreted in response to carbachol consisted of the specific protein (Table 1). This value is similar

TABLE 1

CATECHOLAMINES AND PROTEINS IN PERFUSATES FROM THE STIMULATED GLAND AND IN SOLUBLE LYSATES OF CHROMAFFIN GRANULES

The amounts of catecholamines and protein secreted during stimulation were obtained by subtracting the amounts of each constituent in the control period from the amounts in the stimulation period perfusates. The figures represent the means ($\pm$ S.D.) of n determinations. The term chromogranin A refers to the major component of the soluble proteins from chromaffin granules

|  | $\dfrac{\mu\text{-mole catecholamines}}{\text{mg total soluble protein}}$ | $\dfrac{\mu\text{-mole catecholamines}}{\text{mg chromogranin A}}$ | $\dfrac{\text{mg chromogranin A} \times 100}{\text{mg total protein}}$ |
|---|---|---|---|
| Soluble lysate of granules | 4·8 ±0·6 (n=5) | 10·1±3·9 (n=10) | 47·6±17·8 (n=10) |
| Perfusate upon stimulation |  |  |  |
| 3 min collection | 5·4±1·0 (n=13) | 11·9±5·0 (n=4) | 48·2±20·4 (n=4) |
| 6 min collection | 4·8±1·5 (n=19) | — | — |

to that obtained upon analysis of the soluble lysate of chromaffin granules. In only one experiment was chromogranin A detected in the perfusate collected during control periods; in this instance it was found to be 3% of the total protein. The ratios of catecholamines ($\mu$-mole) to chromogranin A (mg) in the stimulation period perfusate and in the soluble lysate were almost the same. Similar values for these ratios were obtained by Kirshner *et al.* (1966) and by Sage *et al.* (1967).

*Starch gel electrophoresis*

Only one major protein component could be detected in the control perfusate by gel electrophoresis and the electrophoretic mobility of this component was the same as that of bovine serum albumin. Analysis of the perfusate collected upon stimulation showed the presence of several proteins, the electrophoretic mobilities of which were identical to corresponding proteins from the chromaffin granules. In addition there was a band

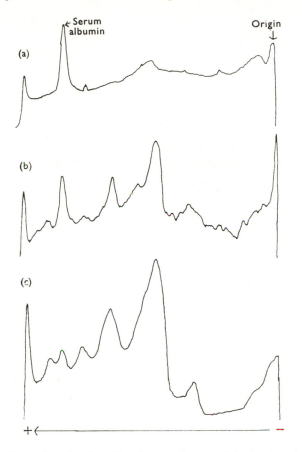

Fig. 4. Starch gel electrophoresis of proteins from perfusates of the bovine adrenal gland and of chromogranins from the soluble lysate of chromaffin granules. After staining the gel with nigrosine (0.05%) the intensities of the bands were measured by transmitted light with a densitometer. The proteins migrated from right to left (a) control period perfusate, (b) stimulation period perfusate, (c) soluble lysate of chromaffin granules.

with the same mobility as serum albumin. Densitometer scans of the starch gels, shown in Fig. 4, illustrate the close similarity between the proteins in the perfusate collected during stimulation and those of the soluble lysate. The major protein band represented 41% of the area under the peaks for the soluble lysate in the scan in Fig. 4 and 43%, of the area in the scan of the stimulation period perfusate gel. Corresponding figures for the next most conspicuous protein band were 23% and 19%.

*Amino acid analyses*

Amino acid analyses of the proteins from stimulation period perfusates showed some similarity between the composition of these proteins and that of the chromogranins (Table 2). The amino acid composition of the protein in the control perfusate was similar to that of serum proteins. The amino acid composition of the proteins secreted in response to carbachol was calculated by subtracting the amount of each amino acid present in the control perfusate from that of each amino acid in the stimulation period perfusate. The calculated amino acid composition had the same characteristics as that of the soluble proteins from chromaffin granules (Table 2).

TABLE 2

#### AMINO ACID ANALYSIS OF PROTEINS IN PERFUSATES AND IN SOLUBLE LYSATE OF CHROMAFFIN GRANULES

The values in each column represent g amino acid/100 g protein. The values in the column headed "increment" were calculated by subtracting the absolute amount of each amino acid/unit volume in the control from the corresponding value of the stimulation period perfusate, and dividing the difference by the increment in total protein/unit volume between the two perfusates. The control period perfusate contained 2 mg. protein and the stimulation period perfusate contained 4·43 mg protein

| Amino acid | Perfusate (control) | Perfusate (stimulated) | Increment between perfusates | Chromogranins of the soluble lysate |
|---|---|---|---|---|
| Glu | 14·2 | 22·5 | 29·3 | 26·6 |
| Arg | 6·2 | 8·0 | 9·5 | 10·7 |
| Lys | 10·0 | 10·2 | 10·4 | 8·6 |
| Pro | 6·1 | 8·3 | 10·1 | 8·0 |
| Asp | 9·8 | 8·5 | 7·4 | 7·7 |
| Leu | 9·0 | 7·0 | 5·4 | 6·8 |
| Ser | 5·6 | 5·7 | 5·8 | 5·2 |
| Ala | 4·7 | 4·3 | 4·0 | 4·2 |
| Gly | 3·3 | 3·8 | 4·2 | 3·8 |
| His | 4·0 | 2·5 | 1·3 | 3·6 |
| Val | 5·4 | 3·3 | 1·6 | 2·7 |
| Thr | 5·2 | 3·0 | 1·2 | 2·3 |
| Phe | 5·1 | 3·0 | 1·3 | 2·3 |
| Tyr | 3·8 | 3·1 | 2·5 | 2·2 |
| Met | 1·9 | 2·0 | 2·1 | 1·8 |
| NH₃ | 1·6 | 2·9 | 3·8 | 1·6 |
| Ile | 2·3 | 1·4 | 0·7 | 1·0 |
| Cys | 1·8 | 0·6 | — | 0·6 |

*Other constituents of the perfusates*

The perfusates contained small amounts of phospholipids, fatty acids and cholesterol. Slight and variable increases in the amounts of these constituents were observed upon stimulation. If the increment for the various lipids ($\mu$-mole) was divided by the amount of catecholamines ($\mu$-mole) secreted, then ratios of 1.2 for phospholipid, 0.9 for cholesterol and 1.2 for fatty acids were found. The corresponding ratios in chromaffin granules were, respectively, 211, 114 and 6. The perfusates from stimulation periods contain, therefore, very small amounts of these constituents relative to the amount of catecholamines. In order to determine whether lysolecithin, a characteristic constituent of chromaffin granules

(Blaschko, Firemark, Smith & Winkler, 1967 ; Winkler, Strieder & Ziegler, 1967), was released during stimulation, quantitative thin-layer chromatography of the phospholipids extracted from the perfusates was performed. No significant secretion of lysolecithin could be detected during stimulation in 3 experiments, even though these perfusates each contained about 20 $\mu$-mole of catecholamines. The recovery of lysolecithin (740 $\mu$g) injected into the perfusion fluid before it reached the gland was 40%.

There was no increase in the amount of lactate dehydrogenase in the perfusate during stimulation with carbachol (Table 3). It can be calculated from the data in Table 3

TABLE 3

LACTATE DEHYDROGENASE ACTIVITY IN BOVINE ADRENAL MEDULLA AND IN PERFUSATES FROM THE BOVINE ADRENAL GLAND

The high speed supernatant from an homogenate of bovine adrenal medulla was obtained by removing the cell particles by centrifugation at $66 \times 10^5$ g-min. Before analysis, the perfusates were concentrated by ultrafiltration at $4°$

|  | Total units of enzyme activity | mg protein | Units of enzyme/mg protein |
|---|---|---|---|
| High speed supernatant (1 ml.) | 8,000 | 4·56 | 1,754 |
| Control period perfusate (415 ml.) | 1,600 | 8·65 | 185 |
| Stimulation period perfusate (415 ml.) | 1,360 | 15·83 | 86 |

that if only 1% of the amount of protein secreted upon stimulation with carbachol had been derived from the cytoplasmic sap it would have been possible to detect this by means of the lactate dehydrogenase assay.

## DISCUSSION

The isolated bovine adrenal gland was used in this work firstly because it has been shown that this preparation will secrete catecholamines (Philippu & Schümann, 1962 ; Banks, 1965), and protein (Banks & Helle, 1965 ; Kirshner *et al.*, 1966 ; Sage *et al.*, 1967) upon stimulation by acetylcholine and carbachol, and secondly because much is known about the biochemistry of the adrenal chromaffin granules of this species. This preparation is therefore well-suited for the study of the question whether catecholamine release is accompanied by the release of other chromaffin granule constituents. Studies have already been made on secretion of adenine nucleotides (Banks, 1966) and of a specific chromaffin granule protein (Banks & Helle, 1965 ; Kirshner *et al.*, 1966 ; Sage *et al.*, 1967) from the bovine adrenal gland.

For further characterization of the protein secreted from the gland it was necessary to find conditions in which the amount of protein in the perfusate prior to stimulation was as low as possible. This was achieved by perfusing the gland for 40 to 60 min before stimulation. The protein occurring in the control perfusate was mainly derived from serum, as shown by starch gel electrophoresis. An increase in the amount of both catecholamine and protein in the perfusate occurred as a result of stimulation with carbachol. The ratios in the perfusates of catecholamine ($\mu$-mole) to the increment of protein (mg) were similar to the corresponding ratios in the soluble lysates of chromaffin granules. Further evidence of a relationship between the release of catecholamine and that of protein was that neither was secreted when calcium was omitted from the perfusion fluid. The dependence of catecholamine secretion on the presence of calcium has already been demonstrated (Douglas & Rubin, 1961 ; Banks, 1965).

The nature of the protein secreted has been studied by immunochemical and biochemical methods. Using a micro-complement fixation technique the presence of the major component (chromogranin A) of the soluble proteins of chromaffin granules was demonstrated in the perfusate. The antigenic protein comprised about half of the protein secreted above the resting level, which is the same as the amount of this protein found by the immunochemical method in lysates of chromaffin granules. By means of Sephadex chromatography (Smith & Winkler, 1967b) and quantitative starch gel electrophoresis (Winkler, Ziegler & Strieder, 1966) it was found that chromogranin A comprised 38 and 49% respectively of the chromogranins. It is, therefore, unlikely that there is a high degree of cross reaction between the antibody to chromogranin A and the other chromogranins.

Analysis, by starch gel electrophoresis, of the perfusates collected during stimulation demonstrated that several proteins were secreted during stimulation. The electrophoretic mobilities of these components are identical to those of the eight soluble proteins of chromaffin granules. As shown by densitometer scans, these eight proteins in the perfusate were present in the same relative proportions as they were in the soluble lysate. Further confirmation of the identity of the proteins in the perfusates with the chromogranins was obtained by the determination of their amino acid composition. The amino acid analysis of the perfusates collected during stimulation revealed a high content of glutamic acid and proline, but a low content of $\frac{1}{2}$ cysteine ; these are characteristic features of the amino acid composition of the chromogranins.

Since Stjärne (1964), Douglas, Poisner & Rubin (1965) and Banks (1966) have already shown that ATP and its metabolites are secreted along with the catecholamines, we conclude that stimulation of the adrenal medulla leads to secretion of all the soluble constituents of the chromaffin granules.

How is the secretion of the soluble constituents of chromaffin granules brought about ? The discharge of the whole chromaffin granule across the plasma membrane is excluded by our observation that only minute amounts of phospholipids and cholesterol, which are major components of the lipids of chromaffin granules, are present in the perfusate. Furthermore, lysolecithin, a phospholipid characteristic of the chromaffin granule was not secreted. A second possibility is that the contents of the chromaffin granule are discharged into the cytoplasm and then diffuse across the plasma membrane ; this is also unlikely because it would involve a marked increase in the permeability of the plasma membrane to proteins of large molecular size (effective hydrodynamic radius of major component$\simeq$62 Å), and would thus allow cytoplasmic proteins to be secreted. However, the starch gel electrophoresis analyses and the lactate dehydrogenase (effective hydrodynamic radius$\simeq$37 Å) estimations showed that cytoplasmic proteins were not secreted. In addition, Kirshner et al. (1966) have reported that the cytoplasmic enzyme phenylethanolamine-N-methyl transferase was not secreted on stimulation.

The remaining possibility is that the secretion of chromaffin granule constituents occurs by a process of exocytosis as was first suggested by de Robertis & Vaz Ferreira (1957).

A similar secretion mechanism was proposed by Palade (1959) for the zymogen granules of the exocrine pancreas. As described by the morphologist, the process of exocytosis involves the fusion of the membrane of the secretory granule with that of the cell. This is the only mechanism that would allow the secretion of both low and high molecular weight components specifically from the chromaffin granules of the adrenal medulla.

SUMMARY

1. The composition of perfusates from isolated bovine adrenal glands has been examined and compared with that of bovine adrenal chromaffin granules. Perfusates were collected during control periods and during periods of stimulation of the gland by carbamylcholine.

2. Stimulation of the glands increased the amount of catecholamines and protein in the perfusates; the secretion of both catecholamines and protein was abolished when $Ca^{2+}$ was omitted from the perfusion fluid.

3. The main protein component (chromogranin A) of chromaffin granules was demonstrated in the stimulation period perfusates by an immunochemical method. This protein, along with the other seven soluble proteins of chromaffin granules, was also detected in these perfusates by means of starch gel electrophoresis. The amino acid composition of the proteins secreted upon stimulation was very similar to that of the soluble proteins (chromogranins) from chromaffin granules.

4. Only small increases in the amounts of phospholipids, cholesterol and fatty acids in the perfusates occurred as a result of stimulation; no increases were observed in the amount of lysolecithin or lactate dehydrogenase.

5. The ratios of the amount of catecholamines both to the total amount of secreted protein and to the amount of chromogranin A in the perfusates were close to the ratios, respectively, of catecholamines to chromogranins and of catecholamines to chromogranin A in isolated chromaffin granules.

6. These results, together with earlier findings, demonstrate that the entire soluble contents of chromaffin granules are secreted from the adrenal medulla upon stimulation. Therefore it is concluded that secretion from the adrenal medulla occurs by means of exocytosis.

We appreciate the interest of Dr. H. Blaschko in this work. Mrs. C. Walker performed the amino acid analyses. This work has been supported by grants from the Medical Research Council and the Royal Society. F. H. S. is a National Science Foundation Postdoctoral Fellow, A. D. S. holds a Royal Society Stothert Research Fellowship and H. W. is a British Council Scholar.

REFERENCES

BANKS, P. (1965). Effects of stimulation by carbachol on the metabolism of the bovine adrenal medulla. *Biochem. J.*, **97**, 555–560.

BANKS, P. (1966). The release of adenosine triphosphate catabolites during the secretion of catecholamines by bovine adrenal medulla. *Biochem. J.*, **101**, 536–541.

BANKS, P. & HELLE, K. (1965). The release of protein from the stimulated adrenal medulla. *Biochem. J.*, **97**, 40–41C.

BARTLETT, G. R. (1959). Phosphorus assay in column chromatography. *J. biol. Chem.*, **234**, 466–468.

BLASCHKO, H., COMLINE, R. S., SCHNEIDER, F. H., SILVER, M. & SMITH, A. D. (1967). Secretion of chromaffin granule protein, chromogranin, from the adrenal gland after splanchnic stimulation. *Nature, Lond.* **215**, 58–59.

BLASCHKO, H., FIREMARK, H., SMITH, A. D. & WINKLER, H. (1967). Lipids of the adrenal medulla: lysolecithin, a characteristic constituent of chromaffin granules. *Biochem. J.*, **104**, 545–549.

COUPLAND, R. E. (1965a). *The Natural History of the Chromaffin Cell.* Longmans, Green, London.

COUPLAND, R. E. (1965b). Electron microscopic observations on the structure of the rat adrenal medulla. 1. The ultrastructure and organization of chromaffin cells in the normal adrenal medulla. *J. Anat.*, **99**, 231–254.

DE DUVE, C. (1963). Endocytosis. In: *Lysosomes*, Ciba Foundation Symposium. Ed. DE REUCK, A. V. S. & CAMERON, M. P., footnote, p. 126. London, Churchill.

DE ROBERTIS, E. & VAZ FERREIRA, A. (1957). Electron microscope study of the excretion of catechol-containing droplets in the adrenal medulla. *Exp. Cell Res.*, **12**, 568–574.

DOUGLAS, W. W. (1966). Calcium-dependent links in stimulation secretion coupling in the adrenal medulla and neurohypophysis. In *Mechanisms of Release of Biogenic Amines*, Ed. EULER, U. S. VON, ROSELL, S. & UVNÄS, B., pp. 267–290. Oxford, Pergamon Press.

DOUGLAS, W. W., POISNER, A. M. & RUBIN, R. P. (1965). Efflux of adenine nucleotides from perfused adrenal glands exposed to nicotine and other chromaffin cell stimulants. *J. Physiol., Lond.*, **179**, 130–137.

DOUGLAS, W. W. & RUBIN, R. P. (1961). The role of calcium in the secretory response of the adrenal medulla to acetylcholine. *J. Physiol., Lond.*, **159**, 40–57.

EULER, U. S. VON & HAMBERG, U. (1949). Colorimetric determination of noradrenaline and adrenaline. *Acta physiol. scand.*, **19**, 74–84.

FOLCH, J., LEES, M. & SLOANE STANLEY, G. H. (1957). A simple method for the isolation and purification of total lipides from animal tissues. *J. biol chem.*, **226**, 497–509.

FULTON, F. & DUMBELL, K. R. (1949). The serological comparison of strains of influenza virus. *J. gen. Microbiol.*, **3**, 97–111.

GOA, J. (1953). A micro biuret method for protein determination; determination of total protein in cerebrospinal fluid. *Scand. J. clin. Lab. Invest.*, **5**, 218–222.

HECHTER, O., JACOBSEN, R. P., SCHENKER, V., LEVY, H., JEANLOZ, R. W., MARSHALL, C. W. & PINCUS, G. (1953). Chemical transformation of steroids by adrenal perfusion; perfusion methods. *Endocrinology*, **52**, 679–691.

KABAT, E. A. & MAYER, M. M. (1961). *Experimental Immunochemistry*. 2nd ed. Thomas, Springfield, Illinois.

KIRSHNER, N., SAGE, H. J., SMITH, W. J. & KIRSHNER, A. G. (1966). Release of catecholamines and specific protein from adrenal glands. *Science, N.Y.*, **154**, 529–531.

MCILVAINE, T. C. (1921). A buffer system for colorimetric comparison. *J. biol. Chem.*, **49**, 183–186.

PALADE, G. E. (1959). Functional changes in the structure of cell components. In: *Subcellular Particles*. Ed. HAYASHI, T., pp. 64–83. Ronald Press, New York.

PHILIPPU, A. & SCHÜMANN, H. J. (1962). Der Einfluss von Calcium auf die Brenzcatechinaminfreisetzung. *Experientia*, **18**, 138–140.

POULIK, M. D. (1957). Starch gel electrophoresis in a discontinuous system of buffers. *Nature, Lond.*, **180**, 1477–1479.

SAGE, H. J., SMITH, W. J. & KIRSHNER, N. (1967). Mechanism of secretion from the adrenal medulla. 1. A microquantitative immunologic assay for bovine adrenal catecholamine storage vesicle protein and its application to studies of the secretory process. *Molec. Pharmac.*, **3**, 81–89.

SHEATH, J. (1965). Estimation of plasma non-esterified fatty acids and triglyceride fatty acids by thin-layer chromatography and colorimetry. *Aust. J. exp. Biol. med. Sci.*, **43**, 563–572.

SKIPSKI, V. P., PETERSON, R. F. & BARCLAY, M. (1964). Quantitative analysis of phospholipids by thin-layer chromatography. *Biochem. J.*, **90**, 374–378.

SMITH, A. D. & WINKLER, H. (1967a). A simple method for the isolation of adrenal chromaffin granules on a large scale. *Biochem. J.*, **103**, 480–482.

SMITH, A. D. & WINKLER, H. (1967b). Purification and properties of an acidic protein from chromaffin granules of bovine adrenal medulla. *Biochem. J.*, **103**, 483–492.

SOBER, H. A., GUTTER, F. J., WYCKOFF, M. M. & PETERSON, E. A. (1956). Chromatography of proteins. 2. Fractionation of serum protein on anion-exchange cellulose. *J. Am. chem. Soc.*, **78**, 756–763.

STJÄRNE, L. (1964). Studies of catecholamine uptake storage and release mechanisms. *Acta physiol. scand.*, **62**, Suppl. No. 228.

WINKLER, H., STRIEDER, N. & ZIEGLER, E. (1967). Über Lipide, insbesondere Lysolecithin, in den chromaffinen Granula verschiedener Species. *Arch. exp. Path. Pharmak.*, **256**, 407–415.

WINKLER, H., ZIEGLER, E. & STRIEDER, N. (1966). Studies on the proteins from chromaffin granules of ox, horse and pig. *Nature, Lond.*, **211**, 982–983.

WRÓBLEWSKI, F. & LADUE, J. S. (1955). Lactic dehydrogenase activity in blood. *Proc. Soc. exp. Biol. Med.*, **90**, 210–213.

ZLATKIS, A., ZAK, B. & BOYLE, A. J. (1953). A new method for the direct determination of serum cholesterol. *J. Lab. clin. Med.*, **41**, 486–492.

# TETRODOTOXIN-RESISTANT ELECTRIC ACTIVITY IN PRESYNAPTIC TERMINALS

By B. KATZ AND R. MILEDI

*From the Department of Biophysics, University College London
and the Stazione Zoologica, Naples*

(*Received 26 February* 1969)

SUMMARY

1. The electric properties of the giant synapse in the stellate ganglion of the squid have been further investigated.

2. During tetrodotoxin (TTX) paralysis, a local response can be elicited from the terminal parts of the presynaptic axons after intracellular injection of tetraethyl ammonium ions (TEA).

3. The response is characterized by an action potential of variable size and duration, whose fall is often preceded by a prolonged plateau. The response, especially the duration of the plateau, is subject to 'fatigue' during repetitive stimulation.

4. The TTX-resistant form of activity is localized in the region of the synaptic contacts, and shows a marked electrotonic decrement even within less than 1 mm from the synapse. It is found only on the afferent, not on the efferent, side of the synapse.

5. During the plateau of the response, the membrane resistance is greatly reduced below its resting value.

6. The response depends on presence of external calcium and increases in size and duration with the calcium concentration. Strontium and barium substitute effectively for calcium. Manganese and, to a lesser extent, magnesium, counteract calcium and reduce the response. The response also declines, and ultimately disappears, if sodium is withdrawn for long periods.

7. The relation of the local TTX-resistant response to the influx of calcium ions and to the release of the synaptic transmitter is discussed.

## INTRODUCTION

It has been shown that abolition of nerve impulses by TTX does not prevent the release of the transmitter from nerve endings in response to locally applied depolarization (Katz & Miledi, 1965, 1966, 1967*a, b, e*;

Reprinted from *The Journal of Physiology* 203: 459–487 (1969) by permission of the publisher.

Bloedel, Gage, Llinás & Quastel, 1966; Kusano, Livengood & Werman, 1967). There is increasing evidence that depolarization leads to transmitter release via inward movement of calcium ions, and that the opening up of 'calcium gates' at specific sites of release is not prevented by TTX (Katz & Miledi, 1967 c, e).

Whether the local influx of calcium is strong enough to reinforce the depolarization has been a matter of conjecture. In general, after TTX dosage, the relation between applied current strength and resulting pre-synaptic depolarization (as well as the ensuing post-synaptic response) is continuously graded and shows no sign of a regenerative effect. But there is an interesting exception: at the frog nerve–muscle junction, addition of a few mM-TEA completely alters the character of the response (Katz & Miledi, 1967 b). One now obtains an explosive type of release which appears abruptly above a certain current strength and results in a very large end-plate potential. In a subsequent paper it will be shown that this triggered form of release occurs even when all the external sodium has been replaced by calcium (cf. Katz & Miledi, 1967 d).

A possible explanation of this finding is that calcium inward current in the presynaptic terminals can reinforce the applied depolarization and become regenerative, provided the counter-current of potassium has been sufficiently reduced by TEA (see Armstrong & Binstock, 1965). To examine this possibility further, similar experiments were made on the synaptic terminals in the stellate ganglion of the squid which are large enough to permit direct measurements with intracellular electrodes. Clear evidence has been obtained for a TTX-resistant local regenerative response, confined to the presynaptic terminals and observed whenever TEA was applied internally and the external calcium concentration was high. The ionic mechanism of the response remains uncertain, but there are several indications that calcium current is involved.

## METHODS

The experiments were made during the summers of 1967 and 1968 on the stellate ganglion of the squid *Loligo vulgaris*. In most cases the 'distal' giant synapse (Young, 1939) formed by an axonic contact between the second-order giant fibre and the largest motor axon (in the hindmost stellar nerve) was used, though occasionally the 'accessory' presynaptic fibre, or a motor axon in one of the short stellar nerves was chosen. The preparation consisted either of a small piece of mantle muscle containing the ganglion, or of the isolated ganglion with its in- and outgoing nerves. The procedure of dissecting and mounting the preparation in a cooled chamber has been described in detail (Miledi, 1967; Katz & Miledi, 1967 e). The temperature of the bath (approx. 20 ml.) was usually about 11° C (varying in different experiments between 7 and 14° C). Oxygenated solutions flowed continuously through the preparation chamber.

Once intracellular electrodes had been inserted in the synaptic region, solution changes were made only slowly, so as to reduce the risk of damage and dislocation of the electrodes.

In a dye dilution test it was found that, with the usual rates of flow, it took approximately 10 min for 50 %, 30 min for 75 %, 1 hour for 90 %, and 2 hours for 99 % change of the bath solution. The alternative method, of removing and reinserting electrodes each time the bath was emptied and changed, could not be used routinely because of the inherent technical difficulties and the time usually required for placing electrodes into the presynaptic terminal. It was necessary, however, to do this in some experiments in which the effects of sodium deficiency, and especially of replacing sodium by calcium, were studied.

Tetrodotoxin (Sankyo) was used in most experiments, in concentrations of $10^{-7}$–$1.1 \times 10^{-6}$. TEA was injected iontophoretically by a method previously described (Katz & Miledi, 1967e). During the present experiments the current pulses used to inject TEA were often of higher intensity than in the previous work. Usually, pulses of about 150 msec duration at a frequency of 5/sec were applied for periods of 10–60 min, the intensity being adjusted so as to limit the depolarization to about 20 mV. At times, the injecting pulses were strong enough to give rise to noticeable post-synaptic responses. This procedure caused the effect of TEA on the presynaptic terminals to appear much more quickly, but it was apt to produce severe deterioration in the post-synaptic response, apparently leading to a drastic, and sometimes complete, failure of transmitter release. We believe that this damaging effect arose not from the injection of TEA as such, but from the frequent application of iontophoretic (depolarizing) pulses which exceeded the intensity required for synaptic transfer. It was found that, in the presence of TEA, frequent repetition of strong pulses produced a prolonged refractoriness of the release mechanism (cf. Fig. 18 below).

As regards the exact positioning of the presynaptic 'current' and 'voltage' electrodes, the precautions described in the previous paper (Katz & Miledi, 1967e) were used; that is, the voltage-recording electrode was placed as close as possible to the beginning of the synaptic contact region, and the current-passing (usually TEA containing) pipette a fraction of a millimetre 'upstream'. This is important, for, as pointed out previously (Katz & Miledi, 1967e), reversal of this position gives spuriously low values of the presynaptic voltage change for a given post-synaptic response.

### RESULTS

#### *The effect of presynaptic TEA injection*

Figures 1 and 2A, B recapitulate the results described in a previous paper (Katz & Miledi, 1967e; see also Kusano *et al.* 1967). The preparation had been treated with a paralytic dose of TTX. The top trace in each recording shows the depolarizing current pulse applied to the presynaptic terminal, the middle trace shows the resulting presynaptic potential change, and the bottom trace the post-synaptic response. The calcium concentration ranged between 11 mM (Fig. 1) and 5.5 mM (Fig. 2A, B). Figure 2A shows the normal behaviour, before application of TEA: the presynaptic membrane resistance falls during the depolarizing pulse so that it is impossible to produce a maintained voltage change of high amplitude. After intracellular injection of TEA (Figs. 1, 2B) the picture is changed: large presynaptic potential changes can now be maintained for the duration of the current pulse, and the phenomena of suppression of transmitter release and its postponement until the end of the pulse are shown up (Figs. 1c; 2B, lower part; cf. Katz & Miledi, 1967e).

### A local electric response in the pre-axon

The time course of the presynaptic potentials has some unusual features which are noticeable in Fig. 2B and quite marked in Fig. 1, namely an inflexion on the rising phase and a more or less prolonged hump during the decline. Similar changes had already been briefly commented on in the earlier paper (Katz & Miledi, 1967e, p. 423). With normal or low calcium concentrations, these features were very variable in extent, but they

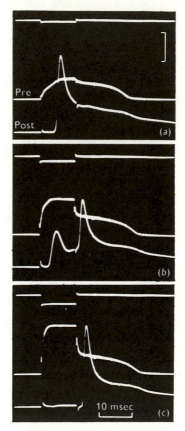

Fig. 1. Pre- and post-synaptic potentials after TEA injection. a, b, c: with three different current intensities applied to the pre-fibre. Calcium concentration 11 mM. In each block, top trace shows current pulse, middle trace presynaptic, bottom trace post-synaptic potential. The vertical scale represents 3·35 μA (top), 100 mV (pre), 20 mV (post). Note: 'upward swing' and delayed fall (hump) of presynaptic potential, and 'suppression' of post-synaptic potential during strong current pulse (partial suppression in b, nearly complete suppression in c). All records in this and following figures were obtained by intracellular recording from TTX-treated stellate ganglia. Position of current electrode at start of synapse; presynaptic recording electrode 0·3 mm down, within synaptic region.

always became striking when the calcium level in the bath was raised to about 50 mM or more. This is shown, for instance, in Fig. 2*C* (see also Figs. 3, 5, 10). Soon after the perfusion fluid was changed to a calcium rich solution, the brief depolarizing pulse evoked a prolonged electric potential change in the presynaptic terminal, accompanied by a greatly increased post-synaptic response. This was a very regular effect, reproducible in all experiments provided (i) a sufficient dose of TEA had been

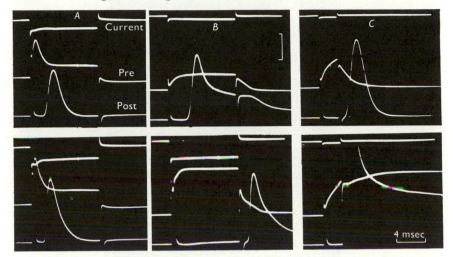

Fig. 2. Effects of TEA and of extra calcium, on pre- and post-synaptic potentials. *A*: 5·5 mM-Ca, no TEA. *B*: 5·5 mM-Ca, after some presynaptic TEA injection. *C*: Ca concentration in bath was raised towards 70 mM and more TEA injected between upper and lower blocks (same current pulse in both cases). In *A* and *B*, different current pulses were used in upper and lower blocks. In each block, the three traces show (from above downwards): current pulse, pre-, and post-synaptic potential. Vertical scale represents: 1·68 μA in *A*, 3·35 μA in *B* and *C*; presynaptic: 40 mV in *A* and *C*, 100 mV in *B*; post-synaptic: 20 mV in *A* and *B*, 10 mV in *C*. Position of presynaptic recording electrode at start of synapse; current electrode 0·28 mm upstream.

injected into the pre-axon (cf. Fig. 5), (ii) the external calcium concentration was moderately high, and (iii) the axon had not been badly damaged or subjected to excessive stimulation. Raising the TTX concentration to $1·1 \times 10^{-6}$ g/l. had little or no effect, even after 2 hr continued perfusion. It appears therefore that under these specific conditions the terminal part of the presynaptic axon gives a local electric response which is highly TTX-resistant, at least compared to the conducted axon spike.

Other features of this presynaptic potential are illustrated in Figs. 3 and 4. In Fig. 3*A* two superimposed oscillograph traces are shown during which identical current pulses were applied. The resulting potential changes diverge, in the characteristic way of a regenerative system at 'threshold'. In Fig. 3*B*, lower trace, the duration of a presynaptic 'response' is shown on a slow time base. Incidentally, this was the longest potential obtained at normal (11 mM) calcium concentration. Figure 4*A* shows the progressive shortening of the presynaptic response during a series of pulses repeated at intervals of 2·5 sec. As with other action potentials of similar shape (e.g. in the heart or crustacean muscle), the

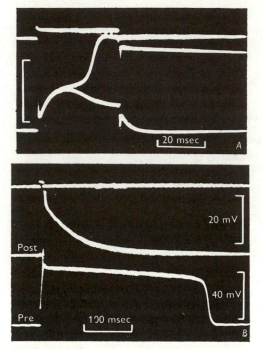

Fig. 3. *A*: 'threshold' of local response. After TEA treatment. 45 mM-Ca. Two successive superimposed traces showing current pulses (upper) and presynaptic potentials (lower trace). Vertical scale represents 1·14 μA and 50 mV. Resting potential 61 mV. *B*: from another synapse (11 mM-Ca), showing on slow time base: current pulse (top), post-synaptic (middle, transient response) and presynaptic potential (bottom, prolonged response). Resting potential (pre): 57 mV. Upper vertical scale represents also 1·83 μA.

response terminates rapidly when the potential has declined to a certain level. The plateau can be cut off much earlier by interposing a hyper-polarizing pulse as shown, for instance, in Fig. 4*B*.

For a further study of this electric response, it was important to devise some convenient way of measuring it. This presents a problem for a potential change which varies with the strength and duration of the applied current. However, with sufficient doses of internal TEA and external calcium, two features of the response become relatively inde-pendent of the applied pulse: these are (i) the duration *T* of the response measured from the end of the pulse to the point of maximum rate of fall (Fig. 6), (ii) the height of the 'plateau' attained several milliseconds after the end of the pulse (i.e. the depolarization $V_a$, or the membrane potential $V_b$, Fig. 6). In any one experiment, the duration $T$ can be made to alter by at least two orders of magnitude; it was therefore sometimes more convenient to use its logarithm (see e.g. Fig. 19 below).

In Table 1, these quantities ($V_a$, $V_b$ and $T$) are listed for a series of experiments at different calcium concentrations. It will be seen that the

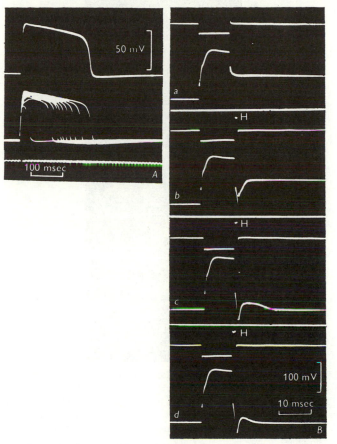

Fig. 4. $A$: effect of pulse repetition, at 2·5 sec intervals. 50 mM-Ca. Upper record shows single, 'unfatigued' presynaptic response to a brief pulse (indicated by the gap in the horizontal bottom line). Middle record shows progressive shortening of response during ten successive pulses. $B$: effect of a brief hyperpolarizing pulse in 'cutting off' presynaptic response. 70 mM-Ca. $a$: response to depolarizing pulse alone. $b$ to $d$: hyperpolarizing pulse (H) added at the end of the depolarizing pulse. The duration of the short H pulse was increased from $b$ to $d$. In $c$ and $d$ the H pulse stopped the response, in $b$ it just failed to do so. Voltage scale also represents 3·35 $\mu$A.

level of the plateau rises (from $-24$ to $+3$ mV), and the duration $T$ lengthens (on the average, from 20 to 470 msec), as the external calcium concentration is increased about tenfold (from 5·5 to 44–70 mM).

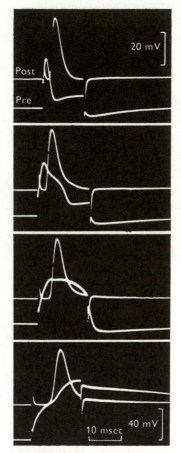

Fig. 5. Effect of progressive TEA injection into pre-axon. Each block shows post-synaptic (top trace) and presynaptic (bottom trace) potentials. 50 mM-Ca throughout. TEA was applied between successive records (from above downwards) in cumulative doses. Vertical scales refer to 'post' (top) and 'pre' (bottom) respectively. Note: appearance of local response, first only during the pulse, later outlasting the pulse.

### The voltage/current relation in the presynaptic terminal

Further information can be obtained by plotting the voltage/current relation of the pre-fibre, under different experimental conditions. In the absence of TEA, the slope of the $V/I$ curve always diminishes with increasing polarization, whether one measures the peak voltage (e.g. Katz & Miledi, 1967e, fig. 3; see also Fig. 20 below) or the final voltage produced by the current pulse (Figs. 7, 9). After TEA injection the $V/I$ relation of the pre-fibre usually shows an 'upward swing', i.e. an increasing slope over a certain range (Figs. 7, 9). This was observed even at normal or reduced calcium concentrations; for instance, in the case of Fig. 8. It may be noted that the upward swing of the $V/I$ curve occurs in the same range of membrane potentials as the inflexions and humps (Figs. 1, 2$B$) in the time course of the potential change.

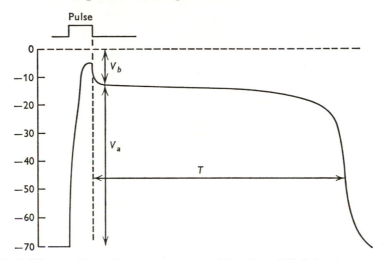

Fig. 6. Diagram illustrating measurements of $V_a$, $V_b$ and $T$. Pulse shown at the top. Dashed horizontal line indicates zero membrane potential. Vertical scale: membrane potential, in mV.

When we first saw these changes, it was difficult to decide whether they were attributable to a regenerative inward current or to an 'anomalous' type of rectification, i.e. to a lowering of potassium conductance, and thus reduced outward current, over a certain range of depolarization. The upswing of the $V/I$ curves, the inflexion during the rise and the hump during the fall of the depolarization could all be explained by either of these alternative mechanisms. Later, we observed the much more pronounced changes in calcium-rich solutions, which suggested that a regenerative process is involved.

### Loss of membrane resistance during the plateau

What finally settled this issue was a measurement of the membrane resistance during the plateau. If the long persistence of the depolarization were due to a lowering of potassium permeability, then the membrane resistance during this period should be higher than in the resting state. If, on the contrary, the resistance during the early period of the plateau is lower than at rest, then this explanation fails, and it becomes more probable that the response arises from inward current of external cations.

That the membrane resistance at the beginning of the plateau is low was already indicated by the high rate, and greatly reduced time constant,

TABLE 1. Effect of calcium concentration on local response. $V_a$ = depolarization measured as indicated in Fig. 6. $V_b$ = membrane potential corresponding to $V_a$. $T$ = duration of response (see Fig. 6). *Distance*, in $\mu$, between presynaptic recording site and start of distal synapse (zero distance means at start, or within, the synaptic region)

| Calcium concentration ... | | | A: 5·5 mM | | B: 11 mM | | B (mean) |
|---|---|---|---|---|---|---|---|
| Distance ($\mu$) | | | 350 | | 100 | 250 | (175) |
| $V_a$ (mV) | | | 46 | | 54·5 | 46 | (50) |
| $V_b$ (mV) | | | −24 | | −13 | −11 | (−12) |
| Calcium concentration C: high (44–70 mM) | | | | | | | |
| Distance ($\mu$) ... | 50 | 50 | 350 | 0 | (80)* | 550* | |
| $V_a$ (mV) | 63 | 79 | 68 | 73 | 56 | 52 | |
| $V_b$ (mV) | −5 | +14 | −2 | +3 | −5 | −4 | |
| | | | | | | | C (mean) |
| Distance ($\mu$) ... | 240 | 100 | 0 | 400 | 0 | 50 | (155) |
| $V_a$ (mV) | 68 | 64 | 70 | 72 | 71 | 63 | (66·5) |
| $V_b$ (mV) | +8 | −4 | +9 | +10 | +10 | +3 | (+3) |

Duration $T$: 5·5 mM-Ca: mean 20 msec (0–68 msec; six observations); 11 mM-Ca: mean 93 msec (25–325 msec; six observations); high Ca: mean 470 (55–1900 msec; 13 observations).

* Omitting accessory axon (bracket) and 550 $\mu$ position: mean $V_a$, 70 mV; mean $V_b$, +4·6 mV.

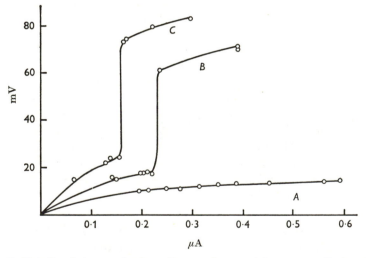

Fig. 7. Relation between steady voltage and current in presynaptic terminal. Pulse duration: 12–15 msec. Approx. 50 mM-Ca throughout. *A*, before TEA injection; *B* and *C*, after two successive doses of TEA, showing the 'jump' from 'subthreshold' to 'superthreshold' levels of depolarization. Position of recording electrode just within synaptic region; current (TEA) electrode 0·2 mm upstream.

with which the membrane potential *falls* to the plateau at the end of a strong pulse (see Figs. 1, 10). This was confirmed more directly by the method of applying repetitive test pulses throughout the period of recording. Figure 11 *A* shows the long-maintained response following a brief depolarizing stimulus. In Fig. 11 *B* brief hyperpolarizing test pulses are

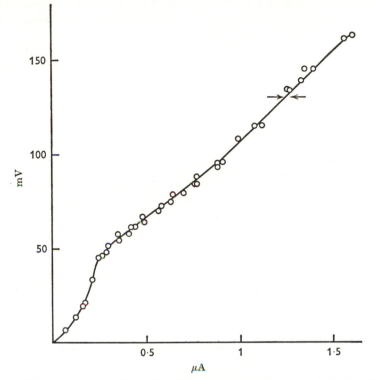

Fig. 8. Voltage/current relation, after TEA treatment in 11 mM-Ca. Pulse duration 18 msec. Arrows show the 'post-synaptic suppression' potential. The resting potential in this terminal was only 52·2 mV. Position of recording electrode 75 μ upstream from synapse; current (TEA) electrode 0·45 mm upstream.

added. From the change in amplitude and time course of the modulating potentials, it is clear that the membrane resistance drops to a low value at the beginning of the plateau and gradually recovers during its later part. Two points require comment: (i) the added test potentials, being in the hyperpolarizing direction, cause the response to be terminated earlier than in its 'unmodulated' form; (ii) the first two or three test pulses following the depolarizing stimulus are reduced in strength. This is an artifact arising from a transient resistance change in the current-passing pipette, and must be allowed for if one compares the amplitudes of the first few modulating potentials. It does not, of course, affect their time course.

In Fig. 11 $C$ simultaneous recordings were made at the synaptic contact region (upper) and 0·625 mm 'upstream' (lower), while the current pulses were applied at a point 1·175 mm upstream from the synapse. The differences between recordings at the two distances will be discussed in the following section.

No accurate estimates could be made from these experiments, but the change in time constant indicates that the loss of membrane resistance

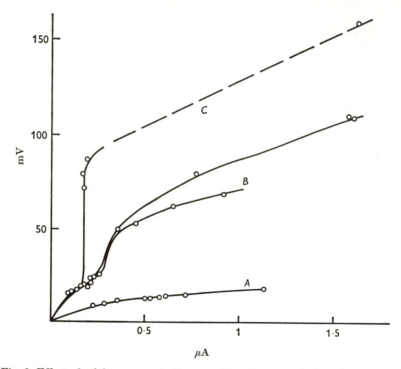

Fig. 9. Effect of calcium concentration on voltage/current relation. $A$: 11 mM-Ca, before TEA injection; $B$, 11 mM-Ca, after TEA injection. The lower curve was obtained first, the upper curve later. $C$: after raising calcium concentration to 70 mM. Ordinate: steady potential change produced by 10 msec current pulse. Abscissa: current intensity. Position of current (TEA) electrode just within synaptic region; recording electrode 0·1 mm further down.

amounted to 80 % or possibly more. This is probably made up in part by increased permeability to external cations whose influx produces the maintained depolarization, and of a residual increase of potassium conductance which was not completely obviated by the TEA injection.

### Localization of the TTX-resistant responses

While the TTX-resistant local response could be obtained regularly from the terminals of presynaptic 'distal' as well as 'accessory' axons, nothing of the kind was ever observed in the post-axon. It may be argued that the larger size and lower input resistance of the post-synaptic fibre make it necessary to inject a greater amount of TEA before the response

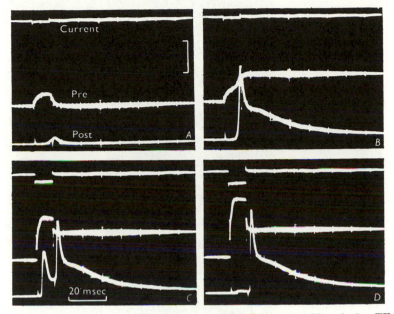

Fig. 10. Pre- and post-synaptic responses in high calcium (70 mM) and after TEA dosage. In each block: current pulse (top), presynaptic (middle), and post-synaptic (bottom) potentials. Four different pulse intensities showing presynaptic 'upswing' from threshold level (in B), and rapid fall to final level (in C and D); also post-synaptic response during pulse (A, B), partial (C) and nearly complete (D) suppression. Vertical scale represents 3·35 $\mu$A, 100 mV (pre) and 20 mV (post).

could become detectable. However, TEA injection periods were made long enough to show up a clear effect on the delayed rectification of the post-fibre. Also, experiments were made on some of the motor axons which run in the smaller stellar nerves (see Miledi, 1967). These axons have an input resistance comparable to that of the presynaptic terminals, yet in spite of prolonged TEA injection no trace of a TTX-resistant response was obtained.

Experiments were then made to find out whether the local response can be initiated anywhere in the pre-fibre, or whether it is confined to the region of the synaptic terminals. To examine this point, three intracellular electrodes were placed into the presynaptic axon at different distances from the giant synapse, the TEA pipette being farthest away.

Results of such experiments are illustrated in Figs. 12–14. Figure 12 was obtained at low calcium concentration (5·5 mm). In $A$ and $B$, recording was at the start of the synapse ($a$) and at 625 $\mu$ upstream ($b$), while the stimulus was applied through the TEA pipette, 1175 $\mu$ from the site of the

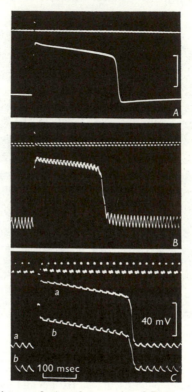

Fig. 11. Membrane resistance during plateau. $A$ and $B$, 55 mm-Ca. Record $A$ shows 'unmodulated' response to brief pulse (monitored in top trace). Record $B$ shows response with hyperpolarizing pulse modulation. $C$: from another preparation. 45 mm-Ca. Simultaneous recording at start of synaptic contact ($a$), and 625 $\mu$ 'upstream' ($b$). The pulse pipette was farther upstream (1175 $\mu$ from $a$). The upper vertical scale applies to all records except $C(a)$, and represents 1·76 $\mu$A and 40 mV. The lower scale (40 mV) refers to record $C(a)$.

synapse. In $A$, the pulse was just 'below threshold'. The difference between the two records reflects mainly the ordinary electrotonic attenuation, from $b$ to $a$. In $B$, a local response develops and outlasts the pulse. The response is clearly larger at $a$ than at $b$, i.e. the attenuation is now in the reverse direction. In $C$, the connexions of the stimulating and the lower recording electrode were interchanged, i.e. the upper record is obtained as before, at the synapse, while the lower record is now 1175 $\mu$ (instead of 625 $\mu$) away. The response is attenuated much more severely, again in the upstream direction.

Similar results, with higher calcium concentrations, are shown in Figs. 13 and 14. In every case the response measured after the end of the current pulse is largest at the synaptic contact, and reduced in size as the recording is moved upstream. Examination of the modulating potentials

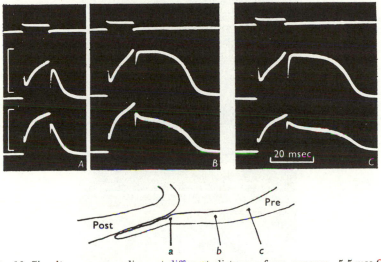

Fig. 12. Simultaneous recordings at different distances from synapse. 5·5 mM-Ca. Top trace in each block shows current pulse. Pulse in $A$ is just 'subthreshold'; in $B$ and $C$ 'above threshold'. Middle trace: recorded at start of synapse (position $a$ in diagram). Bottom trace: in $A$ and $B$, at 625 $\mu$ from synapse (position $b$); in $C$, at 1175 $\mu$ from synapse (position $c$). Upper scale represents 1·83 $\mu$A (top) and 40 mV (middle trace). Lower scale: 40 mV (bottom trace).

in Fig. 11 $C$ shows that the reduction in membrane time constant is more severe at the synapse than at the 625 $\mu$ position upstream, in spite of the fact that the pulses were applied even further upstream. This indicates that the lowering of membrane resistance is most pronounced at the synaptic contact region.

The superimposed tracings in Fig. 14 illustrate even more clearly the electrotonic decrement of a 'subthreshold' depolarization, from $b$ to $a$, and the even more severe *reverse* decrement of the 'superthreshold' response, from $a$ to $b$. It seems possible that the active process may be confined entirely to the synaptic region of the terminals, and that the upstream decrement from $a$ to $b$ is purely passive. It would, however, be difficult to exclude the alternative possibility, namely that some active reinforcement occurs all along the terminal branches, but with a very steep spatial gradient and a high peak of activity in the synapse itself.

### Fractionation of the local response

The pre-axon divides into 8–11 terminal branches (Young, 1939), each of which forms a synaptic contact with the main motor axon of the corresponding stellar nerve. Presumably a local response is elicited at each of these synaptic endings, though the largest terminals (in the last stellar

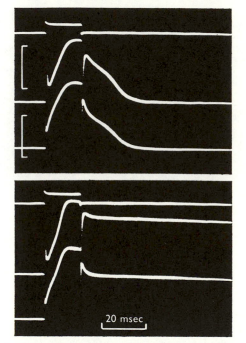

Fig. 13. Effect of calcium on TEA-treated terminal. The bath concentration was changed from 5·5 mM-Ca (top recording) towards 45 mM. The lower block was obtained several minutes after changing the perfusion fluid to higher calcium. Simultaneous recording at start of synapse (middle trace in each block) and 625 $\mu$ upstream (lower trace). Upper scale represents 1·83 $\mu$A and 40 mV (synaptic recording); lower scale 40 mV (upstream recording).

nerves) would make the chief contribution and probably act as pacemaker to the others. Normally, therefore, with the recording electrode placed near the largest synapse, one would expect to obtain a relatively simple wave form of the response dominated by the activity of the nearby 'giant terminal'. Frequently, however, there were indications of a step in the final decline of the potential, suggesting that the response was not cut off simultaneously in all the terminals. Furthermore, during deterioration the response was found in some experiments to break up into two or three

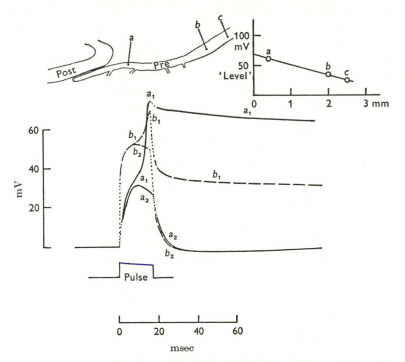

Fig. 14. Superimposed tracings of records obtained at position *a* (0·4 mm from synapse) and *b* (2 mm from synapse). Two pulses, one just below and one above 'threshold', were applied through the TEA pipette, at position *c*. The sub-threshold potentials show a decrement from *b* to *a*, the level of the response shows opposite decrement, from *a* to *b*. Diagram at top left shows positions of intracellular presynaptic electrodes. Inset diagram at top right shows the decrement of response levels, recorded at *a*, *b* and *c*.

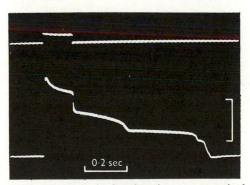

Fig. 15. Fractionation of response in deteriorating axon terminal. Local response to a large pulse is shown. It has several discrete 'steps' on its falling phase. 50 mM-Ca. Resting potential 60 mV. Vertical scale represents 0·88 $\mu$A and 40 mV.

steps of different duration and amplitude. An extreme example of this fractionation is shown in Fig. 15. The explanation is probably that the response deteriorated first at the large terminal nearest the electrode, and its duration there became shorter than at the more distant, smaller terminal branches. The fact that the response breaks into discrete fragments provides further evidence for the conclusion that the activity originates, or at least is concentrated, in discrete synaptic contact areas.

### Presynaptic response and transmitter release

The findings up to this point may be summarized by saying that a regenerative reinforcement of membrane depolarization, resistant to TTX, is found to be localized in the terminal region of the presynaptic axon, i.e. in the area in which transmitter release occurs.

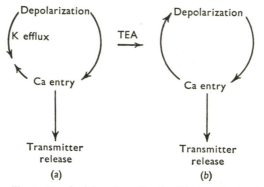

Fig. 16. Diagram illustrating 'calcium hypothesis'. This applies to the presynaptic terminal treated with TTX.

It is natural to look for a link between these two processes, and the most obvious suggestion is the one made at the outset, namely that both, electric reinforcement and transmitter release, depend on influx of calcium which is turned on by the primary depolarization.

The hypothesis, presented diagrammatically in Fig. 16, is that the regenerative effect of calcium entry is normally opposed by potassium efflux (a), and that TEA, by reducing potassium flux, removes this blockage (b). In either situation, with or without TEA, the rate of calcium entry is controlled by the membrane potential, and the calcium influx in turn controls the rate of transmitter release.

*Regeneration and input/output relation.* On this hypothesis the transmitter release is reinforced by the regenerative cycle, but only as a side effect, via the reinforced depolarization. Taking the scheme in its bare outline, there would be no reason why the 'input/output' relation (i.e. the relation between presynaptic potential change and post-synaptic response) should be altered by TEA and its regenerative effect.

In actual fact, however, as pointed out earlier (Katz & Miledi, 1967*b*, *e*; 1968), the transmitter output depends not only on the amplitude of the recorded presynaptic potential, but also on its time course and on the electrotonic decrement between the sites of recording and of transmitter release. Both features are altered by TEA, and it is therefore not surprising that the input/output relation becomes steeper after TEA injection (Fig. 17). This was seen even with small doses of TEA which were not sufficient to produce a clear regenerative potential change. In the case of

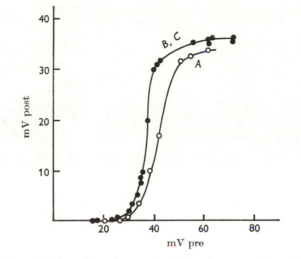

Fig. 17. Effect of TEA on 'input/output' relation of synapse. 50 mM-Ca throughout. *A*, before TEA injection; *B* and *C*, after two and three successive doses of TEA. Pulse duration 12–15 msec. Ordinate: peak amplitude of post-synaptic response. Abscissa: peak amplitude of presynaptic potential. Presynaptic recording electrode just within synaptic region.

Fig. 17, adding more TEA caused no further increase in the slope of the input/output curve, and eventually a decline in the post-synaptic response supervened.

Another important point arises from the results showing the localized nature of the response. Suppose a transient regenerative reinforcement occurs, confined to the distal part of a single terminal. This would be recorded upstream only in greatly attenuated form, but it could lead to a large increase in transmitter release and so produce a steep increment in the observed input/output curve.

In calcium-rich solutions, when a large regenerative response had developed, its relation to transmitter release showed a number of divergent as well as parallel features. In general the 'threshold depolarization' for a local regenerative response was higher than that for transmitter release, so that post-synaptic potentials of small to moderate size could be evoked without presynaptic regeneration, or preceding the latter in time. As the preparation deteriorated, however, the situation sometimes reversed, and it then appeared that a post-synaptic potential could only be elicited when the threshold for presynaptic reinforcement was exceeded.

There was a large difference between pre- and post-synaptic responses in the rate of 'fatigue' or 'inactivation'. This shows up in two ways: (i) the post-synaptic potential usually died out long before the plateau of

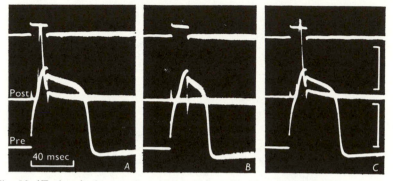

Fig. 18. 'Fatigue' of synaptic transfer. 50 mM-Ca. The three blocks, from left to right, show responses to identical pulses. *A*, rested preparation; *B*, pulse repeated 1·2 sec after *A*; *C*, after 5 min rest. In each block: current pulse (top); post-synaptic response (middle); presynaptic response (bottom). Upper vertical scale: 0·92 $\mu$A and 20 mV (post); lower scale: 40 mV (pre).

the presynaptic response came to an end; (ii) when pulses were repeated at intervals of a few seconds, the presynaptic response shortened in duration (Figs. 4, 18), but the post-synaptic potential was reduced much more drastically, and at times was practically abolished (Fig. 18). The exact site of this striking inactivation cannot at present be ascertained, but very probably it occurs on the presynaptic side and involves a failure of transmitter release. In the terms of our hypothesis, one might suggest that this inactivation is a secondary effect resulting from internal accumulation of calcium during prolonged regenerative current flow.

That the 'inactivation' of the synaptic transfer process (Fig. 18) is not simply due to *post-synaptic* changes (e.g. desensitization) is indicated by the fact that large responses can be repeated at much shorter intervals provided the presynaptic depolarizations are brief pulses (see figs. 17 and 18 in Katz & Miledi, 1967*e*) and not prolonged as in Fig. 18. On the other hand, the synaptic 'fatigue' cannot be attributed to the long-lasting presynaptic potential change *by itself*, for if one raises the potential to the suppression level (and thereby presumably prevents calcium influx) this level can be maintained for several seconds without greatly diminishing the large off-response which occurs at the end of the applied current (unpublished observations). These findings support the suggestion that the presynaptic inactivation probably results from prolonged influx and accumulation of calcium on the inside of the membrane.

## Effects of ionic changes

In order to obtain more evidence on the mechanism of the TTX-resistant response, various changes in the ionic environment were made, and their effects on the level ($V_{a, b}$) and duration ($T$) of the regenerative potential were determined.

*Calcium.* The dependence of the presynaptic reinforcement on the external calcium concentration has already been described and is summarized in Table 1. No great accuracy can be claimed for the values of the levels $V_a$ and $V_b$, as these are affected to some extent by attenuation (over the small distances stated in Table 1) and by other variables such as the internal TEA concentration. Nevertheless, in a qualitative way, these results support the calcium hypothesis. It should be noted that the values of $V_b$ do not represent calcium equilibrium potentials, but levels at which calcium (or other cation) influx is balanced by potassium efflux plus, possibly, chloride influx (see Discussion). The calcium equilibrium level is at a much higher, inside-positive, potential, and on our hypothesis could be estimated by determining the potential at which transmitter release is completely suppressed (see Katz & Miledi, 1967e).

*Strontium and barium.* Both strontium ions and barium ions were effective substitutes for calcium ions and enabled large and prolonged regenerative responses to be produced in the presynaptic terminal. When 50 mM-Sr was added to a calcium-free solution, a response of 0·7 sec duration was obtained; in another experiment, with 80 mM-Sr, the value of $T$ reached 2 sec. With 50 mM-Ba an even larger response, of 6·5 sec duration, was recorded. Strontium and barium are also able, though much less effectively, to substitute for calcium in the release of the transmitter. This aspect will be dealt with in a later paper.

*Magnesium and manganese.* Both magnesium ions and manganese ions were found to act as calcium antagonists and caused the response to be shortened appreciably. The effect of magnesium was comparatively weak, that of manganese quite strong. The concentration of magnesium in the normal bath was 54 mM; raising it to 151 mM, in the presence of 11 mM-Ca, caused $T$ to drop from 124 to 4 msec. In this experiment the recovery (on returning to 54 mM-Mg) was very slow and incomplete: after 75 min $T$ had increased to only 7 msec; perfusion was then switched to a magnesium-free solution which caused $T$ to rise to 100 msec. In another experiment, at half the normal calcium (5·5 mM) and normal magnesium (54 mM), $T$ was 3·3 msec, and increased to 9·6 msec when a magnesium-free solution was substituted.

In two experiments an equimolar concentration of manganese ions was added to a calcium-rich solution (both at 40 or 50 mM). This caused the duration of the regenerative response to drop, reversibly, to a small fraction (from 430 to 19 msec in one, and from 110 to 2·3 msec in the other experiment). Manganese also caused a marked reduction in the synaptic output which will be described elsewhere.

To summarize, the effects of the divalent ions resemble the actions which have been reported for other calcium-dependent processes, in particular the action potential of crustacean muscle (Fatt & Ginsborg, 1958; Hagiwara & Nakajima, 1966) in which strontium and barium are strong synergists, manganese is a strong antagonist, and magnesium has been described as 'inert'.

*Sodium withdrawal.* The calcium hypothesis (Fig. 16) would be greatly strengthened if it could be shown that no other external cation is required, and that the regenerative response still occurs after complete withdrawal of external sodium. A number of experiments were made in which sodium was replaced by either sucrose, or choline or calcium ions.

In one experiment, illustrated in Fig. 19, the isolated ganglion was immersed in a solution whose sodium and magnesium contents had been entirely replaced by calcium. Intracellular electrodes were then inserted. Following the injection of TEA a large local response, of 75 msec duration, was obtained as late as 90 min after the change of the bath, but thereafter the presynaptic response failed. The post-synaptic response had disappeared earlier, within about 1 hr.

In another experiment the preparation was kept in a solution 95 % of whose sodium content had been replaced by choline. In this case a local response of about 10 msec duration could still be recorded after $2\frac{1}{2}$ hours, but then it gradually declined.

In other experiments the intracellular electrodes were introduced in the normal ionic medium, and the effects of changing the perfusion fluid to a sodium-deficient solution were followed. Again, the presynaptic response persisted or even increased in size during the first hour, but it did not survive indefinitely and disappeared after 1–2 hours exposure to the sodium-free solution (see e.g. Fig. 20). The effect always came on slowly, and reversibility after return to high sodium was also slow and usually incomplete. In one case the calcium concentration was raised from 2 to 40 mM, 65 min after the bath had been perfused with a solution containing choline instead of sodium. As a result, a local response began to appear in the pre-fibre within 30 min and built up to over 150 msec in duration during the next 40 min, but declined thereafter.

The interpretation of these results is made difficult in view of the slow clearance of extracellular spaces in the stellate ganglion (see Miledi & Slater, 1966; Katz & Miledi, 1967e). Nevertheless, the delayed abolition and the delayed recovery cannot *both* be attributed to slow extracellular equilibration: for if the delayed extinction were due simply to the long time it takes for the interstitial sodium to fall below a certain level, then this level would be exceeded very quickly and recovery should be rapid on readmission of the high-sodium bath. It is more likely that sodium deprivation has a slow protracted action on the nerve terminal, possibly

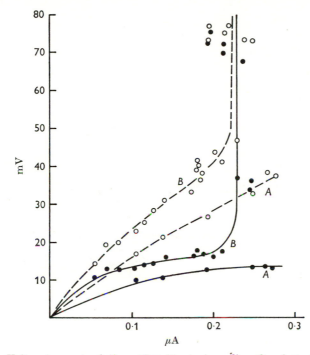

Fig. 19. Voltage/current relation, after 90 min in sodium-free isotonic calcium solution. Filled circles and continuous lines: final potentials (pulse durations 17 msec in *A*, 32 msec in *B*). Open circles and dashed lines: peak potentials. *A*, before TEA; *B*, after TEA injection. Ordinate: presynaptic potential change, mV. Abscissa: current intensity.

(see Blaustein & Hodgkin, 1968) by blocking calcium extrusion and allowing gradual accumulation of calcium to occur inside the terminals.

To summarize, while presynaptic responses could be obtained for a certain length of time in sodium-free solutions, the present experiments on sodium withdrawal complicate the issue, and make the acceptance of the calcium hypothesis more difficult. In view of recent work on the interaction between sodium and calcium fluxes across the axon membrane (Baker, Blaustein, Hodgkin & Steinhardt, 1967; Blaustein & Hodgkin, 1968), one may envisage ways of resolving the difficulties, but further evidence will be needed to test these possibilities.

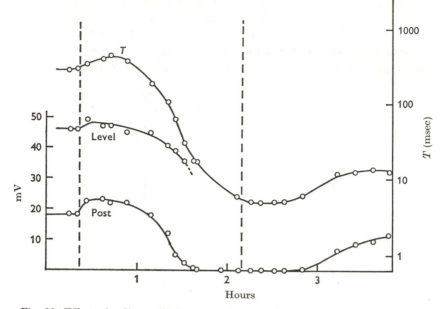

Fig. 20. Effect of sodium withdrawal on duration $T$ (top), level $V_a$ (middle) and post-synaptic response (bottom curve). Ordinate: left scale, mV; right scale, msec (log. scale). Abscissa: time in hours. 11 mM-Ca. TEA injected. At first dashed vertical line, perfusion was switched from sodium to choline. At second dashed line, perfusion returned to sodium.

### DISCUSSION

The observations described in this paper raise a number of interesting problems.

A local electric response has been found which is apparently restricted to the terminal parts of the presynaptic axon, under conditions of complete TTX paralysis of the main parts of the afferent and efferent neurones. The response may, of course, not be totally resistant to TTX, but the doses used were 100 times larger than what is needed to block axonic propagation. Apart from TTX-resistance, the effects and interactions of various divalent cations (Ca, Sr, Ba, Mg, Mn) suggest that the situation is analogous to the electric activity of crustacean muscle fibres in which calcium (or Sr, Ba) inward current appears to be the dominant factor (Fatt & Ginsborg, 1958; Hagiwara & Nakajima, 1966). The situation differs from crustacean muscle in that presence of sodium is needed, at least for long-term maintenance of the presynaptic response.

In the squid axon, Hodgkin & Keynes (1957) observed a small influx of calcium (2–3 % of that of sodium) during periods of impulse activity, and it has been suggested that this may be the basis of the 'calcium action potential' which Watanabe, Tasaki, Singer & Lerman (1967) obtained from the giant axon (after internal perfusion with caesium fluoride and exposure to a 200 mM-CaCl$_2$ solution). This response differs from, and is probably not related to, the one described in the present paper, for it is readily blocked by TTX (Watanabe *et al.* 1967), besides the fact that it occurs in the post-synaptic axon.

A phenomenon somewhat similar to that described here has been observed at the frog nerve–muscle junction (Katz & Miledi, 1967*b*, p. 35, and unpublished results). After TTX-paralysis, treatment with TEA enables one to elicit an 'all-or-none' type of post-synaptic response to a brief pulse applied to the terminal part of the motor axon. This response still occurs after the preparation has been kept for some hours in a sodium-free, isotonic CaCl$_2$ solution. Eventually, however, the response declines irreversibly. There is no doubt that in this case the response survives long beyond the time needed for extracellular equilibration and sodium clearance. The ultimate failure must therefore be attributed to some other change, possibly gradual accumulation of calcium inside the terminals. We have suggested that the refractoriness of transmitter release which follows a large presynaptic response (Fig. 18) may be due to intracellular calcium accumulation, and that recovery depends on elimination and extrusion of calcium from the terminal. There is evidence (Blaustein & Hodgkin, 1968) that calcium extrusion is coupled to sodium influx and becomes greatly reduced when the external sodium concentration is lowered. It is conceivable therefore that the delayed inactivation of the presynaptic response which occurs in a sodium-deficient medium is the result of slow, progressive accumulation of calcium inside the terminal.

An alternative explanation for a somewhat similar case has recently been proposed by Banks, Biggins, Bishop, Christian & Currie (1969). Their argument is based on the fact that the rate of calcium influx through the axon membrane depends on the *intracellular* sodium concentration (Baker *et al.* 1967). In a sodium-free medium there would be a gradual loss of sodium from the cell, which might in turn lead to delayed inactivation of a process which depends on calcium entry.

Thus, while the results can be said to remain compatible with the calcium hypothesis, the description of the roles which sodium and calcium play in the production of the presynaptic response remains uncertain. We shall continue the discussion on the assumption that calcium carries the inward current, alone or as a principal partner, while sodium is required for longer-term maintenance of the process.

The next question to consider is the action of TEA. Without application of TEA no trace of a local response was seen in the TTX paralysed axon; all that was seen was the ordinary 'delayed rectification'. This does not mean that calcium inward current is completely absent, but merely that the effect of calcium influx on the membrane potential is overwhelmed by efflux of potassium. It has been suggested (Beaulieu & Frank, 1967 $a$, $b$) that, at the vertebrate nerve–muscle junction, TEA has a specific action facilitating movement of calcium ions through the membrane. This is indeed a possibility which might be used to explain many of our findings, but it does not seem to be a necessary assumption, for the well-established action of TEA in blocking potassium current appears to be sufficient to account for our results.

To take some simplified quantities, let us suppose the level $V_b$ during the local response (Fig. 6) is at zero, and equidistant from the equilibrium potentials $E_K$ and $E_{Ca}$ (approximately, say, $-0.1$ V and $+0.1$ V respectively). Further, take the potassium conductance $g_K$ of the TEA-treated membrane as 1 mmho/cm$^2$. Then, $g_{Ca}$ during the response is also 1 mmho/cm$^2$, and the inward current of calcium $I_{Ca}$ is approximately 0.1 mA/cm$^2$, balancing a similar outward current of potassium. It will be appreciated that this is small compared to the sodium inward current during the normal action potential, or to the potassium outward current in the absence of TEA. It follows, therefore, that the same intensity of calcium current would have little effect on the shape of the action potential (in the absence of both TEA and TTX); moreover, at the normal calcium concentration (11 mM), $I_{Ca}$ would be lower.

In Fig. 21, an attempt has been made to reconstruct schematically the $V/I$ (steady voltage/current) relation for the TEA-treated axon terminal. The underlying assumptions are shown in the inset. They include some obvious oversimplifications, namely (i) the calcium channel is switched on and off in all-or-none manner; (ii) the resistances in the two parallel channels are fixed, and there is no residual rectification; (iii) arbitrary quantities have been chosen for $E_K$, $E_{Ca}$ and the corresponding resistances. A single 'resting' and two 'active states', for different calcium concentrations have been drawn. Points of interest are ($a$) the intercepts between 'active' slopes and vertical axis which correspond to the levels V attained after the end of the applied pulse, ($b$) the intersections between 'resting' and 'active' slopes which correspond to $E_{Ca}$.

$E_{Ca}$ should, *ex hypothesi*, be estimated from the 'suppression potential' (see p. 479, also Katz & Miledi, 1967$e$). This varied between approximately $+70$ and $+140$ mV in different experiments. Attempts were made to measure this level during changes of the calcium concentration, but the results were disappointing, partly because the suppression potential is a difficult 'end-point' to determine and mainly because it was not easy to maintain sufficient stability during the long experiment. In two out of four experiments, there was a significant increase in the suppression potential with increased calcium concentration; in the others no clear change was observed.

The question now arises whether the calcium current, of $10^{-4}$ A/cm$^2$, which is presumed to underly the regenerative response, can be equated to the influx of calcium at the actual transmitter release sites. We may use the information available at the frog nerve–muscle junction to help us in forming a rough estimate. A single, large terminal arborization in frog muscle has a presynaptic surface of approximately $2 \cdot 5 \times 10^{-5}$ cm$^2$ from which about 250 quantal packets of transmitter are released, after arrival

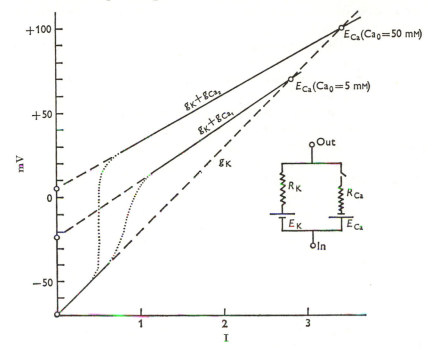

Fig. 21. Theoretical reconstruction of voltage/current relation, making assumptions illustrated in inset diagram. The three slopes represent, successively from below: resting state ($g_K$); active state with 5 mM-Ca ($g_K + g_{Ca_1}$); active state with 50 mM-Ca ($g_K + g_{Ca_2}$). $g_K = 1/R_K$; $g_{Ca} = 1/R_{Ca}$. The significance of the various intersections (marked by circles) is discussed in the text. Ordinate: steady presynaptic membrane potential in mV. Absciscssa: current intensity in relative units. The following values have been chosen: $E_K = -70$ mV, $E_{Ca} = +70$ mV (5 mM-Ca); $+100$ mV (50 mM-Ca). $R_{Ca_1} = 2R_K$ (5 mM-Ca); $R_{Ca_2} = 1 \cdot 25 R_K$ (50 mM-Ca).

of a nerve impulse, within a period of approximately 1 msec. This gives a surface density of transmitter release of about $10^7$ packets/cm$^2$, which may be assumed to apply also to the squid giant synapse (cf. Miledi, 1967, p. 403). If each quantal event requires the simultaneous action of four calcium ions (Dodge & Rahamimoff, 1967), then in our present example 1000 calcium ions can be assumed to have passed through $2 \cdot 5 \times 10^{-5}$ cm$^2$ of presynaptic membrane during 1 msec. This is equivalent to an inward current of only $1.3 \times 10^{-8} \text{A/cm}^2$, i.e. $0.01\%$ of the intensity required for the regenerative presynaptic potential.

It appears that the membrane current associated with the entry of those calcium ions which are *directly* involved in the process of release is immeasurably small. Nevertheless, this very small current may be part of the same process which leads to the reinforcement of the presynaptic potential change. The above calculation merely suggests that, for any one calcium ion which enters the terminal, the probability of it contributing to transmitter release is very low. There are many reasons which could account for this: one possibility arises from the suggestion that simultaneous action of several calcium ions is needed for transmitter release at any point (Dodge & Rahamimoff, 1967; Hubbard, Jones & Landau, 1968). Suppose, in order to be effective, four ions must penetrate a single calcium channel almost synchronously, within a period which is, say, one-tenth of the mean interval between *single* random penetrations. In this case, the expected ratio between single ion entries (which contribute to the electric reinforcement, but not to release) and quadruple entries (which are effective in transmitter release) would be about 10,000:1. Another possibility is that only a very small fraction of the membrane area which is available for calcium entry has the special properties required for the subsequent steps in the release mechanism.

We are indebted to the Director and Staff of the Stazione Zoologica, Naples, for research facilities and the supply of squid, and to the Royal Society for financial support of this work.

## REFERENCES

ARMSTRONG, C. M. & BINSTOCK, L. (1965). Anomalous rectification in the squid giant axon injected with tetraethyl ammonium chloride. *J. gen. Physiol.* **48**, 859–872.

BAKER, P. F., BLAUSTEIN, M. P., HODGKIN, A. L. & STEINHARDT, R. A. (1967). The effect of sodium concentration on calcium movements in giant axons of *Loligo forbesi*. *J. Physiol.* **192**, 43–44P.

BANKS, P., BIGGINS, R., BISHOP, R., CHRISTIAN, B. & CURRIE, N. (1969). Monovalent cations and the secretion of catecholamines. *J. Physiol.* **201**, 47–48P.

BEAULIEU, G. & FRANK, G. B. (1967a). Tetraethylammonium-induced contractions of frog's skeletal muscle. II. Effects on intramuscular nerve endings. *Can. J. Physiol. Pharmac.* **45**, 833–844.

BEAULIEU, G. & FRANK, G. B. (1967b). Tetraethylammonium-induced contractions of frog's skeletal muscle. III. Mechanism of action by calcium release. *Can. J. Physiol. Pharmac.* **45**, 845–855.

BLAUSTEIN, M. P. & HODGKIN, A. L. (1968). The effect of cyanide on calcium efflux in squid axons. *J. Physiol.* **198**, 46–48P.

BLOEDEL, J., GAGE, P. W., LLINÁS, R. & QUASTEL, D. M. J. (1966). Transmitter release at the squid giant synapse in the presence of tetrodotoxin. *Nature, Lond.* **212**, 49–50.

DODGE, F. A. & RAHAMIMOFF, R. (1967). Co-operative action of calcium ions in transmitter release at the neuromuscular junction. *J. Physiol.* **193**, 419–432.

FATT, P. & GINSBORG, B. L. (1958). The ionic requirements for the production of action potentials in crustacean muscle fibres. *J. Physiol.* **142**, 516–543.

HAGIWARA, S. & NAKAJIMA, S. (1966). Differences in Na and Ca spikes as examined by application of tetrodotoxin, procaine and manganese ions. *J. gen. Physiol.* **49**, 793–806.

HODGKIN, A. L. & KEYNES, R. D. (1957). Movements of labelled calcium in squid giant axons. *J. Physiol.* **138**, 253–281.

HUBBARD, J. I., JONES, S. F. & LANDAU, E. M. (1968). On the mechanism by which calcium and magnesium affect the release of transmitter by nerve impulses. *J. Physiol.* **196**, 75–86.

KATZ, B. & MILEDI, R. (1965). Release of acetylcholine from a nerve terminal by electric pulses of variable strength and duration. *Nature, Lond.* **207**, 1097–1098.

KATZ, B. & MILEDI, R. (1966). Input–output relation of a single synapse. *Nature, Lond.* **212**, 1242–1245.

KATZ, B. & MILEDI, R. (1967a). Tetrodotoxin and neuromuscular transmission. *Proc. R. Soc.* B **167**, 8–22.

KATZ, B. & MILEDI, R. (1967b). The release of acetylcholine from nerve endings by graded electric pulses. *Proc. R. Soc.* B **167**, 23–38.

KATZ, B. & MILEDI, R. (1967c). On the timing of calcium action during neuro-muscular transmission. *J. Physiol.* **189**, 535–544.

KATZ, B. & MILEDI, R. (1967d). Ionic requirements of synaptic transmitter release. *Nature, Lond.* **215**, 651.

KATZ, B. & MILEDI, R. (1967e). A study of synaptic transmission in the absence of nerve impulses. *J. Physiol.* **192**, 407–436.

KATZ, B. & MILEDI, R. (1968). The role of calcium in neuromuscular facilitation. *J. Physiol.* **195**, 481–492.

KUSANO, K., LIVENGOOD, D. R. & WERMAN, R. (1967). Correlation of transmitter release with membrane properties of the presynaptic fiber of the squid giant synapse. *J. gen. Physiol.* **50**, 2579–2601.

MILEDI, R. (1967). Spontaneous synaptic potentials and quantal release of transmitter in the stellate ganglion of the squid. *J. Physiol.* **192**, 379–406.

MILEDI, R. & SLATER, C. R. (1966). The action of calcium on neuronal synapses in the squid. *J. Physiol.* **184**, 473–498.

WATANABE, A., TASAKI, I., SINGER, I. & LERMAN, L. (1967). Effects of tetrodotoxin on excitability of squid giant axons in sodium-free media. *Science, N.Y.* **155**, 95–97.

YOUNG, J. Z. (1939). Fused neurons and synaptic contacts in the giant nerve fibres of cephalopods. *Phil. Trans. R. Soc.* B **229**, 465–503.

A. D. SMITH,*† W. P. DE POTTER,* E. J. MOERMAN* and
A. F. DE SCHAEPDRYVER*

# RELEASE OF DOPAMINE β-HYDROXYLASE AND CHROMOGRANIN A UPON STIMULATION OF THE SPLENIC NERVE

ABSTRACT. Two proteins present in noradrenergic vesicles of the splenic nerve (dopamine β-hydroxylase and chromogranin A) are released into the perfusate from the spleen when the splenic nerve is stimulated. Experiments in which drugs were added to the perfusion fluid showed that the proteins were released from terminals of the splenic nerve. There was a correlation between the amounts of the proteins released and the quantity of noradrenaline released; and the release process was dependent upon calcium.

It is suggested that the proteins are released from the large dense-cored vesicles present in the terminals of the splenic nerve, and that secretion from these vesicles occurs by exocytosis.

## Introduction

IN addition to their common origin in the neural crest, the adrenergic neuron and the adrenal chromaffin cell share other features. The pathway of biosynthesis of the catecholamines in the two tissues is identical, and in both types of cell the catecholamines are stored in a membrane-limited particle. Some of the characteristic components of the adrenal chromaffin granule have also been found in the noradrenergic vesicles of neurons. Thus, the neuronal vesicles contain ATP (Schümann, 1958; Euler, Lishajko and Stjärne, 1963; Potter and Axelrod, 1963; De Potter, De Schaepdryver and Smith, 1970), dopamine β-hydroxylase (Potter, 1967; Stjärne, Roth and Lishajko, 1967; Austin, Livett and Chubb, 1967; Hörtnagl, Hörtnagl and Winkler, 1969; De Potter et al., 1970) and the acidic protein chromo-

granin A (Banks, Helle and Mayor, 1969; De Potter et al., 1970).

The identification of specific components of the adrenal chromaffin granule led to the elucidation of the subcellular mechanism involved in the release of catecholamines from the adrenal medulla (for reviews see Douglas, 1968; Smith, 1968; Kirshner, 1969). The secretion of the hormones is accompanied by the quantitative release of the other soluble constituents of the chromaffin granule, i.e. ATP and several soluble proteins (the chromogranins) including chromogranin A and dopamine β-hydroxylase. The release of the soluble proteins of chromaffin granules is not accompanied by that of the lipid components of the granule membrane (Poisner, Trifaró and Douglas, 1967; Malamed, Poisner, Trifaró and Douglas, 1967; Schneider, Smith and Winkler, 1967) or by that of the membrane-bound dopamine β-hydroxylase (Viveros, Arqueros and Kirshner, 1969). These observations, together with electron microscopic evidence (see Diner, 1967) support the hypothesis that the release of catecholamines

* Heymans Institute of Pharmacology, University of Ghent, 9000 Ghent, Belgium.
† Present Address Department of Pharmacology, University of Oxford, Oxford OX1 3QT.

Received 9 June 1970.

Reprinted from *Tissue and Cell* 2: 547–568 (1970) by permission of the publisher, Longman Group Ltd.

from the adrenal medulla takes place by exocytosis, i.e. by fusion of the chromaffin granule membrane with the plasma membrane followed by the formation of an opening into the extracellular space.

The release of noradrenaline from sympathetic neurons requires calcium ions (Huković and Muscholl, 1962; Kirpekar and Misu, 1967) just as does secretion from the adrenal medulla (see Douglas, 1968). Indeed, calcium ions are required for secretion from several tissues, such as exocrine glands, endocrine glands, platelets and polymorphonuclear leucocytes (for reviews see Stormorken, 1969; and Banks, 1970) where there is morphological evidence of release by exocytosis. The work described in this paper was carried out to see whether more direct evidence of exocytosis in sympathetic neurons could be obtained. We have looked for the release from the spleen of two of the proteins which are characteristic components of the noradrenergic vesicle of the splenic nerve. Preliminary reports of some of these observations have been published (De Potter, Moerman, De Schaepdryver and Smith, 1969; De Potter, De Schaepdryver, Moerman and Smith, 1969).

## Methods

### Perfusion experiments

The isolated spleen of the dog was perfused with Tyrode's solution (37°C) at a flow rate of 20 ml/min. as described by Delaunois, Moerman and De Schaepdryver (1968). After perfusion of the spleen for 90 min., the perfusate was collected for a 6 min. control period and also during the next 6 min. when the splenic nerve was stimulated supramaximally at 30 stimuli/sec. Each stimulus lasted 2 msec., and the trains of stimuli were applied for periods of 10 sec., once a minute for 3 min. In some experiments, the perfusate was collected during one or more 6 min. periods following the stimulation period. The spleen was perfused for at least 24 min in between the periods of stimulation. Perfusates were collected in containers standing in an ice-bath.

Calf spleens, together with their vascular and nerve supply, were obtained from the slaughterhouse within 15 min. of the death of the animal, placed on ice and transported to the laboratory. Perfusion with Tyrode's solution (37°C) was carried out in an apparatus similar to that used for dog spleens except that the flow rate was 60 ml/min. After perfusion of the spleen for 2 h, with occasional short periods of stimulation, the perfusate was collected from the vein for a 5 min. control period and during the following 5 min. when the splenic nerve was stimulated supramaximally at 30 stimuli/sec. Each stimulus lasted 2 msec., and trains of stimuli were applied for 20 sec. once a minute for 3 min. The spleen was perfused for at least 30 min. in between periods of stimulation. During the experiments, the perfusion pressure was recorded (Delaunois et al., 1968) in order to obtain an indication of the efficiency of stimulation.

### Analysis of perfusates

An aliquot of each perfusate was mixed with perchloric acid (final concentration 0·4 N), the sediment was removed and the noradrenaline in the supernatant was separated by ion-exchange chromatography (Bertler, Carlsson and Rosengren, 1958; Sharman, Vanov and Vogt, 1962) and estimated fluorimetrically (Laverty and Taylor, 1968). The protein in the precipitate was estimated by the method of Lowry, Rosebrough, Far and Randall (1951).

Enzymic and antigenic activities in the perfusate were estimated on samples which had first been centrifuged (6000 g, for 8 min. at 2°C) to remove any blood cells present, and then concentrated 100–200 fold by ultrafiltration at 2°C. The ultrafiltration apparatus was based on the design described by Sober, Gutter, Wyckoff and Peterson (1956) using Visking dialysis tubing (8/32). After ultrafiltration, the concentrated perfusates were dialysed for 2 h at 2°C against 5 mM potassium phosphate buffer pH 6·0, and then centrifuged at 59,360 $g_{av}$ for 90 min. to remove traces of insoluble matter. Aliquots of the supernatants (0·05–0·2 ml) were assayed for dopamine β-hydroxylase activity using [³H] tyramine as substrate (Friedman and Kaufman, 1965): the composition of the incubation mixture and the units used to express the enzymic activity were given in the preceding paper (De Potter et al., 1970). Dopa decarboxylase activity in the perfusates was determined by the radiochemical method of Laduron and Belpaire (1968a).

Samples of up to 0·2 ml of the concentrated perfusates were assayed for antigenic material which cross-reacted with rabbit antiserum to bovine adrenal chromogranin A. The preparation of the antigen and antiserum was carried out by the methods described previously (Smith and Winkler, 1967; Schneider, Smith and Winkler, 1967); purification and analysis of the antiserum has been described in the preceding paper (De Potter et al., 1970). Perfusates were heated at 56°C for 30 min. prior to assay, in order to destroy any complement. Each sample of the perfusate was tested for anti-complementary activity by carrying out the standard complement-fixation test in the absence of antiserum. The antigenic material is expressed as μg of chromogranin A required to fix the same amount of complement.

Polyacrylamide gel electrophoresis of samples of the concentrated perfusates was done by the method of Clarke (1964) with the modification that the gels were pre-run for 45 min. with the gel buffer in the electrode compartments. After application of the sample, electrophoresis was carried out for 20 min. at 1 mA per tube. The gels were sliced into pieces (0.5 cm), each of which was extracted with 1 ml of 5 mM potassium phosphate buffer, pH 6·0, at 2°C for 18 h. The supernatants were assayed for dopamine β-hydroxylase activity.

Relative sedimentation rates of enzymes in the perfusate and in fractions of bovine splenic nerve were determined by centrifugation of the samples in a stabilising sucrose density gradient (5 ml). The linear gradient ranged from 0·36 M to 0·82 M-sucrose containing 5 mM potassium phosphate buffer pH 6·0. The tubes were centrifuged for 11 h at 99,972 $g_{av}$ in the SW39 head of the Spinco ultracentrifuge. The samples applied to the gradient were mixed with 4000 units of bovine liver catalase, which served as a marker protein. The samples from bovine splenic nerve were obtained by differential centrifugation as described in the preceding paper (De Potter et al., 1970): fraction 3 was used as a source of noradrenergic vesicles, which were lysed by osmotic shock as described in the latter paper.

*Materials*

U[³H] tyramine and 2-[¹⁴C] dopa were purchased from NEN Chemicals, Boston, Mass. ATP (di-sodium) and bovine liver catalase were obtained from Sigma Chemicals, London. Oxoid complement fixation test diluent tablets (BR 16) were used in the immunochemical experiments.

## Results

*Release of noradrenaline, dopamine β-hydroxylase and chromogranin A from the spleen*

*Experiments with dog spleen.* In perfusates collected from the dog spleen during control periods, the amounts of noradrenaline were usually below 2 n moles, close to the limit of sensitivity of the assay method. Dopamine β-hydroxylase activity was also close to, or below, the limit of sensitivity (10 units) of the method. Stimulation of the splenic nerve caused a release of 20 to 36 n moles of noradrenaline and of 38 to 196 units of dopamine β-hydroxylase activity. The results of 4 experiments are given in Table 1. In the fourth experiment the spleen was perfused with calcium-free Tyrode's solution for 24 min. before the second stimulation period: the omission of calcium caused a reversible inhibition of the release of both noradrenaline and dopamine β-hydroxylase.

Analysis of perfusates collected after stimulation of the nerve showed that the release of dopamine β-hydroxylase activity into the perfusate lasted longer than that of noradrenaline (see Fig. 1): the noradrenaline content of the perfusate had fallen almost to the control level in the first collection period after stimulation.

The effect of two drugs on the release of noradrenaline and dopamine $\beta$-hydroxylase was studied. Perfusion of the spleen with hexamethonium bromide (0·1 and 1·4 mM) for 20 min before, as well as during, stimulation of the nerve did not decrease the release of either substance; indeed, the higher concentration of hexamethonium increased the release of both noradrenaline (by 35%) and dopamine $\beta$-hydroxylase (by 40%). When the perfusate contained phenoxybenzamine (0·01 mM) the spleen failed to contract upon stimulation of the nerve, but both noradrenaline and dopamine $\beta$-hydroxylase were still released into the perfusate.

In 9 experiments, the mean ratio of dopamine $\beta$-hydroxylase activity (units) to noradrenaline (n moles) in the perfusate was $3·25 \pm 1·2$ (S.D.). This ratio was also determined in a homogenate of dog splenic nerve: a value of 250 was found.

*Experiments with calf spleen.* The finding that stimulation of the splenic nerve caused the release of dopamine $\beta$-hydroxylase into perfusates of dog spleen led us to look for this enzyme, and for the acidic protein chromogranin A, in perfusates of the calf spleen. The bovine spleen was chosen because we had antiserum to bovine adrenal chromogranin A. Control period perfusates contained undetectable amounts of dopamine $\beta$-hydroxylase activity ($<10$ units) and of antigenic material reacting with antiserum to chromogranin A ($<0·025 \mu$g), and less than 2 n moles of noradrenaline. Perfusates collected during 11 stimulation periods (6 separate spleens) contained 12–82 n-moles of noradrenaline and 73–460 units of dopamine $\beta$-hydroxylase activity. These perfusates also contained antigenic material equivalent to $0·06-0·21 \mu$g of chromogranin A. The substance in the perfusate which reacted with antiserum to chromogranin A no longer did so when the antiserum had been pre-incubated with chromogranin A purified (Smith and Winkler, 1967) from bovine adrenal chromaffin granules.

Calcium was required for the release of noradrenaline and dopamine $\beta$-hydroxylase from the dog spleen, and Fig. 2 shows that this is also so for the calf spleen; furthermore, the release of chromagranin A was inhibited in calcium-free Tyrode's solution. Other treatments failed to block the release of the two proteins or of noradrenaline. The experiment illustrated in Fig. 3 shows that even when a high concentration (3 mM) of hexamethonium bromide was present in the perfusion fluid, the release of the three substances was not prevented: on the contrary, it was potentiated. In another experiment atropine ($29 \mu$M) as well as hexamethonium (3 mM) was added to the perfusion fluid but stimulation of the splenic nerve still released noradrenaline (21 n moles), dopamine $\beta$-hydroxylase (123 units) and chromogranin A ($0·07 \mu$g). Continuous perfusion of the spleen with phenoxybenzamine (0·05 mM) completely prevented contraction of the spleen but, as shown in Fig. 3, did not prevent the release of the two proteins and actually increased the amount of noradrenaline in the perfusate.

Can noradrenaline itself cause the release of dopamine $\beta$-hydroxylase into the perfusate? The experiment illustrated in Fig. 4 was carried out to answer this question. In this experiment the total plasma protein (Folin-reactive) was measured in the perfusates since it had been noticed that, even after prolonged perfusion, some residual blood was expelled into the perfusate when the spleen contracted. Stimulation of the splenic nerve caused the release of large amounts of noradrenaline and of dopamine $\beta$-hydroxylase into the perfusate, together with 20 mg of plasma protein (see Fig. 4). One hour later, the perfusate still contained some protein, but no detectable noradrenaline or dopamine $\beta$-hydroxylase. Noradrenaline (116 n moles) was then injected in four equal doses, which caused the spleen to contract violently. Although the contraction was accompanied by the expulsion of 17 mg of protein, there was only a very small rise in dopamine $\beta$-hydroxylase activity in the

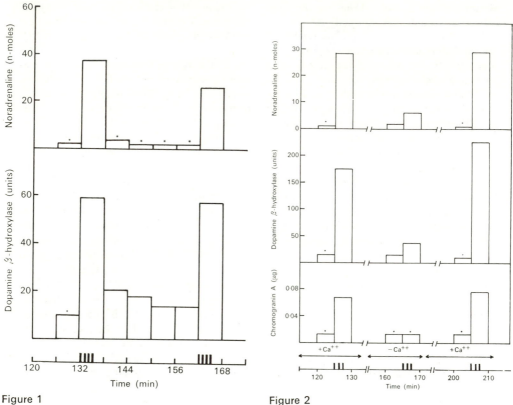

Figure 1

Figure 2

Fig. 1. Release of noradrenaline and of dopamine β-hydroxylase activity from dog spleen. The heights of the columns represent the amounts of enzymic activity and noradrenaline in perfusates collected for 6 min. periods before, during and after stimulation of the splenic nerve at 30/sec. The periods of stimulation are indicated by thick vertical bars on the abscissa. An asterisk above a column shows that the perfusate contained an undetectable amount of the substance; the height of the column represents the least amount which could have been detected.

Fig. 2. Requirement for calcium in the release of noradrenaline, dopamine β-hydroxylase and chromogranin A from calf spleen. The splenic nerve was stimulated at 30/sec at the times indicated by thick vertical lines on the abscissa. The spleen was perfused with calcium-free Tyrode's solution before and during the second stimulation period. An asterisk above a column shows that the perfusate contained an undetectable amount of the substance; the height of the column represents the least amount which could have been detected.

perfusate. Nearly 30% of the infused noradrenaline was recovered in the perfusate. Subsequent stimulation of the splenic nerve caused the release of a large amount of dopamine β-hydroxylase activity.

To see whether there is any correlation between the amounts of each protein released and the amounts of noradrenaline released in the absence of drugs, the results of 9 experiments have been plotted in Fig. 5, and analyzed for significance. There is a highly significant ($P < 0.001$) correlation between the amounts of dopamine β-hydroxylase and noradrenaline in the perfusates, and a similar good correlation ($P < 0.005$) between the amounts of chromogranin A and noradrenaline. The mean of the ratio of dopamine β-hydroxylase activity (units) to noradrenaline (n moles) was $6.77 \pm 1.84$ (S.D.) and that of the ratio chromogranin A ($\mu g$) to noradrenaline was $0.002 \pm 0.001$.

*Dopa decarboxylase.* A sensitive radiochemical method of assay for this enzyme (Laduron and Belpaire, 1968a) was applied to samples (up to 0.2 ml) of concentrated perfusates collected from 4 calf-spleens during stimulation of the splenic nerve, but no activity could be detected: the limit of sensitivity of the method was 0.008 units. These perfusates contained from 17 to 64 n moles of noradrenaline.

*Properties of the dopamine β-hydroxylase in perfusates from the spleen*

The release of large amounts of dopamine β-hydroxylase activity from the calf spleen allowed us to study some of the properties of the enzyme: first, it was necessary to confirm that the assay method was measuring the activity of this enzyme and, second, we wished to see whether there were any differences between the enzyme in the perfusates and that in the noradrenergic vesicles of splenic nerve.

(1) The enzyme in perfusates from dog and calf spleen converted [³H] tyramine to [³H] octopamine. The radioactive octopamine was identified by ion-exchange chromatography (Duch, Viveros and Kirshner,

1968) and the amount of [³H] octopamine formed quantitatively accounted for the radioactivity extracted into toluene in the assay procedure used.

(2) The enzymes in dog and calf spleen perfusates showed the typical properties of dopamine β-hydroxylase in crude tissue extracts (see Kaufman and Friedman, 1965; Duch *et al.*, 1968) viz.: they were activated by ATP, *p*-chloromercuribenzoate and by low concentrations of $CuSO_4$; and were inhibited by pre-incubation without catalase, by high concentrations of $CuSO_4$ or by sodium diethyldithiocarbamate.

(3) The effect of pH on the enzymic activities in the perfusates was compared with that on the enzymic activity in the noradrenergic vesicles of the splenic nerves. As can be seen from Fig. 6, there was a marked similarity between the effect of pH on the activity of the enzymes in the perfusates with that on the enzymic activities in the respective splenic nerves.

(4) The electrophoretic mobility of the dopamine β-hydroxylase in calf spleen perfusate was compared with that of the enzymes in the soluble lysates of ox splenic nerve vesicles and ox adrenal chromaffin granules. Polyacrylamide gel electrophoresis of the soluble lysate of adrenal chromaffin granules gave a pattern very similar to that described by Strieder, Ziegler, Winkler and Smith (1968) and, after sectioning and elution of an unstained gel, the dopamine β-hydroxylase activity was found to correspond to the slowest-running band which just precedes the band given by chromogranin A. The enzymic activity was also recovered in this position in gel electropherograms of soluble lysates of splenic nerve vesicles and of the perfusates.

(5) The sedimentation rate of the dopamine β-hydroxylase from the perfusates was determined relative to that of catalase (mol. wt. 248,000) by centrifugation in a stabilizing sucrose gradient. It can be seen from Fig. 7 that dopamine β-hydroxylase sediments slightly less rapidly than catalase, and that there was no difference between the sedimentation rate of the enzyme in the

perfusate and that in the soluble lysate of noradrenergic vesicles.

Also shown in Fig. 7 is the result of an experiment in which the sedimentation rate of dopa decarboxylase from splenic nerve was measured. This enzyme is located in the particle-free supernatant of homogenates of splenic nerve (De Potter et al., 1970). Dopa decarboxylase sedimented more slowly than did dopamine β-hydroxylase: a similar result has been obtained for the dopa decarboxylase and dopamine β-hydroxylase of adrenal medulla (Laduron and Belpaire, 1968a).

## Discussion

How can we be sure that the two proteins released into the perfusate are chromogranin A and dopamine β-hydroxylase? The identification of one of these proteins as chromogranin A depends entirely on immunochemical evidence. The purity of the protein used as antigen to prepare the antiserum has been established by biochemical methods (Smith and Winkler, 1967) but, as already described for a similar preparation (Sage, Smith and Kirshner, 1967), the antiserum cross-reacted with dopamine β-hydroxylase (De Potter et al., 1970). However, the antibodies to dopamine β-hydroxylase could be precipitated by incubation with the purified enzyme (Sage et al., 1967) and the antiserum used in the present work did not cross-react with dopamine β-hydroxylase (De Potter et al., 1970). The specificity of the antiserum, together with the finding that pre-incubation of the antiserum with purified chromogranin A prevented interaction with the antigenic material in the perfusate, shows that the protein in the perfusate is either chromogranin A or a closely related protein.

Identification of the other protein released into the perfusate as dopamine β-hydroxylase is more readily established because its enzymic activity can be measured. Thus, the protein converted tyramine to octopamine, a property of dopamine β-hydroxylase (Kaufman and Friedman, 1965) and several of the biochemical properties of the enzyme were the same as those of the dopamine β-hydroxylase from splenic nerve and adrenal medulla.

### What is the origin of the proteins released into the perfusate?

Proteins released into the perfusate from the spleen upon stimulation of the nerve could have originated from several sites in the organ: (i) extra-adrenal chromaffin cells, (ii) blood pooled in the venous sinuses and red pulp, (iii) unknown sites in the spleen which respond to noradrenaline released from the nerve, (iv) terminals of the splenic nerve.

Stimulation of the splenic nerve in the dog causes the release of acetylcholine, as well as noradrenaline, into the perfusate (Leaders and Dayrit, 1965) and so the possibility has to be considered that the acetycholine is causing the release of catecholamines, dopamine β-hydroxylase and chromogranin A from chromaffin cells.

There is, however, no morphological evidence for the presence of chromaffin cells in the spleen. The fluorescence histochemical method shows that catecholamines are confined to nerve fibres in the spleen of the dog (Dahlström and Zetterström, 1965) and of the cat (Gillespie and Kirpekar, 1966; Fillenz, 1970). The fluorescent nerve fibres in the cat spleen (Gillespie and Kirpekar, 1966) and more than 90% of the noradrenaline in sheep and dog spleens (Euler and Purkhold, 1951; Laduron and Belpaire, 1968b) disappear after degeneration of the splenic nerve. The residual noradrenaline in the denervated spleen is unlikely to be present in chromaffin cells since, in the dog, it is not released by typical chromaffin cell stimulants such as acetylcholine, nicotine and dimethylphenylpiperazinium (de Burgh Daly and Scott, 1961; Leaders and Dayrit, 1965). Furthermore, biochemical studies on the catecholamine-containing particles of dog spleen (De Potter, 1968; Chubb, De Potter and De Schaepdryver, 1970) have not revealed the presence of any particles with the sedimentation properties of typical chromaffin granules.

As a direct test of the possibility that the noradrenaline and proteins were released from chromaffin cells, hexamethonium was added to the perfusion fluid in some experiments. Far from blocking the release of dopamine β-hydroxylase and chromogranin A, hexamethonium (1·4–3·0 mM) increased

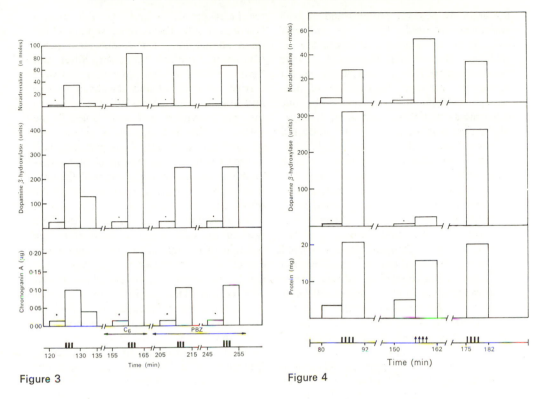

Figure 3

Figure 4

Fig. 3. Effect of hexamethonium and of phenoxybenzamine on the release of noradrenaline, dopamine $\beta$-hydroxylase and chromogranin A from calf spleen. The splenic nerve was stimulated at 30/sec at the times indicated by thick vertical lines on the abscissa. During the times indicated by the symbols $C_6$ and PBZ, hexamethonium (3 mM) and phenoxybenzamine (0·05 mM), respectively, were present in the Tyrode's solution. An asterisk above a column shows that the perfusate contained an undetectable amount of the substance; the height of the column represents the least amount which could have been detected.

Fig. 4. Comparison of the effects of nerve stimulation and infusion of noradrenaline on the release of dopamine $\beta$-hydroxylase from calf spleen. Thick vertical lines on the abscissa indicate periods during which the splenic nerve was stimulated at 30/sec. Vertical arrows on the abscissa indicate the infusion of 29 n-moles of noradrenaline into the spleen. An asterisk above a column indicates that the perfusate contained an undetectable amount of the substance; the height of the column represents the least amount which could have been detected.

287

the amounts of these proteins and of noradrenaline released from dog and calf spleens. It has already been reported by Blakeley, Brown and Ferry (1963) that hexamethonium (28 $\mu$moles/kg body weight) sometimes increased the overflow of noradrenaline from the cat spleen. In our experiments a high concentration of hexamethonium was used in order to produce a complete block of the action of acetylcholine on any chromaffin cells which might have been present. The concentrations used (up to 3 mM) are much higher than those used by other workers. In the dog spleen, hexamethonium (28 $\mu$moles/kg) prevents the contraction of the spleen caused by acetylcholine (de Burgh, Daly and Scott, 1961) and in the cat hexamethonium (28 $\mu$moles/kg) prevented the acetylcholine-induced release of noradrenaline from the spleen (Blakeley et al., 1963). Adrenal chromaffin cells fail to respond to splanchnic nerve stimulation when cats are treated with 1·4 $\mu$moles/kg of hexamethonium (Marley and Paton, 1961) but the presence of atropine (29 $\mu$M) as well as hexamethonium (1·4 mM) appears to be necessary to produce a complete block in the perfused cat adrenal gland (Douglas and Poisner, 1966). In one experiment with the calf spleen, the presence of both hexamethonium (3 mM) and atropine (29 $\mu$M) in the perfusate did not block the release of dopamine $\beta$-hydroxylase or chromogranin A. We conclude that it is unlikely that the chromogranin A and dopamine $\beta$-hydroxylase in the splenic perfusate originate from chromaffin cells.

Although the spleens were perfused with Tyrode's solution for two hours before samples of the perfusate were taken for analysis, a small amount of blood was still present in the tissue and some was ejected when the spleen contracted. Since both chromogranin A and dopamine $\beta$-hydroxylase are released together with catecholamines from the adrenal gland, it is likely that the blood normally contains small amounts of these proteins. It has, in fact, been shown that calf blood contains a protein which cross-reacts with antiserum to chromogranin A and that this protein is released into the adrenal venous blood upon stimulation of the splanchnic nerve (Blaschko, Comline, Schneider, Silver and Smith, 1967). Two kinds of experiment were carried out to see whether the chromogranin and dopamine $\beta$-hydroxylase released from the spleen came from blood pooled in the spleen. In the first type of experiment the spleens (dog and calf) were perfused with Tyrode's solution containing phenoxybenzamine. Although this drug blocked the contraction of the spleen, it did not affect the release of the two proteins. The second type of experiment (see Fig. 4) involved causing the calf spleen to contract by the infusion of noradrenaline: some blood was ejected from the spleen but no more than a trace of dopamine $\beta$-hydroxylase activity was released. These experiments show that most, if not all, of the dopamine $\beta$-hydroxylase released from the spleen does not come from the blood. Furthermore, the experiment in which noradrenaline was added to the perfusate shows that the enzyme is not released from an unknown site in the spleen which is sensitive to the neurotransmitter.

If the dopamine $\beta$-hydroxylase and chromogranin A do not originate from chromaffin cells, from the blood, or from unidentified sites sensitive to noradrenaline, then it is difficult to see where else they could have come from except from the terminals of the splenic nerve. The finding that several of the biochemical properties of the dopamine $\beta$-hydroxylase in the perfusate are identical with those of the enzyme in noradrenergic vesicles of splenic nerve is consistent with this interpretation. However, the similarities between the properties of the enzymes in perfusate and nerve should not be taken as positive evidence for the neural origin of the released dopamine $\beta$-hydroxylase because the adrenal enzyme also has similar properties. Thus, as found in the present work, the nerve and adrenal enzymes have the same mobility in gel electrophoresis and similar pH optima; furthermore, antiserum to adrenal dopamine $\beta$-hydroxylase cross-reacts with sympathetic

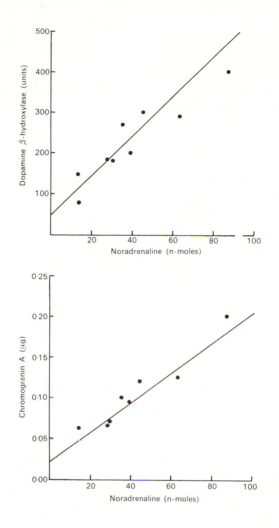

Fig. 5. Correlation between the amounts of dopamine β-hydroxylase, chromogranin A and noradrenaline released from the calf spleen upon stimulation of the nerve. The correlation coefficient for dopamine β-hydroxylase and noradrenaline was 0·95, that for chromogranin A and noradrenaline was 0·92.

nervous tissue (Geffen, Livett and Rush, 1969b).

Perhaps the most convincing evidence for the neural original of the released proteins is that there was such a good correlation between the amounts of the proteins and of noradrenaline in perfusates collected during stimulation of the nerve. This correlation was not only found in the spleens perfused with normal Tyrode's solution, but also when the release was potentiated by hexamethonium and inhibited by lack of calcium. As already pointed out, more than 90% of the noradrenaline in the spleen is present in neurons and so the correlation between the release of noradrenaline and that of the two proteins must either reflect an action of the released noradrenaline on the spleen, which has been excluded, or the common origin of the proteins and the neurotransmitter.

*How are the proteins released from the nerve into the perfusate?*

We not only have to consider how proteins are released from the neuron into the extracellular space, but how they can pass from the extracellular space into the perfusate; the latter question will be discussed first.

In the adrenal medulla, as in other endocrine organs, the proteins secreted from the chromaffin cells probably pass into the blood through fenestrae in the capillary endothelial cells (Elfvin, 1965). Specialized capillaries of this type have not been described in the spleen, and the only other recognized means by which proteins can cross the capillary endothelium are by transport across the cells in vesicles or through endothelial cell junctions (see Karnovsky, 1967). However, in the spleen part of the circulation is open and so material in the red pulp can enter the veins directly without having to cross a layer of smooth muscle and endothelial cells. Fluorescence histochemical studies (Gillespie and Kirpekar, 1966; Fillenz, 1970) have shown that most of the noradrenergic nerves are restricted to smooth muscle of the trabeculae

Table 1. *Release of noradrenaline and dopamine β-hydroxylase from the perfused spleen of the dog.*

| Experiment | Noradrenaline (nmoles) | Dopamine β-hydroxylase (units) |
|---|---|---|
| 1 | 29 | 194 |
| 2 | 36 | 134 |
| 3 | 20 | 110 |
| $4 + Ca^{2+}$ | 33·5 | 170 |
| $- Ca^{2+}$ | 2 | 13 |
| $+ Ca^{2+}$ | 22 | 66 |

Perfusates were collected for 6 min. during stimulation of the splenic nerve at 30/sec. In experiment 4 the perfusate was changed to calcium-free Tyrode's solution after the first stimulation period and 20 min. later the nerve was stimulated again. After the second stimulation period the spleen was perfused with Tyrode's solution for 20 min. before the third stimulation period.

and arteries, and that the nerve bundles lie on the outer edges of the muscles facing the splenic pulp.

Substances released from the nerves will, therefore, enter the red pulp and so could pass into the veins directly via the open circulation (Gillespie, 1966; Fillenz, 1970). This is a particularly easy pathway for large molecules, such as proteins, to pass into the blood-stream.

The release of dopamine β-hydroxylase and of chromogranin A from the nerves into the extracellular space could have been the result of damage to the nerve cell membranes in the perfused spleen. However, this is very unlikely firstly becaused of the correlation in different spleens between the amount of neurotransmitter and the amounts of each protein released and, secondly, because we could not detect the release of any dopa decarboxylase activity. This enzyme is present in the soluble axoplasm of splenic nerve (Stjärne and Lishajko, 1967; De Potter et al., 1970) and a considerable proportion of the dopa decarboxylase of the spleen is in the nerve terminals as shown by the decreased activity (32% of normal) in the spleens of immunosympathectomized rats (Klingman, 1965). The amount of dopa decarboxylase activity that would have been released if all the noradrenaline in the perfusate had come from damaged neurons can be calculated from the ratio of dopa decarboxylase activity to noradrenaline in splenic nerve homogenates (De Potter *et al.*, 1970): in the experiments in which dopa decarboxylase activity was looked for in perfusates, up to 64 n moles of noradrenaline was released and this would have been accompanied by up to 23 units of dopa decarboxylase activity. No enzymic activity was, however, detected and, from the limit of sensitivity of the method, we can say that less than 0·5% of the noradrenaline was released by a process which increased the permeability of the nerve cell membrane to a protein molecule the size of dopa decarboxylase.

From what site within the neuron are the proteins released? The centrifugation experiments described in the preceding paper (De Potter *et al.*, 1970) showed that, in homogenates of splenic nerve, dopamine β-hydroxylase and chromogranin A are found in both a particulate fraction and the final supernatant. However, it was concluded that most of the dopamine β-hydroxylase and all of the chromogranin A in the final supernatant was probably released during fractionation from damaged noradrenergic vesicles. If the vesicle is the predominant, or exclusive site of storage of these two proteins then we have to account for the release of the proteins from the vesicles into the extracellular space upon stimulation of the nerve.

One possible mechanism is for the proteins, together with the noradrenaline, to diffuse across the vesicle membrane into the soluble axoplasm and then across the nerve cell membrane. While this is a possible mode of release for a small molecule like noradrenaline, it is not a likely mechanism for the release of large molecules such as proteins. The experiment in which the sedimentation

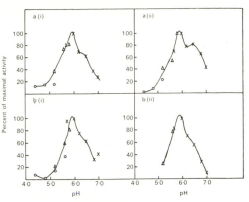

Fig. 6. Effect of pH on the activity of dopamine β-hydroxylase in splenic nerves and splenic perfusates. (a) (i) homogenate of dog splenic nerve, (ii) perfusate from dog spleen. (b) (i) noradrenergic vesicles from bovine splenic nerve, (ii) perfusate from calf spleen. o, 0·05 M sodium acetate buffers; Δ, 0·05 M sodium succinate buffers; x, 0·05 M sodium phosphate buffers.

rate of dopa decarboxylase was found to be less than that of the soluble dopamine β-hydroxylase extracted from vesicles shows that, if both protein molecules have similar conformation, dopa decarboxylase is a smaller molecule than dopamine β-hydroxylase. If the nerve cell membrane has pores in it large enough for dopamine β-hydroxylase to pass through, some leakage of a smaller protein present in the soluble axoplasm would be expected. As discussed above, no dopa decarboxylase activity could be detected in the perfusate. It could be argued that the nerve cell membrane contains specific carriers which transport dopamine β-hydroxylase and chromogranin A (and any other vesicle proteins which may be released) but which do not carry proteins of the soluble axoplasm. This hypothesis runs the risk of multiplying entities beyond necessity. A far simpler hypothesis is that release of the soluble contents of the vesicle occurs by exocytosis. By fusion of the vesicle membrane with the cell membrane a specific opening into the extracellular space will be formed, which excludes the release of any components of the soluble axoplasm.

291

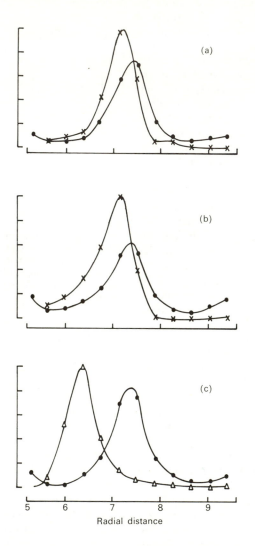

Fig. 7. Comparison of the sedimentation rate of dopamine β-hydroxylase from noradrenergic vesicles with that of dopamine β-hydroxylase released into the splenic perfusate. The curves represent relative enzyme activities, using catalase (●) as a marker, in fractions from sucrose density gradients prepared and centrifuged as described in the methods section. (a) Dopamine β-hydroxylase activity (x) present in perfusates collected from calf spleen during stimulation of the splenic nerve. (b) Dopamine β-hydroxylase activity (x) in soluble lysate of noradrenergic vesicles from bovine splenic nerve (c) Dopa decarboxylase activity (Δ) in particle-free supernatant from bovine splenic nerve.

Table 2. *Relative proportions of chromogranin A and dopamine β-hydroxylase in perfusates from the spleen and in soluble lysates of splenic nerve vesicles.*

| | Dog | | Calf | |
|---|---|---|---|---|
| | Splenic nerve vesicles | Perfusate | Splenic nerve vesicles | Perfusate |
| Dopamine β-hydroxylase/ noradrenaline (units/nmole) | 96 (approx.) | 3·2 | 106 | 6·8 |
| Chromogranin A/noradrenaline (μg/nmole) | — | — | 0·23 | 0·002 |

The value of the ratio of dopamine β-hydroxylase activity to noradrenaline in noradrenergic vesicles of dog splenic nerve was calculated from the ratio found in homogenates of dog splenic nerve assuming a similar distribution of the enzyme to that found in bovine splenic nerve by De Potter *et al.* (1970).

Whereas in the adrenal medulla there is electron microscopic evidence that exocytosis can occur (Coupland, 1965; Diner, 1967) there are no clear pictures of such an event in sympathetic neurons. Even in studies on the adrenal medulla, it has so far not been possible to provide quantitative evidence from electron microscopy that exocytosis is the major mode of release. Evidence for the significance of exocytosis in the adrenal came from biochemical studies (see Introduction) which showed the near identity of the ratio of chromogranins to catecholamines in the perfusate with this ratio in the soluble lysate of isolated chromaffin granules. Adopting a similar approach to the present studies on splenic nerve and perfusates from the spleen, we obtain the data given in Table 2. The ratio of dopamine β-hydroxylase activity to noradrenaline in splenic perfusates is only 3% (dog) and 6% (calf) of that in the soluble lysate of noradrenergic vesicles from the corresponding splenic nerve; the ratio of chromogranin A to noradrenaline in the perfusates is only about 1% of that in the soluble lysate of vesicles.

Interpretation of these figures is complicated because the amounts of proteins and noradrenaline in the perfusates are not necessarily identical with the amounts released from the nerves. The amount of noradrenaline in the perfusate will be less than that released from the nerve due to uptake of noradrenaline into neurons (see Iversen, 1967) and uptake and metabolism by extraneuronal tissues (see Lightman and Iversen, 1969). An estimate of the proportion of the released noradrenaline that is removed by these processes can be obtained from the results of experiments in which phenoxybenzamine was included in the perfusion medium. This drug inhibits the neuronal uptake (Brown, 1965; Hertting, 1965; Iversen, 1965) and extraneuronal uptake (Eisenfeld, Landsberg and Axelrod, 1967; Iversen and Langer, 1969; Lightman and Iversen, 1969) of noradrenaline. In our experiments with dog and calf spleens phenoxybenzamine approximately doubled the amount of noradrenaline recovered in the perfusate after stimulation of the nerve at 30/sec. Similar results were obtained by Blakeley, Brown and Geffen (1969) with the blood perfused cat spleen. It is noteworthy that in the experiment illustrated in Fig. 3 the increased overflow of noradrenaline caused by phenoxybenzamine was not accompanied by a corresponding increase in the amounts of the two proteins released.

It is also likely that we have underestimated the amounts of each protein released from the nerve because, in most experiments, the amounts of protein and noradrenaline were only measured in the six-minute period during which the nerve had been stimulated. The experiments illustrated in Figs. 1 and 3 show that some protein was still present in the perfusates collected after the stimulation periods, whereas the amounts of noradrenaline had fallen to the control level. Possibly this reflects the slower rate of diffusion of the large protein molecules in the splenic pulp. The amount of each protein released from the nerve which was not measured probably does not exceed that amount recovered in the perfusate during the first collection period. It is not possible to estimate the loss of protein, if any by adsorption to the tissue surface or by uptake into cells and so a provisional upper estimate of the amount of protein released from the nerves would be twice the values given in Table 2.

Although a number of assumptions have had to be made, it seems reasonable to conclude that the amounts of noradrenaline and of the two proteins released from the nerve are in each case about twice the amounts found in the perfusates. The ratio of the quantity of protein to the quantity of noradrenaline released from the nerve will, therefore, be similar to this ratio in the perfusates. As pointed out above, these ratios are only 6% (dopamine $\beta$-hydroxylase) and 1% (chromogranin A) of the corresponding ratios in the soluble lysate of noradrenergic vesicles from splenic nerve.

We have already argued that the most likely mode of release of the large molecular weight proteins is by exocytosis; how, then can these ratios be explained? The relative deficiency of chromogranin A to dopamine $\beta$-hydroxylase may be because the former protein is highly acidic and has different hydrodynamic properties (Smith and Winkler, 1967; Kirshner and Kirshner, 1969) from dopamine $\beta$-hydroxylase (Friedman and Kaufman, 1965); these factors may cause

Fig. 8. Diagram representing the types of noradrenergic vesicle in the splenic nerve to illustrate an hypothesis concerning the origin of the noradrenaline and proteins released from the nerve terminals. The large dense-cored vesicles, which are formed in the cell body and which migrate along the axon to the terminals, contain soluble proteins (chromogranin A and dopamine $\beta$-hydroxylase) in addition to noradrenaline. It is suggested that the small dense-cored vesicles, which may originate at the terminal, do not contain these soluble proteins. Stimulation of the nerve causes the release of noradrenaline from both types of vesicle and of the soluble proteins from the large dense-cored vesicles. The most likely mode of release of the contents of the large vesicles is exocytosis. The membrane of the large vesicle may then fragment to give smaller ( ? synaptic) vesicles as it pinches off the nerve cell membrane. The measurements of the sizes of the vesicles are taken from the paper by Geffen & Ostburg (1969) and refer to the splenic nerve of the cat.

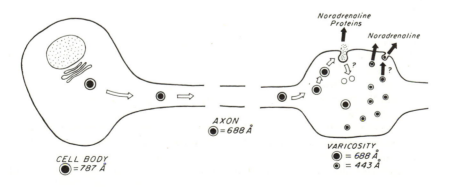

CELL BODY
⬤ = 787 Å

AXON
⬤ = 688 Å

VARICOSITY
⬤ = 688 Å
⊙ = 443 Å

Noradrenaline
Proteins

Noradrenaline

chromogranin A to be more readily bound by the tissues of the spleen. The relative deficiencies in the amounts of both proteins to that of noradrenaline could also be due to tissue binding of the proteins. On the other hand, the observations could reflect events taking place within the nerve terminals. For example: (i) about 6% of the noradrenaline may be released from vesicles by exocytosis, the rest being released by diffusion out of vesicles and across the axoplasm; or, (ii) all the noradrenaline may be released by exocytosis but the fusion of vesicle and cell membrane may be too brief to allow more than 6% of the proteins to be released; or, (iii) up to 6% of the noradrenaline may be released by exocytosis from vesicles which contain soluble chromogranin and dopamine $\beta$-hydroxylase, and the rest of the noradrenaline may be released from a second type of vesicle which does not contain these soluble proteins.

The last hypothesis is supported by morphological and biochemical studies which have shown that not all the noradrenergic vesicles in the terminals of sympathetic neurons are identical with the vesicles in preterminal axons. It should not be forgotten that the ratios of protein to noradrenaline given in Table 2 refer to vesicles isolated from preterminal axons of the splenic nerve.

Electron microscopic observations (Grillo, 1966; Taxi, 1965; Bloom and Aghajanian, 1968; Hökfelt, 1968) have shown that sympathetic nerve terminals contain two kinds of dense-cored vesicles: large (diam. approx. 80 nm) and small (diam. approx. 50 nm), both of which contain catecholamine (Jaim-Etcheverry and Zieher, 1968; Hökfelt, 1968; Tranzer and Thoenen, 1968). In the nerve varicosities of the cat spleen the small dense-cored vesicle is the predominant type (Geffern and Ostberg, 1969; Fillenz, 1970). However, preterminal axons of the splenic nerve contain mainly (Kapeller and Mayor, 1967 and 1969; Hökfelt, 1969) or exclusively (Geffen and Ostberg, 1969; Fillenz, 1970) one type of vesicle which is probably identical with the large dense-cored vesicle of the terminals.

Biochemical studies have also shown that axons of the splenic nerve contain only one type of noradrenergic vesicle (Roth, Stjärne, Bloom and Giarman, 1968; Hörtnagl et al., 1969; De Potter et al., 1970) whereas terminals of sympathetic nerves in the heart (Roth et al., 1968) and spleen (De Potter, 1968; Chubb, De Potter and De Schaepdryver, 1970) contain two kinds of noradrenergic vesicle. In the dog spleen, one type of noradrenergic vesicle equilibrates at the same density in a sucrose gradient as does the noradrenergic vesicle of splenic nerve, and it also contains dopamine $\beta$-hydroxylase activity; the other type of noradrenergic vesicle in the spleen equilibrates at a lower density and does not appear to contain dopamine $\beta$-hydroxylase (Chubb, De Potter and Schaepdryver, 1970). The less dense type of noradrenergic vesicle in the terminals of the splenic nerve is more labile to homogenization than the dense type, and so it is not easy to estimate what proportion of the total noradrenaline is stored in each vesicle; however, at least 40% of the noradrenaline in the spleen is stored in the vesicles in the nerve terminals which lack dopamine $\beta$-hydroxylase activity (Chubb, De Potter and De Schaepdryver, 1970).

As a working hypothesis (Fig. 8) we suggest stimulation of the splenic nerve causes the release of noradrenaline and soluble vesicle proteins by exocytosis from that type of noradrenergic vesicle in the terminal which is identical with the noradrenergic vesicle of splenic nerve axons. The release of noradrenaline from the second type of vesicle in the terminal will not be accompanied by that of chromogranin or dopamine $\beta$-hydroxylase and our observations suggest that most of the noradrenaline is released from this type of vesicle. It is still an open question whether release of noradrenaline from the latter type of vesicle occurs by exocytosis. However, perhaps it is pertinent that the release of noradrenaline from the splenic nerve is entirely dependent upon calcium, just as is the release of the vesicle proteins.

295

*Some implications of secretion by exocytosis*

It was briefly reported by Geffen and Livett (1968) that radioactive protein was released into the splenic perfusate upon stimulation of the nerve several hours after injection of radioactive leucine into the coeliac ganglion of the sheep. Using antisera to sheep adrenal chromogranin A and dopamine β-hydroxylase, Geffen, Livett and Rush (1969a) identified these two proteins in perfusates collected from the sheep spleen during stimulation of the splenic nerve. I. J. Kopin and G. Gewirtz (personal communication) have also demonstrated the release of dopamine β-hydroxylase activity from the cat spleen. These findings are consistent with our observations on dog and calf spleens, and lend further support to the hypothesis of release by exocytosis. The implications of release by exocytosis concern, among other things, (1) the neurotransmitter substance, (2) the dynamics of the neuron and (3) the tissue which is innervated.

(1) Secretion of the neurotransmitter substance by exocytosis (see del Castillo and Katz, 1957) means that it is released directly into the extracellular space, in discrete packets (or quanta), in a highly concentrated form without having to diffuse across the axoplasm or across any membrane. Electrophysiological studies on smooth muscle have raised the possibility that noradrenaline is released in quanta (Burnstock and Holman, 1962; Tomita, 1967) just as is acetylcholine (for a review see Katz, 1969).

(2) If the neuron releases protein as well as the neurotransmitter it must have a means of replacing the protein that is released. Whereas synthesis of most of the noradrenaline released must occur in the nerve terminal (Geffen and Rush, 1968), the synthesis of protein in nerves is mainly, if not entirely, confined to the perikaryon (Droz, 1969). Proteins synthesized in the perikaryon and released at the terminals have to be transported down the axon. It is, therefore, very pertinent that sympathetic nerves can transport proteins from the perikaryon to the terminal at the same rapid rate (Livett,

Geffen and Austin, 1968) as they transport noradrenaline (Dahlström, 1967) and large dense-cored vesicles (Banks, Magnall and Mayor, 1969; Kapeller and Mayor, 1967, 1969; Geffen and Ostberg, 1969). Two of the rapidly transported proteins have been identified in dog splenic nerve as dopamine β-hydroxylase (Laduron and Belpaire, 1968b) and in sheep splenic nerve as dopamine β-hydroxylase and chromogranin A (Geffen, Livett and Rush, 1969b). These two proteins were also shown, by immunohistochemical methods, to be present in the nerve cells in the coeliac ganglion (Geffen *et al.*, 1969b). These findings support the hypothesis that dopamine β-hydroxylase and chromogranin A are synthesized in the perikaryon where they are packaged, together with noradrenaline, in large dense-cored vesicles; these vesicles are then transported down the axon to the terminals where they release their soluble contents by exocytosis. The empty membrane of the large dense-cored vesicle will remain in the terminal: this membrane still contains the insoluble dopamine β-hydroxylase (Hörtnagl *et al.*, 1969; De Potter *et al.*, 1970) and so could be used as a source of this enzyme for the synthesis of noradrenaline. The lack of any electron microscopic evidence for the presence of empty membranes of large dense-cored vesicles raises the possibility that the membrane disintegrates into smaller vesicles after exocytosis, just as is believed to occur in neurosecretory neurons (Normann, 1969; Bunt, 1969).

Sympathetic neurons have a striking ability to conserve the transmitter they release by taking it up again into the terminals (see Iversen, 1967). Can the neuron also recapture some of the protein liberated by exocytosis? If this does occur, then endocytosis is the most likely mode of uptake, and it is noteworthy that electron microscopic studies have shown that nerve terminals can take up exogenous proteins by endocytosis (Brightman, 1968; Zacks and Saito, 1969; Holtzman and Peterson, 1969). Clearly, the fate of the protein after uptake into the neuron will determine whether such a process has any value in the economy of the cell.

(3) The identification of secretory products of a neuron other than the neurotransmitter does, of course, raise the question whether the proteins have any extraneuronal function. Since it is still not known whether the relatively large amounts of chromogranins and dopamine β-hydroxylase released from the adrenal medulla have any function, we can only speculate that the release of these proteins from neurons could be related to some of the long-term 'trophic' effects of nerves on the tissues they innervate.

### Summary

1. Dog and calf spleens were perfused with Tyrode's solution and the splenic nerves were stimulated at 30/sec.
2. Stimulation of the splenic nerve of the dog caused the release into the perfusate of up to 36 n-moles of noradrenaline and of up to 106 units of dopamine β-hydroxylase activity: in 9 experiments the mean ratio of dopamine β-hydroxylase activity to noradrenaline was 3·25. In homogenates of dog splenic nerve this ratio was 250.
3. Stimulation of the splenic nerve of the calf caused the release into the perfusate of up to 82 n-moles of noradrenaline, 460 units of dopamine β-hydroxylase activity, and 0·21 μg of chromogranin A. In 9 experiments the mean ratio of dopamine β-hydroxylase activity to noradrenaline in perfusates was 6·8 and the ratio of chromogranin A to noradrenaline was 0·002; these ratios were 106 and 0·23, respectively, in soluble lysates of noradrenergic vesicles from bovine splenic nerve.
4. Release of noradrenaline and dopamine β-hydroxylase from dog and calf spleen was inhibited by the omission of calcium chloride from the perfusion fluid. The release of chromogranin A from calf spleen was also dependent upon calcium.
5. Concentrations of phenoxybenzamine which prevented contraction of the spleens did not inhibit the release of dopamine β-hydroxylase from dog and calf spleens nor the release of chromogranin A from calf spleens.
6. Infusion of noradrenaline did not release dopamine β-hydroxylase from calf spleen although it caused the spleen to contract.
7. Hexamethonium potentiated the release of dopamine β-hydroxylase and noradrenaline from dog and calf spleens, and the release of chromogranin A from calf spleen.
8. The following properties of the dopamine β-hydroxylase released into the perfusates were identical with those of the enzyme in soluble lysates of noradrenergic vesicles of the splenic nerve: pH optima (dog and calf), mobility in gel electrophoresis (calf) and sedimentation rate (calf).
9. Dopa decarboxylase, an enzyme present in the soluble axoplasm of splenic nerve, could not be detected in perfusates collected during stimulation of the nerve.
10. There was a highly significant correlation between the amounts of dopamine β-hydroxylase and noradrenaline released from the calf spleen, and a similar correlation between the amounts of chromogranin A and noradrenaline.
11. It was concluded that dopamine β-hydroxylase and chromogranin A were released from terminals of the splenic nerve. The hypothesis was proposed that some of the neurotransmitter released from the nerve is secreted by exocytosis, together with the proteins, from a population of noradrenergic vesicles which originate in the perikaryon and are transported along the axon to the terminals.

### Acknowledgements

This work was supported by grants from the Fund for Collective Fundamental Research, Belgium and the Medical Research Council, London. The excellent technical assistance of Miss M. Vanneste and Mrs. B. Baeten is gratefully acknowledged. A. D. Smith is a Royal Society Stothert Research Fellow.

## References

AUSTIN, L., LIVETT, B. G. and CHUBB, I. W. (1967). Biosynthesis of noradrenaline in sympathetic nervous tissue.

BANKS, P. (1970). On the role of calcium ions in the secretion of catecholamines. In: *Calcium in Cellular Function*, pp. (148–162). A. W. Cuthbert (ed.). London: Macmillan Ltd.

BANKS, P., HELLE, K. B. and MAYOR, D. (1969). Evidence for the presence of a chromogranin-like protein in bovine splenic nerve granules. *Molec. Pharmac.*, **5**, 210–212.

BANKS, P., MAGNALL, D. and MAYOR, D. (1969). The re-distribution of cytochrome oxidase, noradrenaline and adenosinetriphosphate in adrenergic nerves constricted at two points. *J. Physiol.*, **200**, 745–762.

BERTLER, A., CARLSSON, A. and ROSENGREN, E. 1958. A method for the fluorimetric determination of adrenaline and noradrenaline in tissues. *Acta physiol. scand.*, **44**, 273–292.

BLAKELEY, A. G. H., BROWN, G. L. and FERRY, C. B. (1963). Pharmacological experiments on the release of the sympathetic transmitter. *J. Physiol.*, **167**, 505–514.

BLAKELEY, A. G. H., BROWN, G. L. and GEFFEN, L. B. (1969). Uptake and re-use of sympathetic transmitter in the cat spleen. *Proc. Roy. Soc.*, *B*, **174**, 51–68.

BLASCHKO, H., COMLINE, R. S., SCHNEIDER, F. H., SILVER, M. and SMITH, A. D. 1967. Secretion of a chromaffin granule protein, chromogranin, from the adrenal gland after splanchnic stimulation. *Nature, Lond.*, **215**, 58–59.

BLOOM, F. E. and AGHAJANIAN, G. K. (1968). An electron microscopic analysis of large granular synaptic vesicles of the brain in relation to monoamine content. *J. Pharmac. exp. Ther.*, **159**, 261–273.

BRIGHTMAN, M. W. (1968). The intracerebral movement of proteins injected into blood and cerebrospinal fluid of mice. *Prog. Brain Res.*, **29**, 19–37.

BROWN, G. L. (1965). The release and fate of the transmitter liberated by adrenergic nerves. *Proc. Roy. Soc.*, *B*, **162**, 1–19.

BUNT, A. H. (1969). Formation of coated and 'synaptic' vesicles within neurosecretory axon terminals of the crustacean sinus gland. *J. Ultrastruct. Res.*, **28**, 411–421.

BURGH DALY, M. DE and SCOTT, M. J. (1961). The effects of acetylcholine on the volume and vascular resistance of the dog's spleen. *J. Physiol.*, **156**, 246–259.

BURNSTOCK, G. and HOLMAN, M. E. 1962. Spontaneous potentials at sympathetic nerve endings in smooth muscle. *J. Physiol.*, **160**, 446–460.

CHUBB, I. W., DE POTTER, W. P. and DE SCHAEPDRYVER, A. F. 1970. Evidence for the existence of two types of noradrenaline storage particles in dog spleen. *Nature, Lond.* (in press).

CLARKE, J. T. (1964). Simplified 'disc' (polyacrylamide gel) electrophoresis. *Ann. N.Y. Acad. Sci.*, **121**, 428–436.

COUPLAND, R. E. 1965. Electron microscopic observations on the structure of the rat adrenal medulla. 1. The ultrastructure and organization of chromaffin cells in the normal adrenal medulla. *J. Anat.*, **99**, 231–254.

DAHLSTRÖM, A. 1967. The intraneuronal distribution of noradrenaline and the transport and lifespan of amine storage granules in the sympathetic adrenergic neuron. *Arch. exp. Path. Pharmak.*, **257**, 93–115.

DAHLSTRÖM, A. B. and ZETTERSTRÖM, B. E. M. 1965. Noradrenaline stores in nerve terminals of the spleen: changes during hemorrhagic shock. *Science*, **147**, 1583–1585.

DELAUNOIS, A. L., MOERMAN, E. J. and DE SCHAEPDRYVER, A. F. 1968. Isolated perfused dog spleen method. *Experientia*, **24**, 307–309.

DEL CASTILLO, J. and KATZ, B. 1957. La base 'quantale' de la transmission neuro-musculaire. *Coll. internat. C.N.R.S.*, Paris, **67**, 245–258.

DE POTTER, W. P. 1968. Doctoral Thesis, University of Ghent.

DE POTTER, W. P., DE SCHAEPDRYVER, A. F., MOERMAN, E. J. and SMITH, A. D. 1969. Evidence for the release of vesicle-proteins together with noradrenaline upon stimulation of the splenic nerve. *J. Physiol.*, **204**, 102P–104P.

DE POTTER, W. P., MOERMAN, E. J., DE SCHAEPDRYVER, A. F. and SMITH, A. D. 1969. Release of noradrenaline and dopamine β-hydroxylase upon splenic nerve stimulation. *Proc. 4th int. Congr. Pharmac.*, *Abstracts*, p. 146, Basel: Schwabe & Co.

DE POTTER, W. P., SMITH, A. D. and DE SCHAEPDRYVER, A. F. 1970. Subcellular fractionation of splenic nerve: ATP, chromogranin A and dopamine β-hydroxylase in noradrenergic vesicles. *Tissue & Cell*, **2** (4), 529-546.

DINER, O. 1967. L'expulsion des granules de la médulla surrénale chez le hamster. *C.r. Séanc. Acad. Sci. Paris*, D **265**, 616–619.

DOUGLAS, W. W. 1968. Stimulus-Secretion Coupling: the concept and clues from chromaffin and other cells. *Br. J. Pharmac.*, **34**, 451–474.

DOUGLAS, W. W. and POISNER, A. M. 1966. Evidence that the secreting adrenal chromaffin cell releases catecholamines directly from ATP-rich granules. *J. Physiol. Lond.*, **183**, 236–248.

DROZ, B. 1969. Protein metabolism in nerve cells. *Int. Rev. Cytol.*, **25**, 363–390.

DUCH, D. S., VIVEROS, O. H. and KIRSHNER, N. 1968. Endogenous inhibitor(s) in adrenal medulla of dopamine β-hydroxylase. *Biochem. Pharmac.*, **17**, 255–264.

EISENFELD, A. J., LANDSBERG, L. and AXELROD, J. 1967. Effect of drugs on the accumulation and metabolism of extraneuronal norepinephrine in the rat heart. *J. Pharmac. exp. Ther.*, **158**, 378–385.

ELFVIN, L.-G. 1965. The ultrastructure of the capillary fenestrae in the adrenal medulla of the rat. *J. Ultrastruct. Res.*, **12**, 687–704.

EULER, U. S. VON, LISHAJKO, F. and STJÄRNE, L. 1963. Catecholamines and ATP in isolated adrenergic nerve granules. *Acta physiol. scand.*, **59**, 495–496.

EULER, U. S. VON and PURKHOLD, A. 1951. Effect of sympathetic denervation on the noradrenaline and adrenaline content of the spleen, kidney and salivary glands in the sheep. *Acta physiol. scand.*, **24**, 212–217.

FILLENZ, M. 1970. The innervation of the cat spleen. *Proc. Roy. Soc. Lond.*, B. **174**, 459–468.

FRIEDMAN, S. and KAUFMAN, S. 1965. 3,4-dihydroxyphenylethylamine β-hydroxylase: Physical properties, copper content, and role of copper in the catalytic activity. *J. biol. Chem.*, **240**, 4763–4773.

GEFFEN, L. B. and LIVETT, B. G. 1968. Axoplasmic transport of ¹⁴C-noradrenaline and protein and their release by nerve impulses. *Proc. int. union physiol. sci.*, **7**, 152.

GEFFEN, L. B., LIVETT, B. G. and RUSH, R. A. 1969A. Immunological localization of chromogranins in sheep sympathetic neurones, and their release by nerve impulses. *J. Physiol.*, **204**, 58–59P.

GEFFEN, L. B., LIVETT, B. G. and RUSH, R. A. 1969B. Immunohistochemical localization of protein components of catecholamine storage vesicles. *J. Physiol.*, **204**, 593–605.

GEFFEN, L. B. and OSTBERG, A. 1969. Distribution of granular vesicles in normal and constricted sympathetic neurones. *J. Physiol.*, **204**, 583–592.

GEFFEN, L. B. and RUSH, R. A. 1968. Transport of noradrenaline in sympathetic nerves and the effect of nerve impulses on its contribution to transmitter stores. *J. Neurochem.*, **15**, 925–930.

GILLESPIE, J. S. 1966. Tissue binding of noradrenaline. *Proc. Roy. Soc. B.*, **166**, 1–10.

GILLESPIE, J. S. and KIRPEKAR, S. M. 1966. The histological localization of noradrenaline in the cat spleen. *J. Physiol.*, **187**, 69–79.

GRILLO, M. A. 1966. Electron microscopy of sympathetic tissues. *Pharmac. Rev.*, **18**, 387–399.

HERTING, G. 1965. The effect of drugs and sympathetic denervation on noradrenaline uptake and binding in tissues. In: *Pharmacology of cholinergic and adrenergic transmission*. W. W. Douglas and A. Carlsson (eds.), pp. 277–288. Oxford: Pergamon Press.

HÖKFELT, T. 1968. *In vitro* studies on central and peripheral monoamine neurons at the ultrastructural level. *Z. Zellforsch. mikrosk. Anat.*, **91**, 1–74.

HÖKFELT, T. 1969. Distribution of noradrenaline storing particles in peripheral adrenergic neurons as revealed by electron microscopy. *Acta physiol. scand.*, **76**, 427–440.

HOLTZMAN, E. and PETERSON, E. R. 1969. Uptake of protein by mammalian neurons. *J. Cell Biol.*, **40**, 863–869.

HÖRTNAGL, H., HÖRTNAGL, H. and WINKLER, H. 1969. Bovine splenic nerve: characterization cf noradrenaline-containing vesicles and other cell organelles by density gradient centrifugation. *J. Physiol.*, **205**, 103–114.

HUKOVIĆ, S. and MUSCHOLL, E. 1962. Die Noradrenaline-Abgabe aus dem isolierten Kaninchenherzen bei sympatischer Nervenreizung und ihre pharmakologische Beeinflussung. *Arch. exp. Path. Pharmak.*, **244**, 81–96.

IVERSEN, L. L. 1965. The inhibition of noradrenaline uptake by drugs. *Adv. Drug. Res.*, **2**, 5–23.

IVERSEN, L. L. 1967. *The uptake and storage of noradrenaline in sympathetic nerves*. Cambridge: Cambridge University Press.

IVERSEN, L. L. and LANGER, S. Z. 1969. Effect of phenoxybenzamine on the uptake and metabolism of noradrenaline in the rat heart and vas deferens. *Br. J. Pharmac.*, **37**, 627–637.

JAIM-ETCHEVERRY, G. and ZIEHER, L. M. 1968. Cytochemistry of 5-hydroxytryptamine at the electron microscope level. 2. Localization in the autonomic nerves of the rat pineal gland. *Z. Zellforsch. mikrosk. Anat.*, **86**, 393–400.

KAPELLER, K. and MAYOR, D. 1967. The accumulation of noradrenaline in constricted sym-

299

pathetic nerves as studied by fluorescence and electron microscopy. *Proc. Roy. Soc.*, *B.*, **167**, 282–292.

KAPELLER, K. and MAYOR, D. 1969. An electron microscopic study of the early changes proximal to a constriction in sympathetic nerves. *Proc. Roy. Soc.*, *B.*, **172**, 39–51.

KARNOVSKY, M. J. 1967. The ultrastructural basis of capillary permeability studied with peroxidase as a tracer. *J. Cell Biol.* (1967), **35**, 213–236.

KATZ, B. 1969. *The release of neural transmitter substances.* Liverpool: Liverpool University Press.

KAUFMAN, S. and FRIEDMAN, S. 1965. Dopamine β-hydroxylase. *Pharmac. Rev.*, **17**, 71–100.

KIRPEKAR, S. M. and MISU, Y. 1967. Release of noradrenaline by splenic nerve stimulation and its dependence upon calcium. *J. Physiol.*, **188**, 219–234.

KIRSHNER, N. 1969. Storage and secretion of adrenal catecholamines. *Adv. Biochem. Psychopharmac.*, **1**, 71–89.

KIRSHNER, A. G. and KIRSHNER, N. 1969. A specific soluble protein from the catecholamine storage vesicles of bovine adrenal medulla. 2. Physical characterization. *Biochim. biophys. Acta*, **181**, 219–225.

KLINGMAN, G. I. 1965. Catecholamine levels and dopa-decarboxylase activity in peripheral organs and adrenergic tissues in the rat after immunosympathectomy. *J. Pharmac. exp. Ther.*, **148**, 14–21.

LADURON, P. and BELPAIRE, F. 1968A. A rapid assay and partial purification of dopa-decarboxylase. *Analyt. Biochem.*, **26**, 210–218.

LADURON, P. and BELPAIRE, F. 1968B. Transport of noradrenaline and dopamine β-hydroxylase in sympathetic nerves. *Life Sci.*, Oxford, **7**, 1–7.

LAVERTY, R. and TAYLOR, K. M. 1968. The fluorimetric assay of catecholamines and related compounds. *Analyt. Biochem.*, **22**, 269–279.

LEADERS, F. E. and DAYRIT, C. 1965. The cholinergic component in the sympathetic innervation to the spleen. *J. Pharmac. exp. Ther.*, **147**, 145–152.

LIGHTMAN, S. L. and IVERSEN, L. L. 1969. The role of uptake in the extraneuronal metabolism of catecholamines in the isolated rat heart. *Br. J. Pharmac.*, **37**, 638–649.

LIVETT, B. G., GEFFEN, L. B. and AUSTIN, L. 1968. Proximo distal transport of [$^{14}$C] noradrenaline and protein in sympathetic nerves. *J. Neurochem.*, **15**, 931–939.

LOWRY, O. H., ROSENBROUGH, N. J., FARR, A. L. and RANDALL, R. J. 1951. Protein measurement with the Folin phenol reagent. *J. biol. Chem.*, **193**, 265–275.

MALAMED, POISNER, A. M., TRIFARO, J. M. and DOUGLAS, W. W. 1968. The fate of the chromaffin granule during catecholamine release from the adrenal medulla. III. Recovery of a purified fraction of electron-translucent structures. *Biochem. Pharmac.*, **17**, 241–246.

MARLEY, E. and PATON, W. D. M. 1961. The output of sympathetic amines from the cat's adrenal gland in response to splanchnic nerve activity. *J. Physiol.*, **155**, 1–27.

POISNER, A. M., TRIFARO, J. M. and DOUGLAS, W. W. 1967. The fate of the chromaffin granule during catecholamine release from the adrenal medulla. II. Loss of protein and retention of lipid in subcellular fractions. *Biochem. Pharmac.*, **16**, 2101.

POTTER, L. T. 1967. Role of intraneuronal vesicles in the synthesis, storage, and release of noradrenaline. *Circulation Res.*, **21** (Suppl. 3), 13–24.

POTTER, L. T. and AXELROD, J. 1963. Properties of norepinephrine storage particles of the rat heart. *J. Pharmac. exp. Ther.*, **142**, 299–305.

NORMANN, T. C. 1969. Experimentally induced exocytosis of neurosecretory granules. *Exp. Cell Res.*, **55**, 285–287.

ROTH, R. H., STJÄRNE, L., BLOOM, F. E. and GIARMAN, N. J. 1968. Light and heavy norepinephrine storage particles in the rat heart and in bovine splenic nerve. *J. Pharmac. exp. Ther.*, **162**, 203–212.

SAGE, H. J., SMITH, W. J. and KIRSHNER, N. 1967. Mechanism of secretion from the adrenal medulla. 1. A microquantitative immunologic assay for bovine adrenal catecholamine storage vesicle protein and its application to studies of the secretory process. *Molec. Pharmac.*, **3**, 81–89.

SCHNEIDER, F. H., SMITH, A. D. and WINKLER, H. 1967. Secretion from the adrenal medulla: biochemical evidence for exocytosis. *Br. J. Pharmac. Chemother.*, **31**, 94–104.

SCHUMANN, H. J. 1958. Über den Noradrenalin- und ATP-Gehalt sympatischer Nerven. *Arch. exp. Path. Pharmak.*, **233**, 296–300.

SHARMAN, D. F., VANOV, S. and VOGT, M. 1962. Noradrenaline content in the heart and spleen of the mouse under normal conditions and after administration of some drugs. *Br. J. Pharmac.*, **19**, 527–533.

SMITH, A. D. 1968. Biochemistry of adrenal chromaffin granules. In: *The Interaction of Drugs and Subcellular Components in Animal Cells*, pp. 239–292 (P. N. Campbell, ed.). London: Churchill Ltd.

SMITH, A. D. and WINKLER, H. 1967. Purification and properties of an acidic protein from chromaffin granules of bovine adrenal medulla. *Biochem. J.*, **103**, 483–492.

SOBER, H. A., GUTTER, F. J., WYCKOFF, M. M. and PETERSON, E. A. 1956. Chromatography of proteins. 2. Fractionation of serum protein on anion-exchange cellulose. *J. Am. chem. Soc.*, **78**, 756–763.

STJÄRNE, L. and LISHAJKO, F. 1967. Localization of different steps in noradrenaline synthesis to different fractions of a bovine splenic nerve homogenate. *Biochem. Pharmac.*, **16**, 1719–1728.

STJÄRNE, L., ROTH, R. H. and LISHAJKO, F. 1967. Noradrenaline formation from dopamine in isolated subcellular particles from bovine splenic nerve. *Biochem. Pharmac.*, **16**, 1729–1739.

STORMORKEN, H. 1969. The release reaction of secretion. *Scand. J. Haemat.*, Suppl. **9**, 1–24.

STRIEDER, N., ZIEGLER, E., WINKLER, H. and SMITH, A. D. 1968. Some properties of soluble proteins from chromaffin granules of different species. *Biochem. Pharmac.*, **17**, 1553–1556.

TAXI, J. 1965. Contribution à l'étude des connexions des neurones moteurs du système nerveux autonome. *Annals. Sci. nat.* (Zool.), **7**, 413–674.

TOMITA, T. 1967. Current spread in the smooth muscle of the guinea-pig vas deferens. *J. Physiol.*, **189**, 163–176.

TRANZER, J. P. and THOENEN, H. 1968. Various types of amine-storing vesicles in peripheral adrenergic nerve terminals. *Experientia*, **24**, 484–486.

VIVEROS, O. H., ARQUEROS, L. and KIRSHNER, N. 1969. Mechanism of secretion from the adrenal medulla. 5. Retention of storage vesicle membranes following release of adrenaline. *Molec. Pharmac.*, **5**, 342–349.

ZACHS, S. I. and SAITO, A. 1969. Uptake of exogenous horseradish peroxidase by coated vesicles in mouse neuromuscular junctions. *J. Histochem. Cytochem.*, **17**, 161–170.

# DEPLETION OF VESICLES
# FROM FROG NEUROMUSCULAR JUNCTIONS
# BY PROLONGED TETANIC STIMULATION

## B. CECCARELLI, W. P. HURLBUT, and A. MAURO

From The Rockefeller University, New York 10021. Dr. Ceccarelli's permanent address is the Department of Pharmacology, University of Milan, Milano 20129, Italy.

ABSTRACT

Curarized cutaneous pectoris nerve muscle preparations from frogs were subjected to prolonged indirect stimulation at 2/sec while recording from end plate regions. At the ends of the periods of stimulation, the curare was removed and the preparations were fixed for electron microscopy or treated with black widow spider venom to determine the degree to which their stores of transmitter had been depleted. After 6–8 hr of stimulation the nerve terminals were almost completely depleted of their stores of transmitter and of their population of vesicles. Most of the transmitter release occurred during the first 4 hr of stimulation, and after this time most (about 80%) of the fibers were depleted of about 80% of their transmitter. The organization of the nerve terminals in 4-hr preparations appeared normal and the terminals still contained many vesicles. When peroxidase was present in the bathing medium, terminals from stimulated preparations showed many vesicles that contained peroxidase, whereas the rested control preparations showed few such vesicles. The fact that after 4 hr the total number of vesicles is not markedly changed while a large fraction (up to 45%) contained peroxidase suggests that in our experiments vesicles were continuously fusing with and reforming from the axolemma.

## INTRODUCTION

Several workers have tried to deplete neuromuscular junctions of their stores of transmitter and of their synaptic vesicles by tetanic stimulation of the nerve (1, 2, 3, 4). Depletion of transmitter has been obtained only when synthesis was inhibited by hemicholinium (2, 3) and, under this condition, a reduction in the number of vesicles occurred only in the regions of the axoplasm immediately adjacent to the axolemma (4). In these previous works the preparations were stimulated for from several minutes to a few hours at frequencies of 10/sec or more. We have stimulated a neuromuscular preparation from the frog for 6–9 hr at a rate of 2/sec in the absence of hemicholinium and have successfully depleted the terminals of their store of transmitter and of their population of vesicles.

## MATERIALS AND METHODS

The cutaneous pectoris muscle of the frog, *Rana pipiens*, was used. The muscles were mounted in the chamber described previously (5) and maintained at about 22°C in a Ringer's solution that contained 116 mM NaCl, 2.0 mM KCl, 1.8 mM CaCl$_2$, 1 mM NaH$_2$PO$_4$, and 2 mM Na$_2$HPO$_4$ (pH 7.0). End plate regions were impaled with micropipettes filled with 3 M KCl. Conventional recording equipment was used and photographic records of the end plate potentials (e.p.p.s) and miniature end plate potentials (m.e.p.p.s) were obtained. The nerve was stimulated with square pulses 0.1 msec in duration and amplitude three to four times threshold.

The muscle twitch was blocked by adding curare to the bath at a concentration of 3 × 10$^{-6}$ g/ml, an

Reprinted from *The Journal of Cell Biology* 54: 30–38 (1972) by permission of the publisher.

end plate region was impaled, and 10–20 min later stimulation was begun at a rate of 2/sec. In our initial experiments the stimulation was interrupted every few hours and the preparation rested for 10–30 min in order to minimize the probability of conduction block developing in the nerve. As an experiment progressed the amplitudes of the e.p.p.s declined and the concentration of curare was reduced until after 6–8 hr the preparation was being stimulated in Ringer's solution. The preparation was rested for 10–20 min and the responses to single shocks were tested. If there was no twitch, or only a weak twitch involving a few muscle fibers, either black widow spider venom (BWSV) was applied or the preparation was fixed for electron microscopy. In other experiments the preparations were stimulated continuously for 2–4 hr before they were washed in Ringer's and then either fixed or treated with venom. In some of these latter experiments horseradish peroxidase (Sigma type VI; Sigma Chemical Co., St. Louis, Mo.) was added to the medium at a concentration of 0.4% during the last 2 hr of stimulation.

When BWSV is applied to unstimulated nerve terminals, it evokes the spontaneous release of several hundred thousand m.e.p.p.s and completely depletes the terminals of their vesicles (6, 7). We used the venom-induced discharge of m.e.p.p.s as a measure of the store of transmitter remaining in the terminal. When the discharge was small we inferred that the terminal was depleted. The venom was prepared by grinding eight venom glands from four spiders (*Latrodectus mactans tredecimguttatus*) in 1.0 ml of 120 mM NaCl and was applied by adding 50–100 μl of the crude homogenate to the 3–4 ml of Ringer's in the bath.

Two solutions were used to fix the muscle for electron microscopy. One contained 2% $OsO_4$ in 0.13 M phosphate buffer (pH 7.4); the other contained 1.0% glutaraldehyde and 2% sucrose in 0.1 M cacodylate buffer (pH 7.4). The solution in the recording chamber was replaced by the fixative and the muscle was cut into small pieces and placed in fresh fixative at 4°C for a total fixation time of 2 hr. Specimens fixed in glutaraldehyde were postfixed for 1 hr in 2% $OsO_4$ in 0.1 M cacodylate buffer. The peroxidase-treated muscles were fixed in glutaraldehyde as described and then treated according to the procedure of Graham and Karnovsky (8) to demonstrate sites of peroxidase activity. All specimens were embedded in Epon 812, cut with a diamond knife, stained with uranyl acetate and lead citrate, and examined with a Hitachi 11B electron microscope.

## RESULTS AND DISCUSSION

Fig. 1 shows some records of e.p.p.s taken during an experiment in which a preparation was stimulated continuously at 2/sec for 4 hr, and Fig. 2

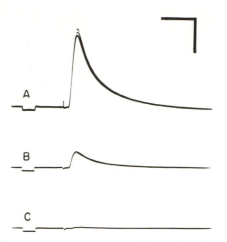

FIGURE 1   Records of e.p.p.s recorded at various times during continuous stimulation at 2/sec in curare, $3 \times 10^{-6}$ g/ml. Each record is a superposition of four successive responses recorded: A, at the beginning of stimulation; B, after 20 min; C, after 4 hr. Calibration: 5 mv and 5 msec.

shows the time course of the change in the amplitude of the e.p.p. during a depletion experiment. After 8 hr of stimulation rather large e.p.p.s were evoked by single shocks in a dilute solution of curare, but the junction was unable to support a tetanus of 2/sec and the e.p.p. fell virtually to zero during 20 min of stimulation. The preparation was rested in Ringer's solution and BWSV was applied.[1]

When BWSV was applied to unstimulated preparations, the m.e.p.p. frequency rose to peak values greater than 500/sec and remained at levels above 50/sec for 30 min or more; about $4 \times 10^5$ m.e.p.p. were released (6). These experiments with unstimulated preparations were carried out in solutions with low concentrations of Ca and high concentrations of Mg, for when the venom was applied to an unstimulated preparation in Ringer's solution, the muscle usually fibrillated violently. In contrast

---

[1] When the frequency of stimulation was increased to 5/sec during the plateau periods, the amplitude of the e.p.p. declined proportionately. This indicates that the rate of transmitter release during the steady state of the plateau periods was relatively independent of the rate of stimulation and it suggests that stimulation at high frequencies does not hasten the depletion of transmitter (9).

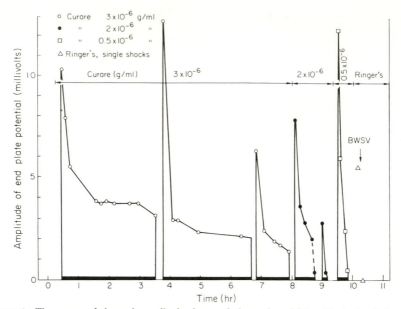

FIGURE 2  Time course of change in amplitude of e.p.p. during prolonged intermittent stimulation at 2/sec. Ordinate: amplitude of e.p.p. in millivolts. Abscissa: time in hours. The initial concentration of curare was $3 \times 10^{-6}$ g/ml (O). The base line is thickened to indicate the periods during which the preparation was stimulated at 2/sec. After stimulation was begun, the e.p.p. declined rapidly to a plateau level that was maintained for several hours. When stimulation was interrupted after about 3 hr the e.p.p. quickly gained its initial amplitude and then fell rapidly to the plateau level when stimulation was resumed. As the experiment progressed the plateau level gradually declined, the recovery of the e.p.p. during the rest intervals became incomplete, and the concentration of curare was reduced first to $2 \times 10^{-6}$ g/ml (●) and then to $0.5 \times 10^{-6}$ g/ml (□). During the period indicated by the dashed portion of the graph the rate of stimulation was raised to 5/sec, and the e.p.p. declined rapidly to zero. Later in the experiment (9.5 hr) relatively large e.p.p.s were evoked by single shocks, but the junction was unable to support a tetanus at 2/sec and the e.p.p. fell virtually to zero in 20 min. Stimulation then was stopped and the curare was removed. After about 10 min in Ringer's the e.p.p. had recovered to about 5 mv (△) and only a few fibers twitched. m.e.p.p.s were clearly visible at this time; their mean amplitude was 0.36 mv and their frequency was 11/sec. At the arrow 50 μl of BWSV were added. 3 min later the m.e.p.p. frequency had risen to its peak value of 134/sec and it had declined to less than 1/sec 9 min later. About $3 \times 10^{4}$ m.e.p.p.s occurred during the discharge. The nerve was stimulated 7 min after the venom had been added, and there was no e.p.p. The membrane potential of this muscle fiber varied between 70 and 90 mv and was lowest at the start.

to the violent reaction of unstimulated preparations, the stimulated preparations showed no fibrillation when the venom was added, and the m.e.p.p. discharge was small. In the fiber illustrated in Fig. 2, only about $3 \times 10^{4}$ m.e.p.p.s were released by the venom. Thus, it is clear that for this fiber the long period of stimulation reduced the venom-evoked discharge of m.e.p.p.s by about 90% and we infer that the store of transmitter in this nerve terminal was severely depleted.

Preparations that had been stimulated at 2/sec

for 6–8 hr were uniformly depleted of transmitter. In several preparations, we explored the surface fibers of the muscle with the micropipette and we rarely found regions that exhibited m.e.p.p.s or e.p.p.s. In some muscles the 5–10 fibers nearest the lateral edge were impaled in Ringer's at the beginning of the experiment and the end plate regions were identified. When these same regions were reimpaled in Ringer's solution after prolonged stimulation, most of them showed neither e.p.p.s nor m.e.p.p.s. When active junctions were found the e.p.p.s were small and the m.e.p.p. frequencies were low. BWSV was applied to 12 preparations while we recorded from known end plate regions. The most vigorous discharge observed was that from the fiber illustrated in Fig. 2; the other fibers gave almost no discharge (fewer than $10^4$ m.e.p.p.s). Thus, it appears that after 6–8 hr of stimulation at 2/sec over 90% of the nerve terminals were depleted of over 90% of their store of transmitter.

However, it was difficult to characterize the physiological state of our preparations after periods of stimulation of 4 hr or less because of the great spread in the results. We recorded from single fibers in 13 preparations stimulated continuously for from 3 to 4.5 hr. The e.p.p.s had failed in five fibers, and in these fibers the venom-induced m.e.p.p. discharges were less than 10% of normal. In two fibers the e.p.p.s were 10% and 30% of normal and the m.e.p.p. discharges were in the normal range. In the other fibers the e.p.p.s had fallen to less than 10% of their initial amplitudes and the m.e.p.p. discharges were 10%–20% of normal. Thus, although there was a broad distribution in the results, it appears that about 80% of the terminals had been depleted of about 80% of their transmitter during 4 hr of stimulation at 2/sec.

We studied the ultrastructure of the neuromuscular junctions in preparations that had been stimulated for 3, 4, or 6–8 hr and in unstimulated controls that had been soaked up to 8 hr in Ringer's solution containing curare. The neuromuscular junctions from control preparations resembled those described in freshly fixed tissue (10). The nerve terminal contained neurofilaments, neurotubules, elements of smooth endoplasmic reticulum, mitochondria, large numbers of synaptic vesicles, and a few coated vesicles (Fig. 3).

After 6–8 hr of stimulation unequivocal changes appeared in all the terminals examined; the terminals were almost entirely depleted of vesicles and appeared to be swollen (Figs. 4 and 5). These changes were observed independently of the fixative used and were due to an absolute decrease in the number of vesicles and not to a simple dilution resulting from the swelling of the terminals. We can conclude, therefore, that the prolonged stimulation of the nerve ultimately resulted in the nearly complete depletion of both the neurotransmitter and the vesicles.

However, the release of transmitter as reflected in the electrophysiological data and the loss of vesicles as seen in the ultrastructural studies were poorly correlated in time. The quantity of transmitter released from a terminal should be proportional to the area under a curve similar to that shown in Fig. 2. In most of our expriments most of the release of transmitter occurred during the first 4 hr of stimulation and, as noted above, most of the terminals were severely depleted of transmitter after 4 hr. However, at this time the general subcellular organization of most terminals still appeared normal and the reduction in the number of vesicles, though present, was not as marked as one would have expected from the physiological results (Fig. 6). This reduction occurred mainly in extensive regions of the terminal well removed from the prejunctional membrane and sometimes also in delimited regions of the terminal close to the prejunctional membrane and directly opposite the junctional folds (Fig. 6).

It is clear that the nerve terminal can secrete large quantities of transmitter without suffering a net loss of vesicles (10, 11). If vesicles must fuse with the axolemma to secrete transmitter, then during vigorous secretion the number of vesicles within the nerve terminal can remain relatively constant only if discharging vesicles are continuously replaced. Replacement of vesicles may occur by transport into the terminal from the axon, by production of new vesicles within the axoplasm of the terminal (possibly from elements of smooth endoplasmic reticulum), or by the formation of vesicles directly from the nerve terminal membrane. In the latter case, discharging vesicles may be recovered, or new vesicles formed by invagination of the plasmalemma of the terminal. Figs. 7–11 provide direct evidence that many synaptic vesicles are formed from the nerve terminal membrane. In these experiments horseradish peroxidase was added to the bathing solution and the figures show that the stimulated preparation contained many synaptic vesicles with reaction product (Figs. 9 and 10) while in the control almost none were found (Figs. 7 and 8) (12). Figs 11 A, B, C show a series of stages in which vesicles opened to the junctional cleft have been penetrated by the marker. Taken together, Figs. 7–11 indicate that the release of a quantum of transmitter is not necessarily associated with the permanent loss of the vesicle membrane. It appears that upon fusion with the axolemma and release of transmitter (Fig. 11) the original vesicle, or a new vesicle derived from the axolemma, returns to the axoplasm (Figs. 9

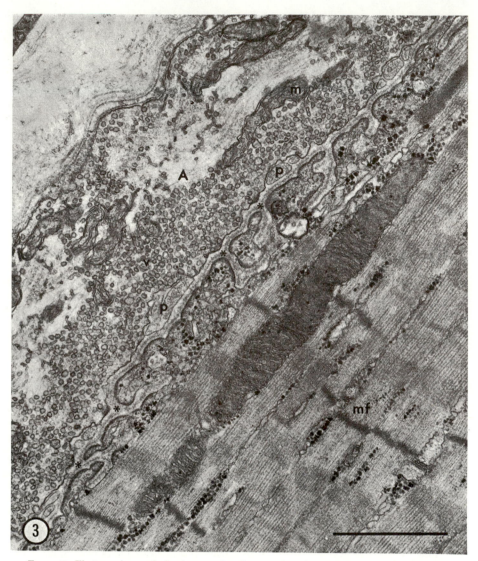

FIGURE 3 Electron micrograph showing a portion of a neuromuscular junction from a control preparation soaked 8 hr in Ringer's solution containing curare at $3 \times 10^{-6}$ g/ml. The axonal ending ($A$) contains numerous mitochondria ($m$), neurofilaments, elements of smooth endoplasmic reticulum, and synaptic vesicles ($v$). Active zones (*), densities on the presynaptic membrane, are often visible opposite the openings of the junctional folds. Projections ($p$) of the glial cell are interposed between the terminal and the end-plate membrane. ($mf$, myofibrils). 1 $\mu$; $\times$ 34,000.

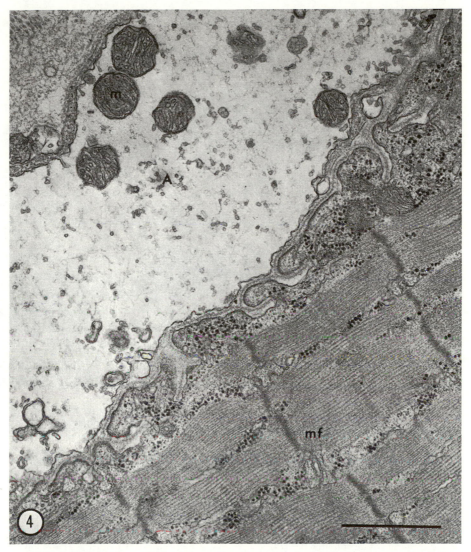

FIGURE 4  Electron micrograph showing a portion of neuromuscular junction from a preparation that had been stimulated for a total time of 8 hr. The axonal ending (A) appears to be swollen and contains mitochondria (m), neurofilaments, and elements of smooth endoplasmic reticulum. Few structures resembling synaptic vesicles are evident. (mf, myofibrils). 1 μ; × 30,000.

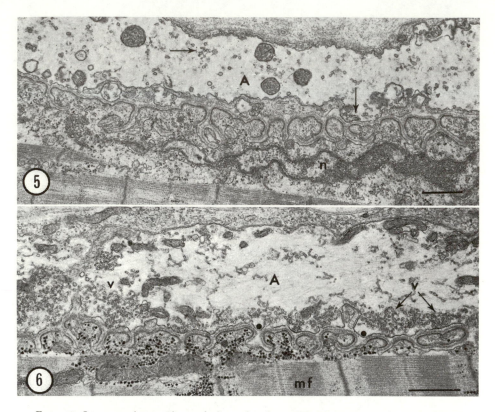

FIGURE 5  Low power electron micrograph of a portion of an end plate from a preparation that had been stimulated for 7 hr at 2/sec. The axonal ending (A) appears to be almost completely depleted. Only a few vesicles remain (arrows). (n, nucleus of muscle fiber). 1 $\mu$; $\times$ 12,500.

FIGURE 6  Electron micrograph showing a portion of a neuromuscular junction from a preparation that had been stimulated continuously for 4 hr. The general organization of the axonal ending (A) appears normal and many synaptic vesicles (v) are present. A reduction in the number of vesicles in regions (A) away from the prejunctional membrane and focal depletion of peripheral vesicles along the prejunctional membrane (●) are evident. (mf, myofibrils). 1 $\mu$; $\times$ 15,000.

and 10), to be possibly reutilized for the storage and subsequent release of transmitter (13).

It is difficult to explain why we succeeded in producing an extensive loss of vesicles by tetanic stimulation of the nerve whereas previous workers did not. The loss of vesicles we observed did not proceed linearly in time and was poorly correlated with the secretion of transmitter. The final massive loss of vesicles illustrated in Figs. 4 and 5 occurred relatively abruptly during the last few hours of prolonged experiments. It appears to represent a terminal stage in the secretion process and it may have been due to the collapse of the unknown mechanisms responsible for the replacement or recycling of vesicle membrane. It is likely that the onset of this collapse depends in a complex manner on many parameters, especially the frequency, duration, and pattern of stimulation.

We wish to thank Dr. George E. Palade for allowing us to use the facilities of his laboratory and for his constant encouragement. We also wish to thank

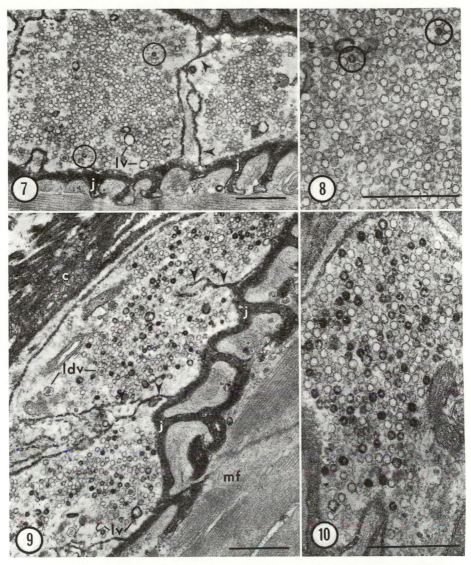

FIGURE 7  Electron micrograph of a portion of an end plate from an unstimulated preparation bathed for 2.5 hr in curare ($3 \times 10^{-6}$ g/ml) plus horseradish peroxidase. Junctional cleft (*j*) and extracellular space delimited by infoldings of the axolemma (arrowheads) contain rich deposits of reaction product. A few vesicles (circles) also contain reaction product. Some large vesicular structures (*lv*) with a peripheral deposit of reaction product are also present. 0.5 $\mu$; $\times$ 29,000.

FIGURE 8  Electron micrograph at high magnification of a portion of another end plate from the same preparation as in Fig. 7. Deposits of reaction product are present in only two synaptic vesicles (circles). 0.5 $\mu$; $\times$ 59,000.

FIGURE 9  Electron micrograph of a portion of an end plate in a preparation stimulated continuously for 3 hr and rested for 0.5 hr (curare, $3 \times 10^{-6}$ g/ml). Horseradish peroxidase was present during the last 2.5 hr of the experiment. This muscle was taken from the same frog as that used for Figs. 7 and 8. Many vesicles contain reaction product. Large vesicular structures (*lv*) with a peripheral deposit of reaction product are present as in the controls. (Arrowheads, infolding of axolemma; *ldv*, large dense core vesicle; *j*, junctional cleft; *c*, collagen fibrils; *mf*, myofibrils). 0.5 $\mu$; $\times$ 35,000.

FIGURE 10  Electron micrograph at high magnification of a portion of another end plate from the same preparation as in Fig. 9. Many vesicles (about 45%) contain reaction product. 0.5 $\mu$; $\times$ 58,000.

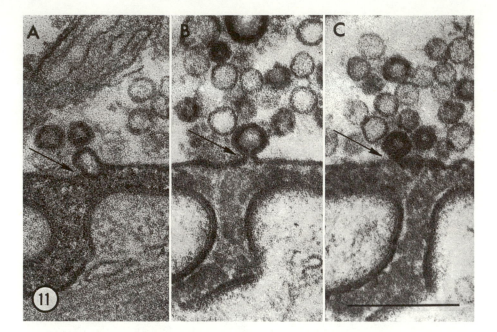

FIGURE 11 High power electron micrographs of portions of three different neuromuscular junctions at the level of the "active zone". The preparations were stimulated for 2 hr at 2/sec in curare ($3 \times 10^{-6}$ g/ml) plus horseradish peroxidase. Junctional clefts contain rich deposits of peroxidase reaction products. The figures show three degrees of association between peroxidase-labeled vesicles and the prejunctional membrane (arrows). In A the membrane of the vesicle is completely fused with the prejunctional membrane; in B the continuity of the two membranes is maintained through a short stalk; and in C the vesicle appears to be in the process of losing contact with the axolemma. 0.25 $\mu$; $\times$ 140,000.

Doctors N. Frontali, A. Grasso, and S. Bettini of the Istituto Superiore di Sanità, Rome, Italy for supplying us with the spiders.

The work was done during the tenure of a fellowship awarded to Dr. Bruno Ceccarelli by the Muscular Dystrophy Associations of America, Inc.

*Received for publication 22 December 1971, and in revised form 27 March 1972.*

REFERENCES

1. BROOKS, V. B., and R. E. THIES. 1962. *J. Physiol. (London).* **162**:298.
2. ELMQVIST, D., W. W. HOFMANN, J. KUGELBERG, and D. M. J. QUASTEL. 1964. *J. Physiol. (London).* **174**:417.
3. ELMQVIST, D., and D. M. J. QUASTEL. 1965. *J. Physiol. (London).* **177**:463.
4. JONES, S. F., and S. KWANBUNBUMPEN. 1970. *J. Physiol. (London).* **207**:31.
5. HURLBUT, W. P., H. E. LONGENECKER, JR., and A. MAURO. 1971. *J. Physiol. (London).* **219**:17.
6. LONGENECKER, H. E., JR., W. P. HURLBUT, A. MAURO, and A. W. CLARK. 1970. *Nature (London).* **225**:701.
7. CLARK, A. W., W. P. HURLBUT, and A. MAURO. 1972. *J. Cell Biol.* **52**:1.
8. GRAHAM, R. C., and M. J. KARNOVSKY. 1966. *J. Histochem. Cytochem.* **14**:291.
9. CAPEK, R., D. W. ESPLIN, and S. SALEHMOG-HADDUM. 1971. *J. Neurophysiol.* **34**:831.
10. BIRKS, R. H., H. E. HUXLEY, and B. KATZ. 1960. *J. Physiol. (London).* **150**:134.
11. HUBBARD, J. I., and S. KWANBUNBUMPEN. 1968. *J. Physiol. (London).* **194**:407.
12. HOLTZMAN, E., A. R. FREEMAN, and L. A. KASHNER. 1971. *Science (Washington).* **173**:733.
13. BITTNER, G. E., and D. KENNEDY. 1970. *J. Cell Biol.* **47**:585.

*Chapter 6*
# TRANSMITTER REMOVAL

After a neurotransmitter is released from a presynaptic nerve terminal, its concentration at the postsynaptic membrane remains high for only a brief period. One factor in its removal is diffusion out of the synaptic cleft, and at a few synapses this appears to be the major factor in reducing the transmitter concentration below physiologically important levels. In addition to diffusion, there are several specific mechanisms for the rapid removal of the transmitter. The enzyme acetylcholinesterase hydrolyzes the transmitter at cholinergic synapses to the physiologically inactive products, choline and acetate. At synapses where norepinephrine and GABA are secreted, specific uptake mechanisms transport the transmitter into surrounding cells.

The physiological importance of the removal of ACh at the vertebrate neuromuscular junction is clear. When acetylcholinesterase is inhibited, repeated stimulation causes accumulation of the transmitter, the ACh receptors become desensitized (see Chapter 7), and neuromuscular transmission fails. The significance of transmitter removal for signaling at the synapses that employ norepinephrine and GABA as transmitters is less certain. Uptake of released norepinephrine does, however, play an important part in the biochemical economy of the synapse, because the transmitter is transported back into the presynaptic terminals and can be secreted again. In an analogous way, the choline produced by the action of acetylcholinesterase at cholinergic junctions is taken up into the terminal and reused for the synthesis of ACh. It has been estimated that half of the choline derived from released ACh is recycled in this way.

Part of the early debate on chemical versus electrical synaptic transmission concerned the apparent difficulty of rapidly removing released ACh from the region of the neuromuscular junction before the arrival of the next impulse. To determine whether acetylcholinesterase plays a role in this process, J. Eccles, B. Katz, and S. Kuffler (1942)

311

examined the effect of the cholinesterase inhibitor eserine on the endplate potential recorded with extracellular electrodes at the frog neuromuscular junction. They demonstrated that eserine potentiated the local postsynaptic response set up by nerve stimulation and that maximal potentiation occurred at the endplate. These findings indicated that ACh was the agent causing the potential and that eserine, by interfering with the hydrolysis of ACh, prolonged its action.

The role of acetylcholinesterase in terminating the action of ACh was further investigated by B. Katz and S. Thesleff in 1957 (reprinted here). They applied both ACh and a reversible acetylcholinesterase inhibitor, edrophonium, by iontophoresis, and followed the response of the muscle by intracellular recording. In suitable doses, edrophonium caused no change in membrane potential, but increased the size of the depolarizing potential produced by ACh. Edrophonium had no effect on the response of the muscle to carbamylcholine, an ACh analogue that is not hydrolyzed by acetylcholinesterase.

Histochemical and autoradiographic techniques have demonstrated that acetylcholinesterase is highly concentrated at the vertebrate neuromuscular junction. A. Roger, et al. (1969) used the stoichiometric reaction of radioactive diisopropylfluorophosphonate (DFP) with acetylcholinesterase to count the enzyme molecules at mouse motor endplates. Incubation of intact muscles with [$^3$H] DFP, followed by autoradiography, yielded an estimate of $3 \times 10^7$ enzyme active sites per endplate.

Several forms of acetylcholinesterase are found in mammalian skeletal muscle, and one of them seems to be specifically associated with the endplate region (Hall, 1973). The endplate enzyme can be selectively detached from the muscle by gentle treatment with collagenase or other proteolytic enzymes. The ease of its removal without alteration of the electrical properties of the membrane suggests that the enzyme resides on the external surface of the cell, either on the exterior of the membrane or on an extracellular structure such as the basement lamina. The superficial location of the enzyme, plus the failure in culture of newly formed neuromuscular junctions to accumulate the endplate enzyme (see Chapter 10), raise interesting questions about its cellular source.

After the importance of enzymic removal of the transmitter had been established for cholinergic junctions, enzymes serving a comparable role at non-cholinergic synapses were sought. In sympathetically innervated tissues, two enzymes, monoamine oxidase and catechol-O-methyl transferase, convert norepinephrine to physiologically inactive products. But inhibitors of neither enzyme enhance the recovery of norepinephrine during stimulation. The mechanism of norepinephrine inactivation thus remained obscure. Investigations by J. Axelrod and colleagues in this country and by B. Stromblad and M. Nickerson in Canada resolved the dilemma. L. Whitby, J. Axelrod, and H. Weil-Malherbe (1961) showed that after injection of radioactive norepinephrine into the circulation, plasma levels of radioactivity fell quickly. The radioactivity in tissues with adrenergic innervation remained at a high level for much longer times. Denervated tissues did not accumulate catecholamines in this way, suggesting that sympathetic nerves were responsible for uptake. D. Wolfe, *et al.* (1962, reprinted here), using autoradiography at the electron microscopic level, directly demonstrated the uptake of catecholamines by nerve terminals.

The properties of the uptake mechanism were further characterized by experiments in which isolated organs, such as heart, were perfused with radioactive norepinephrine (Iversen, 1963). Uptake of the transmitter occurs through a saturable active transport system that enables tissues to accumulate amine to a concentration many times that in the medium. As with other animal cellular transport systems, external sodium ions are required. Cocaine and several other substances block norepinephrine uptake with high affinity (Iversen, 1967). It should be emphasized that uptake occurs across the surface membrane of the terminals and is different from the binding of norepinephrine to vesicles. Norepinephrine that is taken up is retained by the tissue and can be released by nerve stimulation.

In addition, in many tissues there is a second uptake process, called uptake$_2$, which is also saturable, but has a much lower affinity for the transmitter (Iversen, 1965). The pharmacological properties of uptake$_2$ are distinct from those of uptake$_1$, described above. Uptake$_2$ probably represents the transport of norepinephrine into postsynaptic cells or connective tissue. Norepinephrine accumulated by this process is rapidly metabolized.

It has been difficult to obtain detailed information on the role of norepinephrine uptake in terminating the action of the transmitter, partly because of the difficulty of electrophysiological recording from sympathetically innervated tissues. In addition, uptake inhibitors often have secondary effects on the release process or on action potential propagation in the nerve. Complicating matters even more, recent experiments suggest that extracellular norepinephrine may act on presynaptic terminals to depress further transmitter release through a feedback mechanism (see Chapter 5). Inhibition of uptake, by increasing extracellular norepinephrine, may thus decrease the amount of transmitter released and result in no net increase in norepinephrine recovered after trains of stimuli.

Investigation of transmitter removal at synapses employing GABA has followed a course similar to that of studies of noradrenergic junctions. Inhibitors of the enzyme that degrades GABA (GABA-glutamic transaminase) do not affect the physiological response produced by presynaptic nerve stimulation or GABA application, and a highly selective uptake process for GABA has been found in crustacean neuromuscular preparations. This transport system is reminiscent of that found in noradrenergic terminals; it has a high affinity for GABA, is saturable, and requires sodium ions in the bathing medium. A variety of structural analogs of GABA inhibit uptake, but unfortunately they have other effects as well, preventing their use in determining the effect of this uptake system in terminating GABA action.

The sites of GABA uptake in crustacean preparations have been determined through the use of a reaction previously reported as a source of artifact in autoradiographic studies of protein synthesis. This reaction is the covalent attachment of amino acids to macromolecular constituents of tissue by certain aldehyde fixatives. With the aid of a technique based on this reaction, P. Orkand and E. Kravitz (1971, reprinted here) demonstrated that GABA is taken up principally by the Schwann and connective tissue cells in lobster nerve–muscle preparations.

High- and low-affinity uptake systems for GABA have also been found in the mammalian CNS. Autoradiographic studies show that in some CNS regions, uptake occurs chiefly into neuronal elements (Bloom and Iversen, 1971), while in others glial cells are responsible. In a particularly interesting experiment, the uptake of GABA by horizontal cells in fish retina was dramatically stimulated by light, suggesting a relation between uptake and activity (Lam and Steinman, 1971). High affinity uptake systems for other amino acids suspected of being transmitters have also been observed in the mammalian CNS (Logan and Snyder, 1972). If uptake into terminals is specific for substances secreted by the neuron, autoradiographic location of high-affinity uptake systems may be useful in locating terminals that release GABA or other presumed amino acid transmitters (see Chapter 9).

## READING LIST

*Reprinted Papers*

1. Katz, B. and S. Thesleff (1957). The interaction between edro-phonium (tensilon) and acetylcholine at the motor end-plate. *Brit. J. Pharmacol. Chemotherap.* 12: 260–264.

2. Wolfe, D.E., L.T. Potter, K.C. Richardson, and J. Axelrod (1962). Localizing tritiated norepinephrine in sympathetic axons by electron microscopic autoradiography. *Science* 138: 440–442.

3. Orkand, P.M. and E.A. Kravitz (1971). Localization of the sites of γ-aminobutyric acid (GABA) uptake in lobster nerve–muscle preparations. *J. Cell. Biol.* 49: 75–89.

*Other Selected Papers*

4. Eccles, J.C., B. Katz, and S.W. Kuffler (1942). Effect of eserine on neuromuscular transmission. *J. Neurophysiol.* 5: 211–230.

5. Whitby, L.G., J. Axelrod, and H. Weil-Malherbe (1961). The fate of $^3$H-norepinephrine in animals. *J. Pharmacol. Exp. Therap.* 132: 193–201.

6. Iversen, L.L. (1963). The uptake of noradrenaline by the isolated perfused rat heart. *Brit. J. Pharmacol. Chemotherap.* 21: 523–537.

7. Iversen, L.L. (1965). The uptake of catechol amines at high perfusion concentrations in the rat isolated heart: A novel catecholamine uptake process. *Brit. J. Pharmacol. Chemotherap.* 25: 18–33.

8. Iversen, L.L. (1967). *The Uptake and Storage of Noradrenaline in Sympathetic Nerves,* London and New York: Cambridge University Press.

9. Rogers, A.W., Z. Darzynkiewicz, M.M. Salpeter, K. Ostrowski, and E.A. Barnard (1969). Quantitative studies on enzymes in structures in striated muscles by labeled inhibitor methods. I. The number of acetylcholinesterase molecules and of other DFP-reactive sites at motor endplates, measured by radioautography. *J. Cell. Biol.* 41: 665–685.

10. Lam, D.M.K. and L. Steinman (1971). The uptake of [γ-$^3$H] aminobutyric acid in the goldfish retina. *Proc. Nat. Acad. Sci.* 68: 2777–2781.

11. Bloom, F.E. and L.L. Iversen (1971). Localizing $^3$H-GABA in nerve terminals of rat cerebral cortex by electron microscopic autoradiography. *Nature* 229: 628–630.

12. Logan, W.J. and S.H. Snyder (1972). High affinity uptake systems for glycine, glutamic and aspartic acids in synaptosomes of rat central nervous tissues. *Brain Res.* 42: 413–431.

13. Katz, B. and R. Miledi (1973). The binding of acetylcholine to receptors and its removal from the synaptic cleft. *J. Physiol.* 231: 549–574.

14. Hall, Z.W. (1973). Multiple forms of acetylcholinesterase and their distribution in endplate and non-endplate regions of rat diaphragm muscle. *J. Neurobiol.* 4: 343–361.

15. Rieger, F., S. Bon, J. Massoulié, et J. Cartaud (1973). Observation par microscopie électronique des formes allongées et globulaires de l'acétylcholinestérase de gymnote *(Electrophorus electricus). Eur. J. Biochem.* 34: 539–547.

# THE INTERACTION BETWEEN EDROPHONIUM (TENSILON) AND ACETYLCHOLINE AT THE MOTOR END-PLATE

BY

B. KATZ AND S. THESLEFF

*From the Department of Biophysics, University College, London*

(RECEIVED MARCH 28, 1957)

The effect of edrophonium (3-hydroxy-phenyl-dimethylethylammonium chloride) on the motor end-plate and its interaction with acetylcholine and carbachol has been investigated. Use was made of intracellular recording of membrane potential and of ionophoretic micro-application of drugs from single and twin-pipettes.

Small doses of edrophonium potentiate the depolarizing effect of acetylcholine, but not that of carbachol. This action can be observed with doses of edrophonium which have no depolarizing effect by themselves. Large doses of edrophonium have some depolarizing action and, at the same time, inhibit depolarizations produced by carbachol. After treatment with neostigmine, edrophonium fails to potentiate the acetylcholine response. The observations are in agreement with the view that the principal action of edrophonium on the neuromuscular junction is that of a potent and rapidly acting anticholinesterase.

The effects of anticholinesterases on muscle are usually tested under conditions in which the inhibitor/enzyme reaction has been approached or reached equilibrium. In recent experiments (Castillo and Katz, 1957c), a different method was used, brief localized doses of the drug being applied to an end-plate with the help of an ionophoretic micro-technique. Under these conditions, the observed potency of a drug depends on the kinetics, rather than the equilibrium constant, of the reaction. In such experiments it was found that substances like neostigmine, which are strong but slowly acting enzyme inhibitors, produced no potentiation of the acetylcholine response, while less powerful but more rapidly acting esterase inhibitors (choline, decamethonium) caused a marked increase in the acetylcholine effect.

Similar experiments will be described in which edrophonium (3-hydroxy-phenyl-dimethylethyl-ammonium chloride) was allowed to interact with acetylcholine (ACh), by applying the substances from micropipettes placed at close range to an end-plate of the frog's sartorius muscle. The membrane potential of the muscle fibre was recorded with an intracellular electrode inserted within a few hundred microns of the point of drug action.

The effect of edrophonium on neuromuscular transmission in the frog has previously been studied by Nastuk and Alexander (1954), who concluded that the anticurare action of this substance and the modifications which it produced in the shape of the electric end-plate response could be attributed to its anti-esterase activity (see also Smith, Cohen, Pelikan, and Unna, 1952). The present experiments confirm this view and provide additional evidence for the high speed at which the reaction between edrophonium and ACh-esterase proceeds.

## METHOD

The technique has been described in detail in previous papers (Castillo and Katz, 1955, 1957a, c; see also Katz and Thesleff, 1957). The experiments were made on isolated sartorius muscles of *R. temporaria* at about 20° C. The preparations were mounted in a bath of Ringer solution which contained the electrodes for the recording of membrane potentials and for the electrophoretic application of drugs. Single or twin-pipettes were used, containing edrophonium and ACh. or edrophonium and carbachol, in the twin barrels. Edrophonium (Tensilon) was obtained by courtesy of Roche Products. Individual drug pipettes had tip diameters of less than 1 $\mu$ and were filled with a concentrated solution (0.5 to 2.5 M). The discharge of the drug was regulated by "braking" or "releasing" voltages (making the interior of the pipette more negative, or positive, respectively), in the way described in the earlier papers (Castillo and Katz, 1955, 1957a). The current flowing through the drug pipettes was registered on the second beam of the oscilloscope.

Reprinted from the *British Journal of Pharmacology and Chemotherapy* 12: 260–264 (1957) by permission of the authors, the Editor, and the publisher.

## RESULTS

Fig. 1 illustrates the potentiating action of edrophonium. The records show potential changes produced at the end-plate region of a muscle fibre when ACh and edrophonium were discharged from a twin pipette in the immediate neighbourhood. In this experiment ACh was released from one barrel by slightly reducing the steady " braking " current which passed through it. This gave rise to a steady depolarization causing an upward displacement of the baseline from *a* to *b*, and then to *c*. The bottom trace serves to register the current through the pipettes, but the changes in the ACh-pipette were so small (of the order of $10^{-9}$ A.) that no visible displacement in the three successive lines occurred. The brief deflexion which interrupts this trace arose from a pulse through the edrophonium pipette (about $1.4 \times 10^{-8}$ A., duration 13 msec.). The discharge had practically no effect in record *a* when ACh efflux was prevented. In record *b*, when a small efflux of ACh was present producing a steady depolarization of about 0.5 mV, this potential change increased to 3 mV after the edrophonium pulse. In record *c*, a steady ACh potential of 4 mV was increased to 14 mV by the same pulse of edrophonium.

It appeared from these results that a momentary application of edrophonium which, by itself, produced no potential change (record *a*), caused a several-fold increase of the depolarizing effect of ACh. The time course of this potentiation was rapid and had practically subsided within less than one second.

The effect shown in Fig. 1 might be explained by a rapid and quickly reversible anti-esterase action of edrophonium. To test this assumption,

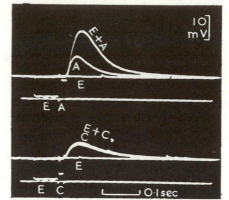

FIG. 2.—Upper part shows potentiation of a brief ACh-potential by a preceding edrophonium pulse. Lower part shows the barely noticeable effect produced by edrophonium on a carbachol potential. In each record, three traces were superimposed. E, edrophonium; A, acetylcholine; C, carbachol. See text for further details. Monitor calibration, 10 mV scale $=6.7 \times 10^{-8}$ A.

two kinds of experiments were made: (*a*) effects of edrophonium were examined when ACh was replaced by a stable depolarizing substance (carbachol); (*b*) the interactions were studied before and after the muscle had been treated with neostigmine.

All the subsequent experiments were made with an assembly of three drug-pipettes, one—a twin pipette—containing edrophonium and carbachol in the two barrels, another separate pipette containing ACh and being placed nearby. This arrangement was chosen to obviate the possibility that any increase in the ACh effect could have been brought about by leakage between the twin barrels. It should be noted that with this set-up, because of the closer proximity of edrophonium and carbachol pipettes, any effect which edrophonium may have on the carbachol response would be more easily detected than interactions between edrophonium and ACh.

In Fig. 2, an example of the results is shown. In the upper part, three records are superimposed in which an edrophonium pulse (E), an ACh pulse (A), and both pulses together (E + A), were applied. The edrophonium pulse by itself produced a minute depolarization, barely rising above the base-line. The ACh dose alone produced the smaller of the two main deflexions. When the ACh pulse was preceded by the edrophonium pulse, the amplitude of the deflexion was more than doubled. In the lower part of the figure a similar series of three records is superimposed, but this time carbachol was used instead of ACh.

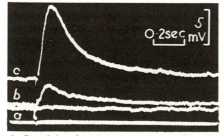

FIG. 1.—Potentiation of steady ACh-potential by a pulse of edrophonium. The pulse is shown in the bottom trace. It had no effect in (*a*) (when ACh-efflux was stopped by a small braking current), but produced a transient large increase of the steady depolarization in (*b*) and (*c*) (when a controlled small efflux from the ACh pipette occurred). See text for further details. The 5 mV scale refers to the membrane potentials (*a* to *c*). Calibration of the " current-monitor " (bottom trace): 5 mV scale $=9.1 \times 10^{-8}$ A.

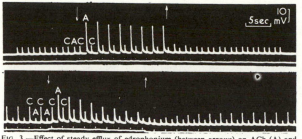

FIG. 3.—Effect of steady efflux of edrophonium (between arrows) on ACh (A) and carbachol (C) potentials. For full description, see text. Monitor calibration, 10 mV scale=8 × 10⁻⁸ A.

The combination of edrophonium + carbachol pulses produced only a very slightly increased effect above that due to the carbachol pulse alone.

That the edrophonium-potentiation is observed specifically with ACh, and not with carbachol, is brought out in a somewhat different fashion in Fig. 3. Here, alternate pulses of ACh and carbachol were applied to the end-plate, and the resulting brief depolarization recorded on slowly moving film. During the interval marked by arrows, the " brake " on the edrophonium barrel was reduced or reversed (signalled by a very small upward displacement of the bottom trace), and a steady efflux of this substance, therefore, occurred. In the upper part of Fig. 3, the pulses of ACh and carbachol had been adjusted initially so that the responses were of approximately the same amplitude. As soon as edrophonium began to be released, a large increase of the ACh-potentials occurred, while the carbachol potentials remained practically unaltered. After the end of the edrophonium application, the ACh-potentials declined within a few seconds to the level of the carbachol responses.

In the lower part of Fig. 3, different dosages were chosen. The pulses had been adjusted so that initially the carbachol potentials were about three times larger than the ACh potentials. The steady edrophonium dose was also increased, to a strength at which it produced a small, but noticeable, steady depolarization. The effect of edrophonium was two-fold. The ACh response was potentiated, its amplitude now exceeding the carbachol potential. The initial increase, however, was not maintained, but the responses gradu-

ally declined during the edrophonium period. This decline affected ACh and carbachol potentials to the same extent, and the ACh potentials remained larger than the carbachol until the efflux of edrophonium was stopped. It is clear, therefore, that the decline was not due to a gradual diminution of the specific ACh potentiation by the drug, but to a progressive " desensitization " of receptors which occurs whenever a depolarizing substance is applied for a prolonged period (see Katz and Thesleff, 1957, for a detailed study of this phenomenon).

It can be concluded from these results that small doses of edrophonium, which by themselves do not appreciably alter the membrane p.d., increase the depolarizing effect of ACh, but not that of carbachol. This supports the view that the effect is brought about by inhibition of ACh-esterase.

When the dose of edrophonium was increased, the potentiation became intensified as shown in Fig. 4 (left part). The method was the same as employed in Fig. 1: an edrophonium pulse was applied during a period of steady ACh depolarization. The bottom traces in each frame show an

ACh                    Carbachol

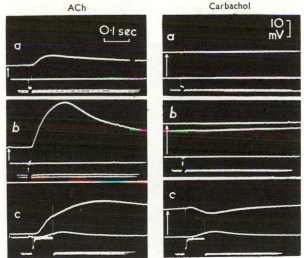

FIG. 4.—Effect of different doses of edrophonium on ACh (left part) and carbachol potentials (right part). The procedure was the same as in Fig. 1, a steady dose of ACh or carbachol being combined with a pulse of edrophonium. The depolarization due to ACh or carbachol is shown by the displacement of the trace in the direction of the arrow. The records in each horizontal row were obtained with the same edrophonium dose, whose strength was increased from *a* to *c*. Note that in *a* and *b*, the edrophonium by itself had no effect on the membrane potential, while it produced a small, transient depolarization in *c*. For further description, see text. Monitor calibration, 10 mV scale — 7.9 × 10⁻⁸ A.

edrophonium pulse, whose coulomb strength was increased from *a* to *c*. In each frame, two records are shown, (1) when ACh efflux has been stopped by a large " braking " current, and (2) when ACh release was allowed to occur. In frame *c*, a very small steady dose of ACh was given, producing only 2 to 3 mV. depolarization ; this was a necessary precaution to avoid excitation and twitching. Potentiation increased, from a factor of 1.7 in *a*, to about 10 times in *c*. In addition, the effect was lengthened considerably.

It will be observed that in *a* and *b*, the edrophonium pulse by itself produced no potential change, while in *c* a transient depolarization of a few mV. was seen. This indicates that there is a substantial margin between the doses of edrophonium which interfere with ACh esterase, and those which combine effectively with the receptors (see also Nastuk and Alexander, 1954). In this respect, edrophonium may be classified as a " specific " anti-esterase, like neostigmine, but unlike decamethonium or choline which have a mixed action on esterase and receptors in the same dosage range (Castillo and Katz, 1957c).

The right-hand part of Fig. 4 shows, for comparison, interactions between edrophonium and carbachol at the same end-plate spot. Each horizontal row of records in Fig. 4 was obtained with identical edrophonium pulses. In the upper right frame, no effect is observed. In the middle frame, there is a barely noticeable trace of inhibition ; in the lower frame, the inhibitory effect of edrophonium on the carbachol-potential is well marked. We are dealing here with an example of competitive interference between two depolarizing drugs, of the kind described in detail by Castillo and Katz (1957c ; see also Ariëns, 1954 ; Stephenson, 1956).

Finally, the observations were repeated after the preparation had been treated for about 30 min. with neostigmine. With a concentration of 10⁻⁶ w/v (neostigmine methylsulphate/Ringer), the potentiating action of edrophonium was greatly reduced. With a two to four times larger dose of neostigmine, the potentiation of the ACh effect had vanished, and the interaction between edrophonium and ACh was now very similar to that observed with edrophonium and carbachol, that is, when relatively large doses were used, edrophonium now *inhibited* ACh as well as carbachol potentials. An example is shown in Fig. 5. The upper records show the depolarization produced by the large edrophonium pulse. The middle frames show an ACh and a carbachol potential, respectively ; the lower frames show the depression of both ACh and carbachol effects when they are preceded by an edrophonium pulse.

Thus, initial treatment with a more slowly-acting, but powerful, anti-esterase abolishes the potentiation, and all that is left is the relatively weak depolarizing action of edrophonium and the associated inhibitory effect due to its competition with more powerful depolarizing agents.

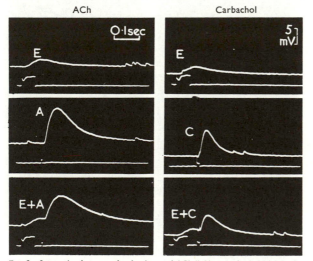

FIG. 5.—Interaction between edrophonium and ACh (left), or carbachol (right), after pre-treatment with neostigmine. The procedure was similar to that in Fig. 2, except that a large dose of edrophonium was used which depolarized by itself. E, edrophonium; A, ACh; C, carbachol. Note that the potentiation of the ACh effect (Fig. 4c, left) has now given place to inhibition, similar to that observed with carbachol. Monitor calibration, 5 mV scale=7.9 × 10⁻⁸ A.

## DISCUSSION

The results fully support the conclusions reached by Nastuk and Alexander (1954) and by Smith *et. al.* (1952), namely that the principal action of edrophonium on neuromuscular transmission is that of an anticholinesterase. Application of this drug potentiates the effect of ACh, but not of its stable analogue, carbachol ; and the potentiation is not seen when the esterase activity has already been inhibited by neostigmine.

The time course of the potentiating effect is rapid. For example, in the experiment illustrated in Fig. 1, the effect of an edrophonium pulse rose to a peak in 85 msec. and fell to one half in about 140 msec. which was only four times slower than a small depolarization produced at the same spot by a similar pulse of ACh from the adjacent pipette. In comparing the time courses of these two effects, a factor of two should be allowed for the enzymatic removal of ACh (see Castillo and Katz, 1957b), and some part of the remaining difference is probably due to slower diffusion rather than to the reaction kinetics. In any case, the bond between edrophonium and esterase must be rapidly reversible, with a time constant of dissociation of less than 0.1 sec. at 20° C. This is very much faster than the dissociation rate of the neostigmine- or eserine-enzyme complex (see Easson and Stedman, 1936; Eccles, Katz, and Kuffler, 1942; Augustinsson and Nachmansohn, 1949; Goldstein, 1951), which have time constants of the order of several minutes and exert their effects too slowly to be usefully investigated with the present method.

Some comment is needed on the relatively small interaction between edrophonium and carbachol. The reduction of a carbachol depolarization by a large pulse of edrophonium can be explained on the asumption that both drugs combine with receptor molecules, but that the edrophonium receptor complex has less " depolarizing efficacy " (see Stephenson, 1956) than the carbachol receptor compound.

With weaker doses of edrophonium, however, a small increase of the carbachol potential was often observed (Fig. 2). This was seen usually when the edrophonium application by itself produced a just noticeable depolarizing effect. It is probable that this small, positive, interaction arises from the fact that two *weak* doses of any depolarizing drug produce a more than additive effect, their dose/response relation having an S-shaped, rather than a linear, start (Katz and Thesleff, 1957).

We are indebted to Mr. J. L. Parkinson for his unfailing help, and to the Nuffield Foundation for financial assistance. It is a pleasure also to thank Dr. F. Hobbiger for valuable discussion. One of us (S. T.) was in receipt of a Travel Grant from the Swedish Medical Research Council.

REFERENCES

Ariëns, E. J. (1954). *Arch. int. Pharmacodyn.*, **99**, 32.
Augustinsson, K. B., and Nachmansohn, D. (1949). *J. biol. Chem.*, **179**, 543.
Castillo, J. del, and Katz, B. (1955). *J. Physiol.*, **128**, 157.
—— —— (1957a). *Proc. roy. Soc. B.*, **146**, 339.
—— —— (1957b). Ibid., **146**, 362.
—— —— (1957c). Ibid., **146**, 369.
Easson, L. H., and Stedman, E. (1936). Ibid., **121**, 142.
Eccles, J. C., Katz, B., and Kuffler, S. W. (1942). *J. Neurophysiol.*, **5**, 211.
Goldstein, A. (1951). *Arch. Biochem. Biophys.*, **34**, 169.
Katz, B., and Thesleff, S. (1957). *J. Physiol.*, **137**, in the press.
Nastuk, W. L., and Alexander, J. T. (1954). *J. Pharmacol.*, **111**, 302.
Smith, C. M., Cohen, H. L., Pelikan, E. W., and Unna, K. R. (1952). Ibid., **105**, 391.
Stephenson, R. P. (1956). *Brit. J. Pharmacol.*, **11**, 379.

# LOCALIZING TRITIATED NOREPINEPHRINE IN SYMPATHETIC AXONS BY ELECTRON MICROSCOPIC AUTORADIOGRAPHY

*D.E. Wolfe, L.T. Potter,*
*K.C. Richardson, J. Axelrod*
*National Institute of Neurological Diseases*
*and Blindness, and National Institute of*
*Mental Health, Bethesda, Maryland*

*Following intravenous infusion of tritiated norepinephrine, rat pineals were prepared for combined autoradiography and electron microscopy. Concentrations of photographic grains were observed only over regions of preterminal autonomic axons containing granulated vesicles, thereby directly demonstrating uptake of norepinephrine into these axons and strongly suggesting that their granulated vesicles contain norepinephrine.*

Electron-microscope studies (*1–5*) have established the presence of characteristic "granulated vesicles" in many autonomic axons. These granulated vesicles are 40 to 50 m$\mu$ wide, contain a 20 to 30 m$\mu$ electron-dense core, and seem to be concentrated in preterminal axoplasm (Fig. 1). It has been suggested that granulated vesicles contain serotonin (*1*), norepinephrine (*2*), or one of several "reducing amines" (*3*). These suggestions rest upon such circumstantial evidence as the morphological analogy between granulated vesicles and chromaffin cell granules possessing a limiting membrane and a dense core, the known concentration of norepinephrine in sympathetic nerves (*6*), and the evidence from centrifugation studies of splenic nerve homogenates that at least 20 percent of the total norepinephrine is associated with "particles" somewhat similar to catecholamine-containing granules obtained from adrenal homogenates (*7*). From one brief reference to an electron microscopic examination of splenic nerve fractions containing particle-associated norepinephrine (*8*), it is uncertain whether the structures observed are identical with the granulated vesicles described above. Electron-microscope studies of autonomic nerves in reserpinized rats (*3, 9*) have not established a definite alteration in the population of granulated vesicles; and, in general, reserpine is too nonspecific a releasing agent to yield precise chemical information about the structures it affects. Thus there is no unequivocal evidence that granulated vesicles in autonomic axons contain norepinephrine, or that they are present only in adrenergic sympathetic fibers.

Recent studies show that tritiated norepinephrine ($H^3$-NE) is rapidly concentrated and retained in certain tissues (*10*). This uptake of $H^3$-NE is prevented by sympathetic denervation (*11*). Once bound in a tissue, $H^3$-NE can be released by sympathetic nerve stimulation and by various sympathomimetic agents (*12*). These findings suggest that $H^3$-NE is taken up into adrenergic sympathetic axons and/or into some anatomically separate structure requiring the presence of sympathetic axons to maintain its capacity to bind $H^3$-NE, such as chromaffin cells (*13*). To decide between these alternative explanations and to obtain more definite information about granulated vesicles in autonomic axons are major aims of the present study. The association of $H^3$-NE with physically separable cytoplasmic particles, and the tendency of catecholamines to form insoluble compounds with fixatives, suggest that the amount of $H^3$-NE lost during fixation, dehydration, and embedding for electron microscopy is small, although direct measurements have not been performed.

Successful localization of $H^3$-NE by the present methods, however, merely requires the preservation of sufficient quantities of tritiated material to yield unequivocal autoradiographs on thin sections of tissue. The attribution of autoradiographic grain clusters specifically to the presence of $H^3$-NE in the underlying tissue section is justified by the demonstration (*10*) that more than 90 percent of a tissue's radioactivity following injection of $H^3$-NE is due to that compound, while its major metabolite, tritiated normetanephrine, contributes an amount of radioactivity that is negligible in the present investigation.

The pineal body was examined because of the richness of its sympathetic innervation (*14*), its known concentration of norepinephrine (*15*), its ability to concentrate $H^3$-NE in vivo in a particulate fraction similar to the particle-associated norepinephrine obtained from rat heart homogenates (*16*), the availability of electron microscopic descriptions of pineal autonomic nerves (*1, 3, 5*), and the knowledge that at least some of the neurites containing granulated vesicles are axons which terminate on pineal parenchymal cells (*5*). Thirty minutes after a slow intravenous infusion of 250 $\mu$c of *dl*-norepinephrine-7-$H^3$ (20 mc/mg), the pineal bodies of adult Osborne-Mendel rats were fixed by perfusion with osmium tetroxide (*17*) and embedded in

323

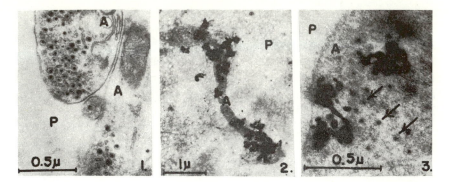

Figs. 1–3. Electron micrographs of sympathetic axons (*A*) in perivascular space (*P*) of rat pineal body after injection of H³-NE. Fig. 1. Clusters of granulated vesicles in sympathetic axons. Fig. 2. Autoradiographic grain concentration over a sympathetic axon. Fig. 3. Specific association of autoradiographic grains with axonal regions containing granulated vesicles (arrows). Figures 2 and 3 are electron microscopic autoradiographs showing opaque, characteristically coiled autoradiographic grains over specimen areas containing H³-NE. The presence of processed photographic emulsion gives a mottled appearance to these two micrographs.

Epon 812. Thin sections were prepared for autoradiography and examination in an RCA EMU 3E electron microscope by methods recently described (*18*), with Ilford L4 nuclear research emulsion and exposure times of 4 to 12 days.

Electron microscopy revealed a very striking localization of photographic grains to areas overlying nonmyelinated axons situated in the perivascular spaces and occasionally between the pineal parenchymal cells (Fig. 2). These axons were single or in bundles and often were encompassed by a basement membrane without an intervening Schwann cell, like autonomic axons elsewhere in the body (*2*). Grain concentrations occurred only over nonmyelinated axons which contained granulated vesicles in the immediate vicinity of grain aggregation (Fig. 3). No grain concentrations were found over pineal parenchymal cells or their perivascular processes, or over any other cells in the perivascular spaces. Cells with granules resembling those in chromaffin cells were not seen.

From these findings we conclude: (i) Circulating H³-NE is taken up into nonmyelinated axons. (ii) No anatomically separate entities such as chromaffin cells or Schwann cells are required for the uptake of H³-NE by these axons. (iii) The autonomic axons incorporating H³-NE are adrenergic sympathetic axons because this capacity, in autonomic nerves elsewhere in the body, is displayed only by elements possessing the defining pharmacological parameters of adrenergic sympathetic axons (*11, 12*). (iv) The constant association of auto-radiographic grain concentration with granulated vesicles directly demonstrates a constant association of $H^3$-NE with granulated vesicles, thereby providing independent evidence for the hypothesis that norepinephrine in sympathetic axons resides in membrane-limited structures, and strengthening the idea that (v) norepinephrine resides in the electron-dense core of the granulated vesicle. (vi) The presence of granulated vesicles can be used as one criterion for the identifi-cation of adrenergic sympathetic axons in electron micrographs. (vii) The absence of autoradiographic grain concentrations over pineal parenchymal cells and the failure to observe typical granulated vesicles in these cells (*1, 5*) suggest that pineal cells neither contain endo-genous nor bind exogenous norepinephrine.

## REFERENCES AND NOTES

1. A. Milofsky, thesis, Yale School of Medicine (1958).
2. K.C. Richardson, *J. Anat. (London),* in press.
3. E. De Robertis and A. Pellegrino de Iraldi, *J. Biophys. Biochem. Cytol.* 10, 361 (1961).
4. M.A. Grillo and S.L. Palay, unpublished data.
5. D.E. Wolfe, unpublished data.
6. U.S. von Euler, *Noradrenaline* (Thomas, Springfield, Ill., 1956); H.J. Schümann, *Arch. Exptl. Pathol. Pharmakol.* 227, 566 (1956).
7. U.S. von Euler, *Acta Physiol. Scand.* 43, 155 (1958); U.S. von Euler and F. Lishajko, *ibid.* 51, 193; ———, *ibid.* 53, 196 (1961); H.J. Schümann, *Arch. Exptl. Pathol. Pharmakol.* 233, 296; ———, *ibid.* 234, 17 (1958).
8. U.S. von Euler, *Adrenergic Mechanisms,* J.R. Vane Ed., (Little, Brown, Boston, Mass., 1960), p. 493.
9. A. Pellegrino de Iraldi and E. De Robertis, *Experientia* 17, 122 (1961).
10. L.G. Whitby *et al., J. Pharmacol. Exptl. Therap.* 132, 193 (1961).
11. G. Hertting *et al., Nature* 189, 66 (1961).
12. G. Hertting and J. Axelrod, *ibid.* 192, 172 (1961); J. Axelrod *et al., ibid.* 194, 297 (1962).
13. J.H. Burn and M.J. Rand, *Brit. J. Pharmacol.* 15, 56 (1960).
14. J.A. Kappers, *Z. Zellforsch. u. mikroskop. Anat.* 52, 163 (1960).
15. N.J. Giarman and M. Day, *Biochem. Pharmacol.* 1, 235 (1958).

16. L.T. Potter, unpublished data.
17. S.L. Palay *et al.*, *J. Cell Biol.* 12, 385 (1962).
18. L. Caro, *J. Biophys. Biochem. Cytol.* 10, 37 (1961); J.P. Revel and E.D. Hay, *Exptl. Cell Res.* 25, 475 (1961).

# LOCALIZATION OF THE SITES OF

# γ-AMINOBUTYRIC ACID (GABA) UPTAKE IN

# LOBSTER NERVE-MUSCLE PREPARATIONS

## PAULA M. ORKAND and EDWARD A. KRAVITZ

From the Department of Anatomy, University of California at Los Angeles School of Medicine, Los Angeles, California 90024, and the Department of Neurobiology, Harvard Medical School, Boston, Massachusetts 02115

## ABSTRACT

The principal sites of γ-aminobutyric acid (GABA) uptake in lobster nerve-muscle preparations have been determined with radioautographic techniques after binding of the amino acid to proteins by aldehyde fixation. Semiquantitative studies showed that about 30% of the radioactive GABA taken into the tissue was bound to protein by fixation. Both light and electron micrographs showed dense accumulations of label over Schwann and connective tissue cell cytoplasm; muscle was lightly labeled, but axons and terminals were almost devoid of label. The possible role of Schwann and connective tissue cells in the inactivation of GABA released from inhibitory axons is discussed.

## INTRODUCTION

Both excitatory and inhibitory neurons directly innervate crustacean skeletal muscle. For this reason, the crustacean nerve-muscle preparation has been extremely valuable for studying the postsynaptic effects of inhibitory nerve stimulation and the interactions between excitatory and inhibitory nerve terminals. The identity and metabolism of the neurotransmitter compounds at these junctions have also been under investigation. Glutamate is the leading candidate for the excitatory transmitter compound (Takeuchi and Takeuchi, 1964), while its decarboxylation product, γ-aminobutyric acid (GABA), is well established as the inhibitory transmitter substance. The evidence presented in support of the transmitter role for GABA includes the demonstration that GABA (*a*) mimics the physiological action of inhibitory nerve stimulation (Boistel and Fatt, 1958; Dudel and Kuffler, 1961; Takeuchi and Takeuchi, 1965), (*b*) is the most active inhibitory compound found in the lobster nervous system (Kravitz et al., 1963),

(*c*) is concentrated in inhibitory neurons (Kravitz and Potter, 1965), and (*d*) is selectively released from inhibitory nerves with stimulation (Otsuka et al., 1966).

In the search for a possible inactivation mechanism for GABA, it was found that an uptake mechanism existed in lobster nerve-muscle preparations (Iversen and Kravitz, 1968). The uptake was specific for GABA; closely related amino acids like glutamate and β-alanine did not interfere. Preparations concentrated GABA to levels several times those of the medium. Uptake was a saturable process, required Na[+], and had an apparent $K_m$ of $6 \times 10^{-5}$ M. When tissues were incubated with GABA-[3]H the major portion (95%) of the radioactivity taken into tissues remained as GABA-[3]H after 1 hr of incubation, and no radioactivity was incorporated into protein.

The latter two observations suggested a possible means of localizing the intracellular site or sites of GABA uptake. It was anticipated that, as a

Reprinted from *The Journal of Cell Biology* 49: 75–89 (1971) by permission of the publisher.

free amino acid, radioactive GABA in the tissue would not survive routine histological procedures. On the other hand, there is an artefact in radio-autography reported by Peters and Ashley (1967) in which free amino acids are bound to tissues by fixatives containing glutaraldehyde. The compounds formed survive dehydration and plastic embedding, and can be visualized by both light and electron microscope radioautography.

The present paper is concerned with the use of aldehyde fixation methods to bind GABA-³H to tissues, and with the localization of the principal sites of GABA uptake.

## MATERIALS AND METHODS

### Nerve-Muscle Preparation

The superficial flexor muscles from the left and right sides of the second and third abdominal segments of 0.5 kg lobster (*Homarus americanus*) were dissected along with their exoskeletal attachments and about 1 cm of the nerve bundle innervating them. The muscles are thin (approximately 1 mm in thickness), allowing adequate contact of tissue with the incubaton medium.

### Incubation Conditions

Muscles were immersed in 5 or 10 ml of saline medium (containing 460 mM NaCl, 15.6 mM KCl, 26 mM $CaCl_2$, 8.3 mM $MgSO_4$, and 13 mM D-glucose) in individual 20-ml beakers. GABA-³H (SA 2 Ci/mmole, New England Nuclear Corp., Boston, Mass.) was added to the medium in final concentrations ranging from $7 \times 10^{-7}$ M to $3.5 \times 10^{-6}$ M. In one experiment, GABA of lower specific activity was used at a concentration of $5 \times 10^{-4}$ M. GABA-³H was purified before use by adsorption to and elution from a Dowex-50-H⁺ column (Dowex Chemical Co., Midland, Mich.) and passing the recovered material over a Dowex-1 acetate column (see Hall and Kravitz, 1967 for experimental details). The preparations were incubated at 15–18°C with shaking for 1 hr, or, in long-term incubations, for 7 hr. After incubation, in order to wash GABA-³H from the extracellular spaces, the muscles were shaken in fresh saline medium without GABA-³H for two periods of 10 min each, or for three periods of 30 min each.

### Fixation

One muscle of each pair was pinned at about rest length to a Sylgard-containing dish (Sylgard 184-Dow Corning Corp. Midland, Mich.), and the fixative was poured over the preparation. Fixation was continued for either 2 or 18 hr. Glutaraldehyde alone, or a variety of mixtures of glutaraldehyde and acrolein (G-A), or glutaraldehyde and paraformaldehyde (G-P) buffered to pH 7.2–7.4 with 0.1 M phosphate (Millonig, 1962), were used. The best fixation for electron microscopy was achieved with a mixture of 1% glutaraldehyde and 4% paraformaldehyde (G-P) in phosphate buffer with 5.7 mM NaCl, 18 mM $CaCl_2$, and 90 mM sucrose. This fixative produced a satisfactory binding of GABA-³H to tissue (see Results), and was used in most experiments. After fixation, the muscles were briefly washed in buffer containing 10% sucrose and dehydrated in a graded methanol series. Muscles used for electron microscopy were postfixed for 2 hr in 2% $OsO_4$ in phosphate buffer before dehydration in methanol and embedding in Epon 812.

### Determination of Radioactivity Surviving Fixation and Dehydration

The fixed and dehydrated muscle and the unfixed muscle of each pair were cut from their skeletal attachments, homogenized in 0.4 N perchloric acid, and centrifuged. The supernatant was collected and the precipitate was washed several additional times with 0.4 N perchloric acid. Samples of the supernatant fraction and precipitates suspended in thixotropic gel (Packard Instrument Co. Inc., Downers Grove, Ill.) were counted in a liquid scintillation spectrometer. Internal standards were added to correct for quenching. Since uptake into the two muscles of a pair is similar (Iversen and Kravitz, 1968), binding of GABA-³H by aldehyde fixation was roughly quantitated by determining the ratio of label in the perchloric acid precipitate of the fixed and dehydrated muscle to the total radioactivity in the extract of the unfixed muscle. In two experiments, samples of the fixative and each change of methanol were counted to search for a loss of label during dehydration.

Liquid scintillation measurements of radioactivity were not done on osmium-treated tissue since the osmium interfered with the counting technique. However, the radioautograms of osmicated and nonosmicated tissues were similar, suggesting that label is not lost in large amounts during postosmication.

### Radioautography

LIGHT MICROSCOPY. Pieces of GABA-³H treated muscle that had been fixed in aldehydes, with or without postosmication, were dehydrated and embedded in Epon 812. Sections 1 or 2 $\mu$ thick were cut with glass knives on a Porter-Blum MT-2 ultramicrotome, and mounted on glass slides. They were dipped into melted Ilford L4 Nuclear Research emulsion (Ilford, Ltd., Ilford, Essex, England) diluted 1:1 with water, dried, and kept in light-tight boxes at room temperature for 2 days–2 wk. After exposure they were developed with Dektol (Eastman Kodak Co., Rochester, N.Y.) and fixed in Kodak acid fixer. In addition, some were stained with 0.1% toluidine blue in 1% Borax.

ELECTRON MICROSCOPY. Sections showing silver to pale gold interference colors were dried on collodion-coated slides which were then dipped into Ilford L4 emulsion. After a 10 day–4 wk exposure, the radioautograms were developed with Kodak Microdol X and fixed in acid fixer. The collodion films were stripped from the slides on distilled water and the tissue sections were picked up on copper grids. After staining with lead citrate (Venable and Coggeshall, 1965) the radioautograms were studied in a Philips 200 electron microscope.

## Electrophoresis of Products of Mixtures of Fixative, Radioactive GABA-H³ and Serum Albumin

1 μl of GABA-³H (SA 2Ci/mmole) containing 1 μCi of isotope was mixed with 1 μl of serum albumin (10 mg/ml) and 10 μl of G-P fixative (see above) in various combinations (see Fig. 1). As soon as possible after mixing, 1 μl samples were removed and spotted in the middle of strips of electrophoresis paper prewet with formate:acetate buffer at pH 1.9. Electrophoresis was performed at room temperature in a Durrum cell (Beckman Instruments, Inc., Fullerton, Calif.) at 250 v for 1.5 hr. The total elapsed time between the mixing of the samples and the start of electrophoresis was about 2 min. Radioactive strips were examined in a Packard Radio-chromatogram Scanner.

## Radioautography of Frozen-Dried Sections

A few control studies were carried out with unfixed cryostat sections (cut at −55°C), 5 μ thick, of radioactive tissue. The sections were dried by cryosorption pumping, attached to emulsion-coated slides, and processed according to the method of Stumpf and Roth (1966).

RESULTS

## Binding of GABA-³H to Tissue by Fixatives

In muscles incubated in GABA-³H without subsequent glutaraldehyde fixation, all of the label was recovered in the supernatant of a perchloric acid extraction; none precipitated with the proteins. After fixation and dehydration, however,

TABLE I

*GABA-³H Uptake and Binding to Tissue by Fixative*

| Muscle | Procedure | dpm taken up | dpm bound to protein | % Bound |
|--------|-----------|--------------|----------------------|---------|
| R 1 | Unfixed | $2.0 \times 10^5$ | | |
| L 1 | G-P fix (1 hr 15 min) | | $5.2 \times 10^4$ | 27 |
| | | | | |
| R 2 | Unfixed | $2.0 \times 10^5$ | | |
| L 2 | G-A fix (1 hr 15 min) | | $4.5 \times 10^4$ | 22 |
| | | | | |
| R 3 | Unfixed | $1.0 \times 10^6$ | | |
| L 3 | G-P fix (2 hr) | | $2.5 \times 10^5$ | 25 |
| | | | | |
| R 4 | Unfixed | $8.4 \times 10^5$ | | |
| L 4 | G-P fix (18 hr) | | $2.6 \times 10^5$ | 31 |
| | | | | |
| L 5 | *G-P fix then add GABA | | $5.3 \times 10^3$ | ~1 |

Muscles R 1–R 4 were incubated 2 hr in 5 ml saline containing GABA-³H. (Pairs 1 and 2 received 1.55 × 10⁷ dpm; pairs 3, 4, and 5 received 3.9 × 10⁷ dpm). After washing 20 min in saline without GABA-³H, they were homogenized in 0.4 N perchloric acid and the extracts were counted. Results are in disintegrations per minute (dpm).

Muscles L 1–L 4, the pairs of R 1–R 4, were incubated and washed in the same way. They were then fixed and dehydrated, homogenized in perchloric acid, and the protein precipitate was counted.

*L 5 was incubated 2 hr in saline without GABA-³H, placed in G-P fixative, and GABA-³H was added. After a 2 hr fixation, the tissue was dehydrated and homogenized in perchloric acid; the precipitate was counted. Its pair was not available for control, but it is compared with the other control muscles, R 1–R 4.

329

a portion of the radioactive material was bound to protein. Table I shows data from representative experiments in which muscles were fixed in glutaraldehyde-containing mixtures for various time periods. The unfixed muscle from the other side of the body was used as a control to measure the total tissue uptake of labeled GABA (see Materials and Methods). In the fixed and dehydrated tissue, 25–31% of the total isotope taken up during incubation was bound to the protein fraction. Of the radioactivity that was lost, 70–90% was found in the fixative and the first rinses of buffer and in the 25% methanol solution; progressively smaller amounts were found in the series of increasing concentrations of methanol.

One muscle (L-5 in Table I) was incubated for 2 hr in saline without labeled amino acid; then G-P fixative was added and was followed by radioactive GABA. Only 2–10% as much radioactive material was bound to the tissue by this procedure compared to the isotope bound in tissues preloaded with isotope.

## Preliminary Kinetics of the GABA Reaction with Fixative and Binding to Protein

A model system was studied, involving GABA-$^3$H, serum albumin, and G-P fixative in a variety of combinations. A sample of each incubation mixture was separated by electrophoresis as quickly after mixing as possible. Protein had no

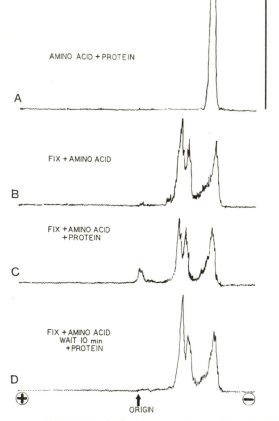

FIGURE 1  Electrophoresis of GABA-$^3$H mixed with serum albumin (A), with G-P fixative (B), and with G-P fixative and serum albumin (C). In Fig. 1 D, GABA-$^3$H was mixed with G-P fixative, and after 10 min serum albumin was added. See text for explanation of results. Scale is 3000 cpm.

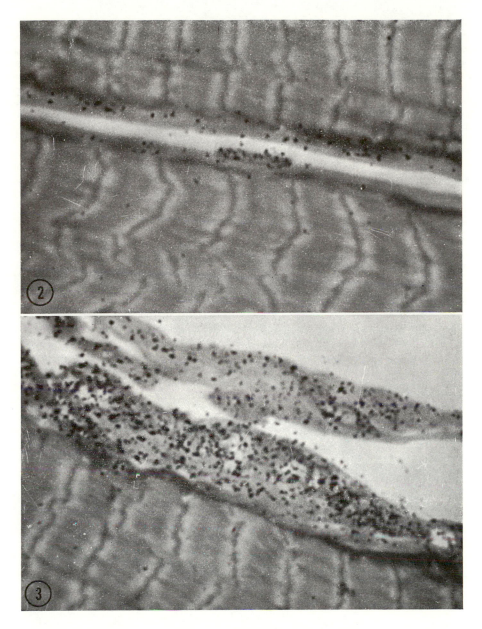

FIGURES 2 and 3  Light microscope radioautograms of GABA-³H uptake in lobster muscle. The focus is on the silver grains lying over the tissue. The muscle is lightly labeled. Most of the silver grains lie on endomysial connective tissue. × 950.

effect on the migration of radioactive GABA (A of Fig. 1). When GABA and aldehyde fixative were mixed, a series of new compounds was formed within 2 min (B of Fig. 1). These compounds were not identified or characterized further, but the distribution of radioactive bands did not change significantly on prolonged incubation before electrophoresis. If protein and radioactive GABA were present when the aldehyde fixative was added, a new band appeared near the origin on the scans of radioactivity of the electrophoresis strips (C of Fig. 1). This is where protein is found under these experimental conditions. Finally, if aldehyde fixative and GABA-$^3$H were preincubated for 2–10 min before adding protein, the radioactive band at the origin was not found (D of Fig. 1).

*Light Microscope Radioautography*

Radioautograms of GABA-$^3$H–treated muscles that had been fixed in mixtures containing glutaraldehyde showed dense accumulations of developed silver grains over connective tissue cell elements (Figs. 2–4). Endomysial fibroblasts were labeled over their nuclei and perinuclear cytoplasm, but grains also lay on connective tissue some distance from cell nuclei (Figs. 2 and 3). Whether these were on extracellular fibers (collagen) or on thin sheets of cytoplasm could not be determined at these magnifications. Round, granulated cells found in the extracellular spaces also accumulated label.

Bundles of axons were frequently seen in the connective tissue stroma of the muscle. Although their dense endoneurial connective tissue wrappings were heavily labeled, and silver grains often immediately abutted the periphery of axons (presumably on Schwann cells), the axons themselves were conspicuously devoid of label (Fig. 4).

The muscle cells themselves were lightly labeled (Figs. 2 and 3); neuromuscular junctions could not be recognized at these magnifications.

A wide variety of experimental variables was introduced: incubation with low ($7 \times 10^{-7}$ M) or high ($5 \times 10^{-4}$ M) concentrations of GABA-$^3$H, short (1 hr) or long (7 hr) incubation periods; short (20 min) or long ($1\frac{1}{2}$ hr) wash periods;

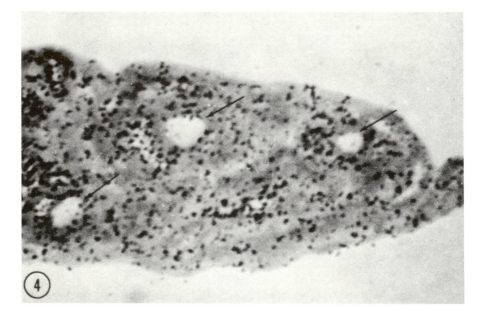

FIGURE 4  Light microscope radioautogram focused on silver grains above intermuscular axons. Endoneurial connective tissue is densely labeled. Silver grains also line the periphery of axons, presumably on Schwann cells. Axons (arrows) are not labeled. $\times$ 950.

fixation with buffered glutaraldehyde, alone or mixed with paraformaldehyde or acrolein for 2 hr or overnight; postfixation with $OsO_4$ or not. In all cases, precisely the same distribution of radioactivity was observed in the radioautograms.

Preliminary control studies of unfixed, frozen-dried sections of radioactive preparations were also performed. While the sections were often lost or badly damaged during development of the emulsions, we were able to see that the label encircled

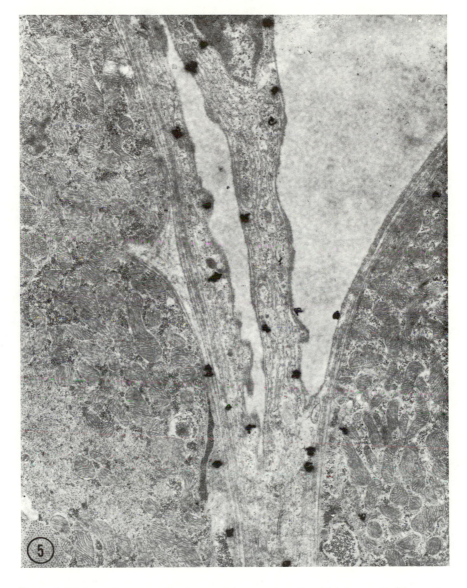

FIGURE 5  Electron microscope radioautogram of transversely sectioned lobster muscle. Silver grains are on connective tissue cell cytoplasm lying between two muscle cells. × 12,500.

the muscle fibers; i.e., at the location of endomysial connective tissue.

## Electron Microscope Radioautography

Electron microscope radioautograms confirmed the light microscope finding that label was concentrated in connective tissue. Furthermore, the higher resolution of the method revealed that developed silver grains most often lay over nuclei and cytoplasm of cells, including the long, thin sheets or finger-like extensions of cytoplasm characteristic of fibroblasts. The extracellular fibrous component (collagen) was rarely labeled (Figs. 5–7).

Lobster muscle fibers have deep clefts or infoldings of the cell membrane running longitudinally along the fiber. There are from two to about five clefts around the circumference of any one fiber. These clefts are wide enough (up to $2\,\mu$) to contain connective tissue elements and neuromuscular junctions. Processes of fibroblasts within these clefts also accumulated labeled GABA (Fig. 6).

In the electron microscope radioautograms, relatively few developed silver grains were found over muscle. No generalizations could be made about their distribution relative to the striation pattern.

The connective tissue accompanying axons in their intermuscular course was, again, heavily labeled (Fig. 8 a). The cytoplasm of Schwann cells immediately surrounding axons also contained GABA-$^3$H in amounts similar to those in fibroblasts in the endoneurium (Fig. 8 b). Silver grains were very rarely found lying over axoplasm.

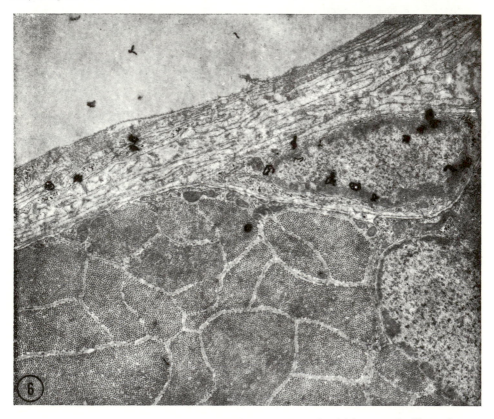

FIGURE 6   Electron microscope radioautogram of transversely sectioned lobster muscle. The nucleus and fingers of cytoplasm of a connective tissue cell are labeled. Neither collagen nor the muscle cell is labeled. × 26,250.

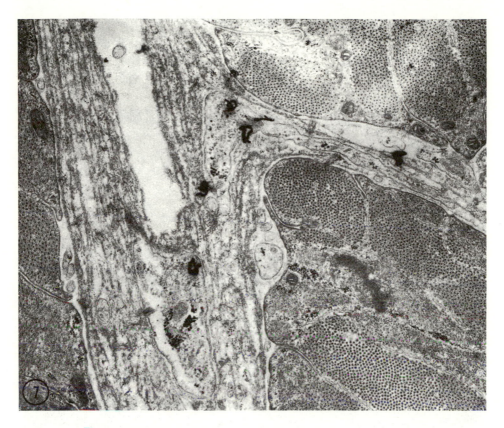

FIGURE 7  Electron microscope radioautogram. Connective tissue cell cytoplasm in the intercellular space and in the cleft of the muscle cell at right is labeled. No silver grains are on collagen or muscle cells. × 26,250.

Although lobster muscle fibers are multiply innervated by both excitatory and inhibitory axons in the muscle that was used, neuromuscular junctions were almost impossible to recognize by ordinary light microscopy and extremely difficult to find in the electron microscope. They were usually small and widely separated, making chance observations rare. In our hands the addition of radioautographic treatment also reduced the usable material. Nevertheless, five nerve terminals were found. In three of these all of the synaptic vesicles were circular in profile, indicating a probable spherical shape (Figs. 10 and 11). Two axon terminals had vesicles that were sometimes circular but more often elliptical or irregular in shape (e.g. Fig. 9). Densely stained particles which resembled glycogen (Revel et al. 1960) were

frequent inclusions in both types of axon terminals. Although these particles were commonly found in connective tissue cells and muscle fibers, there were sometimes especially dense conglomerates in axons near their synapses (Fig. 9).

The Schwann cell cytoplasm overlying neuromuscular junctions and the connective tissue cells outside them were labeled. Sometimes muscle cell cytoplasm beneath the axon terminals also contained label. In most electron micrographs, no grains were seen over the axoplasm of synapses with either spherical or elliptical vesicles (Figs. 9 and 10). However, in two sections label appeared on axon terminals. One of these contained spherical (Fig. 11), the other elliptical, vesicles. Since the number of radioautograms with synapses was small, it was not feasible to determine whether

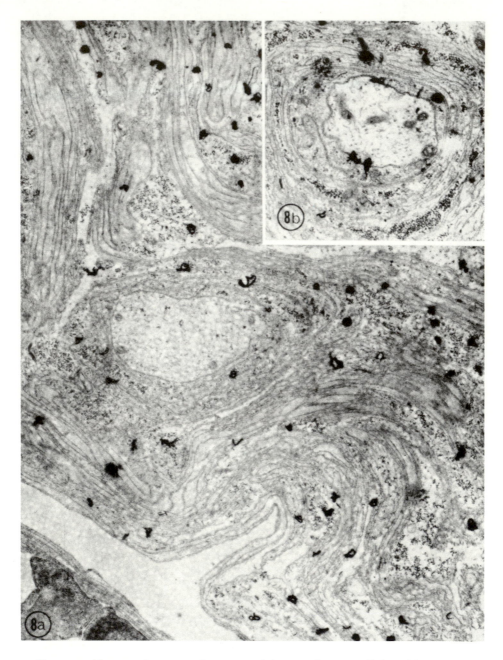

FIGURE 8 a   Electron microscope radioautogram of intermuscular nerve. Endoneurial connective tissue is densely labeled. × 12,500.

FIGURE 8 b   Silver grains lie on Schwann cell cytoplasm. Axons are not labeled. × 16,500.

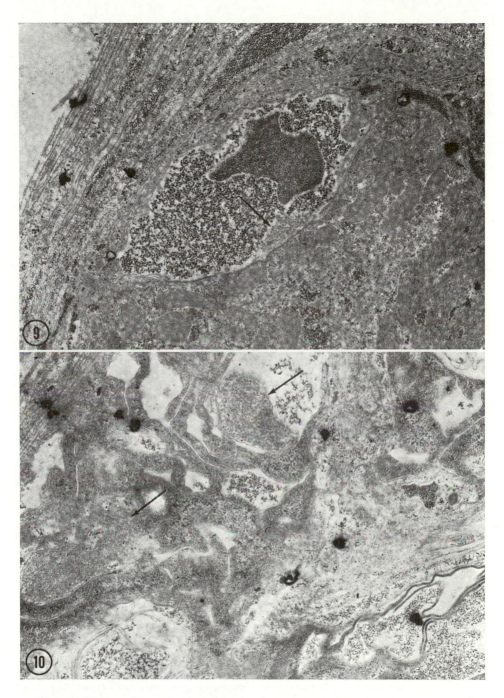

FIGURE 9   Electron microscope radioautogram of lobster neuromuscular junction. This axon terminal contains large amounts of glycogen-like particles including a dense accumulation of particles of smaller size. Ellipsoid synaptic vesicles are indicated by the arrow. The axoplasm is not labeled, but silver grains lie on Schwann and connective tissue cell cytoplasm. × 22,500.

FIGURE 10   Radioautogram of lobster neuromuscular junction. Two parts of the axon terminal appear, each containing spherical vesicles (arrows). Silver grains lie on complicated folds of postsynaptic sarcoplasm and on connective tissue cells. × 22,500.

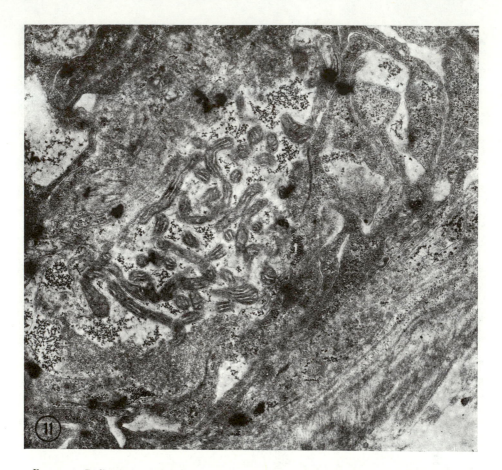

FIGURE 11 Radioautogram of lobster neuromuscular junction. This axon terminal with spherical vesicles is labeled by three silver grains. Other grains lie on postsynaptic sarcoplasm, Schwann cell cytoplasm, and connective tissue. × 22,500.

this finding was greater than background. It is clear, however, that the principal site of uptake around neuromuscular junctions is in connective tissue and Schwann cells. Further study will be necessary to demonstrate clearly whether there are small amounts of GABA taken up into nerve terminals.

## DISCUSSION

### Binding of GABA-³H at Uptake Sites

Previous studies have suggested parallels between the site of GABA uptake and the endogenous GABA content in regions of inhibitory innervation

of tissues. Sisken and Roberts (1964), using frozen-dried whole-mounts of crayfish stretch receptor preparations, observed label in the region of the neuron where inhibitory axons were thought to terminate, but the resolution of this method was not sufficient for precise localization. Iversen and Kravitz (1968) found that the distribution of radioactive GABA taken up by lobster nerve-muscle preparations was similar to the distribution of endogenous GABA measured by enzyme assay. More recently, Morin and Atwood (1969) have shown that crab muscles with a dense inhibitory innervation concentrate more GABA than those with a less dense innervation. Finally, in studies in the vertebrate central nervous system, Neal and Iversen (1969) have shown that radioactive GABA concentrated by rat cortex is found in the synaptosome fraction with a distribution comparable to endogenous GABA.

These studies suggest the possibility that GABA uptake might be into presynaptic inhibitory nerve terminals in a manner analogous to uptake for catecholamines. If this were so, the localization of the uptake site would be a useful marker for the terminals of neurons using GABA as a transmitter compound. This could give more direct evidence concerning the alleged relationship between vesicle shape, whether spherical or elliptical, and transmitter content (Uchizono, 1967). Accordingly, we were disappointed that the surrounding Schwann and connective tissue cells were the principal sites of localization of silver grains.

Between 25 and 30% of the radioactive GABA initially in the preparation was bound to the tissue by aldehyde fixation. It was possible that the silver grains we saw were due to isotope that had moved to the observed sites during fixation, or that the other 70% of the radioactive material selectively washed out of muscle and nerve cells. The control experiments suggest that the latter explanations were not correct. First, silver grains were seen over the cytoplasm of connective tissue cells and not over extracellular collagen. For GABA to have moved to these sites would have necessitated crossing cell membranes during fixation (when presumably transport was inactivated), and would require the presence of substances with a high affinity for binding GABA with fixation only in Schwann and connective tissue cells. When radioactive GABA was added to the medium immediately after fixation of nonradioactive tissue, very few counts were bound. This makes the possibility of some efficient trapping mechanism for radioactivity in the tissue less likely.

The experiments on the kinetics of binding of GABA to the protein by fixative suggest that, for binding, it is necessary for protein and amino acid to be together at the time of fixation. GABA is very rapidly converted to new compounds upon the addition of fixative. These compounds were not characterized or identified in these studies. Within 2 min after the compounds are formed (the shortest time we worked with), very little radioactivity is bound to protein. This suggests that at least two competing mechanisms take place when fixative is added to mixtures of amino acid and

protein: one is the binding of amino acid to protein; the other is the formation of new soluble compounds that can no longer bind to protein. We feel that this latter reaction accounts for the 70% of the radioactive material that washes out of the tissue, and that unless amino acid is bound to protein or other substances close to its intracellular location, it can no longer bind. Still a further suggestion that our observations are correct is the preliminary study of frozen-dried, unfixed tissue. Under these conditions the localization was similar to that observed in the fixed material. These preliminary studies must be expanded, but we have sufficient material to feel secure in the conclusion that the principal sites of uptake are in the surrounding cell types.

We are less secure in regard to the question of whether connective tissue and Schwann cells are the only sites of uptake. Occasional silver grains have been seen on muscle fibers and over nerve terminals. Without proper statistical examination of many samples, we cannot state whether the few grains seen represent radioactive GABA taken into the preparation. The scarcity of nerve terminals makes further studies with other preparations essential to provide a firm answer in this regard.

## Uptake as an Inactivation Mechanism for the Inhibitory Transmitter Compound

In cholinergic synaptic regions, transmitter action is terminated by hydrolysis of the transmitter by acetylcholinesterase (see Katz, 1966). One of the reaction products, choline, is partially transported back into the nerve terminals. During periods of high frequency stimulation, choline uptake plays an important role in replenishing released acetylcholine (Birks and MacIntosh, 1961; Potter, 1970; MacIntosh and Collier, 1969).

At noradrenergic synapses there are two distinct uptake processes for noradrenaline. The first (uptake 1) is into noradrenergic nerve terminals (Hertting and Axelrod, 1961), while the second (uptake 2) is into surrounding cell types (e.g. Gillespie et al., 1970). The two mechanisms are distinct, having different $K_m$'s, and are inhibited by different drugs (Iversen, 1967). Pharmacological studies provide strong support for the suggestion that uptake 1 is involved in the inactivation of noradrenaline in certain tissues. The role of uptake 2 is still questionable.

There is no direct enzymic destruction of GABA

to serve as a transmitter inactivation mechanism in lobster nerve-muscle preparations. The principal fate of exogenous GABA is to be taken into tissues by a transport mechanism and to be slowly metabolized. A kinetic examination of the uptake of GABA yields a curve with only one component, in contrast to the two components of the curve of noradrenaline uptake. Since the principal site of uptake is into Schwann and connective tissue cells, the process is analogous to uptake 2 of noradrenergic synapses.

The anatomical studies provide little evidence, one way or the other, regarding the possible role of uptake in transmitter inactivation. The tissues that are the principal sites of GABA transport surround synapses, so that they could serve to remove released GABA. To demonstrate a possible inactivation role of uptake it will be necessary to find a drug that inhibits uptake without a direct physiological effect of its own, and to show that this compound potentiates the effect of inhibitory nerve stimulation. GABA uptake into surrounding tissues could also serve to protect nerve-muscle preparations from GABA that might accumulate in blood.

We wish to acknowledge the technical assistance of Miss M. Hogan and Mr. J. Gagliardi.

Dr. Orkand was supported by United States Public Health Service Fellowship No. 1 F10 NB 1885-01 NSRB while at Harvard Medical School, and Neuroanatomy Training Program USPHS Grant NB 5464 and Mental Health Training Program 5 T01 MH 06415 at UCLA. Dr. Kravitz is supported by a Career Development Award from the National Institute of Child Health and Human Development (No. K03 HD 05899) and NIH Grants NS 07848 (NINDS) and NS 02253 (NINDS).

*Received for publication 13 July 1970.*

## REFERENCES

BIRKS, R. I., and F. C. MACINTOSH. 1961. Acetylcholine metabolism of a sympathetic ganglion. *Can. J. Biochem. Physiol.* **39**:787.

BOISTEL, J., and P. FATT. 1958. Membrane permeability change during inhibitory transmitter action in crustacean muscle. *J. Physiol. (London).* **144**:176.

DUDEL, J., and S. W. KUFFLER. 1961. Presynaptic inhibition at the crayfish neuromuscular junction. *J. Physiol. (London).* **155**:543.

GILLESPIE, J. S., D. N. H. HAMILTON, and J. A. HOSIE. 1970. The extraneuronal uptake and localization of noradrenaline in the cat spleen and the effect on this of some drugs, of cold and of denervation. *J. Physiol. (London).* **206**:563.

HALL, Z. W., and E. A. KRAVITZ. 1967. The metabolism of γ-aminobutyric acid (GABA) in the lobster nervous system. 1. GABA-glutamate transaminase. *J. Neurochem.* **14**:45.

HERTTING, G., and J. AXELROD, 1961. Fate of tritiated noradrenaline at sympathetic nerve-endings. *Nature (London).* **192**:172.

IVERSEN, L. L. 1967. The Uptake and Storage of Noradrenaline in Sympathetic Nerves. Cambridge University Press, London.

IVERSEN, L. L., and E. A. KRAVITZ. 1968. The metabolism of gamma-aminobutyric acid (GABA) in the lobster nervous system—uptake of GABA in nerve-muscle preparations. *J. Neurochem.* **15**:609.

KATZ, B. 1966. Nerve, Muscle, and Synapse. McGraw-Hill Book Company, New York.

KRAVITZ, E. A., S. W. KUFFLER, and D. D. POTTER. 1963. Gamma-aminobutyric acid and other blocking compounds in crustacea. III. Their relative concentration in separated motor and inhibitory axons. *J. Neurophysiol.* **26**:739.

KRAVITZ, E. A., and D. D. POTTER. 1965. A further study of the distribution of gamma-aminobutyric acid between excitatory and inhibitory axons of the lobster. *J. Neurochem.* **12**:323.

MACINTOSH, F. C., and B. COLLIER. 1969. The source of choline for acetylcholine synthesis in a sympathetic ganglion. *Can. J. Physiol. Pharmacol.* **47**:127.

MILLONIG, G. 1962. Further observations on a phosphate buffer for osmium solutions in fixation. *Proc. 5th Int. Congr. Electron Microsc.* **2**:P8.

MORIN, W. A., and H. L. ATWOOD. 1969. A comparative study of gamma-aminobutyric acid uptake in crustacean nerve-muscle preparations. *Comp. Biochem. Physiol.* **30**:577.

NEAL, M. J., and L. L. IVERSEN. 1969. Subcellular distribution of endogenous (H³) γ-aminobutyric acid in rat cerebral cortex. *J. Neurochem.* **16**:1245.

OTSUKA, M., L. L. IVERSEN, Z. HALL, and E. A. KRAVITZ. 1966. Release of gamma-aminobutyric acid from inhibitory nerves of lobster. *Proc. Nat. Acad. Sci. U.S.A.* **56**:1110.

PETERS, T., and C. A. ASHLEY. 1967. An artefact in radioautography due to binding of free amino acids to tissues by fixatives. *J. Cell Biol.* **33**:53.

POTTER, L. T. 1970. Synthesis, storage and release of (¹⁴C) acetylcholine in isolated rat diaphragm muscles. *J. Physiol. (London).* **206**:145.

REVEL, J. P., L. NAPOLITANO, and D. W. FAWCETT. 1960. Identification of glycogen in electron micrographs of thin tissue sections. *J. Biophys. Biochem. Cytol.* **8**:575.

SISKEN, B., and E. ROBERTS. 1964. Radioautographic studies of binding of $\gamma$-aminobutyric acid to the abdominal stretch receptors of the crayfish. *Biochem. Pharmacol.* **13**:95.

STUMPF, W. E., and L. J. ROTH. 1966. High resolution autoradiography with dry mounted, freeze-dried frozen sections. Comparative study of six methods using two diffusible compounds $^3$H-estradiol and $^3$H-mesobilirubinogen. *J. Histochem. Cytochem.* **14**:274.

TAKEUCHI, A., and N. TAKEUCHI. 1964. The effect on crayfish muscle of iontophoretically applied glutamate. *J. Physiol. (London).* **170**:296.

TAKEUCHI, A., and N. TAKEUCHI. 1965. Localized action of gamma-aminobutyric acid on crayfish muscle. *J. Physiol. (London).* **177**:225.

UCHIZONO, K. 1967. Inhibitory synapses on the stretch receptor neurone of the crayfish. *Nature (London).* **214**:833.

VENABLE, J. H., and R. COGGESHALL. 1965. A simplified lead citrate stain for use in electron microscopy. *J. Cell Biol.* **25**:407.

*Chapter 7*
# ACETYLCHOLINE RECEPTOR

The basic mechanism underlying communication within and between cells in the nervous system is the ability of neurons to regulate the specific ionic permeabilities of their surface membranes. Conduction of regenerative action potentials along axons depends upon the changes in sodium and potassium permeabilities of the membrane that occur in response to changes in transmembrane potential. Energy transduction by sensory receptors occurs by coupling external stimuli to conductance changes. For example, light absorption by the outer segments of retinal rods and cones decreases the ionic conductances of their membranes. In a similar manner, the interaction of a transmitter compound with receptor sites in the postsynaptic membrane produces conductance changes in the postsynaptic cell. The response is excitatory or inhibitory, depending on the particular ions involved and on whether their permeabilities are increased or decreased.

Transmitter–receptor interactions are of interest not only because they are central to the process of synaptic transmission, but also because they appear to be a promising point of entry, particularly for the biochemist, to the general problem of the molecular mechanism by which ionic permeabilities are controlled. If one could understand how an increase in specific ionic permeabilities of a membrane is caused by the binding of transmitter molecules, then one might be able to think in more concrete and useful terms about how ionic permeabilities are controlled by voltage changes, light, and other stimuli.

The transmitter–receptor interactions to be emphasized in this chapter are the interactions of ACh with the receptors of mammalian skeletal muscle and eel electric organ. The electric organ consists of large cells, called electroplax, which receive dense cholinergic innervation and are related embryologically to muscle cells. The muscle and eel receptors will be considered together because the pharmacological

and physiological properties of the two are similar. Electrophysiological recordings with intracellular microelectrodes can be made
easily in both preparations, yielding a rich physiological and pharmacological description of the receptors at these two synapses. The
electric organ has, as an additional experimental advantage, a very
high proportion of receptor-bearing membrane, making it particularly
attractive to the biochemist.

The existence of muscle receptors was first deduced by J.N. Langley
in 1905 from the results of a series of classic and simple experiments.
He observed that both curare and high concentrations of nicotine
could prevent the contraction of denervated muscle caused by ACh,
although the response of the muscle to direct electrical stimulation
remained unaltered. He reasoned that a "receptive substance" must
be interposed between the active agent and the contractile mechanism.

H.H. Dale, in 1914, provided the experimental basis for distinguish-
ing two types of ACh receptors according to the relative abilities of
the pharmacological agents muscarine and nicotine to activate them.
The ACh receptors in the target tissues of the parasympathetic nervous
system are "muscarinic"; the ganglionic receptors of the autonomic
nervous system here and those at the neuromuscular junction are
"nicotinic." Substances that block the two receptors (antagonists) can
also be used to differentiate them. Curare is more effective than
atropine at "nicotinic" synapses, while the reverse is true at "muscarinic" synapses. Further pharmacological distinctions between the
nicotinic ACh receptors of skeletal muscle and those of autonomic
ganglia can be made. For instance, comparison of the relative activities
of a series of compounds in which two ammonium groups are separated by a hydrocarbon chain of variable length shows that in the
ganglia the most active compound in the series is hexamethonium (a
six-carbon chain), while decamethonium (a ten-carbon chain) is
most effective at the neuromuscular junction.

All of the compounds that activate the neuromuscular receptor
(agonists) cause contraction, but their more immediate effect is
to depolarize the muscle membrane by increasing its ionic permeability. Sodium and potassium permeabilities increase by an approximately equal amount, and both permeability changes have the same
time course, suggesting that a single event causes the increased permeation of both ions. The receptor thus has at least two functional parts:
a recognition site (sometimes alone referred to as the receptor) and an
ionic permeation site. Although these two sites may not be parts of
the same molecule, the interactions between them must be fairly

subtle. For instance, different agonists cause different maximal permeability changes.

Perhaps the simplest model for thinking about how the receptor works is one in which an agonist ($A$) binds to the receptor ($R$) to form an agonist–receptor complex ($AR$). The agonist–receptor complex then undergoes transition to an active form ($AR^+$), which is associated with the ionic permeability change.

$$A + R \rightleftharpoons AR \rightleftharpoons AR^+$$

The maximal permeability change caused by an agonist thus would depend upon the equilibrium constant between the agonist–receptor complex and its active form. Antagonists also bind to the receptor, but the antagonist–receptor complex is not converted to an active form.

A. Karlin, and J.-P. Changeux and T. Podleski (1968), have independently pointed out that a two-state model, analogous to that proposed for regulatory enzymes, could also describe the receptor. This model proposes that the receptor, in the absence of transmitter, exists in two conformations, an active or open conformation associated with increased permeability and an inactive or closed form. At rest, the equilibrium would lie far to the side of the closed form. Agonists would bind preferentially to the open form and shift the equilibrium toward the active species, while antagonists would bind preferentially to the closed form. In this model the different affinities of various agonists for the active and inactive forms result in differences in maximal response.

Two additional features must be added to these relatively simple models. Upon prolonged exposure to ACh, muscle receptors become "desensitized," *i.e.*, progressively less sensitive to the transmitter. In an elegant study, B. Katz and S. Thesleff (1957, reprinted here) investigated this process at the frog neuromuscular junction. They recorded intracellularly from the muscle and used iontophoretic application of ACh from a micropipet both to desensitize the receptor and to provide a test pulse of the transmitter. The excellent time resolution offered by this method allowed them to study the kinetics of desensitization and to distinguish between several plausible models.

The second complex feature of the transmitter–receptor interaction, also described in the paper by Katz and Thesleff, is the sigmoid dose–response curve for ACh. Agonists also give sigmoid dose-response curves in eel electroplax (Changeux and Podleski, 1968). These curves could indicate that more than one agonist molecule must bind the receptor to form an active complex, or that a cooperative interaction between different receptor molecules occurs.

Recently, B. Katz and R. Miledi (1971, reprinted here)* have advanced the level of electrophysiological analysis to record events that may represent the interaction of ACh with a single receptor molecule. By analyzing the increased random fluctuation, or noise, in the membrane potential and end-plate current during application of dilute ACh, they obtained information about the size and duration of the elementary permeability event. The duration of this event differs for ACh and carbamylcholine and may represent the lifetime of an active agonist–receptor complex.

Until recently the transmitter–receptor interaction could be reliably measured only by electrophysiological methods; studies on the properties of the receptor thus were limited to intact cells. M. Kasai and J.-P. Changeux (1971, reprinted here) have introduced a preparation, intermediate in complexity between intact cells and the isolated receptor, in which the physiological response produced by ACh can be studied without electrical recording techniques. Membrane vesicles or "microsacs" derived from the innervated face of the eel electroplax increased their permeability to sodium ions in the presence of ACh. Kasai and Changeux demonstrated an extensive correspondence between the effects of various agents on this permeability change and the effects of these substances on the membrane potential changes caused by ACh in the intact electroplax. Microsacs are a particularly useful preparation because both the physiological response and the biochemical properties of the receptor *in situ* can be studied in a series of relatively homogeneous samples.

Another approach to the problem of assaying the receptor, as well as to the problem of identifying it after extraction from the membrane, is chemical modification of the receptor *in situ*. In a series of imaginative experiments, A. Karlin and his coworkers (1969) examined the ability of various chemical agents to modify the ACh response of eel electroplax. Very simple chemical modifications of the receptor produced quite subtle changes in its specificity. For instance, treatment of the electroplax membrane with dithiothreitol, a reagent that reduces disulfide bonds to sulfhydryl groups, abolished the response of the membrane to ACh and carbamylcholine without

*Note: We reprint here only a short paper to illustrate the potential of this method. A more complete account is found in Katz and Miledi (1972). The power spectra given in the paper here represent a plot of the variance in membrane noise vs. the frequency, from which the time constant of the elementary event can be calculated.

otherwise changing its electrical properties. In contrast, the agonist decamethonium was more active after reduction of the membrane, and hexamethonium, normally an antagonist, became an agonist.

Karlin and his colleagues then prepared affinity reagents that combined in the same molecule an alkylating moiety and a quaternary ammonium group resembling that of ACh. These compounds were used to alkylate the sulfhydryl groups exposed in the electroplax membrane after reduction. Because of their structural similarity to ACh, these affinity reagents showed enhanced reactivity for sulfhydryls near the active site of the reduced receptor. Interestingly, several of the affinity reagents produced stable depolarizations of the membrane. The distance from the sulfhydryl group to the active site was estimated by comparing the depolarization produced by different reagents in which the separation between the alkylating group and the quaternary ammonium group was varied.

Next, the receptor was labeled by reaction of a radioactive affinity reagent with the electroplax membrane. Approximately 10 to 20 percent of the radioactivity incorporated into the membrane was estimated to be bound specifically to the receptor. M. Reiter, *et al.* (1972, reprinted here), attempted to identify the labeled receptor by fractionation of the radioactive membrane proteins by polyacrylamide gel electrophoresis in sodium dodecyl sulfate. A single peak of radioactivity, corresponding to a molecular weight of 42,000, was associated with a protein that had enhanced reactivity for the affinity reagent and whose labeling was blocked by several agents that specifically interact with the receptor. Thus, ACh apparently binds to a single polypeptide of 42,000 molecular weight.

In addition to affinity labeling, several other methods have been used to identify the receptor after its removal from the membrane. A number of studies have been made of the reversible binding of cholinergic ligands to membrane fragments and to detergent extracts of electric organ tissue. Changeux and his coworkers have made the most complete effort to correlate specific binding sites with physiological activity. They examined the binding of [$^{14}$C] decamethonium to microsacs and to detergent extracts of eel electric tissue and found that in both cases about half the binding was inhibited by substances known to have affinity for the receptor. The binding curve of [$^{14}$C] decamethonium to microsacs corresponded very closely to the dose–response curve for sodium efflux caused by decamethonium (Kasai and Changeux, 1971). The binding constants of antagonists to the detergent extracts, determined by inhibition of [$^{14}$C] decamethonium binding, also were close to the constants derived from inhibition of the physiological response both in microsacs and in intact tissue. The decamethonium binding site was thus identified as that of the receptor.

By far the most useful reagents for study of the receptor *in vitro* have been a group of protein toxins obtained from the venoms of several snakes. These small, basic proteins bind to the receptor very tightly and specifically. Their use has been largely responsible for the rapid progress made in the study of the receptor during the last few years. C.Y. Lee and his coworkers purified one of these toxins, α-bungarotoxin, from the venom of the Formosan elapid, *Bungarus multicinctus,* and showed that it produced its lethal effect by blocking the ACh receptor of skeletal muscle. The experiments of Lee, Tseng, and Chiu (1967) suggested that the toxin binds selectively to the receptor. They observed that $^{131}$I-labeled α-bungarotoxin binds only to the end-plate regions of normal muscle, but binds to the whole surface of denervated muscle, a distribution in the two tissues that parallels that of ACh sensitivity. More extensive studies have confirmed the specificity of binding of α-bungarotoxin and of the related cobra neurotoxins (Miledi and Potter, 1971; Berg, *et al.,* 1972).

These toxins have been useful in several ways. A number of convenient *in vitro* assays for the receptor are based on its binding to radioactive toxin. The high specific activity of radioactive toxin and the very low dissociation constants of the toxin–receptor complexes (two or more orders of magnitude lower than the constants for most antagonists) make detection of extremely small amounts of receptor possible. In addition, the binding of substances with higher dissociation constants can be measured by their ability to compete with radioactive toxin. This method of measuring dissociation constants is particularly useful in a tissue like vertebrate skeletal muscle where the receptor concentration is very low. Another useful application of the toxin is autoradiography of tissue to which radioactive toxin has been bound, allowing the density and distribution of the receptor in the membrane to be studied (Barnard, 1971; Hartzell and Fambrough, 1972). Finally, affinity columns, constructed by coupling toxins to Sepharose beads, have provided a powerful method for receptor purification.

The availability of a variety of techniques for identification and study of the ACh receptor *in vitro* has led to rapid progress in its purification in a number of laboratories. Recently, E. Reich and his coworkers (1973) have purified the ACh receptor from eel electric organ to apparent homogeneity. The purified receptor contains no detectable lipid phosphorus and only a trace of cholinesterase activity. In several preparations, a minimum of one mole of toxin was bound per 90,000 grams of protein. The physical and pharmacological properties of the intact receptor protein are currently under investigation.

One presently unanswered question is whether the "receptor," purified with reference to its transmitter-binding site, also contains the channels or carriers responsible for increased ionic permeability of the membrane. Although a definitive answer to this question will require incorporation of the purified receptor into a natural or artificial membrane system, it may be possible to use specific drugs to study the ionic permeability site *in vitro*. For example, some of the effects of xylocaine and perhydrohistrionicotoxin on the ACh receptor suggest that these agents may interact directly with the ionic permeability site (Steinbach, 1968; Albuquerque, *et al.*, 1973).

In view of these developments, the field of receptor biochemistry has an air of expectancy about it. While physiological methods continue to provide important information, as the paper by Katz and Miledi illustrates, to these are now added the possibility of studying the properties of the receptor in solution and in reconstituted membrane systems.

## READING LIST

*Reprinted Papers*

1. Katz, B. and S. Thesleff (1957). A study of "desensitization" produced by acetylcholine at the motor end-plate. *J. Physiol.* 138: 63–80.
2. Katz, B. and R. Miledi (1971). Further observations on "acetylcholine noise." *Nature New Biol.* 232: 124–126.
3. Kasai, M. and J.-P. Changeux (1971). *In vitro* excitation of purified membrane fragments by cholinergic agonists. I. Pharmalogical properties of the excitable membrane fragments. *J. Membrane Biol.* 6: 1–23.
4. Reiter, M.J., D.A. Cowburn, J.M. Prives, and A. Karlin (1972). Affinity labeling of the acetylcholine receptor in the electroplax: electrophoretic separation in sodium dodecyl sulfate. *Proc. Nat. Acad. Sci.* 69: 1168–1172.

*Historical Papers*

5. Langley, J.N. (1905). On the reaction of cells and of nerve-endings to certain poisons, chiefly as regards the reaction of striated muscle to nicotine and to curari. *J. Physiol.* 33: 374–413.
6. Dale, H.H. (1914). The action of certain esters and ethers of

choline, and their relation to muscarine. *J. Pharmacol. Exp. Therap.* 6: 147–190.

*Other Selected Papers*

7. Takeuchi, A. and N. Takeuchi (1960). On the permeability of end-plate membrane during the action of transmitter. *J. Physiol.* 154: 52–67.
8. Lee, C.Y., L.F. Tseng, and T.H. Chiu (1967). Influence of denervation on localization of neurotoxins from clapid venoms in rat diaphragm. *Nature* 215: 1177–1178.
9. Changeux, J.-P. and T.R. Podleski (1968). On the excitability and cooperativity of the electroplax membrane. *Proc. Nat. Acad. Sci.* 59: 944–950.
10. Steinbach, A.B. (1968). Alteration by Xylocaine (Lidocaine) and its derivatives of the time course of the end-plate potential. *J. Gen. Physiol.* 52: 144–161.
11. Karlin, A. (1969). Chemical modification of the active site of the acetylcholine receptor. *J. Gen. Physiol.* 54: 245S–264S.
12. Barnard, E.A., J. Wieckowski, and T.H. Chiu (1971). Cholinergic receptor molecules and cholinesterase molecules at mouse skeletal muscle junctions. *Nature* 234: 207–209.
13. Kasai, M. and J.-P. Changeux (1971). *In vitro* excitation of purified membrane fragments by cholinergic agonists. III. Comparison of the dose–response curves to decamethonium with the corresponding binding curves of decamethonium to the cholinergic receptor. *J. Membrane Biol.* 6: 58–80.
14. Miledi, R. and L.T. Potter (1971). Acetylcholine receptors in muscle fibers. *Nature* 233: 599–603.
15. Berg, D.K., R.B. Kelly, P.B. Sargent, P. Williamson, and Z.W. Hall (1972). Binding of $\alpha$-bungarotoxin to acetylcholine receptors in mammalian muscle. *Proc. Nat. Acad. Sci.* 69: 147–151.
16. Hartzell, H.C. and D.M. Fambrough (1972). Acetylcholine receptors. Distribution and extrajunctional density in rat diaphragm after denervation correlated with acetylcholine sensitivity. *J. Gen. Physiol.* 60: 248–262.
17. Katz, B. and R. Miledi (1972). The statistical nature of the acetylcholine potential and its molecular components. *J. Physiol.* 224: 665–699.
18. Albuquerque, E.X., E.A. Barnard, T.H. Chiu, A.J. Lapa, J.O. Dolly, S.-E. Jansson, J. Daly, and B. Witkop (1973). Acetylcholine receptor and ion conductance modulator sites at

the murine neuromuscular junction: Evidence from specific
toxin reactions. *Proc. Nat. Acad. Sci.* 70: 949–953.

19. Moody, T., J. Schmidt, and M.A. Raftery (1973). Binding of
acetylcholine and related compounds to purified acetylcholine
receptor from *Torpedo californica* electroplax. *Biochem.
Biophys. Res. Comm.* 53: 761–772.

20. Klett, R.P., B.W. Fulpius, D. Cooper, M. Smith, E. Reich, and L.
Possani (1973). The acetylcholine receptor. I. Purification
and characterization of a macromolecule isolated from *Electrophorus electricus. J. Biol. Chem.* 248: 6841–6853.

# A STUDY OF THE 'DESENSITIZATION' PRODUCED BY ACETYLCHOLINE AT THE MOTOR END-PLATE

By B. KATZ and S. THESLEFF

*From the Department of Biophysics, University College London*

(*Received* 1 *April* 1957)

It has been accepted for many years that acetylcholine (ACh) undergoes two kinds of reactions at the motor end-plate: it combines with a receptor molecule (which leads to an increase of ion permeability in the end-plate membrane), and it combines with a hydrolytic enzyme situated side-by-side with the receptor. Both reactions probably proceed in two steps and involve the formation of unstable intermediate compounds before the hydrolysis, or the depolarizing reaction, occurs (see, for example, Augustinsson, 1948; Ariëns, 1954; Stephenson, 1956; del Castillo & Katz, 1957$b$). Competitive inhibitors are presumed to act by forming a relatively stable compound, either with the receptor or with the esterase.

These simple concepts have helped to explain the action of many end-plate drugs, and also to elucidate the apparently complex interactions between different depolarizing agents, for example, between ACh and decamethonium (del Castillo & Katz, 1957$b$), or ACh and edrophonium (Katz & Thesleff, 1957). However, the picture of two simple, parallel events at the end-plate fails to account for an important secondary effect of ACh and its depolarizing analogues, namely the profound desensitization which develops when the drug concentration is maintained for a sufficiently long time. Recent experiments (Thesleff, 1955) have shown that the neuromuscular block produced by ACh and by its stable counterparts ($C_{10}$, succinylcholine) is due mainly to desensitization, that is, a condition in which the end-plate has become refractory to depolarizing agents, and from which it recovers only slowly after complete withdrawal of the drug. It has been suggested that this change arises from gradual transformation of the drug-receptor compound into an inactive form. In order to obtain some information on the kinetics of desensitization and recovery processes, we have used the ionophoretic micromethods described by Nastuk (1953) and by del Castillo & Katz (1955$a$). It seemed possible that the time course of the events might come well within the practical range of this method, and the results described in this paper have borne out this expectation.

## METHODS

The technique has been fully described by del Castillo & Katz (1957a). Use was made in most experiments of twin micropipettes, with an additional central 'spacing' barrel, the two outer barrels being filled with a concentrated solution of ACh or of a stable choline derivative.

Superficial end-plates of the frog sartorius were used, at a temperature of about 20° C. The membrane potential of the muscle fibre was recorded by inserting a separate micro-electrode within a few hundred microns of the point of drug application. To diminish the risk of twitching, the spike threshold was artificially raised in most experiments by using a high calcium concentration in the Ringer's solution (9 mM-$CaCl_2$). Control experiments were made with normal Ringer's solution (116 mM-NaCl, 2 mM-KCl, 1·8 mM-$CaCl_2$) and also with phosphate-buffered Ringer's solution (about pH 7) which showed that the drug effects were not altered in any obvious way by the special composition of the calcium-rich Ringer's solution.

The experimental procedure was to move the drug pipette to an effective position at which the application of a brief, positive, voltage pulse to the pipette resulted in a transient depolarization of rapid time course (cf. del Castillo & Katz, 1955a). Having located such a spot, the sensitivity of the receptors was tested by applying a series of brief pulses of constant intensity, repeated every 1–2 sec. When the responses were found to be sufficiently stable, a 'conditioning' dose was added, consisting usually of a prolonged steady release of the drug from the other barrel. It was applied by closing a switch which reduced the 'braking' voltage on the 'conditioning' barrel by a known voltage step (of the order of one or a few tenths of a volt). The amplitude of the test-responses showed a gradual decline during the steady drug application and recovered after the withdrawal of the conditioning dose. Further details and modifications of this method will be described at the appropriate places below.

Compared with more conventional forms of drug application, the present method has a number of drawbacks as well as advantages. Complications arise from the localized nature of the application and from uncertainties about absolute and relative quantities discharged by the ionophoretic pulses. These difficulties have already been discussed elsewhere (del Castillo & Katz, 1955a; 1957a), but they appear with even greater force when one attempts to use the present results for a quantitative kinetic analysis. Unavoidably, receptors at different distances from the pipette are subjected to different drug concentrations, and this circumstance, together with the non-linear dose-response relation indicated by Fig. 9, makes a proper evaluation of some results very difficult. Secondly, the relation between the dose and the applied voltage, or the current flowing through the pipette, is bound to deviate from direct proportionality so that even relative amplitudes of the doses cannot be stated with any degree of precision. It follows, therefore, that a theoretical analysis of the results cannot be taken very far and will have to be restricted mainly to a discussion of general trends.

On the other hand, the method of local microapplication offers great technical advantages. It is very rapid; diffusion times are reduced to a fraction of a second, and much faster events can therefore be studied than before. Moreover, the removal of the drug is automatic, there is no need for periods of washing or long rests between successive tests, and many different applications can therefore be made to one receptive area. When the response of a given spot finally deteriorates, it is often only necessary to move the drug pipette to another spot on the same end-plate in order to repeat or continue the experiment.

## RESULTS

Fig. 1 illustrates the type of effect investigated in these experiments. The records in the upper part were obtained in a preliminary experiment in which a *single* ACh pipette was used for the application of the test pulses as well as of the conditioning dose. The records show that the depolarization produced by a steady efflux of ACh is not maintained, and that, immediately after the withdrawal of the conditioning dose, the effect of the test pulses is greatly reduced and then gradually recovers.

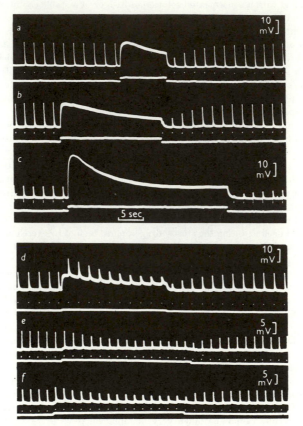

Fig. 1. Desensitization and recovery of end-plate receptors. Upper part: single ACh-pipette. Brief test doses were applied before and after the steady conditioning dose. Currents through pipette are registered in lower trace of each recording. (Calibration of monitor trace: *a* and *c*, voltage scale $= 1\cdot2 \times 10^{-8}$ A; *d*, $3\cdot1 \times 10^{-8}$ A; *e*, $10^{-8}$ A; *f*, $1\cdot6 \times 10^{-8}$ A.) Lower part: twin-pipettes were used, test pulses and conditioning currents being passed through separate channels.

The single pipette technique has certain disadvantages. Test pulses must be stopped while the steady 'brake' is reduced, because the dose delivered by the pulse increases, and may lead to twitching, when the braking current in the same pipette is lowered (see del Castillo & Katz, 1955*a*). In the absence of test pulses, however, one has no direct indication of the progress of desensitization. The time course of the slow potential change produced by the conditioning dose itself does not provide a reliable measure, because it arises from an action on a more diffuse area, and at a lower average concentration than that affecting the near-by receptors whose recovery is being tested by brief pulses.

To overcome such difficulties, twin pipettes were used, test and conditioning doses being delivered by separate barrels. Examples of double-barrel applications are shown in the lower part of Fig. 1. These records give a better indication of the onset of desensitization. It is interesting that marked depression of the pulse response occurred even with conditioning doses which caused only a small steady depolarization, of the order of 1 mV. This was regularly observed, provided the drug pipette had been closely applied to a sensitive spot.

Figs. 2 and 3 show examples from two experiments in which conditioning doses of varying intensities were applied to a receptor spot. The degree and speed of desensitization, as revealed by the test pulses, increase with the dose, while the recovery time is not greatly altered. Series of records of this kind were obtained in about twenty experiments, and an attempt will be made to analyse the relations between dose, final intensity of desensitization, and time course of onset and recovery.

Even with the double-barrel technique it was clear that pulse responses did not sum directly with the depolarization produced by the steady dose. With weak conditioning currents there was often more than simple addition, the pulse response showing a small initial increase of its amplitude and a slowing of its time course. This effect will be examined in some detail below. In spite of this complication, there was no real difficulty in measuring the rate at which successive pulse responses declined during relatively weak conditioning doses.

Desensitization started sometimes after a delay of a few seconds, though frequently the decline followed an approximately exponential curve from the start. The steepest part of the curve was chosen for determining the half-time of the process.

When large conditioning doses were applied, the measurement was more difficult. This is because test responses superimposed on large depolarizations suffer more serious distortion, due to saturation effects of various kinds (electrically, the local depolarization is limited in extent (del Castillo & Katz, 1954; Martin, 1955), chemical saturation of receptors being an additional factor). When high-speed records were made of the test responses, it was found that during a large ACh-depolarization the pulse potentials were not only smaller but considerably slower than normally, and the slowing continued to progress during the conditioning period. Immediately after withdrawal of the conditioning dose, the test response was shortened in time course and further reduced in height before recovery took place. A probable explanation of these complicated phenomena is that the shape of the test response, superimposed on a large drug dose, is dominated increasingly by contributions of more distant receptors which are subjected to a more

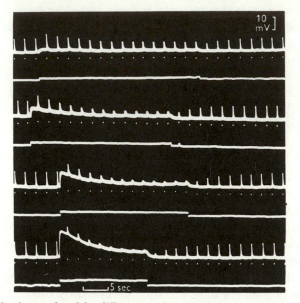

Fig. 2. Desensitization produced by different conditioning doses of ACh, at a single end-plate spot. Strength of dose increases successively from above down. Monitor calibration (10 mV scale) = $1\cdot2 \times 10^{-8}$ A.

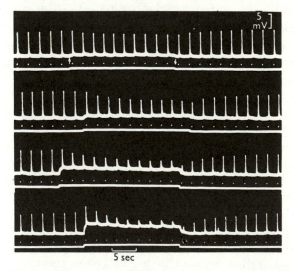

Fig. 3. Desensitization by different doses of ACh, from another end-plate. Monitor calibration (5 mV scale) = $1\cdot4 \times 10^{-8}$ A. Arrows indicate duration of conditioning dose in top record.

moderate concentration, and therefore do not suffer the same degree of saturation or desensitization as the close-range receptors (see also del Castillo & Katz, 1955 *a*). It is clear in the cases illustrated in Figs. 4 and 5 (lower part) that desensitization becomes nearly complete within less than 8 sec, but the half-time of the process cannot be derived accurately from the superimposed test responses.

The method adopted in most experiments was to use superimposed test responses only with weak and moderate doses, with which the first test response, immediately after the start of the conditioning current, was not greatly diminished. With larger doses the time course of desensitization was determined by varying the duration of a conditioning dose of given intensity

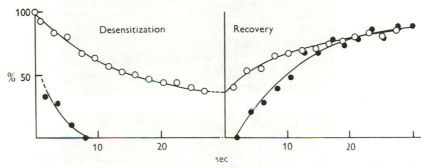

Fig. 4. Amplitude of test responses, during and after application of two conditioning doses. Initial depolarization produced by conditioning dose was 3·4 mV (○) and 20·7 mV (●).

and observing the test response immediately after its withdrawal. Records and plotted results are illustrated in Figs. 5 and 6. When the two methods of determining the time course were checked against each other, with intermediate conditioning doses, reasonable agreement was found. Checks were also made, using different, low range, intensities of *test* pulses with a given conditioning dose; these showed no significant difference in the time courses.

An example of the quantitative information derived in this way is shown in Table 1. Although the accuracy of these measurements was low, certain features were consistent:

(i) Desensitization was noticeable with depolarizations of the order of 0·5 mV and became nearly complete with doses which produced depolarizations of the order of 10 mV.

(ii) The time course of recovery appeared to be independent of the conditioning dose or the degree of desensitization. Occasionally, however, and especially after prolonged large doses, recovery was slowed or incomplete. Even when the initial rate of recovery was high, it often failed to reach completion, and there was always a tendency of the test responses to decline during successive sets of observations. Whether this was due to a slow second

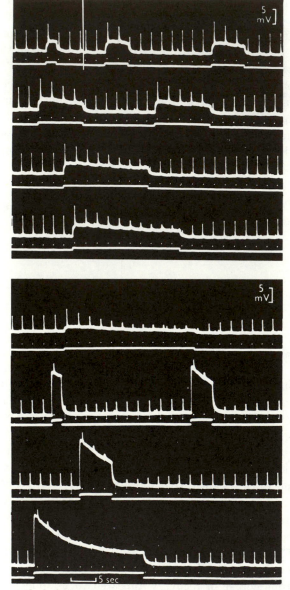

Fig. 5. Alternative method of determining time course of desensitization, by varying the duration of a conditioning dose of given strength. Two examples are shown. The development of desensitization is seen by the reduction in amplitude of the test response, immediately after the end of each conditioning period. In the lower part, the effect of a weaker dose is shown for comparison (top record).

component of the recovery process could not be decided with the present technique. The average half-time of recovery in these experiments was about 5 sec.

(iii) The time course of onset showed an interesting relation to the dose. With moderate doses which led to a final desensitization of 20–70%, the half-time of development was of the same order as, and often slower than, that of recovery (e.g. Fig. 1e). With large doses, however, which led to nearly complete suppression of the response, the rate of development exceeded that of the recovery, half-times being of the order of 1–2 sec.

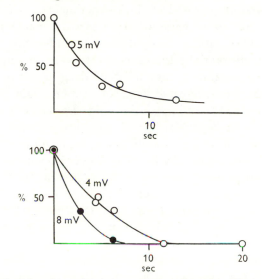

Fig. 6. Examples of results obtained by the method illustrated in Fig. 5. Ordinates: relative amplitude of test response, immediately after a conditioning period. The amplitude was measured either directly or, when necessary, by extrapolating the recovery curve to the falling edge of the conditioning potential. Abscissae: duration of conditioning dose. Initial depolarization produced by the conditioning doses is shown on the curves.

TABLE 1. Effects of varying conditioning doses

Eight different doses were used, applying positive voltage steps of 0·15–1·1 V to the conditioning barrel.

| Initial depolarization produced by conditioning dose (mV) | Reduced amplitude of test response (% of 'unconditioned' response) | Half-time of onset of desensitization (sec) | Half-time of recovery (sec) |
|---|---|---|---|
| ca. 0·2 | 93 | — | — |
| ca. 0·3 | 75 | 6·7 | ca. 2·4 |
| ca. 0·6 | 50 | 7·2 | ca. 2·5 |
| 1·45 | 22 | 4·5 | 2·5 |
| 4·4 | ca. 8 | 2·4 | 4·8 |
| 10 | ca. 2 | ca. 1·5 | ca. 4·8 |
| 15·6 | 0 | ca. 1 | 3·5 |
| 24 | 0 | ca. 0·7 | ca. 3·2 |

In addition to acetylcholine, carbachol and succinylcholine were used as depolarizing drugs and were found to possess very similar actions, with similarly fast time courses of desensitization and recovery. Several experiments were made on denervated muscles, the nerve having been divided 3–4 weeks previously. These experiments did not reveal any unusual features; critical spots of high drug-sensitivity could be located in the 'neural' regions, and fast desensitization and recovery effects were observed similar to those in normal muscle.

One of the surprising features was the rapidity with which the desensitization developed and disappeared in these experiments. Before accepting this finding, a search had to be made for artifacts which might possibly simulate such results. The observations clearly did not depend on any peculiarity of the twin-pipette, for substantially the same effects were obtained with single, as well as with two separately manipulated, drug pipettes. It was further considered whether an undetected local contraction might produce results of this kind. This seemed very improbable, but the possibility remained that, during very localized depolarization of receptive membrane spots, minute movements could occur in this critical region, too small to detect visually and yet influencing the sensitivity by altering the distance between receptors and pipette. There are several reasons for regarding a movement artifact as extremely unlikely and as incapable of eliciting results of the consistency observed here. An important point was that very similar results were obtained under conditions in which contractility is known to be greatly reduced or absent. Thus, in muscles placed in a solution made hypertonic by adding about $0.2$M-NaCl to the Ringer's solution, typical desensitization and recovery curves were observed, although contractile responses are known to be very weak under these conditions (Hodgkin & Horowicz, 1957). Even more decisive were experiments made in an isotonic $K_2SO_4$ solution (cf. del Castillo & Katz, 1955$b$) in which the fibre membrane had been completely depolarized. With the help of an additional internal electrode, 'catelectrotonic' potentials (inside-positive) were produced, and ACh was then applied to the end-plate in the usual way, causing a 'depolarization' of the electrotonic potential. An example is shown in Fig. 7, which confirms earlier observations (del Castillo & Katz, 1955$b$) and also illustrates the fact that desensitization still occurs at approximately the same speed as in normal Ringer's solution. These observations were made under conditions, and in a range of membrane potentials, well outside those at which a mechanical response can be obtained from a frog's sartorius muscle. The suggestion of a contraction artifact can therefore be safely dismissed.

### The non-linear dose–response relation

It was noticed that a test pulse, superimposed at the beginning of a small conditioning depolarization, produced often *more* than a simple additive effect. Although this phenomenon was not very conspicuous, it seemed of considerable interest. We thought at first that it might have arisen from an artifact, namely, possible electric leakage between the two barrels, in spite of the use of an intermediate 'spacing' tube (see del Castillo & Katz, 1957a). To eliminate this possibility altogether, the experiments were repeated with two separate pipettes, and even then the effect could still be obtained. It appears then that a steady small dose of ACh can in some way facilitate the action of a superimposed ACh-pulse, or in other words that the relation between dose and depolarization has an 'S-shaped' rather than linear start. This cannot be explained by the excitatory properties of the fibre membrane, for the phenomenon was observed with potential changes well below the range in which the non-linear effect of a local response becomes conspicuous; moreover, the

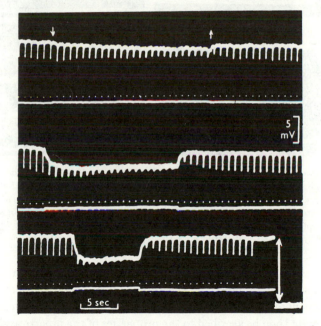

Fig. 7. ACh-desensitization and recovery, observed in isotonic $K_2SO_4$. The membrane potential had initially been displaced electrotonically, from near zero to about 15 mV, inside positive. At the end of the bottom record, the electrotonic current is withdrawn. In this figure, ACh responses are 'inverted', because the membrane potential is of opposite direction to that in the other experiments. Conditioning doses of three intensities are used, causing the usual effects. The conditioning period in the top record is indicated by arrows. Monitor calibration (5 mV scale) $= 1.1 \times 10^{-7}$ A.

phenomenon was most noticeable at the time of withdrawal of a conditioning dose when the depolarizations were considerably smaller than at the beginning of the dose.

A more-than-linear summation of this kind might conceivably be due to partial saturation of cholinesterase activity by the steady dose, but this was not a likely explanation because the phenomenon was still seen in experiments in which carbachol was used (with two separate pipettes), and after the preparation had been treated with neostigmine $3 \times 10^{-6}$. Particularly clear-cut examples of this kind are shown in Fig. 8.

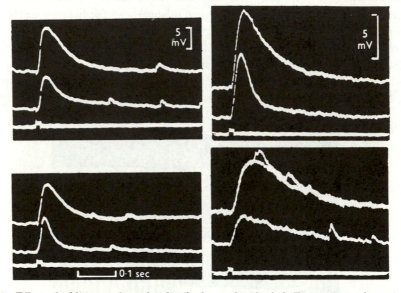

Fig. 8. Effect of adding steady and pulsatile doses of carbachol. Two separate drug pipettes. Neostigmine methylsulphate $3 \times 10^{-6}$. In each record, two successive traces were obtained, with and without a steady drug depolarization produced by steady release of carbachol from one pipette. In the right half of the figure, the upper pair of traces was observed during initial application of the steady dose, the lower pair during its withdrawal. Monitor calibration (left 5 mV scale) $= 7.3 \times 10^{-8}$ A for all records.

Further evidence was sought by examining the relation between the strength of a carbachol pulse and the amplitude of the depolarization produced by it. This cannot be done with a single drug pipette because departures from linearity might then be ascribed to the properties of the pipette and to variation of the transport number with the intensity of the pulse. Our procedure was to use a twin-pipette and apply approximately equal doses from each barrel, separately and simultaneously. Starting with very small doses, the dose-response relation was traced in increasing steps. The observed relation had an 'S shaped' rather than linear start, there being more than addition of effects for small pulses, and less than linear summation for large pulses (Fig. 9). The shape of the relation cannot be explained by subthreshold membrane excitation, for this would cause an upward curvature near threshold, at depolarizations of more than 30 mV.

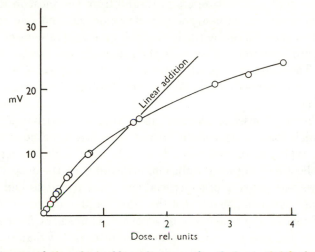

Fig. 9. Dose-response relation, obtained by an 'increment' method, using brief pulses from a twin carbachol pipette. Starting with a very small depolarization from one pipette (lowest plot), approximately the same dose (producing approximately the same depolarization) was applied by the other pipette. The response to *combined* application was plotted, as ordinate, against the *sum* of the single responses (abscissa). The procedure was then repeated with larger doses, each time choosing a step which was within the already determined portion of the dose-response relation. In this way, the relation was traced up to a depolarization of 24 mV, and followed by a reverse series. The 45° line corresponds to linear addition of effects.

## DISCUSSION

The desensitization effects described in this paper are qualitatively similar to those previously obtained with the more usual methods of drug application, but differ quantitatively, especially in their time scale. Both onset and recovery are fast compared with the time courses observed before, and it is indeed one of the advantages of the ionophoretic method that it is capable of following events of such rapidity. It has been shown by Fatt (1950) that the rate of development of the desensitization process increases markedly with the drug concentration, and one might therefore suppose that the localized concentration attained with the ionophoretic technique is higher than usually employed with bulk applications of ACh, even though the resulting membrane depolarization in our experiments was less. The value of the depolarization is of little use in estimating the drug concentration, for with highly localized application a given potential change of the fibre membrane may arise either from a low drug concentration acting over a wide area, or from a high concentration acting on a small area of receptors. It is, however, of interest that appreciable desensitizations were obtained with doses which produced little more than 0·5 mV initial depolarizing effect, that is, a potential change of the same order as the amplitude of a brief miniature e.p.p. There is good evidence for the view that a miniature e.p.p. results from the most localized form of 'ACh-application' which can possibly be achieved, and one may therefore conclude that the ACh concentrations which were used in some of our desensitization experiments were not outside the range of concentrations which occur normally. The 'unphysiological' feature in our experiments is, of course, the prolonged maintenance of the ACh concentration, for seconds rather than milliseconds.

While the rapid onset of desensitization might be attributed to the attainment of high local drug concentrations, the fast time course of recovery cannot be explained in this way. It may be that with the usual prolonged 'bulk' application protracted diffusion, into and from the deeper layers of the tissue, slows the recovery of superficial end-plate receptors and disguises the existence of a fast component. On the other hand, our present method while capable of revealing a fast phase of recovery, is unsuitable for the detection of very slow changes (with a time scale of minutes rather than seconds), which might be disguised by a minute drift of the pipette location. It is possible, therefore, that the present experiments merely disclose a fast phase of the recovery process which is complementary to the results of previous work.

Ideas about the mechanism of desensitization are at present bound to remain speculative. Nevertheless, it is of interest to try certain simple hypotheses and see whether they can be fitted to the observations. Del Castillo & Katz (1957*b*) had put forward the following working hypothesis:

$$\text{ACh} + \text{R} \underset{\text{inter-}\atop\text{mediate}\atop\text{step}}{\overset{(1)}{\rightleftharpoons}} \text{AChR} \underset{\text{depolar-}\atop\text{ization}}{\overset{(2)}{\rightleftharpoons}} \text{AChR}' \overset{(3)}{\underset{\text{desensiti-}\atop\text{zation}}{\longrightarrow}} \text{ACh} + \text{R}', \qquad (1)$$

where R is the receptor molecule in its initial, reactive, form. Reaction (1) is a postulated intermediate step which precedes the 'depolarizing' reaction (2). We are not, at present, concerned with the evidence bearing on the existence of the intermediate compound, and for simplicity the depolarizing reaction will be treated as a single reversible process, of sufficient speed to be at equilibrium during the relatively slow desensitization. Del Castillo & Katz suggested that desensitization results from gradual transformation of the receptor into a non-reactive form R' which reverts slowly to R after the withdrawal of the drug. This is one of several simple hypotheses which may be put forward.

The following alternative schemes have also been considered (symbols: *S*, conditioning drug concentration; $A$, free receptors; $SA$, 'effective' drug-receptor compound; $SB$, 'refractory' compound).

$$S+A \underset{}{\overset{\text{Fast}}{\rightleftharpoons}} SA \underset{}{\overset{\text{Slow}}{\rightleftharpoons}} SB \tag{2}$$

$$\tag{3}$$

These schemes represent two successive (2), or simultaneous (3) reactions, a depolarizing reaction which reaches equilibrium very rapidly, and a desensitizing reaction which proceeds much more slowly.

These hypotheses lead to certain common predictions, namely that the final degree of desensitization $I$ is given by an equation of the type

$$I = \frac{1}{1 + \dfrac{k_2\,(1+aS)}{k_1 aS}},$$

and its development and decay follow exponential time courses with rate constant

$$\frac{1}{\tau} = \frac{k_1 aS}{1+aS} + k_2,$$

$k_1$ being the forward, $k_2$ the reverse rate constant of the desensitizing step; $a$ being the affinity constant of the fast depolarizing step. For the case of two parallel reactions ((3) above), $k_1$ should be replaced by $k_1/a$.

The significant result is that on these hypotheses, the *onset* of desensitization (when $S$ is finite) must always be faster than the recovery (when $S=0$), and that complete, or nearly complete, desensitization would occur only when the rate of onset is infinitely, or very much, faster than that of recovery. For 50 % desensitization, the rate of development should be twice that of the recovery. These predictions are clearly at variance with what has been consistently observed. Half-desensitization was found to develop at a rate about equal to, or lower than, that of the subsequent recovery. At doses which produced nearly complete desensitization, the onset was usually faster, but not more than five times faster, than recovery. These schemes, therefore, cannot be accepted as suitable working hypotheses. What is apparently needed is a reaction in which the recovery process, from $B$ to $A$, is slowed by the presence of the drug. A scheme which will fit the results reasonably well is the following

$$
\begin{array}{ccc}
 & a & \\
S+A & \overset{}{\underset{}{\rightleftharpoons}} & SA \\
\text{(slow)}\ k_2 \uparrow \scriptstyle(\text{fast}) & & \downarrow k_1\ \text{(slow)} \\
 & b & \\
S+B & \underset{(\text{fast})}{\rightleftharpoons} & SB
\end{array}
\tag{4}
$$

where $a$ and $b$ are affinity constants.

On this hypothesis, the receptor can exist in two forms, effective ($A$) and refractory ($B$). The drug combines rapidly and reversibly with both forms, but the combined receptor is transformed irreversibly from $A$ to $B$ with rate constant $k_1$, while the free receptor reverts to form $A$ with rate constant $k_2$. (A system of this kind would require energy supply in order to be maintained in a steady state: e.g. if the change from $SA$ to $SB$ involves degradation of energy, a metabolic 'drive' would be needed for the recovery reaction.)

On this hypothesis, desensitization $I$ is given by

$$I = \frac{1}{1 + \dfrac{k_2 (1 + aS)}{k_1 aS (1 + bS)}}$$

and the exponential rate constant by

$$\frac{1}{\tau} = \frac{k_1 aS}{1 + aS} + \frac{k_2}{1 + bS}.$$

We found that the observed results can be fitted moderately well if the affinity of the drug to receptor $B$ is much higher than to receptor $A$. In this case, a dose may produce relatively little depolarization and yet lead to a profound desensitization; moreover, the rate of onset may be low compared to the rate of recovery when the drug has been completely removed.

We have at present no means for a rigorous quantitative test, because the values of $S$ are not known. If one makes the oversimplifying assumption that the initial depolarization produced by the conditioning dose is proportional to $S$, then the average result, from an analysis of 19 experiments, was: $b/a$ (ratio of affinity constants) $= 20$ (varying between 5 and 100); $1/k_1 = 1\cdot4$ sec (half-time 1 sec, varying between 0·5 and 2 sec); $1/k_2 = 7$ sec (half-time 5 sec, varying between 2 and 7 sec). Examples are shown in Figs. 10 and 11.

It may be preferable to choose a reversible version of hypothesis (4), one which allows the attainment of thermodynamic equilibrium. The scheme would then be as follows:

$$
\begin{array}{ccc}
& a & \\
S + A & \overset{}{\underset{}{\rightleftharpoons}} & SA \\
\text{(fast)} & & \\
(\text{slow}) \, k_2 \; \Big\Vert \, k_4 \quad k_3 \; \Big\Vert \, k_1 \, (\text{slow} & & \\
S + B & \overset{}{\underset{}{\rightleftharpoons}} & SB \\
& b & \\
& \text{(fast)} &
\end{array}
\qquad (5)
$$

Equilibration requires that

$$\frac{b}{a} = \frac{k_1 k_2}{k_3 k_4}.$$

Desensitization $I$ would be given by

$$I = \frac{1}{1 + \dfrac{k_2\,(1+aS)}{k_4\,(1+bS)}},$$

and the over-all rate constant by

$$\frac{1}{\tau} = \frac{k_1 aS + k_4}{1+aS} + \frac{k_3 bS + k_2}{1+bS}.$$

Our data do not allow us to discriminate between hypotheses (4) and (5). The last scheme can also be fitted reasonably well, with $k_1 \gg k_3$, $b \gg a$, and

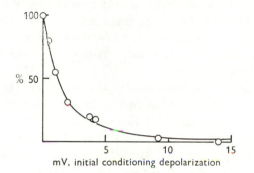

Fig. 10. Relation between final desensitization and initial depolarization produced by varying conditioning doses. Ordinates: amplitude of 'desensitized' test responses, as % of normal responses. The curve was calculated from hypothesis (4), with $b/a = 10$, $1/k_1 = 0.7$ sec, $1/k_2 = 4.2$ sec, and $aS = 1$ for 12.5 mV.

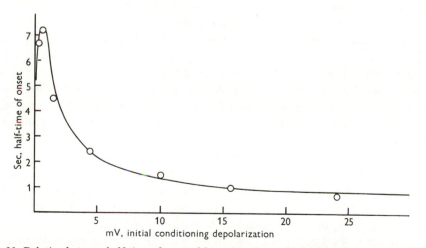

Fig. 11. Relation between half-time of onset of desensitization and initial depolarization produced by varying conditioning doses. This was an exceptionally 'good' result: usually the half-time values were scattered to a much greater extent. The curve was calculated from hypothesis (4), with $b/a = 86$, $1/k_1 = 0.7$ sec, $1/k_2 = 5.2$ sec, and $aS = 1$ for 17.1 mV.

367

$b/a > k_1/k_2$. An interesting feature of hypothesis (5) is that the free receptors are distributed, even in the absence of a drug, between states $A$ and $B$, that is a proportion of receptors is present in a refractory form, and on account of its very high affinity ($b/a \gg 1$) will preferentially absorb small quantities of applied ACh.

To sum up, schemes of the type (4) and (5) may be regarded as possible working hypotheses. Although the available results are not accurate enough to provide a secure basis for a kinetic theory, they do at least allow us to reject certain types of hypothesis such as (1) to (3).

Some further comment is required on the finding of an 'S-shaped' dose-effect relation (Fig. 9), and the observation that a small steady dose may facilitate the action of an added pulse of the drug. An S-shaped relation could be the result of a reaction in which two (or more) drug molecules become attached to a receptor molecule, and the efficacy of the compound increases with the number of attachments.

Another possible explanation arises from scheme (5). The reaction between drug and receptor takes place presumably in the post-junctional folds of the muscle membrane (Couteaux, 1955; Robertson, 1956) whose lumen is not more than a few hundred Ångström units wide and which appear to be lined with receptor and esterase molecules. Applied drugs must diffuse into these spaces and react there with the surface receptors. If there are a large number of $B$-type receptors, of high affinity to the drug, but no depolarizing power, then the effect of a small dose would be mainly to occupy and partially to saturate these sites. If a second dose is added, a smaller fraction of the drug molecules would be absorbed by sites $B$, and therefore a larger fraction become available for the depolarizing action, than if this dose had been given alone.

Whatever the cause of this 'facilitation', it differs from the more conspicuous effect which certain choline derivatives produce when they are allowed to interact with ACh (del Castillo & Katz, 1957 b). In these cases there was evidence for a specific interference with the enzymic destruction of ACh, because the potentiation was abolished and reversed by pre-treating the muscle with an esterase inhibitor, or by using stable depolarizers (carbachol or succinyl-choline) instead of ACh.

### SUMMARY

1. Ionophoretic microapplication has been used to study the desensitization which depolarizing drugs produce at the motor end-plate. Steady 'conditioning' and brief 'test' doses of a drug were applied, from the two barrels of a twin-pipette, to sensitive end-plate spots of the frog.

2. When a relatively small dose of acetylcholine, producing a depolarization of 0·5–1 mV, is maintained for 10–20 sec, an appreciable loss of sensitivity occurs (sometimes exceeding 50 %). Conditioning doses which produce an initial depolarization of 10–20 mV can cause nearly complete desensitization

of local receptors within a few seconds. After withdrawal of the dose, the sensitivity starts to recover with a half-time of the order of 5 sec.

3. The variations in intensity and time course of the desensitizing process have been examined with different doses, different depolarizing drugs (acetylcholine, carbachol, succinylcholine) and in different ionic environments (Ringer's solution, isotonic $K_2SO_4$).

4. The kinetics of the process have been discussed assuming that the receptor molecules can change from an 'effective' to a 'refractory' state.

5. The dose–effect relation has been examined for small depolarizations produced by ionophoretically applied drug pulses. It is found to have an S-shaped, rather than linear, start.

We are indebted to Mr J. L. Parkinson for his unfailing help, and to the Nuffield Foundation for financial assistance. One of us (S.T.) was in receipt of a Travel Grant from the Swedish Medical Research Council.

## REFERENCES

ARIËNS, E. J. (1954). Affinity and intrinsic-activity in the theory of competitive inhibition. Part I. Problems and theory. *Arch. int. Pharmacodyn.* **99**, 32–49.

AUGUSTINSSON, K.-B. (1948). Cholinesterases. A study in comparative enzymology. *Acta physiol. scand.* **15**, Suppl. 52, 1–182.

COUTEAUX, R. (1955). In: Microphysiologie comparée des éléments excitables. *Colloq. int. Cent. nat. Rech. sci.* (in the Press).

DEL CASTILLO, J. & KATZ, B. (1954). Quantal components of the end-plate potential. *J. Physiol.* **124**, 560–573.

DEL CASTILLO, J. & KATZ, B. (1955a). On the localization of acetylcholine receptors. *J. Physiol.* **128**, 157–181.

DEL CASTILLO, J. & KATZ, B. (1955b). Local activity at a depolarized nerve-muscle junction. *J. Physiol.* **128**, 396–411.

DEL CASTILLO, J. & KATZ, B. (1957a). A study of curare action with an electrical micro-method. *Proc. Roy. Soc.* B, **146**, 339–356.

DEL CASTILLO, J. & KATZ, B. (1957b). Interaction at end-plate receptors between different choline derivatives. *Proc. Roy. Soc.* B, **146**, 369–381.

FATT, P. (1950). The electromotive action of acetylcholine at the motor end-plate. *J. Physiol.* **111**, 408–422.

HODGKIN, A. L. & HOROWICZ, P. (1957). The differential action of hypertonic solutions on the twitch and action potential of a muscle fibre. *J. Physiol.* **136**, 17P.

KATZ, B. & THESLEFF, S. (1957). The interaction between edrophonium (Tensilon) and acetylcholine at the motor end-plate. *Brit. J. Pharmacol.* **12**, 260–264.

MARTIN, A. R. (1955). A further study of the statistical composition of the end-plate potential. *J. Physiol.* **130**, 114–122.

NASTUK, W. L. (1953). Membrane potential changes at a single muscle end-plate produced by transitory application of acetylcholine with an electrically controlled microjet. *Fed. Proc.* **12**, 102.

ROBERTSON, J. D. (1956). The ultrastructure of a reptilian myoneural junction. *J. biophys. biochem. Cytol.* **2**, 381–394.

STEPHENSON, R. P. (1956). A modification of receptor theory. *Brit. J. Pharmacol.* **11**, 379–393.

THESLEFF, S. (1955). The mode of neuromuscular block caused by acetylcholine, nicotine, decamethonium and succinylcholine. *Acta physiol. scand.* **34**, 218–231.

# Further Observations on Acetylcholine Noise

IN a recent communication we reported that the end-plate depolarization produced by a steady dose of acetylcholine (ACh) is accompanied by a significant increase in voltage noise across the membrane[1]. We have continued to analyse this phenomenon on the assumption that the average depolarization as well as the superimposed voltage fluctuations arise from the same molecular "shot effects", that is, from summation and statistical variation in the number of ACh-operated ionic membrane gates which open and shut during any given time interval.

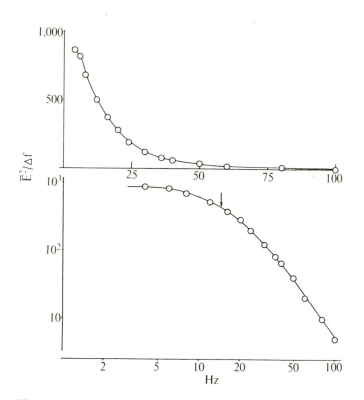

**Fig. 1** Power spectrum of intracellularly recorded ACh-noise. Temperature 5.5° C. Linear plot ($\bar{E}^2/\Delta f$, in relative units against frequency, in Hz) in upper part; double-log plot in lower part. Arrow indicates half-maximal power density.

Reprinted from *Nature New Biology* 232: 124–126 (1971) by permission of the publisher.

Additional experiments were made using intracellular as well as focal external recording from frog motor end-plates to determine the variance and spectral power distribution of the recorded voltage fluctuations (Figs. 1 and 2). Extracellular focal recording from an end-plate provides important direct information on the time course of the elementary conductance change and the associated elementary current pulse (Figs. 2–4). Unlike the "intracellular" voltage noise, the power spectrum of the external ACh noise is not limited by the membrane time constant, but rather by the time course of the elementary current pulses arising from the ACh–receptor reaction. The individual current pulses might be of rectangular, rather than exponentially decaying shape, but if their durations vary in random fashion, the mean effect would not be easy to distinguish from that of an exponential pulse. We have, therefore, analysed both intracellular and extracellular recordings on the simple tentative assumption of an exponentially decaying average shape.

This communication summarizes our principal results. The average "shot amplitude" of the ACh potential, recorded intracellularly, is calculated to be approximately 0.22 μV at 22° C, and 0.51 μV at 3° C, the increased size at low temperature arising from increased duration of the underlying elementary current pulse. At 22° C, frequency analysis of the extra-

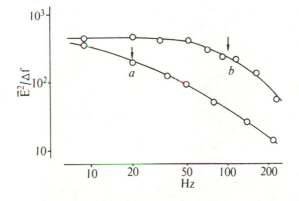

**Fig. 2** Power spectra of intracellular (*a*) and focally recorded extracellular (*b*) ACh noise. Temperature 22 and 25° C respectively. Half-power points indicated by arrows. Note the differences between these two spectra, and also the differences in slope between intracellular spectra obtained at 22° C and 5.5° C (compare Figs. 1 and 2).

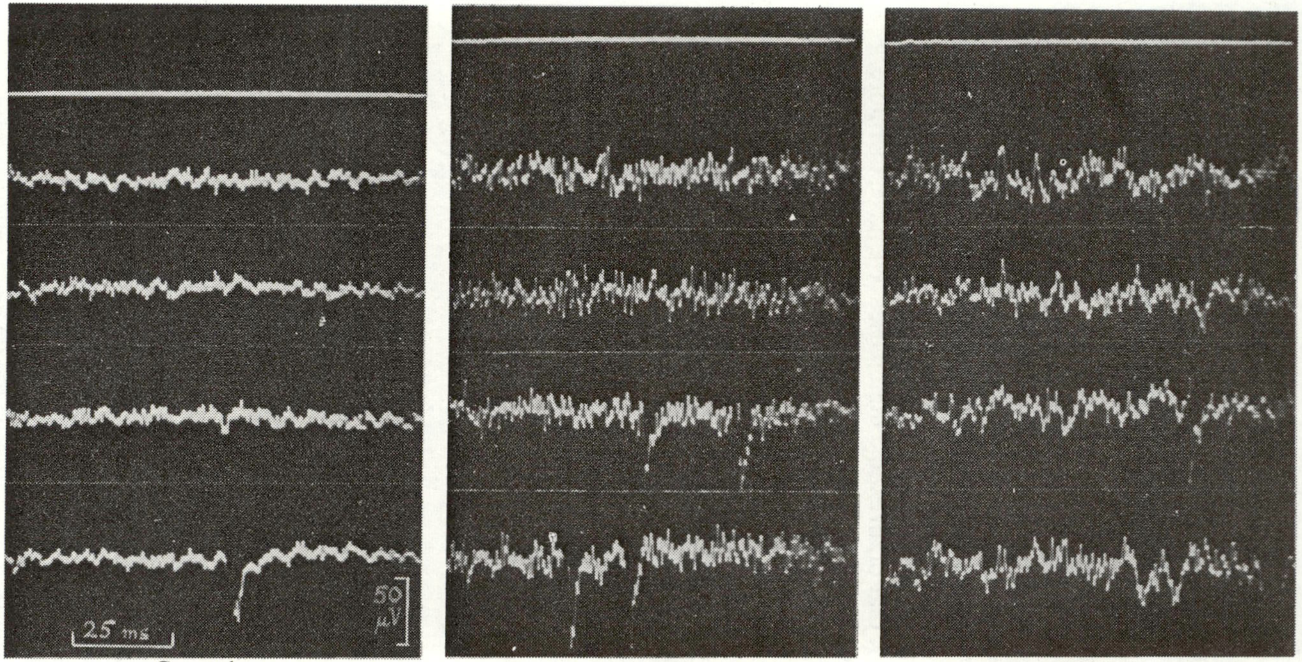


Control Carbachol ACh

**Fig. 3** Sample records (magnetic tape reproduction) of focal extracellular noise during carbachol and acetylcholine applications. Temperature 21° C. The membrane depolarization was monitored by simultaneous intracellular recording. It was approximately 5 mV during both carbachol and ACh applications, and is indicated by the displacement of the horizontal line at the top of each column. The very large rapid deflexions (for example, in the bottom traces of control and carbachol records) arose from external miniature end-plate potentials which saturated the tape amplifier.

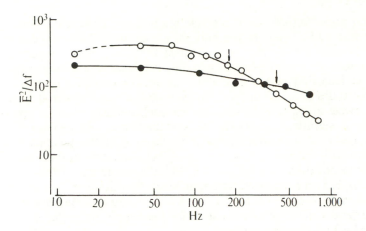

**Fig. 4** Extracellular noise power spectra during ACh (○) and carbachol (●). Temperature 24° C. Double-log plots as in Fig. 2. Half-power points (arrows): 180 Hz and 410 Hz, for ACh and carbachol respectively.

cellularly recorded noise power indicates that the average duration, or relaxation time constant, of the ionic channel is of the order of 1 ms. This is not very different from the time constant of decline of external miniature end-plate potentials (m.e.p.p.) recorded in the absence of anti-cholinesterases. It is possible that the ACh–receptor reaction is much briefer and merely initiates the "ionic gating" process which we measure and which lasts for about 1 ms. Alternatively, it is also possible that this time corresponds to the period of molecular receptor occupation. If this is the case, it would follow that, in normal neuromuscular transmission, hydrolysis prevents individual ACh molecules from acting, on the average, more than once. The greatly prolonged duration of external m.e.p.p.s which is observed after inhibition of ACh-esterase presumably results from repeated action of individual ACh molecules opening several ionic channels in succession.

The current-carrying capacity of a single channel at 22° C is of the order of $10^{-11}$ A for approximately 1 ms, the net charge transfer is equivalent to about $5 \times 10^4$ univalent ions, and the channel conductance of the order of $10^{-10}$ mho. After curare application (d-tubocurarine chloride 1 to $5 \times 10^{-6}$ g/ml. which reduced the size of m.e.p.p.s to less than 1/10), there was little, if any, change in the calculated "shot amplitude"; that is to say, although a much larger dose of ACh was now required to produce a given depolarization, the noise accompanying the depolarization was approximately the same before and after curare treatment.

An interesting observation was made when ACh effects were

compared with those of a stable cholinester, carbachol, which is not hydrolysed by the end-plate esterase. The two drugs were applied to the same end-plate region from separate barrels of a twin pipette, and the resulting membrane noise was recorded with intracellular or focal extracellular micro-electrodes (Figs. 3 and 4). Analysis of the noise power spectra showed, unexpectedly, that the "carbachol-channel" stays open for a significantly briefer period than the "ACh-channel". Correspondingly much smaller voltage noise fluctuations are recorded intracellularly, for a given depolarization, with carbachol than with ACh. At 22° C, the elementary carbachol pulse has an average duration, or relaxation time, of only about 0.4 ms (one-third of that of ACh) which may be indicative of a larger dissociation rate constant for the depolarizing step of the carbachol–receptor reaction.

We thank Professor G. D. Dawson and Mr M. Jarvis of the Department of Physiology for help with computer programming.

B. Katz
R. Miledi

*Biophysics Department,*
*University College London,*
*Gower Street,*
*London, WC1*

Received June 2, 1971.

[1] Katz, B., and Miledi, R., *Nature*, **226**, 962 (1970).

# In Vitro Excitation of Purified Membrane Fragments
# by Cholinergic Agonists

## I. Pharmalogical Properties of the Excitable Membrane Fragments

MICHIKI KASAI and JEAN-PIERRE CHANGEUX

Département de Biologie Moléculaire, Institut Pasteur, Paris, France

Received 31 December 1970; revised 12 May 1971

*Summary*. Excitation of membrane fragments by cholinergic agonists is measured *in vitro* by a filtration technique. Membrane fragments which contain high levels of the enzyme acetylcholinesterase and presumably originate from the innervated excitable faces of electroplax are first purified from homogenates of electric organ of *Electrophorus electricus* by centrifugation in a sucrose gradient. Then the fragments, which make closed vesicles or microsacs, are equilibrated overnight with a medium containing $^{22}Na^+$. After equilibration of the inside of the microsacs with the outside medium, the suspension is diluted into a nonradioactive medium. The $^{22}Na^+$ content of the microsacs as a function of time is then followed by rapid filtration on Millipore filters. In the presence of cholinergic agonists, the time course of $^{22}Na^+$ release changes: the rate of $^{22}Na^+$ release increases. This increase is blocked by *d*-tubocurarine and is absent with microsacs derived from the non-innervated inexcitable membrane of the electroplax. The response to cholinergic agonists is thus followed on a completely cell-free system, in a well-defined environment. The dose-response curves to cholinergic agents obtained *in vitro* agree, quantitatively, with the dose-response curves recorded *in vivo* by electrophysiological methods. In particular, the dose-response curve to agonists is sigmoid, the antagonism between *d*-tubocurarine and carbamylcholine competitive, and the antagonism between tetracaine and carbamylcholine noncompetitive. The effects of two different affinity labeling reagents on the response to agonists and on the catalytic activity of acetylcholinesterase are followed in parallel on the same microsac preparation. The effects of dithiothreitol and of gramicidin A on the microsacs are studied and are found to be similar to those observed *in vivo* with the isolated electroplax.

Up to now the excitability of biological membranes has been almost exclusively studied with whole cells using electrophysiological techniques. Although this approach has yielded considerable information and will certainly continue to do so, the molecular basis of this important regulatory mechanism remains largely unknown. New methods and simpler preparations are required.

Reprinted from *The Journal of Membrane Biology* 6: 1–23 (1971) by permission of the publisher.

First attempts to obtain a subcellular excitable preparation included those of Oikawa, Spyropoulos, Tasaki and Teorell (1961) and of Baker, Hodgkin and Shaw (1961) who showed that squid giant axons are still excitable after removal of the cytoplasm when perfused internally with a physiological solution. Experimentation with this preparation presents difficulties however; the external surface of the excitable membrane is covered by Schwann cells, an important fraction of neural cytoplasm embeds the internal surface (Hoskin, 1966), and electrical measurements are still essential.

In this series of papers, we shall describe and analyze the main properties of an entirely *acellular* system which appears particularly convenient for the study of chemical excitation. It consists of membrane fragments which are purified from crude homogenates of electric organ of *Electrophorus electricus*. In our preparation, these membrane fragments form closed vesicles, or "microsacs", of very small size (average diameter, 0.1 µm and the permeability of these microsacs to radioactive ions can easily be followed by rapid filtration on Millipore filters in a well-defined ionic environment. The principle advantage of this preparation resides in the fact that the microsacs which derive from the excitable membranes of electric tissue retain their excitability *in vitro*: they respond to cholinergic agonists by an increase of permeability to cations. We are thus able to follow chemical excitation (references in Nachmansohn, 1959, 1971) on a completely acellular system in a well-defined environment by a simple, direct and quantitative measure of ion flux.

In the first paper, we shall be concerned with the general description of the system and its pharmacological properties. We shall compare extensively the sensitivity of the excitable microsacs to a variety of effectors — including cholinergic agents — with that of the excitable membrane of the isolated electroplax. In general, the *in vitro* and the *in vivo* data agree, and, moreover, the *in vitro* measurements are more reliable and quantitative than the electrical potential measurements on the whole cell.

In paper II of this series, the ionic permeability of the excitable microsacs and the effects of cholinergic agonists and ionic environment on this permeability are analyzed in some detail. In paper III, we compare quantitatively the selective increase of permeability and the amount of cholinergic agonist specifically bound to the cholinergic receptor integrated in the microsacs Finally, paper IV describes the ultrastructure, at high resolution, of two classes of microsacs.

A preliminary presentation of this work has already been published (Kasai & Changeux, 1970).

## Materials and Methods

The electric eels, *Electrophorus electricus*, were bought alive from Paramount Aquarium (Ardsley, New York), and were stored in Paris in the Tropical Aquarium of the Musée des Arts Africains et Océaniens (thanks to the generous help of Mr. Goussef and Mr. Denise).

Membrane fragments which originate from the *innervated faces* of the electroplax were purified, as a concentrated suspension, on the basis of their high acetylcholinesterase (AcChE) content, following a method described by Changeux, Gautron, Israel and Podleski (1969). A 10 g portion of fresh electric organ was cut with scissors in fragments of approximately 1 cm$^3$ and suspended in 50 ml of 0.2 M sucrose in distilled water. The suspension was homogenized with a Virtis apparatus in a 250 ml glass vessel, carefully maintained at 0 °C with crushed ice, for 1 min and 30 sec at 75 % of maximal speed. The homogenate was then centrifuged at $5.000 \times g$ (6,500 rpm) for 20 min in a rotor L of a Servall centrifuge. The supernatant fluid was collected and centrifuged at high speed in a SW 25 rotor of a Beckman LH 20 ultracentrifuge. In general, the 30 ml centrifuge tube contained, from the bottom to the top, 5 ml of 1.0 M sucrose, 5 ml of 0.4 M sucrose, and 20 ml of low-speed supernatant, carefully layered on top of each other. Sometimes 25 ml of low-speed supernatant was disposed on 5 ml of 1.4 M sucrose. In this latter case, the suspension of membrane was more concentrated but was contaminated by soluble cytoplasmic proteins. The gradients were centrifuged for 5 to 7 hr at $64,000 \times g$ (25,000 rpm) immediately after preparation. Fractions of 1 ml were collected after perforation of the bottom of the tubes with a needle. The specific activity of AcChE and the response to carbamylcholine was measured in each fraction. The fourth and (or) fifth tubes collected usually had the highest activity in AcChE and contained the most excitable fragments. A detailed profile of AcChE, protein, flux and excitability in a typical sucrose gradient after centrifugation is given in Fig. 7 of paper II of this series. The recovery of AcChE in the membrane fragments was generally 80 to 100 % of the total amount of AcChE added on top of the gradient.

The specific activity of AcChE in the fraction used in the flux experiments usually ranged between 0.5 and 3 moles acetylthiocholine (AcTCh) hydrolyzed per hr per g protein. The concentration of AcChE was between 3 and 5 moles of AcTCh hydrolyzed per hr per liter of microsacs suspension, and the concentration of membrane proteins in the suspension was between 2 and 5 mg per ml. In the method formerly used by Changeux *et al.* (1969), 5 instead of 20 ml of low-speed supernatant was added on top of the sucrose gradient. As a consequence, the total quantity and the concentration of membrane fragments in the recovered fractions were much lower, although the specific activity of AcChE in the purified fractions sometimes reached 7 moles of AcTCh hydrolyzed per hr per g protein.

Success in the flux measurements was found to depend on the concentration of AcChE-rich microsacs in the membrane fractions. This concentration is directly related to the concentration of AcChE-rich microsacs in the low-speed supernatant, which is itself determined by the homogenization procedure and the quality of the organ. Increasing the speed of the blade of our old Virtis apparatus from 75 % up to 90 % gave marked improvement in the recent purifications of excitable membrane fragments.

As mentioned later, flux experiments appeared to be highly reproducible within a preparation. However, the absolute values of the rates measured vary significantly from one preparation to the other. As a consequence, we shall identify a given group of experiments carried out with a particular preparation of microsacs by the number of the preparation (from 1 to 24).

Microsacs which originate from the *non-innervated membrane* were isolated following the procedure originally described by Bauman, Changeux and Benda (1970) on the basis of their high content in the $Na^+$, $K^+$-activated, ouabain-sensitive ATPase. Homogenization and low-speed centrifugation were carried out in the same manner as for the excitable microsacs. The low-speed supernatant was then centrifuged at high speed in the following manner: 20 ml of low-speed supernatant was layered on a discontinuous gradient of 5 ml of 1.4 M sucrose and 5.0 ml of 1.0 M sucrose in a 30 ml lusteroid tube. The gradients were then centrifuged in a SW 25 rotor for 3 hr at 25,000 rpm in a Beckman preparative ultracentrifuge. The ATPase-rich fragments accumulated at the interface between 1.4 and 1.0 M sucrose. They were collected after perforation of the bottom of the tube, pooled, and then diluted twofold with distilled water and recentrifuged, for the same length of time and at the same speed, above a bottom layer of 5 ml of 1.4 M sucrose. The purified microsacs formed a thin layer at the interface between the supernatant and the 1.4 M sucrose solution; they were again collected after perforation of the bottom of the tube. Recovery of ATPase in this fraction was approximately 50% of the total ATPase added on top of the first sucrose gradient. The specific activity of ATPase in these fragments was 300 to 500 μmoles of ATP hydrolyzed per hr per mg protein at 37 °C, and that of AcChE was 0.080 moles of AcTCh hydrolyzed per hr per g protein at 27 °C.

AcChE was assayed with AcTCh as the substrate by the method of Ellmann, Courtney, Andress and Featherstone (1961). The assay mixture contained $5 \times 10^{-4}$ M AcTCh, $5 \times 10^{-4}$ M dithiobis-dinitrobenzoic acid in $5 \times 10^{-2}$ M sodium phosphate buffered at pH 7.0. The total volume was 1.0 ml. The assay was carried out at 27 °C in a Zeiss PMQ spectrophotometer. The reaction was started by the addition to the assay mixture of, for example, 10 μliters of membrane suspension diluted 100-fold in $5 \times 10^{-2}$ M sodium phosphate buffer, pH 7.0. The increase of optical density was recorded at 412 nm.

*Protein concentration* was estimated by the method of Lowry, Rosebrough, Farr and Randall (1951), using bovine serum albumin as the standard.

*Sucrose concentrations* were measured by refractometry with a Zeiss Abbe's refractometer.

*Measurement of the permeability* of the microsacs to $^{22}Na^+$ was routinely performed in the following manner: 1 ml of membrane suspension in 0.7 to 0.8 M sucrose containing 2 to 5 mg of membrane protein per ml was mixed with 0.3 ml of an aqueous solution of $^{22}NaCl$ (prepared by the Radiochemical Centre, Amersham, Great Britain) containing 0.1 mC/ml of $^{22}Na^+$ with a specific activity close to 75 mC/mg. To the radioactive solution was then added 3 M NaCl (approximately 20 μliters) and enough distilled water (approximately 0.2 ml) to make the solution $8 \times 10^{-6}$ M $^{22}NaCl$, $10^{-2}$ M nonradioactive NaCl, and 0.5 M sucrose. The pH of the suspension was, in the absence of added buffer, close to 7.0. The suspension was then stored at 4 °C, in the refrigerator, for 10 to 20 hr (overnight). The flux measurement was started by the 50-fold dilution of the radioactive microsacs suspension (0.1 in 5.0 ml) into a nonradioactive "dilution buffer" at room temperature (22 °C) containing $1.7 \times 10^{-1}$ M KCl, $2 \times 10^{-3}$ M $CaCl_2$, $1 \times 10^{-3}$ M sodium phosphate, pH 7.0, with (or without) the cholinergic effector. In these conditions the osmotic pressure of the dilution medium was slightly lower than that of the equilibrium medium. At given times 1.0 ml samples were rapidly filtered on Millipore filters (HAW P 02500, 25ea, HA 0.45 μ, white plain, 25 mm) and washed three times with 3 ml of cold (0 °C) dilution buffer. Under these conditions 95% of the microsacs remain on the Millipore filter although their size is much smaller than that of the pores of the filter. The Millipore filters were then dried and soaked in 10 ml of scintillation counting medium containing 3 g of PPO and 0.3 g of POPOP in 1 liter of toluene. The flasks were counted for 10 min in either a Packard scintillation counter model 3003 on channel 3 with a gain of 25% and a window width of 0.050 to infinity or in an Intertechnique "spectromètre à scintillation liquide" ABAC SL 40 on channel C with a window width of 0 to 10. The counting efficiency was 60 to 70%. The radioactivity remaining on the Millipore filter in the absence of microsacs (from 50 to 200 cpm depending on the batch of Millipore) was always subtracted from the total number of counts. Since the dilution of the concentrated microsacs suspension was always finite (approximately 50-fold), the equilibrium concentration of $^{22}Na^+$ in the microsacs after dilution was expected to be that of the diluted suspension. Therefore we routinely subtracted as well the number of counts corresponding to the total radioactivity remaining on the Millipore divided by the dilution factor. The radioactivity remaining on the filters which was associated with the presence of microsacs varied from one experiment to another from 200 to 2,000 cpm. This amount was always a linear function of the concentration of microsacs present in the dilution medium.

In the great majority of experiments, the permeability measurements were carried out on microsacs prepared from fresh electric tissue. Interestingly, microsacs which still present permeability properties and excitability can be prepared from frozen tissue following the standard procedure.

## Results

### *The in Vitro Response of Purified Membrane Fragments to Cholinergic Agonists*

In the eel electroplax, the surfaces of the cell which are excitable are distinct from those which carry the active transport of $Na^+$ and $K^+$ (reference in Nachmansohn, 1959, and in Changeux, Podleski, Kasai & Blumenthal, 1970). The active transport takes place at the level of the rostral part of the cell surface: the non-innervated membrane. The enhanced flux of ions caused by excitation is exclusively restricted to the caudal surface of the electroplax which receives the nerve terminals and is referred to as the innervated membrane. As shown by Bauman *et al.* (1970), fragments which belong to each of these two classes of cytoplasmic membranes are easy to separate, *in vitro*, by ultracentrifugation of crude homogenates of electric tissue. They are purified on the basis of their different enzymatic compositions. Fragments of the non-innervated membrane are expected to be rich in the active transport enzyme – the ouabain-sensitive, $Na^+$, $K^+$-activated ATPase. On the other hand, fragments of the innervated membrane should have a high content in AcChE, which is commonly associated with excitability and which, in fact, is present almost exclusively on the innervated surface of the cell (*see* Benda, Tsuji, Daussent & Changeux, 1970). Indeed, fragments with high levels of ouabain-sensitive ATPase but low levels of AcChE are found to migrate to a higher density of sucrose ($d=1.14$; 1.15 M) than those with low levels of ATPase but high levels of AcChE ($d=1.09$; 0.65 M).

Both classes of membrane fragments make closed vesicles, or microsacs, but their permeability behavior and their sensitivity to cholinergic agents are different.

Our first step in the study of the sensitivity of these fragments to cholinergic agonists was the measure of their permeability to cations: we selected $^{22}Na^+$ as a particularly convenient radioisotope. The experimental procedure that we routinely used (*see* Methods) had two steps: (1) an overnight incubation in the presence of $^{22}Na^+$ to equilibrate the microsacs with the radioactive permeant, and (2) a dilution of the equilibrated suspension into a nonradioactive "dilution medium".

The $^{22}Na^+$ content of the microsacs as a function of time was then measured by rapid filtration of the diluted suspension on Millipore filters (Fig. 1). The curves of equilibration obtained are characterized by the following two parameters:

(1) *The time for half equilibration* ($\tau_0$). This time was, in general, close to 20 min for $^{22}Na^+$, but depended on the nature of the permeant ion. A significant variation of $\tau_0$ from one membrane preparation to another was encountered (from 15 to 24 min), but with a given preparation of microsacs the error of $\tau_0$ was always smaller than 5%.

(2) *The apparent volume* ($V_{app}$). The extrapolation of the curve of equilibration at zero time gives an amount of radioactivity ($R_0$) which corresponds to $^{22}Na^+$ either trapped within the microsacs or irreversibly bound to their membrane. Extrapolation back to zero time was, in a few cases, done by fitting the experimental points by the equation $N(t) = N_0 \left( \dfrac{t_0}{t + t_0} \right)^v$, where $t$ is the time, and $v$ a constant ($0.45 \pm 0.05$). In general, extrapolation was done by eye and gave almost the same results. We define the apparent volume as the quantity:

$$V_{app} = \frac{R_0}{R \times p}$$

where $p$ is the mass of membrane proteins filtered on the Millipore, and $R$ is the radioactivity of the solution of incubation per unit volume. This quantity represents a volume per unit mass and more rigorously might be called a specific volume. The apparent volume usually ranged between 0.5 and 2 μliters/mg protein. In the experiment reported in Fig. 1, the apparent volume was 1.1 μliters/mg protein.

In paper II of this series, we shall extensively study and discuss the transport properties of the microsacs. Briefly, we show that the amount of radioactivity which remains on the Millipore filter after overnight equilibration with $^{22}Na^+$ corresponds to $^{22}Na^+$ trapped within the microsacs. The time course of $^{22}Na^+$ release from the microsacs is shown to be insensitive to $10^{-3}$ M ouabain and thus corresponds to a passive efflux of $^{22}Na^+$. Using a very simple filtration technique, we are able to measure the permeability of membrane fragments to $Na^+$ in a well-defined environment.

Fig. 1a shows that the AcChE-rich microsacs are excitable *in vitro*. After overnight equilibration with $^{22}Na^+$, the microsacs were diluted in the presence of a cholinergic agonist, $10^{-4}$ M carbamylcholine (Carb). Under these conditions, the apparent volume did not change but the rate of $^{22}Na^+$

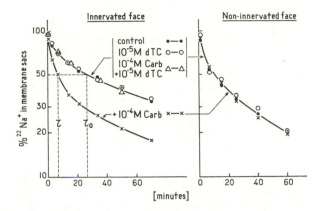

Fig. 1. Specific effect of a cholinergic agonist, carbamylcholine (Carb), on the efflux of $^{22}Na^+$ from excitable microsacs. *Left:* Excitable AcChE-rich microsacs derived from innervated membranes. dTC is the abbreviation for *d*-tubocurarine. *Right:* Non-excitable ATPase-rich microsacs derived from non-innervated membranes. — The method of preparation of the membrane fragments and the measurement of $^{22}Na^+$ efflux are described in the text. The concentration of proteins in the suspension filtered on Millipore filters was 89 µg/ml (innervated face) and 46 µg/ml (non-innervated face). The specific activity of AcChE in the preparation of excitable microsacs (no. 1) was only 0.8 mmoles of AcTCh/hr/mg protein at 27 °C. $\tau$ and $\tau_0$ are the times for half equilibration in the presence and in the absence of cholinergic agonist respectively

exit increased three- to fourfold. This increase was blocked by $10^{-5}$ M *d*-tubocurarine (*d*-tubo) which, in the absence of Carb, had no significant effect on $^{22}Na^+$ efflux. The observed effect thus corresponds to a permeability response of the microsacs to Carb. In order to evaluate the specificity of the response to Carb, we then studied the behavior of the ATPase-rich microsacs. Fig. 1 illustrates that, after overnight equilibration, the ATPase-rich microsacs, like the AcChE-rich ones, retained $^{22}Na^+$ and released it upon dilution. The rate of equilibration was somewhat faster than that of the AcChE-rich microsacs but did not change in the presence of cholinergic agonists or antagonists. As expected from their origin, the ATPase-rich microsacs are *not* excitable *in vitro*. Only the microsacs which are derived from the innervated face of the electroplax are excitable.

### Quantitative Comparison of the Dose-Response Curves to Cholinergic Agonists Obtained in Vitro and in Vivo

In the preceding paragraph, we have seen that, in a *qualitative* manner, the physiological response to cholinergic agonists still operates, *in vitro*, on isolated membrane fragments. An important question is then to what

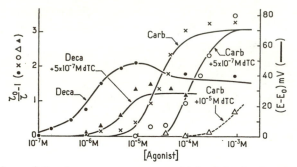

Fig. 2. Comparison of the dose-response curves obtained *in vivo* by measuring steady-state membrane potentials with a single isolated electroplax and *in vitro* by following $^{22}Na^+$ efflux. Carb and Deca represent carbamylcholine and decamethonium, two specific cholinergic agonists of the electroplax *in vivo*. dTC is the abbreviation for *d*-tubocurarine, a typical cholinergic antagonist. The electrophysiological data are from Changeux and Podleski (1968). Preparation no. 1

extent is there *quantitative* agreement between the data obtained *in vitro* and those obtained *in vivo* by electrophysiological techniques?

We used as a measure of the *in vivo* response the measurements of the electric potential of the isolated electroplax of Changeux and Podleski (1968) recorded intracellularly, by the technique of Higman, Podleski and Bartels (1964). We have taken as the measure of the response to a given dose of cholinergic agonist the difference $(E-E_0)$ between the resting potential $(E_0)$ and the *steady-state* potential $(E)$ observed after a 1 to 5 min bath application of cholinergic agonist. In Fig. 2 we have reported these data as a continuous line and superimposed on them (dots) the *in vitro* results.

*In vivo*, as *in vitro*, the experiments were performed at room temperature and in a dilution medium with ionic strength $(\Gamma/2=0.177)$ very close to that of the physiological Ringer's solution $(\Gamma/2=0.180)$. We have taken as the measure of the *in vitro* response the relative increase of the rate of $^{22}Na^+$ exit: $\frac{\tau_0}{\tau}-1$, $\tau_0$ and $\tau$ being the times for half equilibration of $^{22}Na$ between the inside and the outside of the microsacs in the absence and in the presence of cholinergic agonists, respectively. In order to allow quantitative comparison between both sets of results, we have normalized all the data to the same maximal response to decamethonium (Deca).

The general shapes and positions of the dose-response curves are very similar. Almost the same midpoints and thus the same "apparent affinities" are obtained with the two agonists tested, Carb and Deca. In addition, both *in vitro* and *in vivo*, the maximal response (or "intrinsic activity") to Carb is larger than that to Deca. Moreover, *d*-tubo, a typical cholinergic antagonist, acts quantitatively in exactly the same manner *in vitro* and *in vivo*. In the presence of *d*-tubo, the dose-response curves to Carb and Deca are shifted to the right and almost the same apparent inhibition constant for *d*-tubo is measured. Podleski and Changeux (*unpublished results*) have noticed that, with the isolated electroplax, the antagonism between *d*-tubo and Carb is simply competitive, whereas that between *d*-tubo and Deca is accompanied by a decrease of the maximal response to Deca, i.e. is not strictly competitive. Interestingly, *d*-tubo presents, both qualitatively and quantitatively, the same behavior *in vitro*.

The agreement is good enough to allow a comparison of some characteristic details of the shape of the dose-response curves. For instance, as first found by Higman *et al.* (1964), and further confirmed and extended by Changeux and Podleski (1968), the dose-response curves to various agonists recorded *in vivo* with the isolated electroplax systematically deviate from simple Langmuir isotherms. Their early parts show a slight but significant convexity to the abscissa (or sigmoid shape); they are converted into straight lines in the double logarithmic plot of Hill (Brown & Hill, 1922), and in this plot their slopes (or Hill coefficient) are systematically different from one (Fig. 3a). Depending on the agonist considered, the Hill coefficients range from 1.6 to 2.0 (Changeux & Podleski, 1968). Fig. 3 and the Table show that the same effects are present *in vitro*. The Hill coefficients measured in these conditions are very close, if not identical, to those reported *in vivo*. Further confirmation of the presence of cooperative effects in the response to cholinergic ligands was offered by the analysis of the shape of the dose-response curve to an antagonist, *d*-tubo, measured in the presence of a fixed concentration of Carb ($10^{-4}$ M) as the agonist. Fig. 3b shows that, here again, the shape of the response curve to increasing concentration of *d*-tubo is sigmoid and has a Hill coefficient of 1.5. Apparent cooperative effects are thus present with both cholinergic agonists and cholinergic antagonists. Additional evidence in favor of this conclusion is offered by the occurence *in vitro* of the same conversion of shape of the dose-response curve to a given agonist in the presence of another agonist as observed by Changeux and Podleski (1968) on the isolated electroplax. Indeed, Fig. 4 shows that the early part of the dose-response curve to Carb is concave to the abscissa in the absence of Deca, but convex in its presence. The two curves cannot be converted by simple translation in a semilogarithmic plot. The effects of Carb and Deca are not additive but cooperative.

Finally, in the Table we have compared the results obtained with a variety of cholinergic agonists and antagonists on the microsacs with those available in the literature for the same compounds on the isolated

Table. *Parameters characteristic of the dose-response curves to various cholinergic agonists and antagonists obtained in vivo and in vitro*

| Agonists | In vivo | | | | | In vitro | | | |
|---|---|---|---|---|---|---|---|---|---|
| | Temp. (°C) | $K_{app}$ (M) | $R_{max}$ (mV) | $\dfrac{R_{max}}{R_{max\,Deca}}$ | $n_H$ | Temp. (°C) | $K_{app}$ (M) | $\dfrac{R_{max}}{R_{max\,Deca}}$ | $n_H$ |
| Decamethonium (C. & P.) | 22 | $1.2 \times 10^{-6}$ | 50 | 1 | $1.63 \pm 0.02$ | 22 | $1.2 \times 10^{-6}$ | 1 | 1.7 |
| | | | | | | 4 | $1.2 \times 10^{-6}$ | 1 | 1.7 |
| Carbamylcholine (C & P.) (H.P & B.) | 22 | $2.6 \times 10^{-5}$ $3.0 \times 10^{-5}$ | 69.5 60.0 | 1.39 1.20 | $2.0 \pm 0.1$ $1.8 \pm 0.1$ | 22 | $3.3 \times 10^{-5}$ $4 \times 10^{-5}$ $5 \times 10^{-5}$ | 1.56 1.87 1.68 | 1.7 1.5 1.7 |
| | | | | | | 4 | $1.2 \times 10^{-4}$ $1.0 \times 10^{-4}$ | 1.6 1.65 | 1.5 1.7 |
| Phenyltrimethyl ammonium (C. & P.) | 22 | $1.2 \times 10^{-5}$ $1.3 \times 10^{-5}$ | 50 50 | 1 1 | $1.77 \pm 0.05$ $1.66 \pm 0.05$ | 22 | $2 \times 10^{-5}$ | 1.57 | 1.7 |
| | | | | | | 4 | $4 \times 10^{-5}$ | 1.57 | 2.0 |
| Acetylcholine $+5 \times 10^{-5}$ M eserine (M.B. & W.) | 22 | $3 \times 10^{-6}$ | | | | 22 | $4 \times 10^{-6}$ | 1.70 | 1.6 |
| Acetylthiocholine $+5 \times 10^{-5}$ M eserine (M.B & W.) | | $5 \times 10^{-5}$ | | | | 22 | $1.3 \times 10^{-4}$ | 1.55 | 1.0 |

Excitation *in Vitro*. I

| Antagonists | In vivo | | In vitro | |
|---|---|---|---|---|
| | Temp. (°C) | $Ki_{app}$ | Temp. (°C) | $Ki_{app}$ |
| *d*-Tubocurarine (agonist carbamylcholine) (C. & P.) (H. P. & B.) | 22 | $1.6 \times 10^{-7}$ | 22 | $1.5 \times 10^{-7}$ |
| | | | 4 | $1.6 \times 10^{-7}$ |
| *d*-Tubocurarine (agonist decamethonium) (C. & P.) | 22 | $1.6 \times 10^{-7}$ | 22 | $1.5 \times 10^{-7}$ |
| | | | 4 | $1.5 \times 10^{-7}$ |
| Flaxedil (agonist carbamylcholine) (C. & P.) | 22 | $3.0 \times 10^{-7}$ | 22 | $3.3 \times 10^{-7}$ |
| | | | 4 | $3.5 \times 10^{-7}$ |
| Hexamethonium (K. & W.) | 22 | $3.0 \times 10^{-5}$ | 22 | $6.2 \times 10^{-5}$ |

$K_{app}$ is the apparent dissociation constant of the considered agonist: it is the concentration of agonist which gives a response which is half that of the maximal response $R_{max}$. The presence of cooperative effects is neglected in this estimate. $Ki_{app}$ is determined from the curve of antagonism of the response to a fixed concentration of agonist at increasing concentration of antagonist. In the *in vitro* measurements, the concentrations of agonist were $a = 10^{-4}$ M Carb, and $A = 3 \times 10^{-6}$ M Deca. The concentration of antagonist giving 50 % inhibition of the response ($I_{50}$) was measured, and $Ki_{app}$ was estimated from these measurements by the relation: $Ki_{app} = \dfrac{I_{50}}{1 + \dfrac{A}{K_{app}}}$. We took for Carb:

$K_{app} = 4 \times 10^{-5}$ M, and for Deca: $K_{app} = 1.20 \times 10^{-6}$ M. The term $n_H$ is the slope of the straight line obtained by plotting the data in the system of coordinates of Hill (Brown & Hill, 1923). The *in vivo* data are from Changeux and Podleski (1968) (C. & P.), Higman, Podleski and Bartels (1964) (H. P. & B.), Mautner, Bartels & Webb (1966) (M. B. & W.), and Karlin and Winnik (1968) (K. & W.).

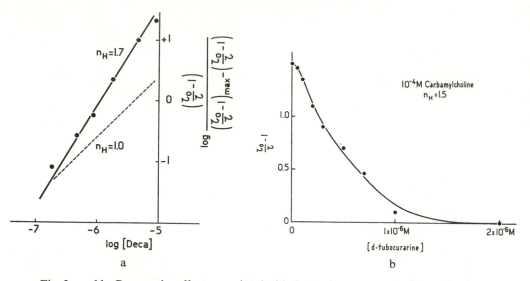

a    b

Fig. 3a and b. Cooperative effects associated with the *in vitro* response to decamethonium (Deca) (a) and the antagonism by *d*-tubocurarine of the response to Carb (b). (a) Hill plot of the same data as for Fig. 1. (b) Overnight incubation was carried out in the presence of $10^{-2}$ M NaCl, $5 \times 10^{-1}$ M sucrose, and $^{22}Na^+$. The concentration of proteins was 5.1 mg/ml. The suspension was supplemented 30 min before dilution with $10^{-4}$ M Carb. The suspension was then diluted 80-fold in $1.7 \times 10^{-1}$ M KCl, $2 \times 10^{-3}$ M $CaCl_2$, $10^{-3}$ M Na-phosphate buffer, pH 7.0, supplemented with $10^{-4}$ M Carb, and the indicated concentration of *d*-tubocurarine. The apparent $K_i$ for *d*-tubocurarine was found to be $1.3 \times 10^{-7}$ M with $K_D = 4 \times 10^{-5}$ M for Carb. Preparation no. 13

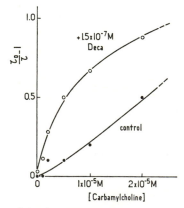

Fig. 4. Conversion of shape of the dose-response curve to Carb by Deca. The concentrated suspension of microsacs (no. 3) containing 4.4 mg of protein per ml, was incubated overnight with $^{22}Na^+$ in the standard conditions. Before dilution the suspension was preincubated with $1.5 \times 10^{-7}$ M Deca for 50 min. Dilution was carried out in the standard dilution medium in the presence of $1.5 \times 10^{-7}$ M Deca and the indicated concentration of Carb. In the presence of $10^{-4}$ M Carb, the maximal responses recorded were 1.8 and 2.0 in the presence and in the absence, respectively, of $1.5 \times 10^{-7}$ M Deca

electroplax. There is quantitative agreement between the two series of results.

A slight but significant discrepancy should, however, be mentioned. As shown in Fig. 2 and in the Table, there is a difference between the *absolute values* of the maximal responses to Carb recorded *in vitro* and *in vivo*. When the curves are normalized to the same maximal response to Deca, the maximal response to Carb measured *in vitro* is 20 to 40% larger than that measured *in vivo*.

### In Vitro Study of Some Characteristic Properties
### of the Excitable Membrane of the Electroplax

In this section we shall be concerned with some characteristic properties of the innervated membrane of the electroplax which are related only *indirectly* to the typical response to cholinergic agonists. Here again, we shall see that the *in vitro* behavior of the excitable microsacs is almost exactly the same as that of the excitable membrane *in situ*.

*Noncompetitive Antagonism Between Carb and Tetracaine.* Podleski and Bartels (1963) have reported that tetracaine blocks the response to Carb in a manner different from that of *d*-tubo. In the presence of tetracaine, the maximal response to Carb is lower; this antagonism between Carb and tetracaine is not competitive. Fig. 5 shows that this was found to be true also with the isolated membrane fragments, and that the concentration of local anesthetic which blocked the response *in vitro* was very similar

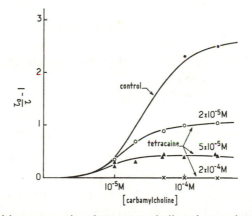

Fig. 5. Noncompetitive antagonism between a cholinergic agonist (Carb) and a local anesthetic (tetracaine). Overnight incubation was carried out in the standard conditions: the concentration of proteins was 6.6 mg/ml. The suspension was supplemented 10 min before dilution with tetracaine at the indicated concentration. The concentrated suspension was diluted 94-fold in the standard dilution medium supplemented with the indicated concentration of Carb and tetracaine. Preparation no. 6

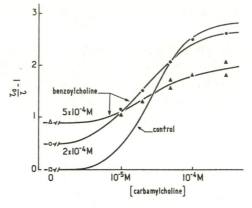

Fig. 6. Mixed agonistic and antagonistic effects of benzoylcholine. Exactly the same conditions as for Fig. 4 except that benzoycholine was used instead of tetracaine. Preparation no. 6

to that which blocks the response *in vivo*. About $4 \times 10^{-5}$ M tetracaine was needed to reduce the response to $10^{-4}$ M Carb by 50% *in vivo*; the same result was obtained *in vitro* with $2 \times 10^{-5}$ M tetracaine. *In vivo*, as *in vitro*, tetracaine behaves like a noncompetitive antagonist.

*Mixed Agonistic and Antagonistic Effects of Benzoylcholine.* Bartels (1965) has shown that, *in vivo*, benzoylcholine might act like either an agonist or an antagonist. It is an agonist since it causes the depolarization of the excitable membrane of the isolated electroplax. However, the maximal response, or intrinsic activity, of benzoylcholine is considerably lower than that of Carb or even Deca ($E_{max} - E_0 = 25$ mV, about 40% of the maximal response to Carb). It is an antagonist as well since, at saturating levels, it antagonizes the response to Carb as long as the Carb response is larger than its own maximal response. Fig. 6 shows that this particular behavior could be repeated *in vitro* and thus that benzoylcholine has mixed agonistic and antagonistic effects on the excitable membrane.

*Covalent Binding of Affinity Labeling Reagents.* A variety of affinity labeling reagents have been used by several groups of workers to identify the cholinergic receptor macromolecule. The first to be tested on the isolated electroplax was *p*-(trimethylammonium) benzene diazonium fluoroborate (TDF), a compound initially designed by Fenton and Singer (1965) to label the active sites of antibodies directed against the phenyl trimethylammonium hapten. As shown by Changeux, Podleski and Wofsy (1967), TDF acts on the isolated electroplax as an irreversible antagonist. Fig. 7 shows that it

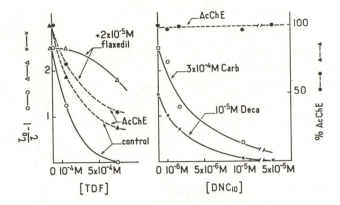

Fig. 7. Compared effects of two affinity labeling reagents on the *in vitro* response of excitable microsacs to Carb and Deca and on the activity of AcChE present in the same microsacs. TDF is for trimethyl ammonium benzene diazonium difluoroborate, DNC 10 M for dinaphthyl decamethonium mustard (*see* Rang & Ritter, 1969). Overnight incubation was carried out in the presence of $10^{-2}$ M NaCl, $5 \times 10^{-1}$ M sucrose and $^{22}$Na$^+$. The concentration of protein was 4.4 mg/ml. The experiment was started by the addition to the microsac suspension, equilibrated at 22°, of TDF or DNC 10 M at the indicated concentration. The length of exposure was 10 min for DNC 10 M and 20 min for TDF. When TDF was used, the microsac suspension was adjusted to pH 8.0 by addition of Tris-HCl buffered at pH 8.0 up to a final concentration of $10^{-2}$ M Tris. The suspension was then diluted 70-fold in the usual dilution medium supplemented with either $3 \times 10^{-4}$ M Carb (TDF and DNC 10 M) or $10^{-5}$ M Deca (DNC 10 M only). AcChE was assayed in the diluted suspension. In the case of the TDF experiment, exposure to TDF of the concentrated suspension was performed either in the presence of $2 \times 10^{-5}$ M flaxedil or in its absence (control). Preparation no. 11

has the same action *in vitro*. Furthermore, in agreement with the observation of Changeux *et al.* (1967), flaxedil, a reversible antagonist, both *in vivo* and *in vitro* protects against the irreversible blockade by TDF of the response to Carb. The use of TDF to isolate the receptor protein meets, however, with a serious problem of specificity. As shown by Wofsy and Michaeli (1967) and by Meunier and Changeux (1969), TDF reacts as well with the catalytic site of AcChE and even with some "allosteric" sites on the same enzyme (Changeux, 1966). It would be possible to distinguish without ambiguity between these various classes of sites if the kinetics of reaction of TDF with each class of site was measurable. A considerable advantage of the microsac assay is that such a measurement is feasible. We have followed in parallel the effect of TDF on the activity of AcChE present in the fragments and the abolition of the permeability response to Carb. Fig. 7 shows that, in the presence of TDF, both the activity of AcChE and the response to Carb were strongly inhibited. As expected, TDF reacted with both the cholinergic receptor site and the catalytic site of AcChE. However, the TDF concentration dependence of the rates of the two reactions differed strikingly. This difference was amplified in the presence of an antagonist such as flaxedil, which presents a high affinity for the cholinergic receptor site and a low affinity for the catalytic center of AcChE. Indeed, $2 \times 10^{-6}$ M flaxedil strongly protected against the inactivation of the response to Carb, but had only little effect, at the concentration used, against the inactivation of AcChE. The catalytic center of AcChE and the active site of the cholinergic receptor are, unambiguously, distinct structures (*see* Podleski, 1967, and Changeux *et al.*, 1969).

This last conclusion is supported by studies carried out with another affinity labeling reagent discovered by Rang and Ritter (1969), the dinaphthyl decamethonium mustard (DNC 10 M). This compound is again, like TDF, an irreversible curare *in vivo*. Fig. 7 shows that it plays the same role *in vitro*. Interestingly, as shown in the same figure, the mustard had strictly no effect on the catalytic activity of AcChE. DNC 10 M is thus a much more specific labeling reagent of the cholinergic receptor site than TDF.

*In Vitro Alteration by Dithiothreitol of the Response of the Microsacs to Cholinergic Agents.* Karlin and associates (Karlin & Bartels, 1966; Karlin & Winnik, 1968) have shown that *in vivo* exposure of the innervated membrane of the electroplax to dithiothreitol (DTT), a reducing agent, is accompanied by characteristic perturbations of the cell response to cholinergic agents. In particular, the amplitude of the response to Carb decreases, and hexamethonium, a typical antagonist, becomes an agonist after DTT treatment. The same observation could be repeated *in vitro* (Fig. 8). After *in vitro* exposure of the microsacs to $10^{-3}$ M DTT, the response to Carb decreased and hexamethonium then behaved like Carb: it increased the efflux of $Na^+$ ions.

Again, the microsacs react in exactly the same manner as the excitable membrane of the cell. The molecular mechanisms which account for the process of excitation are thus integrally preserved after isolation and purification of the microsacs.

*Effect of Gramicidin A on the Permeability of the Microsacs.* Podleski and Changeux (1969) have shown with the isolated electroplax that the polypeptide antibiotic, gramicidin A (Gra), causes an irreversible increase in the permeability of the innervated membrane to $Na^+$ ions.

Fig. 9 illustrates that *in vitro* exposure of microsacs to Gra was accompanied, as well, by an increase of $^{22}Na^+$ release. In addition, Gra was active

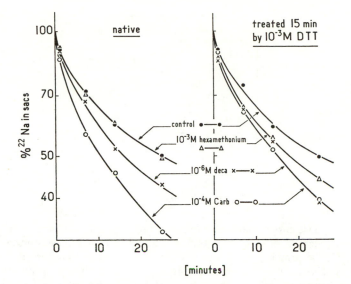

Fig. 8. Effect of dithiothreitol (DTT) on the response of excitable microsacs to hexamethonium, Carb and Deca. The concentrated suspension of microsacs containing 4.9 mg of protein per ml was exposed overnight to $^{22}$Na$^+$ in the presence of $10^{-2}$ M NaCl and $5 \times 10^{-1}$ M sucrose. The experiment was started the next morning by adding DTT to the concentrated microsac suspension, equilibrated at 15 °C at a final concentration of $10^{-3}$ M DTT in the presence of $10^{-2}$ M Tris buffer, pH 8.0. The mixture was then diluted 60-fold in the standard dilution medium supplemented with the indicated concentration of Carb, Deca or hexamethonium. Preparation no. 2

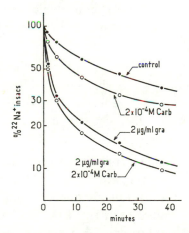

Fig. 9. Sensitivity of the excitable microsacs to $2 \times 10^{-4}$ M Carb after exposure to gramicidin A (Gra). The concentrated suspension of microsacs (preparation no. 6) containing 6.6 mg/ml of membrane protein was incubated overnight with $^{22}$Na$^+$ in the standard conditions. It was preincubated with 16.7 µg/ml Gra for 10 min and then diluted 84-fold in the standard dilution medium supplemented or not with Carb; the final concentrations of Carb or Gra are indicated on the figure

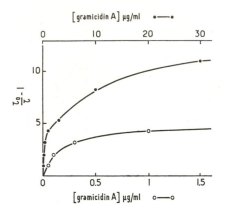

Fig. 10. Dose-response curve of excitable microsacs to Gra. The two curves correspond to two different scales for the Gra concentration. The concentrated suspension containing 6.1 mg of membrane protein per ml was first equilibrated with $^{22}Na^+$ in the standard conditions and subsequently diluted 60-fold in the standard dilution medium with or without Gra at the indicated concentration. Preparation no. 4

in the same concentration range both *in vitro* and *in vivo* (Fig. 10). Interestingly, at high levels of Gra, the rates of $^{22}Na^+$ release became much larger than those measured at saturating concentrations of Carb. This suggests that, in agreement with the interpretation of Podleski and Changeux (1969), new channels or pores for $Na^+$ ions, which are distinct from those associated with the cholinergic receptor appear after exposure of the microsacs to Gra.

In the presence of Gra, the microsacs still responded to Carb but, again in agreement with the Podleski and Changeux results, the amplitude of the response to Carb was markedly reduced (Fig. 9). However, in contrast with these authors' findings, the *apparent* cooperative effects observed *in vivo* have not yet been detected *in vitro* (Fig. 10).

Finally, in order to test the reversibility of the effect of Gra, we carried out the dilution experiment represented in Fig. 11. The microsacs were first exposed to 0.3 µg/ml Gra and then diluted 20-fold. The rates of $^{22}Na^+$ release of a suspension of microsacs treated by Gra were exactly the *same* *before* dilution and *after* dilution; dilution did not reverse the effect of Gra. We thus confirm the result of Podleski and Changeux (1969) that Gra acts as an *irreversible* membrane effector. This effect is strikingly different from the action of Carb, which, as extensively discussed in paper II, is always reversible.

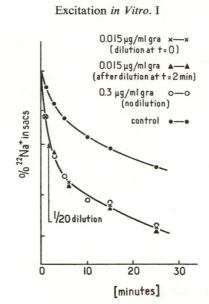

Fig. 11. Irreversible effect of Gra on the permeability of the microsacs to $^{22}$Na$^+$. A concentrated suspension of microsacs containing 4.8 mg of protein per ml was exposed overnight to $^{22}$Na$^+$ in the standard incubation medium, then diluted 20-fold in the standard dilution medium supplemented or not with Gra at the indicated concentration. The diluted suspension was then diluted a second time, 20-fold, at $t = 0$ and $t = 2$ min (indicated by the vertical arrow). Preparation no. 7

## Discussion

Membrane fragments purified from the electric organ of *E. electricus* respond *in vitro* to cholinergic agonists by an increase of permeability to $^{22}$Na$^+$. This effect is blocked specifically by cholinergic antagonists. The dose-response curves measuring $^{22}$Na$^+$ efflux *in vitro* superimpose almost exactly with those recorded *in vivo* by measuring steady-state electrical potentials. The same apparent affinities for the cholinergic effectors, as well as the same shapes for the response curves, are found with the two methods. The competitive and noncompetitive effects observed *in vivo* between cholinergic agonists and antagonists are the same with the isolated microsacs.

A slight discrepancy was noticed, however, when the maximal responses to various agonists *in vitro* were compared with those recorded *in vivo*. For instance, when the dose-response curves to Carb and Deca are normalized to the maximal response to Deca, the maximal response to Carb is significantly larger *in vitro* than *in vivo*. The question is then, which of these two measurements is the more reliable? The electrical potential measurements could plausibly give an underestimation of the maximal response to Carb. Indeed, at high concentration of Carb, the membrane potential

393

decreases down to −15 mV, a domain of potential where the membrane permeability might change without being accompanied by parallel changes of electrical potential. It is very likely that, under these conditions, the flux measurements become more reliable than the measurements of electrical potential.

We have never been able to demonstrate without ambiguity the phenomenon of receptor desensitization with the excitable microsacs. As clearly shown in paper II of this series, the effect of cholinergic agonists (at the concentrations tested) is entirely reversible. The peak in sensitivity, which seems to occur in the dose-response curve to Deca around $10^{-5}$ M (10 times its apparent dissociation constant) (Fig. 2), might be considered as an indication of receptor desensitization. However, alternative interpretations, e.g., a weak antagonistic effect of Deca, cannot be ruled out.

The sigmoid shape of the dose-response curve to various agonists, which was extensively studied by Changeux and Podleski (1968) on the isolated electroplax, is preserved *in vitro* with the microsacs. The apparent cooperativity observed *in vitro* rules out electrical artifacts as a cause of this observation and makes more plausible a theoretical structural cooperativity in the assembly of the cholinergic receptors. These might possibly be grouped in oligomeric clusters within the excitable membrane. On the other hand, we have not been able to show *in vitro* that cooperative effects accompany the irreversible action of Gra.

A local anesthetic, tetracaine, blocks the response of the microsacs to Carb in a noncompetitive manner. This result, which confirms the observation of Podleski and Bartels (1963) on the isolated electroplax, might be accounted for by several different interpretations. Podleski and Bartels, for instance, following Keynes and Martins-Ferreira (1953), have distinguished two classes of excitable membranes in the innervated face of the electroplax: a subsynaptic membrane and a conductive membrane. The noncompetitive effect of tetracaine would be due to its preferential action on the conducting membrane. An alternative interpretation is that the local anesthetic binds to a site *on* the cholinergic receptor protein, or in its immediate vicinity, which is, at least partially, *distinct* from the active site of the receptor macromolecule.

A similar interpretation might be valid for benzoylcholine, which behaves, *in vitro*, as *in vivo*, both as an agonist and as a noncompetitive blocking agent. Benzoylcholine would bind to both the active site of the cholinergic receptor where it acts as an agonist and to the "local anesthetic receptor site" where it acts, like tetracaine, as a noncompetitive antagonist.

The simple fact that the preparation consists of a suspension of small membrane fragments has proved to be extremely convenient for quantitative biochemical and physicochemical studies. For example, the catalytic activity of AcChE and the permeability response to cholinergic agonists can be measured in parallel on the same membrane fragments. Experiments in which the effect of affinity labeling reagents was followed on both the activity of AcChE and the response to cholinergic agonists strongly support the conclusion that the catalytic site of AcChE and the receptor site of the receptor protein are entirely distinct entities.

In relation to the effect of affinity labeling reagents, we would like to mention some recent results of Changeux, Kasai and Lee (1970). These authors have demonstrated that a snake venom toxin, α-bungarotoxin, is *in vivo* as well as *in vitro* a highly specific and irreversible reagent of the cholinergic receptor site. By using the excitable microsacs, they have even been able to offer a quantitative estimate of the number of α-bungarotoxin sites, and thus of cholinergic receptor sites, per mass of membrane proteins. The microsac preparation is thus particularly convenient for a quantitative binding study (*see* paper III).

In addition, the microsac suspension presents several important advantages over all the physiological preparations used up to now: (1) the membrane fragments constitute a well-defined subcellular preparation; (2) the environment of the excitable membrane fragments can be controlled *ad libitum* on both faces; and (3) the permeability to a single ionic species and the permeability changes caused by the cholinergic agonists can be measured quantitatively.

It is expected that this technique shall be extended to the study of the excitatory process in tissues other than the electric tissue of the eel. Neuroblasts or myoblasts in culture, or suspensions of neurons isolated from brain, might be convenient biological materials for this purpose. The only technical prerequisite is a sufficiently concentrated suspension of membrane fragments consisting of closed vesicles.

We thank Drs. T. Podleski, J. Patrick, P. Ascher, R. Walter, I. Schwartz and R. Olsen for helpful criticism and comments, and Dr. H. Rang for the gift of a sample of DNC 10 M. The research in the Department of Molecular Biology at the Pasteur Institute has been aided by grants from the U.S. National Institutes of Health, the Centre National de la Recherche Scientifique, the Délégation Générale à la Recherche Scientifique et Technique, the Fondation pour la Recherche Médicale Francaise, the Collège de France, and the Commissariat à l'Energie Atomique.

## References

Baker, P. F., Hodgkin, A. L., Shaw, T. I. 1961. Replacement of the protoplasm of a giant nerve fibre with artificial solutions. *Nature* **190**:885.

Bartels, E. 1965. Relationship between acetylcholine and local anesthetics. *Biochim. Biophys. Acta* **109**:194.

Bauman, A., Changeux, J.P., Benda, P. 1969. Purification of membrane fragments derived from the non-excitable surface of the eel electroplax. *F. E. B. S. Letters* **8**:145.

Benda, P., Tsuji, S., Daussent, J., Changeux, J.P. 1969. Localization of acetylcholinesterase by immunofluorescence in eel electroplax. *Nature* **225**:1149.

Brown, W.E., Hill, A.V. 1922—1923. The oxygen dissociation curve of blood and its thermodynamical basis. *Proc. Roy. Soc. (London) B.* **94**:297.

Changeux, J.P. 1966. Response of acetylcholinesterase from *Torpedo marmorata* to salts and curarizing drugs. *Mol. Pharmacol.* **2**:369.

— Gautron, M., Israël, M., Podleski, T.R. 1969. Séparation de membranes excitables à partir de l'organe électrique d'*Electrophorus electricus*. *Compt. Rend. Acad. Sci. (Paris)* **269**:1788 D.

— Kasai, M., Lee, C.Y. 1970. The use of a snake venom toxin to characterize the cholinergic receptor protein. *Proc. Nat. Acad. Sci.* **67**:1241.

— Podleski, T.R. 1968. On the excitability and cooperativity of the electroplax membrane. *Proc. Nat. Acad. Sci.* **59**:944.

— — Kasaï, M., Blumenthal, R. 1970. Some molecular aspects of membrane excitation studied with the eel electroplax. *In:* Excitatory Synaptic Machanisms. P. Andersen and J.K.S. Jansen, editors. p. 123. Universitetsforlaget, Oslo.

— — Wofsy, L. 1967. Affinity labeling of the acetylcholine receptor. *Proc Nat. Acad. Sci.* **58**:2063.

— Thiéry, J., Tung, Y., Kittel, C. 1967. On the cooperativity of biological membranes. *Proc. Nat. Acad. Sci.* **57**:335.

Ellman, G.L., Courtney, K.D., Andress, V., Featherstone, R. 1961. A new rapid colorimetric determination of acetylcholinesterase activity. *Biochem. Pharmacol.* **7**:88.

Fenton, J.W., Singer, S.J. 1965. Affinity labeling of antibodies to the *p*-azophenyltrimethylammonium hapten and a structural relationship among antibody active sites of different specificities. *Biochem. Biophys. Res. Commun.* **20**:315.

Higman, H., Podleski, T.R., Bartels, E. 1969. Apparent dissociation constants between carbamylcholine, *d*-tubocurarine and the receptor. *Biochim. Biophys. Acta* **79**:187.

Hoskin, F. 1966. Anaerobic glycolysis in parts of the giant axon of the squid. *Nature* **210**:856.

Karlin, A., Bartels, E. 1966. Effects of blocking sulfhydryl groups and of reducing disulfide bonds on the acetylcholine-activated permeability system of the electroplax. *Biochim. Biophys. Acta* **126**:525.

— Winnik, M. 1968. Reduction and specific alkylation of the receptor for acetylcholine. *Proc. Nat. Acad. Sci.* **60**:668.

Kasaï, M., Changeux, J.P. 1970. Démonstration de l'excitation par des agonistes cholinergiques à partir de fractions de membranes purifiées, *in vitro*. *Compt. Rend. Acad. Sci. (Paris)* **270**:1400 D.

Keynes, R.D., Martins-Ferreira, H. 1953. Membrane potentials in the electroplates of the electric eel. *J. Physiol.* **119**:315.

Lowry, O.H., Rosebrough, N.J., Farr, A.L., Randall, R.J. 1951. Protein measurement with the Folin phenol reagent. *J. Biol. Chem.* **193**:265.

Mautner, H.G., Bartels, E., Webb, G.D. 1966. Sulfur and selenium isologs related to acetylcholine and choline. IV. Activity in the electroplax preparation. *Biochem. Pharmacol.* **15**:187.

Meunier, J.C., Changeux, J.P. 1969. On the irreversible binding of *p*-(trimethylammonium) benzene diazonium fluoroborate to acetylcholinesterase from electrogenic tissue. *F. E. B. S. Letters* **2**:224.

Nachmansohn, D. 1959. Chemical and Molecular Basis of Nerve Activity. Academic Press, New York and London.

Nachmansohn, D. 1971. Proteins in bioelectricity. Acetylcholine-esterase and -receptor. *In*: Handbook of Sensory Physiology, vol. 1. W. R. Loewenstein, editor. p. 18. Springer-Verlag. Berlin.

Oikawa, T., Spyropoulos, C. S., Tasaki, I., Teorell, T. 1961. Methods for perfusing the giant axon of *Loligo pealii*. *Acta Physiol. Scand.* **52**:195.

Podleski, T. R. 1967. Distinction between the active sites of acetylcholine receptor and acetylcholinesterase. *Proc. Nat. Acad. Sci.* **58**:268.

— Bartels, E. 1963. Difference between tetracaine and *d*-tubocurarine in the competition with carbamylcholine. *Biochim. Biophys. Acta* **75**:387.

— Changeux, J. P. 1969. Effects associated with permeability changes caused by gramicidin A in electroplax membrane. *Nature* **221**:541.

Rang, H. P., Ritter, J. M. 1969. A new kind of drug antagonism; evidence that agonists cause a molecular change in acetylcholine receptors. *Mol. Pharmacol.* **5**:394.

Wofsy, L., Michaeli, D. 1967. Affinity labeling of the anionic site of acetylcholinesterase. *Proc. Nat. Acad. Sci.* **58**:2296.

# AFFINITY LABELING OF THE ACETYLCHOLINE RECEPTOR IN THE ELECTROPLAX: ELECTROPHORETIC SEPARATION IN SODIUM DODECYL SULFATE

*Michael J. Reiter, David A. Cowburn,*
*Joav M. Prives, and Arthur Karlin*

Department of Neurology,
College of Physicians and Surgeons,
Columbia University, New York, N.Y. 10032

*Communicated by S.J. Singer, February 28, 1972*

*Electroplax, single cells dissected from electric tissue of* Electrophorus, *are labeled in a two-step procedure: reduction by dithiothreitol followed by alkylation by the affinity label 4-(N-maleimido)-α-benzyltri[methyl-³H]methylammonium iodide, either alone or in combination with [2,3-¹⁴C]N-ethylmaleimide. Electrophoresis in sodium dodecyl sulfate on polyacrylamide gel of an extract, prepared with this detergent, of single-labeled or of double-labeled cells results in a major peak of ³H activity, with a mobility corresponding to a polypeptide of molecular weight 42,000. In addition, in the double-labeled samples, there is a unique peak in the ratio of ³H to ¹⁴C that is coincident with the ³H peak. The electrophoretic patterns of extracts of cells in which affinity alkylation of the reduced receptor has been suppressed by dithiobischoline, an affinity oxidizing agent, by cobra-toxin, an irreversible ligand, or by hexamethonium, a reversible ligand, show a considerably diminished peak of ³H activity in the region of molecular weight 42,000. This is the predominant difference between the electrophoretic patterns of extracts of unprotected and of protected cells. Furthermore, extracts of cells protected with*

Abbreviations: MBTA, 4-(*N*-maleimido)-α-benzyltrimethylammonium iodide; NEM, *N*-ethylmaleimide; SDS, sodium dodecyl sulfate.

Reprinted from *Proceedings of the National Academy of Sciences* 69: 1168–1172 (1972) by permission of the publisher.

398

*dithiobischoline before labeling with both tritiated affinity label and [¹⁴C] N-ethylmaleimide do not show the peak in the ³H to ¹⁴C ratio seen in the absence of protection. Thus, by several diverse criteria, the peak of ³H activity corresponding to a molecular weight of 42,000 contains affinity-labeled acetylcholine receptor or receptor subunit.*

The receptor for acetylcholine in the electroplax of *Electrophorus electricus* appears from physiological evidence to be reduced *in situ* by dithiothreitol, and a sulfhydryl group thereby formed appears to be subsequently alkylated with considerable specificity by 4-(*N*-maleimido)-α-benzyltrimethylammonium iodide (MBTA) (1). It appears that MBTA alkylates the reduced receptor *in situ* 1000-fold as rapidly as does the neutral *N*-ethylmaleimide (NEM), due to the affinity of the benzyltrimethylammonium moiety for the receptor (1). Corroborating the physiological evidence is the result that the extent of reaction of 4-(*N*-maleimido)-α-benzyltri[methyl - ³H] methylammonium iodide ([³H] MBTA) with the dithiothreitol-reduced electroplax under physiological conditions is decreased either by the application before alkylation by [³H] MBTA of dithiobischoline, an affinity-oxidizing agent of the reduced receptor (2), or by the presence, during the alkylation, of hexamethonium, a reversible ligand of the receptor (3–5). These decrements in the extent of the labeling reaction approach asymptotic limits with increasing concentrations of [³H] MBTA, and the quantity of receptor in the electroplax has been estimated from these limits (4, 5). Comparison of the extent of labeling of the protectible SH-groups (presumably receptor) and of non-protectible SH-groups corroborates the inferred 1000-fold greater rate of reaction of MBTA with receptor SH-groups; the 10–20% overall specificity of the labeling results from the about 10⁴-fold greater quantity of available nonreceptor SH-groups (5).

The present work suggests that a single polypeptide component of the electroplax has the properties previously inferred for the receptor; i.e. after reduction, its rate of reaction with MBTA compared with NEM is enhanced, and it is protected by dithiobischoline and by hexamethonium against alkylation by MBTA. In addition, a third protecting agent, cobratoxin, has been introduced. This polypeptide component of the venom of *Naja naja siamensis* is structurally very similar to the neurotoxins from other elapid snakes. Such neurotoxins appear from physiological evidence to block irreversibly the acetylcholine receptor in vertebrate neuromuscular junctions and electroplax synapses (6–8; and manuscript in preparation). Cobratoxin appears to block the labeling by [³H]MBTA of the same component as does dithiobischoline and hexamethonium.

## MATERIALS AND METHODS

*Labeling.* Single cells (electroplax) dissected from the organ of Sachs of *Electrophorus electricus* were labeled (5) with [methyl-$^3$H] MBTA (2 Ci/mmol). In each experiment, two groups of about 15 cells each were treated in parallel. One group was labeled without protection (*A*) and one group was labeled with protection (*B, C,* or *D*) as follows: both groups were treated with 0.2 mM dithiothreitol in a Tris-Ringer's solution [165 mM NaCl, 5 mM KCl, 2 mM CaCl$_2$, 2 mM MgCl$_2$, 2 mM Tris (pH 8.0)] for 10 min, then washed for 10 min in a phosphate-Ringer's solution [as above, except 1.5 mM phosphate (pH 7.1) replaces Tris] containing 10 mM glucose (RG buffer); thereafter, one group was treated according to Procedure *A* and one according to *B, C,* or *D:*

(*A*)  RG buffer (20 min); 12 nM [$^3$H] MBTA (10 min);

(*B*)  RG buffer (5 min); 0.5 $\mu$M dithiobischoline (5 min); RG buffer (10 min); 12 nM [$^3$H] MBTA (10 min);

(*C*)  RG buffer (15 min); 1 mM hexamethonium (5 min); 12 nM [$^3$H] MBTA in 1 mM hexamethonium (10 min);

(*D*)  0.28 $\mu$M cobratoxin (10 min); RG buffer (10 min); 12 nM [$^3$H] MBTA (10 min).

Finally, both groups were washed for 25 min with five changes of RG buffer, blotted, and weighed. All solutions other than dithiothreitol were made up in phosphate—Ringer's solution (pH 7.1). Purified cobratoxin from *Naja naja siamensis* was a gift from Drs. D. Cooper and E. Reich. Groups of cells were double-labeled in parallel according to schemes *A* and *B*, except that alkylation was by a mixture of 12 nM [$^3$H] MBTA and 9.6 $\mu$M [2,3-$^{14}$C] NEM (2 Ci/mol).

*Extraction of Single-Labeled Cells.* To each group of blotted, single-labeled cells, an equal volume of 2% sodium dodecyl sulfate (SDS)—10 mM dithiothreitol—20 mM Tris-acetate (pH 8.0) was added. This mixture was then kept at 50° for 2 hr and centrifuged; the supernatant was removed for counting and electrophoresis.

*Fractionation and Extraction of Double-Labeled Cells.* About 1 g each of double-labeled cells from procedures *A* and *B* were treated in parallel as follows: the cells were dispersed with a Ten Broeck tissue grinder in Ringer's solution (pH 7.1) (final volume 8 ml); the homogenate was sedimented in a Spinco 65 rotor for 15 min at 50,000 rpm (4°).

The pellet was suspended in 8 ml of 1 mM sodium-EDTA (pH 7.2) and sedimented as before. The pellet was then suspended in 1 ml of 1% SDS–5 mM dithiothreitol–10 mM Tris-acetate (pH 8.0), maintained at 50° for 2 hr with frequent mixing, and sedimentated at 30,000 rpm for 15 min (20°). Samples of the supernatant were electrophoresed.

*Polyacrylamide Gel Electrophoresis.* Gels were prepared in 1% SDS–100 mM Tris-acetate (9), and were run for 1 hr with the buffer containing 1% SDS–2 mM DTT–100 mM Tris-acetate (pH 8.0) before use for an analysis. Typically, 0.2 ml of extract, to which sucrose and bromphenol blue had been added, was layered on the gels, which were then run at a constant current of 3 mA/tube until the bromphenol blue front had migrated to within 1–2 cm of the end of the gel. Duplicate or triplicate gels were run for each extract. After removal from the tubes, gels were fractionated according to the technique of Maizel (10).

Molecular weight standards were prepared by treatment of bovine serum albumin (Sigma Chemical Co.), ovalbumin (Sigma Chemical Co.), and cytochrome *c* (Boehringer-Mannheim) with [$^{14}$C] dimethylsulfate (40–58 Ci/mol) (11). The labeled and unlabeled proteins had indistinguishable electrophoretic mobilities in SDS.

*Counting.* The gel fractions were dried at 50°, then digested in 0.2 ml of water and 1 ml of NCS (Amersham/Searle) at 50° for 2 hr. Aliquots of extracts were similarly made up to 0.2 ml with water, 1 ml of NCS was added, and the resulting solutions were digested at 50° for 2 hr. 10 ml of PPO–dimethyl POPOP–toluene were added, and all vials were counted in a Packard scintillation spectrometer for 20 min. Counting efficiencies were 20% for $^{3}$H alone, and 17 and 46% for $^{3}$H and $^{14}$C together. The single-label and double-label counting data were processed by a computer program similar to that described in ref. 12.

## RESULTS

### Single-labeled cells

Electrophoresis of the SDS extract of electroplax labeled without protection according to procedure *A* results in a major peak of $^{3}$H activity that is considerably diminished in extracts of electroplax labeled with protection according to procedures *B, C,* and *D* (Fig. 1). Similar results are obtained on 5% (Fig. 2) and on 7.5% acrylamide

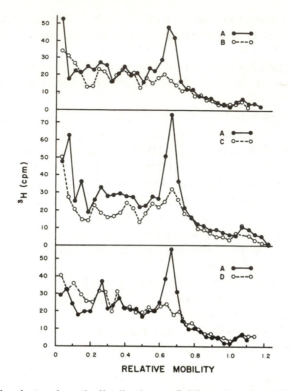

Fig. 1. The electrophoretic distribution on 7.5% acrylamide gel, in 1% SDS, of [³H] activity in extracts of [³H] MBTA-labeled electroplax. Typical parallel gels from three experiments are shown. In each experiment, one group of electroplax cells was labeled (see *Methods*) according to procedure $A$ (dithiothreitol, [³H] - MBTA) and one group according to either procedure $B$ (dithiothreitol, dithiobis-choline, [³H] MBTA), $C$ (dithiothreitol, hexamethonium, [³H] MBTA in hexa-methonium), or $D$ (dithiothreitol, cobratoxin, [³H] MBTA). The labeled electro-plax were extracted in SDS–dithiothreitol–Tris-acetate solution and 200-$\mu$l samples of the extracts, containing about 500 $\mu$g of protein and 1200 net cpm, were layered over 12 × 0.6-cm gels. Mobility is calculated relative to that of the bromphenol blue front.

gels (Fig. 1). The predominant difference between the electrophoretic distributions of the extracts of unprotected ($A$) and of protected ($B$, $C$, and $D$) cells is in the region of the major peak, as shown by the average differences between distributions of percent of total ³H activity per vial (Fig. 3). In extracts of cells protected with hexa-methonium ($C$) and with cobratoxin ($D$) there are, in addition, dif-ferences at the top of the gels, where the percent ³H activity in $A$ is greater than in $C$, and less than in $D$.

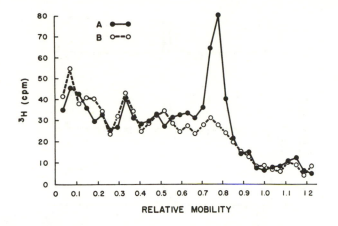

Fig. 2. The electrophoretic distributions on 5% acrylamide gel in 1% SDS of $^3$H activity in extracts of electroplax labeled with [$^3$H]MBTA according to procedures *A* and *B*. Details as in Fig. 1.

The SDS extracts contain 80% of the total radioactivity of the cells. The difference in radioactivity between the extracts of unprotected and protected cells accounts for 90% of the total differences between the two groups of cells. The average recovery of radioactivity on the gels is 90 ± 10%.

## Double-labeled cells

From previous work, it was expected that NEM would have no specificity for receptor SH-groups (1) and would serve as a general label for cellular SH-groups. In addition, if dithiobischoline specifically reoxidizes the SH-groups of the reduced receptor (2, 5), then this agent should have an insignificant effect on the labeling of SH-groups by [$^{14}$C]NEM, since only a small fraction of the total available SH-groups are receptor SH-groups (5). In fact, cells labeled by procedure *A* and by procedure *B* with a mixture of 12 nM [$^3$H]MBTA and 9.6 $\mu$M [$^{14}$C]NEM differ by 13 ± 4% ($n$ = 6) in $^3$H activity, not an appreciably different result than that obtained with [$^3$H]MBTA alone. (The extents of reaction in *A* are 1.4 × 10$^{-14}$ mol of [$^3$H]MBTA/mg of cells and 1.7 × 10$^{-11}$ mol of [$^{14}$C]NEM/mg of cells.) Dithiobischoline has no significant effect on the labeling by [$^{14}$C]NEM, and the presence of [$^{14}$C]NEM has no effect on the depression by dithiobischoline of the labeling by [$^3$H]MBTA. After disruption of double-labeled cells in Ringer's solution, about 80% of the $^3$H activity is sedimentable, whereas about 80% of the $^{14}$C activity is soluble. Sus-

403

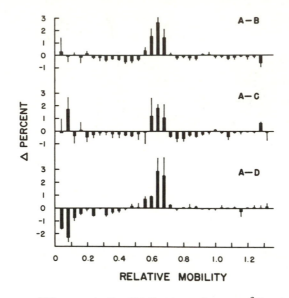

Fig. 3. Average differences in the distributions of percent $^3$H activity between gels from extracts produced by procedure $A$ and by procedures $B, C,$ and $D$. All experiments in which gels from procedure $A$ and $B$ $(n = 12)$, $C$ $(n = 4)$, or $D$ $(n = 5)$ (7.5% acrylamide) were run in parallel are included. In the original data, the number of fractions to the bromphenol blue front ranged from 24 to 29. For the purposes of averaging the distributions, a new distribution was calculated for each gel by interpolation; the radioactivity was partitioned into fractions that each corresponded to a mobility range of 0.04; i.e. the front in the new distribution is in fraction number 25. For each experiment, the calculated distributions of radioactivity of replicate gels were then summed fraction by fraction, and the sums were divided by the overall total radioactivity to yield the average distribution of percent of total radioactivity. The fraction by fraction differences between the average distribution by procedure $A$ and the average distribution by procedures $B, C,$ and $D$ were calculated for each experiment. These differences were then averaged over comparable experiments. The mean difference and standard error of the mean or range are presented. The sum of the differences $(100 - 100\%)$ is zero.

pension of the particulate fraction in 1 mM EDTA solubilizes an additional 1% of the $^3$H activity and 2% of the $^{14}$C activity. Finally, 80% of the $^3$H activity and 75% of the $^{14}$C activity sedimentable after EDTA treatment are solubilized by 1% SDS. This extract is enriched about 4-fold with respect to $^3$H to $^{14}$C ratio over whole cells.

The gel-electrophoretic distribution of $^3$H activity of the SDS extract of the particulate fraction of unprotected double-labeled cells $(A)$ shows a major peak at the same position as in comparable single-labeled gels, and this peak is considerably diminished in the

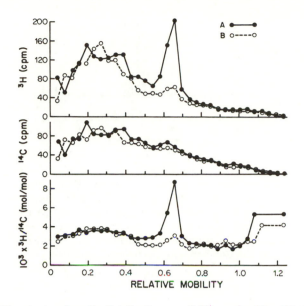

Fig. 4. The electrophoretic distributions on 7.5% acrylamide gel in SDS of
[3H] activity, [14C] activity, and [3H] to [14C] ratio in extracts of electroplax labeled with
[3H]MBTA and [14C]NEM according to procedures A and B. Electroplax
labeled with (B) and without (A) protection by dithiobischoline (see *Methods*)
were homogenized in Ringer's solution, and a particulate fraction was prepared.
The particulate fraction was extracted with SDS–dithiothreitol–Tris-acetate
solution, and 200-$\mu$l samples of the extract, containing about 250 $\mu$g of protein,
2400 net cpm of [3H], and 1800 net cpm of [14C], were layered over 12 × 0.6-cm
gels. The distributions of typical gels run in parallel are shown. The statistical
counting error at the end of the gel, where there are few counts, is relatively
large, and where the coefficient of variance of the [3H] to [14C] ratio exceeded 20%,
the counts of successive fractions were combined for the calculation of the
ratio (compare ref. 12). This combination step was only necessary in the last
few fractions of the gels. The coefficient of variance of the ratio at the peak is
5% in procedure A and 7% in procedure B.

extract of the particulate fraction of protected cells (B) (Fig. 4).
Insignificant differences are seen in the distributions of [14C] activity.
There is only one significant peak in the ratio of [3H] to [14C]. It is coincident with the [3H] peak, and is virtually eliminated by dithiobischoline. An elevation in [3H] to [14C] ratio seen just past the bromphenol
blue front is associated with less than 1% of the total [3H] activity,
and may be due to hydrolysis of reacted [3H]MBTA. The average differences in the distributions of [3H] to [14C] suggest that the only significant effect of dithiobischoline is to eliminate the preferential labeling
by [3H]MBTA of a component in the major peak (Fig. 5).

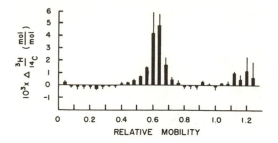

Fig. 5. Average differences in the $^3$H to $^{14}$C ratio on double-labeled gels from extracts prepared by procedures $A$ and $B$. The $^3$H and $^{14}$C distributions of all gels such as those in Fig. 4 were partitioned as in Fig. 3. Within an experiment the new distributions of the replicate gels were averaged, and the average $^3$H to $^{14}$C ratios and the differences in the ratios between procedures $A$ and $B$ were calculated. These differences were then averaged over three comparable experiments. The mean and the standard error of the mean is presented.

### Molecular weight

For a given concentration of acrylamide, there is, over a wide range, a linear relationship between log of molecular weight and electrophoretic mobility of many reduced proteins in SDS-containing buffers (13, 14). The mobility of the major $^3$H peak relative to that of bromphenol blue is compared to the mobilities of $^{14}$C-labeled molecular weight standards treated similarly to the extracts and coelectrophoresed on 5, 7.5, and 10% acrylamide gels (Fig. 6). Assuming that the components of the peak are reduced polypeptides saturated with SDS (15), we obtain molecular weight estimates, respectively, of 39,900, 42,500, and 43,300, with a mean of 42,000, for the three concentrations of acrylamide.

### DISCUSSION

The labeling of the electroplax by [$^3$H]MBTA has been analyzed by polyacrylamide gel electrophoresis in SDS, a technique that separates proteins into molecular weight classes. A major peak of $^3$H activity, with a mobility corresponding to a polypeptide of molecular weight 42,000, is found in the electrophoretic distribution of the SDS extract of [$^3$H]MBTA-labeled electroplax. The activity found in this peak region is depressed in extracts of electroplax labeled after protection with three diverse agents (Figs. 1, 2, and 3). Two of these, dithio-

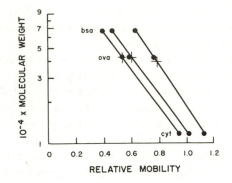

Fig. 6. Molecular weight estimation of the major peak (+). Electroplax labeled with [³H]MBTA according to procedure *A* were extracted with SDS–dithiothreitol–Tris-acetate solution, and the extract was coelectrophoresed with ¹⁴C-labeled bovine serum albumin (*bsa*), ovalbumin (*ova*), and cytochrome *c* (*cyt*), treated similarly. Mobility is given relative to that of bromphenol blue. From left to right, the acrylamide concentrations are 10, 7.5, and 5%.

bischoline (2, 5) and cobratoxin (ref. 8 and unpublished results), are applied at the low concentrations at which they are physiologically effective, and probably highly specific for the receptor. The third agent, hexamethonium, is applied at the relatively high concentration required for this reversible ligand to retard the irreversible reaction of [³H]MBTA with the receptor, and is probably less specific in its interactions (5). The differences between procedure *A* and *C* at the top of the gels (Fig. 3) may be due to the protection by hexamethonium of some high-molecular-weight nonreceptor proteins, a possibility also suggested by the higher than expected overall protection against labeling afforded by hexamethonium (5). The difference in the same region, but in the opposite direction, between gels of extracts treated by procedures *A* and *D* (Fig. 3) may be due to the facilitation by cobratoxin of the reaction of [³H]MBTA with some high molecular weight components, or to the prevention by cobratoxin of the dissociation of labeled receptor in SDS. Notwithstanding the possibly incomplete specificity of the protecting agents, the predominant and overlapping effect of dithiobischoline, hexamethonium, and cobratoxin is on a component of the major peak. Furthermore, a component of the major peak is preferentially labeled with the affinity-alkylating agent [³H]MBTA relative to the non-affinity-alkylating agent [¹⁴C]NEM, and this preferential labeling is uniquely eliminated by application before labeling of dithiobischoline (Fig. 4 and 5). Significant preferential labeling is found only in the major peak area. By several different criteria, therefore, a component of the major peak is affinity-labeled receptor or receptor subunit.

The polypeptide nature of this labeled component is supported by the consistency of the molecular weight estimates obtained at three different gel concentrations when colinearity with protein standards is assumed (13–15, and compare ref. 16). The chemistry of the labeling process suggests that a disulfide is being reduced and alkylated, and the physiological effects of the reduction and of several affinity reactions suggest that the disulfide is about 1 nm from the negative subsite of the acetylcholine-binding site of the receptor (1, 4, 5). Thus, it is likely that the specifically labeled polypeptide component is either the receptor or a receptor subunit containing all or part of the acetylcholine-binding site.

The portion of the radioactivity of the major peak that is due to labeled receptor can be estimated from the distributions expressed in percent of total activity, to minimize differences in loading and in recovery. If we assume that all labeled receptor in gels from extracts prepared by procedure $A$ is in the major peak, that gels of extracts prepared by procedure $B$ contain no labeled receptor, and that the distributions of labeled nonreceptor components are equivalent in extracts prepared by procedures $A$ and $B$, then the fraction of radioactivity in the peak from an extract labeled by procedure $A$ that is labeled receptor is given by $(a - b)/a(1 - b)$, where $a$ and $b$ are the fraction of the total $^3H$ activity in the peak region in parallel gels from extracts prepared by procedures $A$ and $B$, respectively. The three vials that contained the maximal counts in the peak from procedure $A$ contain $17.2 \pm 0.6\%$ ($n = 15$) of the total recovered activity in procedure $A$, and the three corresponding vials in procedure $B$ contain $11.1 \pm 0.3\%$ ($n = 15$) of the total recovered activity in procedure $B$. The average fraction of $^3H$ activity in the procedure $A$ peak (3 vials) due to labeled receptor is $40 \pm 3\%$.

The results of the fractionation of double-labeled cells support the expectation that $[^3H]MBTA$, being positively charged, penetrates the cell membrane relatively slowly, reacting predominantly with externally accessible components, whereas $[^{14}C]NEM$ penetrates rapidly, reacting with both external and internal components. The $[^{14}C]NEM$-labeled components of the total particulate fraction are likely to be representative of the membrane proteins of the cell capable of reacting with maleimide. The receptor accounts for a small fraction of the total of such proteins migrating to the region of the major peak. On the assumption that, except for the contribution of the receptor on gels from extracts prepared by procedure $A$, the distribution of the $^3H$ to $^{14}C$ ratio is equivalent on gels prepared by procedures $A$ and $B$ (see Fig. 5), the ratio of $^3H$-labeled receptor to $^{14}$C-labeled protein in the peak is given by the $^{3}$H to $^{14}$C ratio in the peak from procedure $A$ minus the $^{3}$H to $^{14}$C ratio in the corresponding region in the peak from procedure $B$. For the peak vial, the average difference is $6.1(\pm 1.6) \times 10^{-3}$ mol of [$^{3}$H] receptor/mol of [$^{14}$C] protein. (The peak difference seen in Fig. 5 is slightly less due to the peak-broadening effect of the averaging of distributions.) The overall purification of [$^{3}$H] receptor relative to [$^{14}$C] protein can be estimated from the differences in the $^{3}$H to $^{14}$C ratio from procedures $A$ and $B$ at the different stages: $0.1 \times 10^{-3}$ for whole cells; $0.4 \times 10^{-3}$ for the SDS extract of the particulate fraction; and $6 \times 10^{-3}$ mol of $^{3}$H/mol of $^{14}$C for the peak vial. Therefore, the purifications achieved are 4-fold by fractionation of the cells, 15-fold by gel electrophoresis, and 60-fold overall.

Others have identified the receptor as a component that tightly binds elapid snake neurotoxins similar to cobratoxin (17, 18). A component to which $\alpha$-bungarotoxin is tightly bound has been extracted from the electric tissue of *Torpedo* with Triton X-100. In SDS, two components, which have approximate molecular weights as determined by gel filtration of 88,000 and of 180,000 (17), bind the toxin. A component to which the $\alpha$-toxin of *Naja nigricollis* is tightly bound has been solubilized from the electric tissue of *Electrophorus* with deoxycholate, and is said to have a molecular weight of about 50,000 by SDS–gel electrophoresis (18). The latter molecular weight estimate is close to ours after the molecular weight of one toxin molecule [6800 (19)], presumably still bound, is subtracted. As previously noted, a molecular weight of about 40,000 for the receptor protomer is consistent with its occupancy of 5% of the subaxonal membrane area in the electroplax (5).

We are indebted to Mrs. Clara Silaghy for expert technical assistance and to Drs. D. Cooper and E. Reich for purified cobratoxin. This research was supported in part by U.S. Public Health Service Grant NS 07065, by National Science Foundation Grant GB 15906, and by a gift from the New York Heart Association, Inc. A.K. is a Career Scientist of the Health Research Council of the City of New York. M.R. and D.A.C., in part, were supported by USPHS training grant MH 10315.

# REFERENCES

1. Karlin, A. (1969) *J. Gen. Physiol.* 54, 245s–264s.
2. Bartels, E., Deal, W., Karlin, A., & Mautner, H. (1970) *Biochim. Biophys. Acta* 203, 568–571.

3. Karlin, A. & Winnik, M. (1968) *Proc. Nat. Acad. Sci. USA* 60, 668–674.
4. Karlin, A., Prives, J., Deal, W. & Winnik, M. (1970) in *Ciba Foundation Symposium on Molecular Properties of Drug Receptors*, eds. Porter, R., & O'Connor, M., (J. & A. Churchill, London), pp. 247–261.
5. Karlin, A., Prives, J., Deal, W. & Winnik, M. (1971) *J. Mol. Biol.* 61, 175–188.
6. Lee, C.Y. (1970) *Clin. Toxicol.* 3, 457–472.
7. Changeux, J.-P., Kasai, M. & Lee, C.Y. (1970) *Proc. Nat. Acad. Sci. USA* 67, 1241–1247.
8. Lester, H.A. (1971) *J. Gen. Physiol.* 57, 255.
9. Shapiro, A.L., Vinuela, E. & Maizel, J.V., Jr. (1967) *Biochem. Biophys. Res. Commun.* 28, 815–820.
10. Maizel, J.V., Jr. (1966) *Science* 151, 988–990.
11. Kiehn, E.D. & Holland, J.J. (1970) *Biochemistry* 9, 1716–1728.
12. Yund, M.A., Yund, E.W. & Kafatos, F. (1971) *Biochem. Biophys. Res. Commun.* 43, 717–722.
13. Weber, K. & Osborn, M. (1969) *J. Biol. Chem.* 244, 4406–4412.
14. Chrambach, A. & Rodbard, D. (1971) *Science* 172, 440–451.
15. Reynolds, J.A. & Tanford, C. (1970) *J. Biol. Chem.* 245, 5161–5165.
16. Bretscher, M.S. (1971) *Nature New Biol.* 231, 229–232.
17. Miledi, R., Molinoff, P. & Potter, L.T. (1971) *Nature* 229, 554–557.
18. Meunier, J.-C., Olsen, R., Menez, A., Morgat, J.-L., Fromageot, P., Ronseray, A.-M., Boquet, P. & Changeux, J.-P. *C.R. Acad. Sci.* 273D, 595–598.
19. Karlsson, E., Eaker, D.L. & Porath, J. (1966) *Biochim. Biophys. Acta* 127, 505–520.

*Chapter 8*
# AXONAL TRANSPORT

Most neurons are highly asymmetric cells, whose axons may extend up to a meter or more from the cell body. Owing to this characteristic neuronal geometry, the volume of the cytoplasm in the axon and terminal arborizations may be orders of magnitude greater than that in the cell body. No extramitochondrial protein synthesis is known to occur in these extremities; proteins for production and maintenance of this large volume of cytoplasm derive almost entirely from the cell body. The early observation that neuronal perikarya, like secretory cells, contain profuse rough endoplasmic reticulum is now understood. The cell body must synthesize and export proteins for a large and extended volume of cytoplasm. Indeed, in a sense neuronal cell bodies can be regarded as carrying on an intracellular secretory function in supplying the axon and terminal extremities with essential cellular components.

Experimental evidence for such a process originated with the classical experiments of Paul Weiss and his coworkers. A portion of his 1948 paper with H. Hiscoe is reprinted here. The object of their experiments was to determine whether neuronal processes grow only from the cell body, or along their entire length, using nutrients and substrates supplied locally. The experimental design was simple: if growth proceeds from the cell bodies, then ligation of the axons should interrupt the transport of growth-supporting material from somata. Several days after ligation, the nerves became enormously distended proximally to the ligation and greatly narrowed distally. Weiss and Hiscoe interpreted these changes as resulting from interruption, by the ligature, of a normal physiological process: the proximodistal flow of axoplasm from the cell bodies to the terminals of the neurons. Upon removal of the ligature, the dammed-up axoplasm was liberated, and movement of material along the axon resumed at a rate of about one to two mm per day. This was taken to be the normal rate of axonal flow.

In subsequent years debate persisted on whether the damming and subsequent recession represented a normal physiological movement of material or some unnatural axonal response to injury. With the advent of ratioisotopic techniques, investigators re-examined the question of axonal flow by measuring the movement of radioactive tracers from cell bodies down axons. A most conclusive demonstration of this was reported by B. Droz and C. LeBlond (1963, reprinted here). Animals were given a single injection of à radioactive amino acid and, at various times thereafter, nervous tissue was removed, and the disposition of labeled proteins in spinal motor neurons was examined by autoradiography. Shortly after the injection, all the isotope was found in cell bodies; at longer intervals, the radioactivity decreased in the cell bodies and began to appear in the initial portions of the axons and, later still, in the axon proper. The approximate rate of movement agreed with the rate found by Weiss and Hiscoe. One of the important observations made by Droz and LeBlond was that the radioisotope moves in the axon as a discrete peak, a finding that eliminated diffusion as a mechanism for axonal transport.

The basic experiment of Droz and LeBlond has been refined and applied to a number of different systems by other workers. An important modification has been the labeling of limited populations of neurons by micro-injection of radioactive precursors close to their cell bodies. This allows both a more selective localization of labeled cells and a considerably greater cellular uptake of isotope than were achieved with the intraperitoneal injections used by Droz and LeBlond. These more recent studies have shown that in addition to the slow rate of movement of materials down axons (one to two mm per day), fast rates exist, ranging from 50 to 2000 mm per day. Furthermore, materials also move in a retrograde (nerve terminal to cell body) direction. Several laboratories are actively investigating the kinds of materials moved by neurons at the different rates in the two directions. The only well-characterized protein that has been shown to move at the slower rate is tubulin, the subunit of microtubules.

At what rate do the components necessary for transmitter synthesis, packaging, and release move down axons? This question has been explored particularly with noradrenergic neurons. The sequence of synthetic and degradative enzymes in the catecholamine pathway is described in Chapter 3. Because the packaging of the transmitter, norepinephrine, involves at least one of these enzymes, dopamine $\beta$-hydroxylase, as well as other soluble proteins known as the chromogranins, we can examine the rate of movement of granule components down axons and compare their transport with that of various enzymes not associated with granules. Early work by A. Dahlström demonstrated that ligation of noradrenergic nerves caused accumulation, on the proximal side of the ligation, of material exhibiting the specific histochemical fluorescence of catecholamines. Treatment with reserpine reduced the amount of catecholamine that accumulated, suggesting that it may be present in vesicles. Further confirmation that particles containing norepinephrine may be transported comes from electron microscopic studies showing large numbers of dense-cored vesicles on the proximal side of the ligation.

A direct demonstration of norepinephrine transport in neurons was described by B. Livett, L. Geffen, and L. Austin (1968, reprinted here), who injected [$^{14}$C] norepinephrine into a sympathetic ganglion and observed movement of isotope as a discrete peak down the axon. The rate of movement, found by this and other methods, is about 50 to 120 mm per day. Very recently, tyrosine hydroxylase, DOPA decarboxylase, and dopamine β-hydroxylase have also been found to move down axons rapidly (Jarrott and Geffen, 1972; Dairman, Geffen, and Marchelle, 1973). The rate of movement of tyrosine hydroxylase and DOPA decarboxylase was only about one-third that of the presumed vesicle constituents, dopamine β-hydroxylase and norepinephrine. The mitochondrial enzyme monoamine oxidase and several other intracellular enzyme markers did not move at a fast rate. One obvious explanation is that the catecholamine-synthesizing enzymes and vesicle contents move down axons at a rapid rate in several different units, at least one of which may be associated with the large dense-cored granules seen in these axons.

Transport of ACh has been demonstrated by the elegant experiments of H. Koike, M. Eisenstadt, and J. Schwartz (1972), who injected radioactive choline into the cell bodies of single cholinergic and non-cholinergic *Aplysia* neurons. In the cholinergic neurons, radioactive ACh was rapidly formed and was transported down the axons at a rate of approximately 17 mm per day. About half of the ACh in the axons was associated with sedimentable particles, perhaps corresponding to synaptic vesicles. In mammals, ligation experiments have shown that acetylcholinesterase is rapidly transported down axons (Jarrott and Geffen, 1972).

Besides the particles containing transmitters, other cellular organelles move along axons. Time-lapse movies of neurons in cell culture clearly demonstrate the bidirectional movement of mitochondria within axons. This process was systematically investigated by P. Banks, D. Mangnall, and D. Mayor (1969), who ligated nerves at two points and, after several days, assayed for the mitochondrial enzyme, cyto-

413

chrome oxidase. In contrast to norepinephrine, which accumulates only on the proximal side of a constriction, the distribution of cyto-chrome oxidase indicated an accumulation of mitochondria on both sides of the two constrictions, a finding that was confirmed by elec-tron microscopic observations. These experiments supported the earlier visual observation that mitochondria move in both directions. The rate of mitochondrial flux was estimated to be about 15 mm per day. This rapid movement of mitochondria appears to conflict with the slow transport of the mitochondrial enzyme, monoamine oxidase, mentioned above. No explanation for the difference in transport velocities has been provided.

There are retrograde movements of other substances along axons. Acetylcholinesterase accumulates distally to a ligation, as well as proximally. Moreover, when nerve terminals are selectively exposed to peroxidase or labeled proteins, these substances later appear in the corresponding cell bodies (LaVail and LaVail, 1972). How these proteins are taken up, and whether their translocation occurs by diffusion or by a specific transport mechanism, are not yet known.

Thus materials move through axons both centrifugally and centri-petally at varying velocities. Only preliminary clues are at hand regarding the mechanism by which any of these transport processes operates, or concerning the fate of various substances that reach axonal terminals. S. Ochs (1972) showed that the mechanism for fast transport is present entirely within axons, and that the cell soma is not necessary. Furthermore, his studies indicated that an energy supply and oxidative metabolism are essential for fast transport.

A number of studies support the increasingly attractive hypothesis that microtubules play an important role in fast axonal transport. P. Banks, *et al.* (1971, reprinted here), showed that in axons incu-bated *in vitro,* the movement of norepinephrine is blocked by the drugs colchicine and vinblastine, which disrupt axonal microtubules, leaving the movement of mitochondria unaffected. In one case, U. Jarlfors and D. S. Smith (1969) observed a very close physical associa-tion between vesicles and microtubules in electron micrographs of the lamprey nervous system. The involvement of microtubules in other intracellular movements, such as those of mitosis, adds plausibility to the idea of participation of microtubules in axonal transport. Other cellular organelles might also play a role in intracellular movement of material. For example, the smooth-surfaced endoplasmic reticulum seen in axons and nerve terminals is thought to communicate with membrane systems in the cell body. The lumen of the reticulum might be a special channel for movement of certain materials between cell body and terminals.

We can say even less about the fate of transported material at neuronal terminals. Evidence exists that certain proteins (those associated with granules) are released and can be collected in fluids perfusing tissues. Other proteins are degraded at terminals, while some may be returned to the cell soma. A particularly interesting possibility is that specific substances could be released by neurons and selectively taken up by cells with which they form synapses. For example, B. Grafstein (1971) has injected tritiated amino acids into one mouse eye and demonstrated isotopic transport both to the lateral geniculate and to the corresponding visual cortex. She interpreted her findings to mean that labeled material was released from optic axonal terminals, taken up by geniculate neurons, and then transported through their axons to the striate cortex. While the accuracy of this interpretation and the generality of its implications remain uncertain, the results suggest the important possibility that cells communicate with each other at the level of selective transynaptic exchange of proteins.

Despite many unanswered questions about axonal transport, it is clear that neurons have mechanisms for movement of molecules back and forth between cell soma and axonal terminals. The vigorous efforts now under way to elucidate the mechanisms and functions of axonal transport processes should soon lead to better understanding of the types of information exchanged between different parts of the same cell.

## READING LIST

*Reprinted Papers*

1. Weiss, P. and H.B. Hiscoe (1948). Experiments on the mechanism of nerve growth. *J. Exp. Zool.* 107: 315–396 (only pp. 315–329 plus references are included here).
2. Droz, B. and C.P. LeBlond (1963). Axonal migration of proteins in the central nervous system and peripheral nerves as shown by autoradiography. *J. Comp. Neurol.* 121: 325–346.
3. Livett, B.G., L.B. Geffen, and L. Austin (1968). Proximo-distal transport of [14C] noradrenaline and protein in sympathetic nerves. *J. Neurochem.* 15: 931–939.
4. Banks, P., D. Mayer, M. Mitchell, and D. Tomlinson (1971). Studies on the translocation of noradrenaline-containing vesicles in postganglionic sympathetic neurones *in vitro.* Inhibition of movement by colchicine and vinblastine and evidence for the involvement of axonal microtubules. *J. Physiol.* 216: 625–639.

*Other Selected Papers*

5. Kapeller, K. and D. Mayor (1967). The accumulation of nor-adrenaline in constricted sympathetic nerves as studied by fluorescence and electron microscopy. *Proc. Roy. Soc. B.* 167: 282–292.

6. Banks, P., D. Mangnall, and D. Mayor (1969). The redistribution of cytochrome oxidase, noradrenaline and ATP in adrenergic nerves constricted at two points. *J. Physiol.* 200: 745–762.

7. Jarlfors, U. and D.S. Smith (1969). Association between synaptic vesicles and neurotubules. *Nature* 224: 710–711.

8. Geffen, L.B. and B.G. Livett (1971). Synaptic vesicles in sympathetic neurons. *Physiol. Rev.* 51: 98–157.

9. Grafstein, B. (1971). Transneuronal transfer of radioactivity in the central nervous system. *Science* 172: 177–179.

10. Karlsson, J.O. and J. Sjöstrand (1971). Transport of microtubular protein in axons of retinal ganglion cells. *J. Neurochem.* 18: 975–982.

11. Jarrott, B. and L.B. Geffen (1972). Rapid axoplasmic transport of tyrosine hydroxylase in relation to other cytoplasmic constituents. *Proc. Nat. Acad. Sci.* 69: 3440–3442.

12. Koike, H., M. Eisenstadt, and J.H. Schwartz (1972). Axonal transport of newly synthesized acetylcholine in an identified neuron of *Aplysia. Brain Res.* 37: 152–159.

13. LaVail, J.H. and M.M. LaVail (1972). Retrograde axonal transport in the central nervous system. *Science* 176: 1416–1417.

14. Ochs, S. (1972). Fast transport of materials in mammalian nerve fibers. *Science* 176: 252–260.

15. Dairman, W., L. Geffen, and M. Marchelle (1973). Axoplasmic transport of aromatic L-amino acid decarboxylase (EC 4.1.1. 26) and dopamine $\beta$-hydroxylase (EC 1.14.2.1) in rat sciatic nerve. *J. Neurochem.* 20: 1617–1623.

# EXPERIMENTS ON THE MECHANISM
# OF NERVE GROWTH [1]

PAUL WEISS AND HELEN B. HISCOE

*Department of Zoology, University of Chicago, Illinois*

TWENTY-NINE FIGURES

## INTRODUCTION

The extreme elongation of its cytoplasm makes the neuron uniquely suited for the study of the relative roles of nucleus and cytoplasm in cell growth. For the last 6 years, one of the authors (P. W.) has carried on research on this problem with results that have shed new light on protoplasm synthesis in general. Cursory reference to these results was made on previous occasions (Weiss, '43b, p. 19; Weiss and Davis, '43, p. 277; Weiss, '44a, '44b, '47), but a full account has been purposely held up pending the conclusion of additional experimental tests. These have now been completed, but at the same time, the volume of significant data has grown to such proportions as to call for monographic treatment. Since the prospects for such a monograph are still rather indefinite, it seemed desirable to present at least a condensed record of the main results with illustrative examples. This summary account is given in the present paper.

The volume of an axon may be many hundred times that of the cell body (perikaryon) containing the nucleus. How this comparatively enormous mass can be maintained in the adult nerve fiber, and restored in the regenerating nerve fiber, is a basic problem of growth. The axon is enveloped by sheath cells over its full length and is in active exchange with sur-

[1] This work was aided by the Dr. Wallace C. and Clara A. Abbott Memorial Fund of The University of Chicago and by a grant from the United States Public Health Service.

Reprinted from the *Journal of Experimental Zoology* 107: 315–329 and refs. 392–395 (1948) by permission of the publisher.

rounding blood and endoneurial fluid. The general notion is that the axon thus draws from its environment nutrients, which, in the presence of certain undefined "trophic influences" of the nucleus, can be assimilated in situ to form new protoplasm. In this view, the axon would grow over its entire length from local resources. Contrary to this supposition, the experiments to be reported here have furnished evidence that the axon grows from its base in the nucleated cell body; that synthesis of new protoplasm occurs exclusively at the nuclear ·site; and that this is equally true for the incremental growth of immature or regenerating axons and for the anabolic renewal of the cytoplasm in mature axons. The evidence rests mainly on experiments in which the "supply line" between nucleus and the more outlying parts of the axoplasm was throttled in various degrees by a constricting ring of artery placed around the whole nerve.

## METHODS AND TERMINOLOGY

Most experiments were done with nerves of white rats (totaling over 300), with corroborating results in rabbits, chickens, and monkeys.[2] Since the nerve fibers were examined individually, the actual number of test cases amounts to more than 100,000. In this report, only those observations will be considered which have been fully verified throughout the course of our research and which can be safely repeated. The following terminology will be used:

Perikaryon: the nucleated body of the nerve cell.

Axoplasm: the cytoplasm of the axon (A, fig. 1).

Plasma membrane: the outer surface film of the axon, usually closely adhering to the inner surface of the myelin sheath.

Neurokeratin: the protein framework of the myelin sheath.

Schwann cells: the sheath cells enveloping the myelin sheath, but lying inside the fibrous sheath of the nerve fiber (S, fig. 1).

[2] In an earlier phase, Dr. A. Cecil Taylor collaborated in these experiments and his assistance is gratefully acknowledged.

Neurilemmal tube: the fibrous sheath which contains the nerve fiber (including the sheath of Henle or Key-Retzius); abbreviated "tube" (T, fig. 1).

Internode: the segment of a nerve fiber lying between two nodes of Ranvier.

Ovoids: the oval vacuoles in nerves undergoing Wallerian degeneration, containing axon and myelin debris.

Nerves were studied either in paraffin sections or in teased preparations. The former were either fixed in Bouin's solution and impregnated with silver according to Bodian or fixed in formalin and stained with osmic acid. Teased preparations were made either from living fibers immersed in Ringer's solution or from fixed specimens impregnated with silver

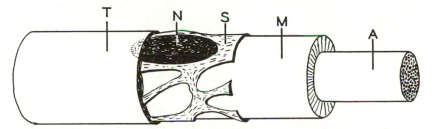

Fig. 1 Diagram of the components of a nerve fiber. A, Axis cylinder. M, Myelin sheath. S, Schwann cell. N, Nucleus of the Schwann cell. T, Fibrous sheath or "tube."

according to Bielschowsky. The stained fibers were teased in glycerin and embedded in the same medium or in Gurr's water mounting medium. Nerve fiber calibers were measured in tracings of either teased fibers or cross sections of whole nerves, either by planimetry or by diameter determinations as described previously (Weiss, Edds and Cavanaugh, '45).

Since all experiments deal with constricted nerve fibers and their characteristic deformations, it will be expedient to use standard designations for the different regions of the experimental nerves in their relation to the constricted zone (fig. 2). An arrow marks the proximo-distal direction of the nerve. The constricted zone is referred to as C, and the parts of the nerve lying proximally and distally to it as P and D, respectively.

P is subdivided into $P_a$, $P_b$ and $P_c$, indicating different degrees of axon alteration: heaviest alteration in $P_c$, minor disturbance in $P_b$, and normal unaffected appearance in $P_a$. Similarly, in the distal stump, the part near C may be distinguished as $D_a$ from the more peripheral part $D_b$. All illustrations are oriented with the proximo-distal direction from left to right or from top to bottom.

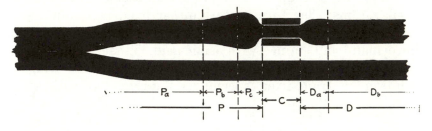
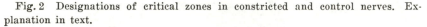

Fig. 2  Designations of critical zones in constricted and control nerves. Explanation in text.

### RESULTS

The diagram, figure 3, summarizes the essential features of the experiments for the case of single regenerating fibers. Rows A to E review the main phases of ordinary nerve regeneration after simple crushing. Interruption of the axon B leaves a proximal stump connected with, and a distal stump severed from, the perikaryon; the distal stump disintegrates. In C, the proximal stump begins to elongate by the active advance of its amoeboid tip. This elongation, usually referred to as "outgrowth," is primarily a phenomenon of protoplasmic movement, rather than growth in the sense of increase of protoplasmic mass. Its mechanism has been dealt with in previous publications (Weiss, '41, '44c, '45) and need not concern us here. The regenerating branch is originally only 1 micron or less in diameter, its cross section therefore only a small fraction of that of the old fiber stem (e.g., less than 1 hundredth in the case of a 10 μ fiber). In D, the advancing tip has reached and become connected with the peripheral end organ, and the new axon portion has gained in width. This enlargement continues long after terminal connections are reestablished, until finally, in E, the whole fiber has recovered nearly its original caliber. This increase of the originally slender protoplasmic filament to a multiple of its size (in the above example, 100 times), is an expression of extensive growth, that is, production of new axoplasm. This phase of the regeneration process has been our basic test object. We can alter it controllably by narrowing the space available to

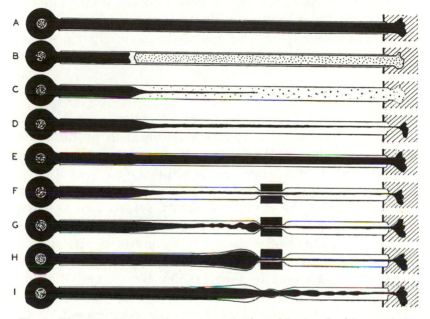

Fig. 3 Diagram of stages of nerve regeneration without and with constriction. Explanation in text.

the fiber for expansion, as is shown in rows F to I of the diagram.

Reduction of the lumen of the fiber tube, as in F, does not interfere with the distad advance and terminal reconnection of a regenerating fiber, which is slender. But as soon as this fiber, as it continues to expand, attains the dimensions of the constricted zone, a remarkable difference appears between those parts lying at the distal and at the proximal sides of the narrow neck. The distal segment ceases to grow and remains permanently undersized, while the proximal segment not only continues to enlarge, but near the entrance into the constricted zone, enlarges excessively. Two stages of this process are shown in rows G and H. One gets the impression that a column of axoplasm is pressing distad and becomes dammed up where its channel narrows. This impression is strengthened by observations on released constrictions: some of the dammed material then moves into the distal portion, which widens accordingly, as illustrated in row I.

With this schematic description of the basic experiments as background, we may now turn to a more detailed account.

## 1. The effect of constriction

Short segments (cca. 1 mm long) of artery with a lumen smaller than the nerve diameter were used to produce constriction (Weiss and Davis, '43; Weiss and Taylor, '44b). When distended, these rings can be slipped over the cut nerve end and placed in the desired position. Their subsequent contraction produces the effects commonly referred to as nerve compression or constriction. Since this compression is localized, it is physically absurd to compare its effects with those of static pressure acting uniformly on an enclosed system, as is occasionally done (Denny-Brown and Brenner, '44b). The difference lies in the fact that localized pressure produces a shift of substance from the compressed to the non-compressed area. The extent of this movement depends on the physical properties (mobility, elasticity, etc.) of the compressed system and its restraining environment; in the present instance, the axon and its tube, the former more plastic, the latter more rigid. The arterial collar, in closing down on the nerve, squeezes underlying nerve content into the adjacent free portions. This involves, besides blood and endoneural fluid, neuroplasm and myelin (see below, section 6). For the individual nerve fiber, this implies a gradual reduction of diameter throughout the constricted zone, and slight dilation at either end of the constriction. As the yielding nerve content accommodates itself to the arterial lumen, the local pressure declines and eventually disappears. So-called "pressure block" of nerve conduction produced by arterial cuffs (Weiss and Davis, '43) is due not to maintained "pressure," but to the displacement of axonal substance.

Constriction thus acts stepwise: local increase of pressure causes escape of substance into zones of lower pressure thus producing reduction of diameter, which, in turn, automatically relieves the excess pressure. The high plasticity and elasticity of nerve fibers is clearly demonstrated by their incomplete redistension after temporary constriction of only a few hours duration. The salient permanent feature of constriction is thus the local narrowing of the fiber tube which it entails.

The degree of narrowing suffered by a given nerve fiber varies not only with the degree of compression of the whole nerve, but also with (a) the topography of the fiber; (b) the consistency of the surroundings; (c) the fiber diameter. The compressing force reaches maxima at the ends of the constricting sleeve, but with the short rings used in our studies, this longitudinal differential is negligible. In more detail, these relations are as follows.

*(a) Topographic variation of the compression effect.* The effect is not evenly distributed over the whole cross section of the nerve, but is strongest at the surface and declines rapidly toward the interior. This gradient can be readily demonstrated by the following model experiment imitating the conditions of nerve constriction (fig. 4): A bundle of rubber tubes to represent nerve fibers is arranged in concentric circles. Their lower ends are closed, the upper ends connected to glass manometers. They are partly filled with indicator fluid. Constriction of the bundle is produced by a metal bracelet with overlapping edges. During the constriction, the water columns rise in direct proportion to the volumes of fluid displaced, which, in turn, are proportional to the respective reductions of diameters. The diagram shows the average displacement for 15 separate determinations. Dis-

regarding the minor deviations due to inequalities in the packing of the tubes and in the constricting force, it is evident that the tubes, and comparably the nerve fibers, are the more compressed, the nearer the surface they lie. The innermost elements are least affected. This gradation has been verified in our experimental nerves and will be dealt with in section 2.

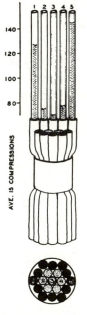

Fig. 4  Model of differential displacement of the content of a bundle of tubes under local compression. The water levels indicate the average displacement in 12 outer, 6 intermediate and 1 innermost tube computed from 15 separate experiments.

*(b) Variation of the compression effect with the proportion of interstitial tissue.* Since interstitial fluid around a nerve fiber can shift more easily than the content of the fiber, it acts as a shock absorber. The nerve sheaths (epineurium, perineurium) likewise have a cushioning effect. Accordingly, a given amount of constriction will affect the nerve fibers the more, the smaller the interstices, that is, the denser the packing of the fibers, and the less the amount of enveloping tissue.

*(c) Variation of the compression effect with fiber size.* In general, the larger fibers of a constricted nerve suffer a greater proportional reduction of diameter than do the smaller ones. Originally deduced from the fact that the

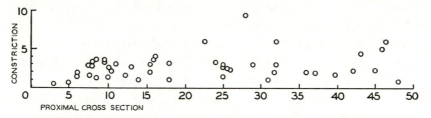

Fig. 5 Constriction in fibers of different size. Cross section of the constricted part of fiber plotted over cross section of the normal proximal stem of the same fiber, for 47 teased fibers.

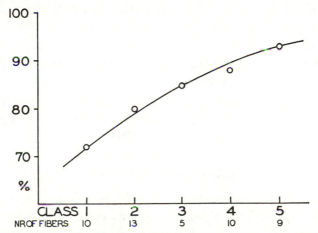

Fig. 6 Degree of constriction in relation to fiber size. Relative loss of diameter of fibers of different size classes plotted over original diameter, for the same fibers as in figure 5. Class 1 includes fibers between 1.6 and 2.4 $\mu$; subsequent classes follow in steps of 0.8 each.

largest fibers are the first to cease conducting during progressive constriction (Gasser and Erlanger, '29; Weiss and Davis, '43), the greater relative involvement of the larger fibers has now been confirmed by direct measurements. The graphs reproduced in figures 5 and 6 are based on a sample of 47 individual fibers teased from 3 different nerves (fixed and stained) after constrictions of long standing. In figure 5, the cross section of the constricted part of each fiber is plotted over the cross section of a far proximal, normal segment of the same fiber. One notices a remarkable uniformity of the calibers in the constriction irrespective of the original fiber caliber. What fluctuation there is, can be ascribed to local conditions such as outlined in (a) and (b), rather than to original fiber size. The fact that fibers of all sizes thus approach a common lower size level, implies that the larger ones have lost relatively more than the smaller ones. This is directly shown in figure 6. This graph gives the average percentage reduction of cross sectional area in the constriction ($100 \frac{P-C}{P}$, where P and C are the cross sectional areas at $P_a$ and C, respectively) for the various size classes of fibers. It can be seen that there is a steady increase in the degree of constriction with increasing caliber. The same conclusion can be reached from comparing the constriction of the total cross section of a nerve with the reduction of its 150 largest fibers; in a sample case ($R_2 56$), these reductions amounted to 20% and 65%, respectively, demonstrating the relatively heavier involvement of the larger fiber classes.

## 2. Standard experiment

As the standard experiment, we choose the one diagrammed in figure 2 F–I; i.e., placing a constriction around one of a pair of nerves (tibial and peroneal), at the same time initiating regeneration by a crush farther proximally. After intervals varying from 4 to 35 weeks, the regenerated nerves are examined for recovery of fiber size at different levels. Figure 7 shows samples from a typical case ($R_2 59$; 35 weeks p. op.) at the indicated levels P and D at identical magnifications. The 2 left panels represent the regenerated fibers of the unconstricted control nerve. By comparison, the right panels show the great disparity of size of the regenerated fibers in the constricted nerve proximally and distally to the

426

constriction. The fibers are very much undersized at level D, while excessively dilated at $P_c$.

Figure 8 shows the histogram of the 150 largest fiber cross sections of the case illustrated in figure 7 at corresponding

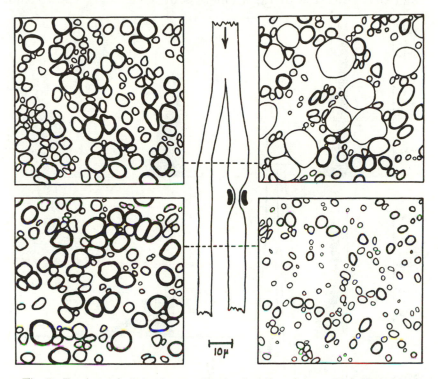

Fig. 7   Tracings of photomicrographs, showing fiber sizes at the indicated levels of a control peroneal nerve (left) and a constricted tibial nerve (right), both regenerated from a high crush for 35 weeks.

levels ($P_c$ lies a little closer to the constriction in fig. 8 than in fig. 7). One notes the inverse relation between fiber sizes proximal and distal to the constriction. Histograms of all other cases are essentially similar to this one. Instead of presenting them in detail, we have computed the total areas of the 150 largest fiber cross sections at levels $P_f$, $P_c$, and $D_b$ for 7 pairs of nerves. These data are summarized in the

427

graph, figure 9. All show marked surpluses and deficits of fiber volume at levels $P_c$ and $D_b$, respectively.

The subnormal size of fibers distal to a constriction was first noted by Weiss and Taylor ('44b). It was recognized then that since the distal diameters of such fibers showed no

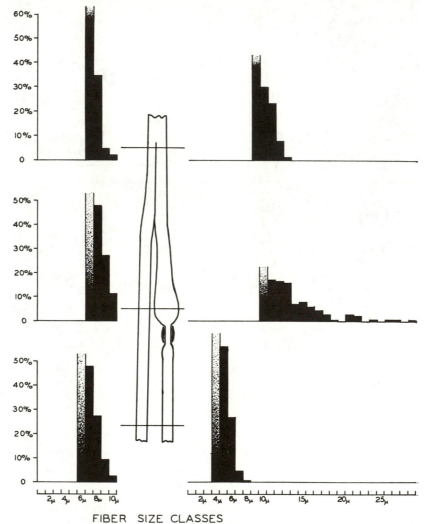

FIBER SIZE CLASSES

Fig. 8 Histograms of the 150 largest fibers at the indicated levels of the nerves illustrated in figure 7. (35 weeks p. op.)

further increase after 4 weeks of regeneration up to 15 weeks, their growth was not just retarded, but fully arrested. This conclusion has been substantiated by the present series with observations extending over an even longer period, up to 35 weeks (see figs. 9 and 18). The distal parts of the fibers never widen appreciably above the caliber imposed upon them in the constricted zone, and this size deficit is permanent. Actual

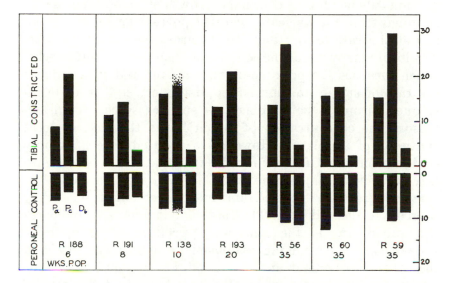

Fig. 9   Total areas of the 150 largest fiber cross sections of 7 pairs of constricted and control nerves at levels $P_a$, $P_c$ and $D_b$. Regeneration times indicated at bottom of graph — 1 unit = 1000 $\mu^2$. Note (1) the greatly reduced fiber size in the constricted nerves at level $D_b$, showing no increase with longer regeneration periods; (2) the excessive fiber size at level $P_c$, tending to increase with time; (3) over-all reduction of fiber size during earlier weeks due to atrophy of disconnection, followed by recovery.

values will be given below. Myelinization was found to vary directly with the diameter; that is, the distal segments of reduced size possess a correspondingly thin myelin sheath (see figure 4 in Weiss and Taylor, '44b). Control series, in which the constricted nerves were either left disconnected from their peripheral fields or were reconnected by arterial splices, proved that as far as the part of the nerve lying distally to the constriction is concerned, the results were essentially the same in both conditions.

The explanation of these results is unequivocal. The constriction divides the nerve into 2 parts of unequal growth — an unimpaired proximal one, and a distal one whose size is limited in direct proportion to the reduced lumen of the fiber at its narrowest point. This relation indicates that the distal portion depends for its continued growth on something that is supplied from the nucleated central portion and transported distad at a rate proportional to the cross section of the tube. The local narrowing at the constriction acts as a ''bottleneck'' which throttles the proximo-distal transfer and thus reduces the rate of supply to the farther distal levels. The material in question might be axoplasm as such or some growth accessory the concentration of which limits the rate of local synthesis of axoplasm. However, a reduced rate of supply could not of itself account for the fact that the deficit in size is a permanent one, for the distal fiber part would merely be slower in reaching normal dimensions, but ought eventually to grow to the full size. The fact that it does not, indicates that fiber size is the stationary product of 2 opposite processes, one consuming axoplasm at a uniform rate and the other replacing it at the rate at which supplies become available. Constriction evidently does not affect the rate of consumption, which will depend on local factors, but only reduces the rate of replacement. In consequence, the distal fiber volume comes to a steady state at a lower size level than proximally.

The decision of whether what moves down the fiber is axoplasm as such or merely growth accessories for its local synthesis, is of fundamental importance, because it contains the answer to the general problem of whether a cell grows from a circumscribed source, especially the nucleus, or ubiquitously throughout the cytoplasm. While the distal growth deficit in constricted nerve fibers can be reconciled with either view, the character of the compensatory surplus on the proximal side of the constriction, the ''damming'' phenomenon, points to the perikaryon as the sole production site of neuroplasm.

(End of reprinted portion of paper.)

## LITERATURE CITED

BODIAN, DAVID 1947 Nucleic acid in nerve-cell regeneration. Symposia, Soc. f. Exp. Biol., no. 1, pp. 163–178.

BODIAN, DAVID, AND R. C. MELLORS 1945 The regenerative cycle of moto-neurons, with special reference to phosphatase activity. J. Exp. Med., 81: 469–488.

CAJAL, S. RAMON Y 1928 Degeneration and Regeneration of the Nervous System. Translated and edited by Raoul M. May, Oxford University Press, London: Humphrey Milford.

CAREY, E. J., E. M. DOWNER, F. B. TOOMEY AND E. HAUSHALTER 1946 Morpho-logic effects of DDT on nerve endings, neurosomes, and fiber types in voluntary muscles. Proc. Soc. Exp. Biol. and Med., 62: 76–83.

CAVANAUGH, MARGARET 1948 Atrophy of sensory neurons deprived of peripheral connections. Anat. Rec., 100: 736.

COOK, D. D., AND R. W. GERARD 1931 The effect of stimulation on the degen-eration of a severed peripheral nerve. Am. J. Physiol., 97: 412–425.

DENNY-BROWN, D., AND CHARLES BRENNER 1944a Paralysis of nerve induced by direct pressure and by tourniquet. Arch. Neurol. Psychiat., 51: 1–26.

———— 1944b Lesion in peripheral nerve resulting from compression by spring clip. Arch. Neurol. Psychiat., 52: 1–19.

DUNCAN, DONALD, AND WALTER HEARNE JARVIS 1943 Observations on repeated regeneration of the facial nerve in cats. J. Comp. Neur., 79: 315–327.

DUSTIN, A. P. 1917 Les lésions posttraumatiques des nerfs. Contribution a l'histopathologie du système nerveux périphérique chez l'homme. Am-bulance de ''L'Océan,'' 1: 71–161.

ERLANGER, J., AND H. S. GASSER 1937 Electrical Signs of Nervous Activity. Philadelphia. Univ. Pa. Press., 221 pp.

GASSER, H. S., AND J. ERLANGER 1929 The role of fiber size in the establish-ment of a nerve block by pressure or cocaine. Am. J. Physiol., 80: 522.

GERARD, R. W. 1932 Nerve metabolism. Physiol. Rev., 12: 469–592.

GREENMAN, M. J. 1913 Studies on the regeneration of the peroneal nerve of the albino rat: Number and sectional areas of fibers: Area relation of axis to sheath. J. Comp. Neur., 23: 479–513.

GROAT, R. A., AND H. KOENIG 1946 Centrifugal deterioration of asphyxiated peripheral nerve. J. Neurophysiol., 9: 275–284.

GUTMANN, E., AND F. K. SANDERS 1943 Recovery of fiber numbers and diameters in the regeneration of peripheral nerves. J. Physiol., *101:* 489–518.

HAMBERGER, CARL-AXEL, AND HOLGER HYDÉN 1945 Cytochemical changes in the cochlear ganglion caused by acoustic stimulation and trauma. Acta Oto-laryngol., *61* (suppl.), 5–89.

HAMMOND, W. S., AND J. C. HINSEY 1945 The diameters of the nerve fibers in normal and regenerating nerves. J. Comp. Neur., *83:* 79–89.

HARRISON, R. G. 1910 The outgrowth of the nerve fiber as a mode of protoplasmic movement. J. Exp. Zool., *9:* 787.

HELD, HANS 1909 Die Entwicklung des Nervengewebes bei den Wirbeltieren. Leipzig.

HISCOE, HELEN B. 1947 Distribution of nodes and incisures in normal and regenerated nerve fibers. Anat. Rec., *99:* 447–476.

HOLMES, W., AND J. Z. YOUNG 1942 Nerve regeneration after immediate and delayed suture. J. Anat., *77*, part 1, 63–96.

HOWE, H. A., AND D. BODIAN 1941 Refractoriness of nerve cells to poliomyelitis virus after interruption of their axones. Bull. Johns Hopkins Hosp., *69:* 92–133.

HYDÉN, HOLGER 1943 Protein Metabolism in the Nerve Cell During Growth and Function. Acta Physiol. Scand., *6* (suppl. 17), 5–136.

LEEGAARD, CHR. 1880 Über die Entartungsreaktion. Deutsch. Arch. f. Klin. Med., *26:* 459–522.

LEWIS, W. H. 1945 Axon growth and regeneration. Anat. Rec., *91* (suppl.), 25.

MATSON, D. D., EBEN ALEXANDER AND PAUL WEISS 1948 Experiments on the bridging of gaps in severed peripheral nerves of monkeys. J. Neurosurg.

MURALT, A. L. VON 1946 Die Signalübermittlung im Nerven. Basel, Birkhäuser.

NAGEOTTE, J., AND L. GUYON 1918 Différences physiologiques entre la neuroglie des fibres motrices et celle des fibres sensitives, dans les nerfs périphériques mise en evidence par la régénération. C. r. Soc. Biol., Paris, *81:* 571–574.

OPPENHEIMER, J. M. 1941 The anatomical relationships of abnormally located Mauthner's cells in Fundulus embryos. J. Comp. Neur., *74*, no. 1, 131.

———— 1942 The decussation of Mauthner's fibers in Fundulus embryos. J. Comp. Neur., *77*, no. 3, 577–587.

PARKER, G. H., AND V. L. PAINE 1934 Progressive nerve degeneration and its rate in the lateral-line nerve of the catfish. Am. J. Anat., *54:* 1–25.

ROSENBLUETH, A., AND E. C. DEL POZO 1943 The centrifugal course of Wallerian degeneration. Am. J. Physiol., *139:* 247–254.

SANDERS, F. K., AND J. Z. YOUNG 1944 The role of the peripheral stump in the control of fiber diameter in regenerating nerves. J. Physiol., *103:* 119–136.

———— 1945 Effect of peripheral connexion on the diameter of nerve fibers. Nature, *155:* 237.

SCHOENHEIMER, R., S. RATNER, D. RITTENBERG AND M. HEIDELBERGER 1942 The interaction of antibody protein with dietary nitrogen in actively immunized animals. J. Biol. Chem., *144:* 545.

SIMPSON, S. A., AND J. Z. YOUNG 1945 Regeneration of fiber diameter after cross-unions of visceral and somatic nerves. J. Anat., *79:* 48–65.

STROEBE, H. 1893 Experimentelle Untersuchungen über Degeneration peripherer Nerven nach Verletzungen. Beitr. path. Anat., *13:* 160–278.

THORELL, BO 1947 Studies on the formation of cellular substances during blood cell production. Acta Med. Scand., (suppl. CC).

VOGT, CECILE, AND OSKAR VOGT 1947 Lebensgeschichte, Funktion und Tätigkeitsregulierung des Nucleolus. Ärztliche Forschung, *1:* 8–14 and 43–50.

WEISS, PAUL 1936 Selectivity controlling the central-peripheral relations in the nervous system. Biol. Rev., *11:* 494–531.

———— 1941 Nerve patterns: The mechanics of nerve growth. Third Growth Symposium, Growth (suppl.), *5:* 163–203.

———— 1943a Endoneurial edema in constricted nerve. Anat. Rec., *86:* 491–522.

———— 1943b Nerve regeneration in the rat, following tubular splicing of severed nerves. Arch. of Surg., *46:* 525–547.

———— 1944a Damming of axoplasm in constricted nerve: a sign of perpetual growth in nerve fibers. Anat. Rec., *88* (suppl.), 464.

———— 1944b Evidence of perpetual proximo-distal growth of nerve fibers. Biol. Bull., *87:* 160.

———— 1944c The technology of nerve regeneration: A review. Sutureless tubulation and related methods of nerve repair. J. Neurosurg., *1:* 400–450.

———— 1945 Experiments on cell and axon orientation in vitro; the role of colloidal exudates in tissue organization. J. Exp. Zool., *100:* 353–386.

———— 1947 Protoplasm synthesis and substance transfer in neurons. Proc. XVII International Physiol. Congress, Oxford, p. 101.

———— 1948a Differential Growth. In: Conference on Chemistry and Physiology of Growth. Princeton University Press.

———— 1948b Growth and differentiation on the cellular and molecular levels. Proc. 6th Internat. Congr. Exp. Cytol., Stockholm.

WEISS, PAUL, AND AGNES S. BURT 1944 Effect of nerve compression on Wallerian degeneration in vitro. Proc. Soc. Exp. Biol. and Med., *55:* 109–112.

WEISS, PAUL, AND HALLOWELL DAVIS 1943 Pressure block in nerves provided with arterial sleeves. J. Neurophysiol., *6:* 269–286.

WEISS, PAUL, AND M. V. EDDS, JR. 1945 Sensory-motor nerve crosses in the rat. J. Neurophysiol., *8:* 173–193.

WEISS, PAUL, M. V. EDDS, JR., AND M. CAVANAUGH 1945 The effect of terminal connections on the caliber of nerve fibers. Anat. Rec., *92:* 215–233.

WEISS, PAUL, AND A. C. TAYLOR 1944a Further experimental evidence against "neurotropism" in nerve regeneration. J. Exp. Zool., *95:* 233–257.

———— 1944b Impairment of growth and myelinization in regenerating nerve fibers subject to constriction. Proc. Soc. Exp. Biol. and Med., *55:* 77–80.

WEISS, PAUL, H. WANG, A. C. TAYLOR AND M. V. EDDS, JR. 1945 Proximo-distal fluid convection in the endoneurial spaces of peripheral nerves, demonstrated by colored and radioactive (isotope) tracers. Am. J. Physiol., *143*: 521–540.

YOUNG, J. Z. 1944a Contraction, turgor and the cytoskeleton of nerve fibers. Nature, *153*: 333.

———— 1944b Surface tension and the degeneration of nerve fibers. Nature, *154*: 521.

———— 1945a The History of the Shape of a Nerve Fiber. In: Growth and Form. Essays presented to d'Arcy Thompson, pp.. 41–93. Oxford, Clarendon Press.

———— 1945b Structure, degeneration and repair of nerve fiber. Nature, *156*: 132.

YOUNG, J. Z., E. GUTMANN, L. GUTTMANN AND P. B. MEDAWAR 1942 The rate of regeneration of nerve. J. Exp. Biol., *19*: 14–44.

# Axonal Migration of Proteins in the Central Nervous System and Peripheral Nerves as Shown by Radioautography

B. DROZ and C. P. LEBLOND

*Department of Anatomy, McGill University, Montreal, Canada*

The "axonal flow" theory holds that the nerve cell body is continuously forming new cytoplasm which enters the axon and travels along its length. This theory was formulated by Weiss and collaborators (Weiss and Hiscoe, '48) to account for the accumulation of material in front of a nerve constriction and for the high concentration of enzymes appearing in the proximal stump of a sectioned nerve (Sawyer, '46; Hebb and Waites, '56; Friede, '59). For instance, since the so-called neurosecretory substance of the hypothalamus accumulates in the central stump of the severed pituitary stalk, this substance is believed to migrate down into the posterior pituitary (Scharrer and Scharrer, '54).

Techniques that do not damage the nerves have been used in a search for direct evidence in support of the axonal flow theory. Thus, radioactive substances were given, which it was hoped would be taken up into the nerve cell body and flow down the axon: phosphate-$P^{32}$ (Samuels et al., '51; Ochs and Burger, '58; Ochs et al., '62), glucose-$C^{14}$ (Waelsch, quoted by Weiss, '60), and labeled amino acids (Waelsch, '58; Koenig, '58b; Schultze and Oehlert, '58; Verne and Droz, '60). However, the radioactive substances used were taken up not only by nerve cell bodies, but also by Schwann cells. Hence the difference in radioactivity in successive segments of nerve trunks was small and Weiss ('60) commented that, while the results obtained "were expected to lend deeper insight into the processes involved, this expectation has thus far remained disappointingly unfulfilled." In fact, several authors hold the view that there is no axonal migration at all (Schultze and Oehlert, '58; Koenig and Koelle, '60; Miani, '60).

At the present time, an experimental approach is needed which will either prove or disprove the axonal flow theory. It was thought that the attempts at tracing amino acids into the proteins of neurons might be repeated, but in such a way that the radioactivity of individual axons could be distinguished from that of glial cells. This aim might be achieved with tritium labeled amino acids, since a high radioautographic resolution is obtained with tritium.

The first step was to make sure of the *sites of protein synthesis*. That such synthesis takes place continuously in the central nervous system was shown biochemically by the incorporation of labeled amino acids into the protein fraction (Friedberg et al., '48; Gaitonde and Richter, '56; Palladin, '57; Vladimirov, '57; Lajtha et al., '57). Radioautography after injection of a labeled amino acid indicated that the protein synthesis takes place in the body of nerve cells (Cohn et al., '54; Fisher et al., '56; Flanigan et al., '57; Leblond et al., '57; Koenig, '58a; Oehlert et al., '58; Droz and Verne, '59). However, these experiments were carried out using amino acids labeled with isotopes which do not allow good radioautographic resolution (such as sulfur$^{35}$) and the animals were sacrificed several hours after injection, that is, too late to be sure that the newly-formed proteins had not migrated out of their sites of synthesis (Warshawsky et al., '63). It was, therefore, decided to reinvestigate the problem using mainly tritium labeled amino acids and sacrificing the animals very soon after injection, so that newly-formed proteins would still be at their site of synthesis.

Once the sites of synthesis of protein were known with certainty, it was possible

Reprinted from the *Journal of Comparative Neurology* 121: 325–346 (1963) by permission of the publisher.

TABLE 1

*Experimental groups*

| Experiment number | Amino acid | | Animals used | | | | Injection | | Time between injection and sacrifice (given for each group) |
|---|---|---|---|---|---|---|---|---|---|
| | Name | Specific activity | Type | Weight | No. of groups | No. of animals per group | No. | Total dose | |
| | | *mc/mM* | | *g* | | | | *μc/gm body wt* | |
| I | leucine-H³ | 3570 | male rats | 120±5 | 4 | 2 | 1 | 2.5 | 2,5,10,30 minutes |
| II | leucine-H³ | 3570 | female rats | 77±3 | 5 | 4 | 1 | 2.5 | 7,15,30,90,240 minutes |
| III | leucine-H³ | 29 | male rats | 120±5 | 4 | 4 | 1 | 2.5 | 4 h.; 1,5,7,30 days |
| IV | arginine-H³ | 270 | male mice | 20±2 | 8 | 2 | 1 | 10 | 0.16,0.5,4,12 h.; 1.5,4,12,30 days |
| V | methionine-S³⁵ | 42 | male rats | 50±5 / 50±5 | 5 / 3 | 1 / 1 | 1 / 5¹ | 10 / 10 | 0.5 h.; 1,4,10,17 days / 1,4,17 days |
| VI | methionine-S³⁵ | 42 | male mice | 25±2 / 25±2 | 6 / 3 | 1 / 1 | 1 / 5¹ | 10 / 10 | 0.5,3,12 h.; 1,4,17 days / 1,4,17 days |
| VII | leucine-H³ | 5400 | male rats | 45±5 / 45±5 | 1 / 5 | 1 / 1 | 1 / 9¹ | 20 / 30 | 0.5 h. / 1.1,2,4,8,16 days |
| VIII | leucine-H³ | 5400 | female rats | 250±5 | 5 | 1 | 8¹ | 30 | 1,2,4,8,16 days |

¹ The multiple injections in Experiments V–VIII were done every three hours during a given day. The time between injection and sacrifice was measured from the first injection.

436

to examine whether the new, radioactive protein underwent *migration*. This was done as follows. The regions that showed no radioactivity immediately after injection of the tritium labeled amino acid were examined at later and later time intervals to find out if they ever became radioactive. Any region which did so was then examined at high magnification in the hope of identifying the structure — particularly the axons — in which the radioactivity was present.

## MATERIAL AND METHODS

Eight experimental series were used, consisting of animals given single or multiple intraperitoneal injections of a labeled amino acid dissolved in saline. The key experiments were carried out with tritium ($H^3$) labeled leucine in rats. Confirmatory experiments were done with arginine-$H^3$ and methionine-$S^{35}$ in rats and mice. The animals of an experiment were injected and divided into groups of one or several animals each. All the animals of a group were killed at the same time after injection (table 1).

Under light anesthesia, the animals were sacrificed by section of the abdominal aorta. The brain, spinal cord and semilunar ganglion were removed. In experiments IV–VIII, the sciatic nerve and the maxillary branch of the trigeminal nerve were also preserved. Fixation was in Bouin's for 48 hours. After fixation, the brain was cut into two halves along the midline. One side was used for longitudinal parasagittal sections and the other side for transverse sections at four levels: rhinencephalon, hippocampus, cerebellum and medulla oblongata.

After histological processing, stained and unstained 4-μ sections were radioautographed by the coating technique (Kopriwa and Leblond, '62). The exposure was usually three or six months.

The radioautographic reactions, that is, the groups of silver grains appearing in the emulsion overlying the radioactive site, were recorded either by photography or by

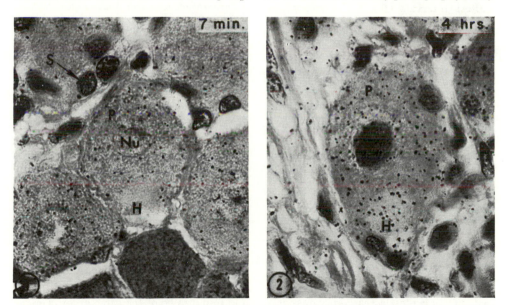

Figs. 1 and 2   Hematoxylin-eosin stained radioautographs of semilunar ganglion of 80-g rats given a single injection of leucine-$H^3$ and sacrificed after seven minutes (fig. 1) and four hours (fig. 2). (*Experiment II.*) × 980.

At seven minutes (fig. 1), the silver grains are scattered over nucleus (Nu) and perikaryon (P) with the exception of the axon hillock (H). A few grains may be seen over satellite cells (S).

At four hours (fig. 2), the silver grains also extend to the axon hillock (H).

counting grains. In the latter case, the structure over which grains were to be enumerated, was usually outlined on paper with the help of a camera lucida and the grains drawn in and counted. The outlined structures were then cut out and weighed. It was thus possible to calculate the concentration of grains per unit area of the investigated structure in the section.

## RESULTS

### Cell bodies (Experiments I–VII)

When radioautographs were examined at early time intervals after a single injection of leucine-H³ into rats, distinct accumulations of silver grains were lacking at the two- and five-minute intervals, but appeared over all cell bodies at the seven-minute interval (fig. 1) and increased in amount there until the one and one-half hour interval (fig. 4). The silver grains could be assigned to the nucleus and perikaryon of neurons, including the base of large dendrites (fig. 3), but they were absent over the axon hillock, at least at the earliest intervals (fig. 1). Silver grains were also present over the cell bodies of neuroglia, although less abundant than over neurons (fig. 3), as well as over satellite cells of ganglia (fig. 1), Schwann cells of peripheral nerves, cells of blood vessels, meninges, etc. Finally, the presence of an early reaction over the cell bodies of neurons and glial cells was confirmed with arginine-H³ in mice (exp. IV) and methionine-S³⁵ in rats (exp. V, figs. 15, 19) and mice (exp. VI, figs. 23, 27). It is concluded that radioactivity appears in neurons and glial cells within seven minutes after injection of labeled amino acids.

Neuronal radioactivity showed changes in pattern with time, as some label eventually appeared in the axon hillock (fig. 2); but the concentration of radioactivity rose more slowly in this area than in the perikaryon (fig. 4).

After reaching a maximum between 1.5 and 4 hours after injection of any one of the three amino acids used, the radioactivity of cell bodies decreased progressively, as may be seen in figures 12–14, 20–22, 24–26, 28–30 (exp. V and VII). Grain counts over the perikaryon of Purkinje cells (solid curves, fig. 5) and semilunar ganglion cells (fig. 6) as well as over pyram-

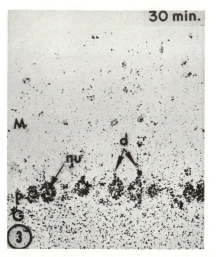

Fig. 3  Unstained radioautograph of cerebellar cortex of a 45-g rat sacrificed 30 minutes after a single dose of leucine-H³ (*Experiment VII*) × 230.

The Purkinje cell layer (P) shows a strong radioautographic reaction, which may be assigned to the perikaryon and nucleolar region (nu) of Purkinje cells. The base of the dendrites (d) of the Purkinje cells also shows a radioautographic reaction. A moderate reaction is seen over the cells of the granular layer (G). In the molecular layer (M), the scattered weak reactions are due to scattered oligodendrocytes and neurons.

idal cells in the hippocampus (fig. 7) confirmed the decrease in radioactivity with time.

Since the decay of a substance metabolized under steady state conditions is exponential, the logarithm of its concentration plotted versus time yields a straight line. However, the plots from the three cell types in figures 5–7 appeared to be curved lines. An analysis of these curves (detailed in the legend of figs. 5–7) suggested that they arise from the combination of two straight lines. Each one of the two lines would represent the decay of one radioactive substance. The turnover time of the two substances was calculated by the method of Zilversmit et al. ('43) and found to be of the same order of magnitude in the three cell types under consideration (table 2), that is, one of the two substances had a turnover time of about a day (0.9–1.4 days) and the other, of about two weeks (13.7–17.3 days).

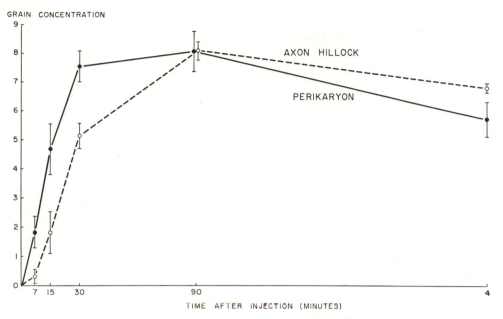

Fig. 4   Plot of grain concentration in perikaryon and axon hillock (with standard errors) versus time (*Experiment II*).
Radioactivity appears earlier and rises faster in perikaryon than in axon hillock.

### Neuropile and white matter
### (Experiments V–VIII)

Regions of the central nervous system which contain few cell bodies, such as the molecular layer and white matter of *cerebellum*, showed only scattered reactions 30 minutes after injection of leucine-H³ into young rats (fig. 11). With the passage of time, however, abundant, widespread radioactivity appeared in both the molecular layer (figs. 12, 13) and white matter (fig. 14). The same pattern was obtained with multiple injections of leucine-H³ into adult rats or a single injection of methionine-S³⁵ into young rats (figs. 15–18) or adult mice, except for a reduced reaction of the white matter in these cases. Examination under high power did not reveal which microscopic component contained the radioactivity appearing in these layers at late intervals.

In the *hippocampus*, the radioautographic reactions which at the 30-minute interval were restricted to cell bodies, particularly those of the pyramidal layer (fig. 19 Am), were found at 1 and 4 days over the alveus hippocampus (figs. 20, 21 H) and stratum radiatum (R) and by 17 days over the fimbria (fig. 22 F), by which time the cells contained so little radioactivity that they appeared as a negative of their early picture (fig. 19 vs. 22). Again, it was not possible to make sure which structure contained the late-appearing radioactivity.

In the *spinal cord*, the neuropile lacked radioactivity at the 30-minute interval but contained it by 12 hours (figs. 23, 24), though again the radioactive structures of this region were not identified. However, the radioactivity which made its appearance in the white matter of the lumbar spinal cord at one day after leucine-H³ injection in young and adult rats (figs. 31, 32) could be definitely assigned to axons running transversally from the gray matter to the ventral roots (fig. 33). Furthermore, by the 16-day interval, many of the axons running longitudinally in the white matter had also become radioactive, particularly in the ventral and lateral funiculus of the lumbar spinal cord. Similar observations

TABLE 2

*Characteristics of labeled proteins in three types of nerve cells, as estimated from the decay of the radioactivity concentration (figs. 4–6) after a single injection of labeled amino acid*

| Neuron | Site | Injected amino acid | Short-lived substance (exportable protein) | | Long-lived substance (sedentary protein) | |
|---|---|---|---|---|---|---|
| | | | Turnover time | Per cent of label at time 0 | Turnover time | Per cent of label at time 0 |
| | | | *days* | | *days* | |
| Purkinje cell | Cerebellum | Leucine-H$^3$ | 1.4 | 67 | 13.7 | 33 |
| Pyramidal cell | Hippocampus | Leucine-H$^3$ | 0.9 | 43 | 17.3 | 57 |
| Ganglionic cell | Semilunar ganglion | Arginine-H$^3$ | 1.1 | 81 | 13.7 | 19 |

were made at other levels of the spinal cord and in the medulla oblongata. Thus, axons from the nucleus reticularis medius became radioactive 16 days after injection (figs. 34, 35).

In the *semilunar ganglion*, the radioactivity was mainly present in the cell bodies at 30 minutes (fig. 27 N), but extended to the groups of nerve fibers by 12 hours (fig. 28 F). Examination under the high power of the microscope at this time showed that the axons of the nerve fibers had become radioactive. At the end of one day and later, this radioactivity was almost gone (fig. 29 F).

*Peripheral nerves*
(Experiments VII, VIII)

The axons in the lumbar plexus (L$_5$, L$_6$) and sciatic nerve were unlabeled during the first few hours after leucine-H$^3$ injection. At one day, the axons of the ventral roots of the lumbar plexus were labeled in young and adult rats (fig. 32 V).

The sciatic nerve was examined in longitudinal and transverse sections. Thus, in young rats, a "proximal" set of sections was taken 1.6 mm beyond the junction of the L$_5$-L$_6$ branches of the lumbar plexus (about 8–9 mm from spinal cord). A "distal" set was taken 20.0 mm beyond the junction (about 26–28 mm from spinal cord). The results revealed that no significant radioactivity was present in the axons at one day (fig. 8), though Schwann cells were radioactive (fig. 36). At four days, radioactivity was seen in all axons of the proximal region but in none of the distal region (fig. 10). In contrast, at 16 days, axonal radioactivity was found in the distal region only (figs. 10 and 37).

Longitudinal sections revealed that the radioactivity extended over a certain length of each axon (up to 12 mm) as shown in figure 10. At four days, the "front" of the radioactive portion was in the proximal region. At eight days, the "rear" was in this location (fig. 9). By 16 days, the front of the radioactive portion had reached the distal region (fig. 10). A

Figures 5–7

Fig. 5 (top) Labeled proteins in Purkinje cells of the cerebellar cortex after leucine-H$^3$ injection into rats (*Experiment III*).

Fig. 6 (middle) Labeled proteins in Ammon's pyramidal cells of the hippocampus after leucine-H$^3$ injection into rats (*Experiment III*).

Fig. 7 (bottom) Labeled proteins in Ganglionic cells of the semilunar ganglion after arginine-H$^3$ injection into mice (*Experiment IV*).

The log of radioactivity concentration (x) is plotted against time after injection (t). The curve (solid black line) shows a decrease with time.

The curve has a straight line portion (slope $-k_2$), which may be extrapolated to time O, thus yielding the dotted line. This line in turn may be subtracted from the corresponding portion of the original curve. The difference yields a straight line, depicted in the diagram as a broken line (slope $-k_1$).

Thus, the radioactivity decay curve may be considered to consist of two components, a rapidly decaying one ($k_1$) and a slowly decaying one ($k_2$), such that:

$$x = x_1 e^{-k_1 t} + x_2 e^{-k_2 t}$$

in which $x_1$ and $x_2$ are graphically determined by extrapolating back to zero time.

Since $k_1$ and $k_2$ measure the rate of decay of the two components, their turnover times are respectively $\frac{1}{k_1}$ and $\frac{1}{k_2}$. These are listed in table 2. (By the method used, the turnover time of the rapidly decaying substance is a minimal value.)

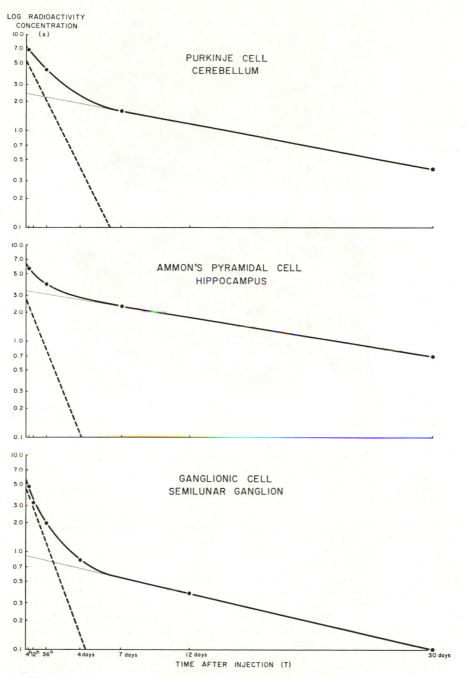

Figs. 5–7   Decay curves of labeled proteins in the body of three types of neurons.

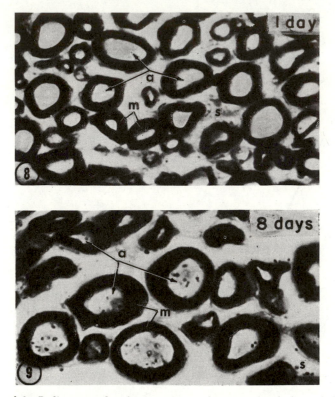

Figs. 8 and 9   Radioautographs of sciatic nerve taken immediately beyond the junction of L₅-L₆ roots ("proximal" region) at one day (fig. 8) and eight days (fig. 9) after the first of multiple injections of leucine-H³ into 45-g rats (*Experiment VII*). The axons were fixed in osmic acid and not otherwise stained. The sections were coated with two layers of celloidin before dipping into emulsion. × 1,500.

The myelin sheath (m) takes up osmic acid and appears dark. The axons (a) fill up the space within the myelin sheath, and are little or not stained. Associated material, including Schwann cells, may be detected (s).

Silver grains are not seen over the axons at one day (fig. 8), but are definite at eight days on many axons (fig. 9).

rough estimate of the migration rate of the radioactive material is 1.5 mm per day.

Similar axonal migration was also observed in other nerves of young rats. Thus, in the dorsal root of the lumbar spinal cord, radioactive material was seen at the end of one day over the axons close to the spinal ganglion, extending later in two directions, that is, towards the sciatic nerve as well as towards the spinal cord. The maxillary branch of the trigeminal nerve showed axonal migration of radioactive material away from the semilunar ganglion at a rate of approximately 3 mm per day.

In *adult rats*, the radioactive material reached the ventral roots of the spinal cord in about a day (thus covering a 0.7 mm distance, figs. 31–33). By the 16-day interval, the label was not present in the axons of the sciatic nerve, but extended in the axons of the L₅-L₆ roots of the lumbar plexus up to 10–14 mm from the spinal cord. The rate of migration in adult rats was, therefore, of the order of 0.8 mm per day.

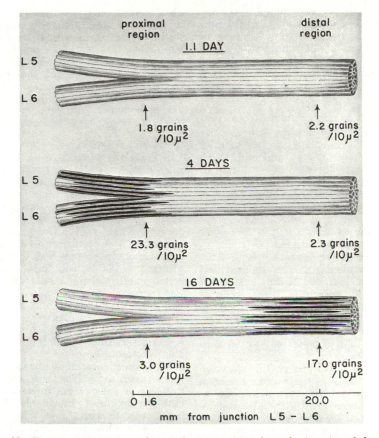

Fig. 10  Diagrams representing the sciatic nerve arising from the junction of the L₅ and L₆ roots (at left). The heavy black lines seen in the second diagram (four days after injection of leucine-H³) and third diagram (16 days after injection) indicate the location of the axonal radioactivity observed at these two time intervals. Grain counts were made on transverse section of the nerve at 1.6 mm (proximal region) and 20.0 mm (distal region) from the junction. The grain counts were expressed per 10 μ² of axon and given below each diagram.

It may be seen that axonal radioactivity is not significant at 1.1 days, appears in the proximal region at four days and in the distal region at 16 days after injection of leucine-H³.

## DISCUSSION

For a rather short time after their injection — a few hours at most — the labeled amino acids, leucine and methionine, were found free in the circulation (Borsook et al., '50; Leblond et al., '57) and in brain tissue (Appel et al., '60). Thus, free labeled methionine reaches a peak in brain at 15–20 minutes after injection; and its amount then declines in such a way that two hours after injection, the content is only one-sixth of the peak (Appel et al., '60).

As long as free labeled amino acids are present in the circulation, they are incorporated into the proteins which are being synthesized and thus become labeled. Such proteins may then be detected in sections by radioautography (Droz and Warshawsky, '63).

The pattern of radioautographic reaction — and, therefore, the distribution of

443

labeled proteins — was found to be the same whether labeled leucine, methionine or arginine is used (as may be seen by comparing figs. 11–14 with 15–18, or by looking at the diagrams in figs. 5, 6 and 7). Presumably, each one of the three amino acids was taken up into the same newly-synthesized proteins.[1]

### Sites of protein synthesis

By seven though not by five minutes after leucine-H³ injection, many structures were radioactive (fig. 1) and had, therefore, just been the site of synthesis of labeled protein. Briefly, these sites were the nucleus and perikaryon of all neurons, including the base of large dendrites (fig. 3). Neither the axon hillock (fig. 1) nor the axon proper (figs. 8, 34, 36) gave evidence of protein synthesis.

In view of the prominent role of RNA in protein synthesis, it is of interest that RNA has been observed in the nucleus and perikaryon of neurons and glial cells as well as in large dendrites, but not in axon hillock nor in axons proper (M. Amano, private communication). Hence, the distribution of RNA corresponds to the sites of protein synthesis.

Though previous authors did not sacrifice their animals as early after injection of labeled amino acid as we did, our results are in agreement with their conclusion that proteins are being synthesized continuously in the cell body of neurons and neuroglia (Cohn et al., '54; Fisher et al., '56; Flanigan et al., '57; Leblond et al., '57; Oehlert and Schultze, '57; Koenig, '58a; Droz and Verne, '59).

### Fate of newly-formed cellular proteins

From four hours after injection of a labeled amino acid on, the concentration of labeled protein decreased in neurons (figs. 5–7). The rate of decay was such as to suggest that two newly-synthesized proteins — or at least two classes of such proteins — were present, one turning over in about a day and the other in about two weeks (table 2). The cells of thyroid gland (Nadler et al., '60) and pancreas (Warshawsky et al., '63) and the visual cells of the retina (Droz, '63) also contained two classes of proteins: "export-able" ones (such as thyroglobulin, pancreatic enzymes, and opsin, respectively) which rapidly migrate away from their site of synthesis, and "sedentary" ones which turn over slowly within the cell. On this basis, it was felt that in neurons too, the protein with a one-day life might be an "exportable" one leaving the perikaryon, whereas the protein with a two-week life might be a "sedentary" one.

### Axonal migration

Radioactive proteins were found in the axon hillock within the hour following labeled amino acid injection (figs. 2, 4) and in neighboring axons by 12 hours (semilunar ganglion, fig. 28). Furthermore, the axons of ventral horn cells in the spinal cord contained radioactive proteins at the end of the first postinjection day (figs. 31–33). Since no protein was synthesized in axons, it must be concluded that the labeled protein arising in a given cell body had migrated into its own axon and indeed had done so within the day after leucine-H³ injection. This evidence supports the suggestion that the cellular material with a mean life of about a day was an "exportable" protein.

With time, migration of labeled protein in the axon away from the cell body continued. In young rats injected with leucine-H³, the labeled proteins which had been seen at the 1-day interval in the axons emerging from ventral horn cells were traced at 2 days along the ventral root, at 3 and 4 days in the lumbar plexus, and at 16 days about 20 mm farther on (fig. 10), that is, almost at the back of the knee (Droz and Leblond, '62).

The appearance of labeled proteins in axons was seen in many parts of the nervous system (figs. 34, 35). Even when the radioactivity of individual axons was not distinguishable, migration of proteins from cell bodies down the length of axons could be implied. Thus, the successive presence of radioactivity in the pyramidal cells of the hippocampus (fig. 19), alveus (fig. 20) and fimbria (fig. 22) indicated passage of

---

[1] In each experiment the amount of radiation absorbed by nervous tissue remained below the threshold at which radiation damage occurs in nerve cells (Zeman, '61). Indeed, all animals appeared healthy, even the young rats given 30 μc leucine-H³ per gm body weight in Expt. VII, since they gained weight at the rate of 5 g per day during the experiment, that is, at the usual rate in our colony.

labeled protein from the cell bodies into the axons which occupy the alveus and farther on the fimbria. (The proteins appearing in the white matter of the cerebellum (fig. 14) may be in the axons of Purkinje cells or in those of afferent fibers.)

In the *adult rat*, migration was slower, since the labeled protein had not progressed beyond the branches of the lumbar plexus at 16 days. Rough estimates indicated that the migration rate was approximately twice as rapid in young (about 1.5 mm per day) as in adult rats (about 0.8 mm per day).

### Significance of axonal migration

The results of this investigation provide what is believed to be the first direct proof of the "axonal flow" theory. *It is now clear that the continuous migration of protein from nerve cell bodies into axons and down the length of the axons is a general phenomenon, which occurs in central and peripheral neurons of young and adult animals.*

The proteins migrating in axons may be free in the axoplasm, present in some cell organelles (vesicles, mitochondria) or in all components of the axoplasm. The fine location of the labeled protein is not shown by the data. Neither is it known whether the movement is due to the peristaltic contractions of nerve fibers observed in young mouse ganglia explanted with their nerves (Weiss et al., '62).

Evidence of protein migration in axons was obtained not only in young, but also in adult mice (figs. 23–30) and in 250-g female rats (figs. 31–33). On repeated weighing of these adult animals before and after injection, it was conclusively shown that they were not gaining weight. Presumably, they were in "steady state" with regard to axonal proteins. Consequently, those proteins which enter the axons must have replaced proteins that were somehow lost. A simple explanation is that axonal proteins break down under the influence of proteolytic enzymes. Indeed, such enzymes have been found to be present in brain tissue: cathepsin (Kies and Schimmer, '42; Ansell and Richter, '54), peptidases (Hanson and Tendis, '55) and dipeptidase (Pope, '59). Since the dipeptidase activity appears to be located in nerve cell bodies of neurons and glial cells (Pope, '59), this enzyme might account for the turnover of the sedentary protein in cell bodies. Other enzymes would be responsible for the catabolism of the exportable protein in axons.

In the case of rapidly growing rats, such as those weighing 45 g, the body weight of which had nearly doubled 8 days after injection and nearly tripled after 16 days, there was a lengthening of nerve fibers (by about 6.5 mm in the sciatic nerve) as well as an increase in their diameter (visible by comparing figs. 8 and 9 or 36 and 37). Hence the migrating proteins might have been used not only for renewal, but also for growth. This dual requirement may explain the more rapid rate of axonal migration in young as compared with adult animals. Nevertheless, an essential feature of the protein migration appears to be the replacement of preexisting axonal proteins. The nerve cell body which supplies the necessary material for renewal of axonal proteins may thus carry out "the trophic function" (Bodian, '62) recognized long ago by physiologists.

### SUMMARY

The dynamic condition of proteins in nerve cells and processes was examined in the central nervous system and peripheral nerves of growing and adult rats and mice. The animals received single or multiple injections of labeled amino acids (methionine-$S^{35}$, leucine- or arginine-$H^3$) and were sacrificed at various time intervals up to 30 days thereafter. Since immediately after injection of a labeled amino acid, the label appears in proteins undergoing synthesis, sections of brain, spinal cord, semilunar ganglion and sciatic nerve were radioautographed for detection of any protein so labeled.

Within minutes after injection of any one of the amino acids used, a radioautographic reaction appears over the nucleus and perikaryon (including the base of large dendrites), but not over the axon hillock nor over the axon proper of central and ganglionic neurons. It is concluded that protein is synthesized in the nucleus and perikaryon, including the base of large dendrites, but probably not in dendritic arborizations and certainly not in axon hillock or in central and peripheral axons.

The radioactivity of the perikaryon eventually decreases. Analysis of the decay suggests that it consists of two categories of proteins. One is probably a slowly turning over protein, referred to as "sedentary," which is presumably catabolized in situ, the other a rapidly turning over protein, referred to as "exportable," which is presumed to migrate into cell processes.

Shortly after labeled proteins appear in cell bodies, they may be detected in the axon hillock, and later still in the axon proper. Such protein migration occurs in central and peripheral axons. Labeled proteins may be traced from the ventral horn neurons of the lumbar spinal cord into the sciatic nerve in rats weighing 45 g. One day after injection, the labeled protein is in the axons as they cross the white matter and enter the ventral root; at 2 days, it is well in the ventral root, at 4 days at the junction of the $L_5$ and $L_6$ roots of the lumbar plexus, and at 16 days about 20 mm more distal in the sciatic nerve (approximately behind the knee). The rate of migration is of the order of 1.5 mm per day.

In full grown rats, a similar sequence takes place but at a slower rate, circa 0.8 mm per day.

It is suggested that the proteins migrating from the perikaryon along the axon replace proteins broken down in the axoplasm.

ACKNOWLEDGMENTS

This work was done with the support of a Block Term grant of the Medical Research Council of Canada. The authors are much indebted to Drs. N. J. Nadler for the mathematical interpretation and Y. Clermont for general suggestions, Dr. Beatrix M. Kopriwa for assistance with the radioautographic work, Dr. P. Pinheiro and Mr. H. Warshawsky for providing material, Miss Ritha Paradis for help with the histological work, Mr. J. Burton and Mr. D. Wright for counting grains in radioautographs.

LITERATURE CITED

Ansell, G. B., and D. Richter 1954 The proteolytic activity of brain tissue. Biochim. Biophys. Acta, 13: 87–89.

Appel, K. R., E. Appel and W. Maurer 1960 Konzentration und Austauschrate des freien Methionins im Gehirn der Ratte. Bioch. Zschr., 332: 293–306.

Bodian, D. 1962 The generalized vertebrate neuron. Science, 137: 323–326.

Borsook, H., C. L. Deasy, A. J. Haagen-Smit, G. Keighley and P. H. Lowy 1950 Metabolism of C14-labeled glycine, L-histidine, L-leucine and L-lysine. J. Biol. Chem., 187: 839–848.

Cohn, P., M. K. Gaitonde and D. Richter 1954 The localization of protein formation in the rat brain. J. Physiol., 126: 7P.

Droz, B. 1963 Dynamic condition of proteins in the visual cells as shown by radioautography with labeled amino acids. Anat. Rec., 145: 157–167.

Droz, B., and C. P. Leblond 1962 Migration of proteins along the axons of the sciatic nerve. Science, 137: 1047–1048.

Droz, B., and J. Verne 1959 Incorporation du 35S de la méthionine radio-marquée dans les cellules ganglionnaires végétatives in vivo et in vitro. Acta Neurovegetativa, 20: 372–384.

Droz, B., and H. Warshawsky 1963 Reliability of the radioautographic technique for the detection of newly synthesized protein. J. Histochem. Cytochem., 11: 426–435.

Fisher, J., J. Kalousek and Z. Lodin 1956 Incorporation of methionine (Sulphur-35) into the central nervous system. Nature, 178: 1122–1123.

Flanigan, S., E. R. Gabrielli and P. D. MacLean 1957 Cerebral changes revealed by radioautography with S35-labeled L-methionine. Arch. Neurol. Psych., 77: 588–594.

Francis, G. E., W. Mulligan and A. Wormall 1959 Isotopic tracers. The Athlone Press, London.

Friedberg, F., H. Tarver and D. M. Greenberg 1948 The distribution pattern of sulphur-labeled methionine in the protein and the amino acid fractions of tissues after intravenous administration. J. Biol. Chem., 173: 355–361.

Friede, R. 1959 Transport of oxidative enzymes in nerve fibers, a histochemical investigation of the regenerative cycle in neurons. Exp. Neurol., 1: 441–446.

Gaitonde, M. K., and D. Richter 1956 The metabolic activity of the proteins of the brain. Proc. Roy. Soc. B, 145: 83–99.

Hanson, H., and N. Tendis 1955 Darstellung von Zellbestandteil-Präparationen aus Hirngewebe und ihre Peptidase-Aktivität im Vergleich zu Niere und Leber. Zschr. ges. inn. Med., 9: 224–232.

Hebb, C. O., and G. Waites 1956 Choline acetylase in antero- and retrograde degeneration of a cholinergic nerve. J. Physiol., 132: 667–671.

Kies, M. W., and S. Schwimmer 1942 Observations on proteinase in brain. J. Biol. Chem., 145: 685–691.

Koenig, E., and G. B. Koelle 1960 Acetylcholinesterase regeneration in peripheral nerve after irreversible inactivation. Science, 132: 1249–1250.

Koenig, H. 1958a An autoradiographic study of nucleic acid and protein turnover in the mammalian neuraxis. J. Biophys. Biochem. Cytol., 4: 785–792.

———— 1958b The synthesis and peripheral flow of axoplasm. Trans. Am. Neurol. Assoc., pp. 162–164.

Kopriwa, B. M., and C. P. Leblond 1962 Improvements in the coating technique of radioautography. J. Histochem. Cytochem., 10: 269–284.

Lajtha, A., S. Furst and H. Waelsch 1957 The metabolism of the proteins of the brain. Experientia, 13: 168–172.

Leblond, C. P., N. B. Everett and B. Simmons 1957 Sites of protein synthesis as shown by radioautography after administration of S35-labeled methionine. Am. J. Anat., 101: 225–256.

Miani, N. 1960 Proximodistal movement along the axon of protein synthesized in the perikaryon of regenerating neurons. Nature, 185: 541.

Nadler, N. J., C. P. Leblond and J. Carneiro 1960 Site of formation of thyroglobulin in the mouse thyroid as shown by radioautography with leucine-H3. Proc. Soc. Exp. Biol. Med., 105: 38–41.

Oehlert, W., B. Schultze and W. Maurer 1958 Autoradiographische Untersuchung der Grösse des Eiweissstoffwechsels der verschiedenen Zellen des Zentralnervensystems. Beitr. pathol. Anat., 119: 343–376.

Ochs, S., and E. Burger 1958 Movement of substance proximo-distally in nerve axons as studied with spinal cord injections of radioactive phosphorus. Am. J. Physiol., 194: 499–506.

Ochs, S., D. Dalrumple and G. Richards 1962 Axoplasmic flow in ventral root nerve fibers of the cat. Exp. Neurol., 5: 349–363.

Palladin, A. V. 1957 The use of radioisotopes in the study of protein, nucleic acid and glycogen metabolism in the brain and the peripheral nerves. Internat. Conf. Radioisotopes in Scient. Res. UNESCO, RIC 166; Pergamon Press, London.

Pope, A. 1959 The intralaminar distribution of dipeptidase activity in human frontal isocortex. J. Neurochem., 4: 31–41.

Samuels, A. J., L. L. Boyarsky, R. W. Gerard, B. Libet and M. Brust 1951 Distribution, exchange and migration of phosphate compounds in the nervous system. Am. J. Physiol., 164: 1–15.

Sawyer, C. H. 1946 Cholinesterases in degenerating and regenerating peripheral nerves. Am. J. Physiol., 146: 246–253.

Scharrer, E., and B. Scharrer 1954 Neurosekretion. In: Handbuch der mikroskopischen Anatomie des Menschen. W. von Möllendorf and W. Bargmann. Springer Verlag, Berlin, p. 953–1066.

Schultze, B., and W. Oehlert 1958 Autoradiographische Untersuchungen des Eiweissstoffwechsels in den Zellen des Zentralnervensystems des Kaninchens und des Ratte. Strahlentherapie, 38: 68–80.

Verne, J., and B. Droz 1960 Déplacement de la radioactivité dans le ganglion cervical supérieur après injection de 35S-méthionine. Experientia, 16: 77–78.

Vladimirov, G. E. 1957 The renewal of amino acids in brain proteins. Internat. Conf. Radioisotopes in Scient. Res. UNESCO, RIC 167b; Pergamon Press, London.

Waelsch, H. 1958 Some problems of metabolism in relation to the structure of the nervous system. Proc. IVth Internat. Congr. Biochem., Vienna; IN: Biochemistry of the Central Nervous System, Pergamon Press, London, pp. 36-45.

Warshawsky, H., C. P. Leblond and B. Droz 1963 Synthesis and migration of proteins in the cells of the exocrine pancreas as revealed by specific activity determinations from radioautographs. J. Cell Biol., 16: 1–24.

Weiss, P. 1960 The concept of perpetual neuronal growth and proximo-distal substance connection. IVth Internat. Neurochem. Symp., Pergamon Press, London, pp. 220–242.

Weiss, P., and H. B. Hiscoe 1948 Experiments on the mechanism of nerve growth. J. Exp. Zool., 107: 315–396.

Weiss, P., A. L. Taylor and P. A. Pillai 1962 The nerve fiber as a system in continuous flow: microcinematographic and electronmicroscopic demonstration. Science, 136: 330.

Zeman, W. 1961 Radiosensitivities of nervous tissues. In: Fundamental Aspects of Radiosensitivity, Brookhaven Symp, in Biol., 14: 176–199.

Zilversmit, D. B., C. Entenman, M. C. Fishler and I. C. Chaikoff 1943 The turnover rate of phospholipids in the plasma of the dog as measured with radioactive phosphorus. J. Gen. Physiol., 26: 333–360.

447

PLATE 1

EXPLANATION OF FIGURES

Figs. 11–14   Unstained radioautographs of *cerebellum* of 45-g rats injected with leucine-H³ and sacrificed at various time intervals thereafter (*Experiment VII*).  × 30.

11   Thirty minutes after injection of a single dose, the radioautographic reaction is intense over Purkinje cells (P) and moderate over granular layer cells (G). In the molecular layer (M) and in the white matter (W) the discrete reaction is due to scattered oligodendrocytes or neurons.

12   At 1.1 days after the first of a series of multiple injections, a strong radioautographic reaction persists over Purkinje and granular layer cells. The molecular layer is covered with silver grains showing a gradient decreasing from the base of this layer towards the periphery.

13   At the four-day interval, the radioautographic reaction has declined over Purkinje and granular layer cells, whereas the molecular layer shows a fairly intense and homogeneous reaction. At this time, a diffuse radioautographic reaction appears over the white matter.

14   At the 16-day interval, the radioautographic reaction is still fairly intense over the molecular layer and reaches a maximum over the white matter. Note the difference with figure 11.

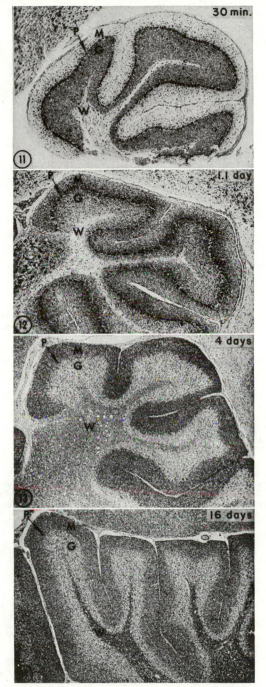

Figs. 15–18 Unstained radioautographs of cerebellum of mice injected with a single dose of methionine-S$^{35}$ and sacrificed at various time intervals thereafter (*Experiment VI*). $\times$ 14.

M: molecular layer; P: Purkinje cell layer; G: granular layer; W: white matter; Ch: choroid plexus.

The pattern of radioautographic changes with time is similar to that seen with leucine-H$^3$ in figures 11–14.

Figs. 19–22 Unstained radioautographs of hippocampus of 50-g rats injected with a single dose of methionine-S$^{35}$ and sacrificed at various time intervals thereafter (*Experiment V*). $\times$ 27.

19 At 30 minutes, the radioautographic reaction is intense over the nerve cell bodies of pyramidal cells (Am) and the cells of the fascia dentata (D). The reaction is rather weak over the alveus hippocampi (H) and over the stratum radiatum (R) which contain respectively the axons and the dendrites of the pyramidal cells. The weak reaction seen over these structures and over the fimbria is due mainly to glial cells.

20 At one day after injection, the radioautographic reaction is still strong over pyramidal cells (Am) and the cells of the fascia dentata (D), but now a moderate reaction is seen over the alveus hippocampi (H) and stratum radiatum (R), especially in the proximity of nerve cell bodies. At lower left, there is an intense radioautographic reaction over the choroid plexus (Ch).

21 At four days, the reaction has considerably decreased over pyramidal cells and the cells of the fascia dentata, but not over the alveus hippocampi. The fimbria (F) shows now an increased and diffuse radioautographic reaction.

22 At 17 days, the group of pyramidal cells (Am) and the cells of the fascia dentata (D) appear as light bands, whereas the radioautographic reaction is strong over the fimbria (F).

450

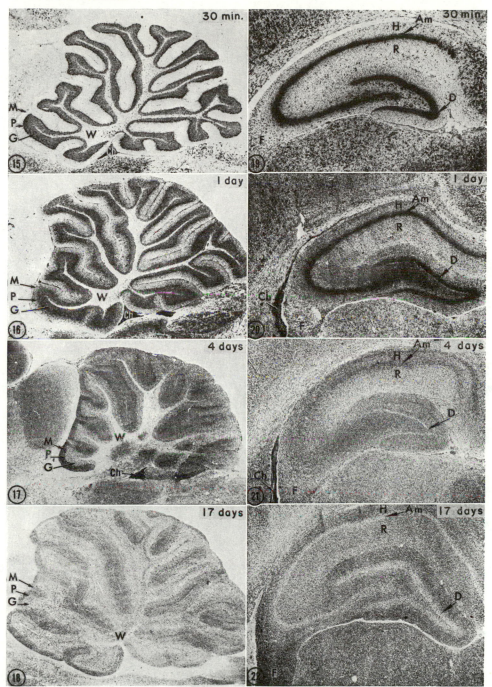

Figs. 23–26  Unstained radioautographs of the *spinal cord* of 25-g mice injected with a single dose of methionine-S[35] and sacrificed at various time intervals thereafter (*Experiment VI*). × 47.

23  At 30 minutes, the radioautographic reaction is intense over the nerve cell bodies (n) of the gray matter (G). The reaction is weak or doubtful over the neuropile, the white matter (W) and the dorsal root (D).

24  At 12 hours, the radioautographic reaction is still intense over the nerve cell bodies of the spinal cord (and of the spinal ganglia, SG). A diffuse reaction has now appeared over the neuropile of the gray matter, as well as over the dorsal root (D).
In the white matter, the discrete reaction is due to glial cells and blood vessels.

25  At one day, the radioautographic reaction of neurons has decreased. The reaction of dorsal (D) and ventral root (V) is moderate.

26  At four days, the radioautographic reaction is homogeneous over the gray matter.


Figs. 27–30  Unstained radioautographs of the *semilunar ganglion* of the trigeminal nerve of 25-g mice injected with a single dose of methionine-S[35] and sacrificed at various time intervals thereafter (*Experiment VI*). × 47.

27  At 30 minutes, an intense radioautographic reaction is seen over the neurons (n), while nerve fibers (f) are little or not reactive.

28  At 12 hours, the radioautographic reaction is still intense over neurons (n), and has considerably increased over nerve fibers (f).

29, 30  At one day and four days, the radioautographic reaction has considerably decreased over neurons and fibers.

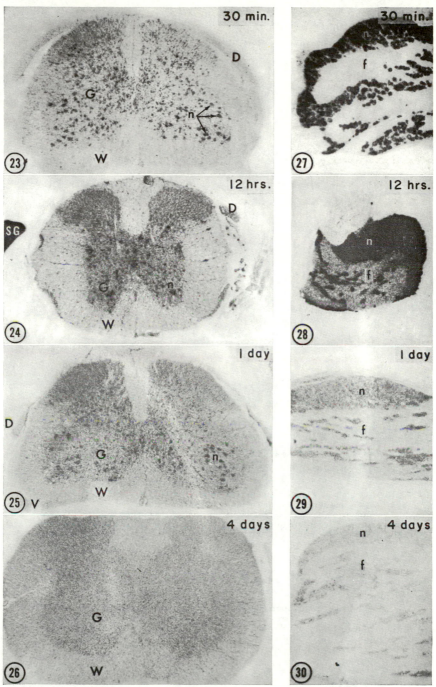

## PLATE 4

### EXPLANATION OF FIGURES

Figs. 31–33 Radioautographs of *spinal cord* of a 250-g rat sacrificed one day after the first of multiple injections of leucine-$H^3$ (*Experiment VIII*).

31 Unstained radioautograph showing at left the ventral horn of the gray matter (G) which contains strongly radioactive motor neurons appearing as black spots (n). In center, the white matter (W) is crossed from left to right by radioactive axons (a). The neuron at n seems to continue into an axon (indicated by the lower arrow a). × 100.

32 As in figure 31, with labeled axons (a) extending from the ventral horn of the gray matter (G), across the white matter (W) into the ventral root (V). The 3 arrows at right point to minute black dots which are axons in cross section. × 100.

33 Radioautograph stained with hematoxylin-eosin showing wavy labeled axons (oblique arrow a) coming from the ventral horn and going to the ventral root (V). Silver grains may be seen over individual axons in the ventral root (vertical arrows, a), while the axons seen in cross section in white matter are unlabeled (ua). × 340.

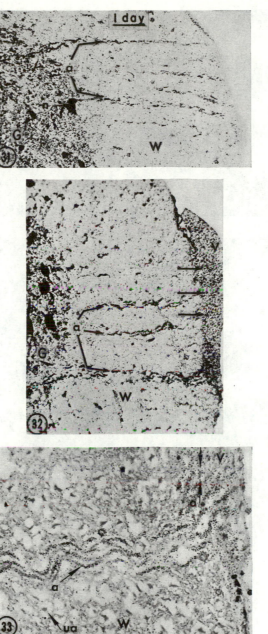

455

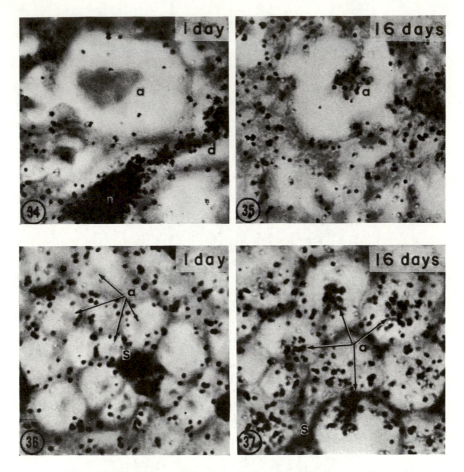

Figs. 34–37  Hematoxylin-eosin stained radioautographs at 1 day and 16 days after the first of multiple injections of leucine-$H^3$. Axons are indicated by the letter a.  $\times$ 1,500.

34–35   Medulla oblongata of the adult rat (*Experiment VIII*) showing axons in the nucleus reticularis medius. The pictures illustrate a large, unreactive axon at 1 day (fig. 34) and a reactive one at 16 days (fig. 35). At lower center in figure 34, a strongly reactive neuron (n) is continued by a reactive process believed to be a dendrite (d).

36–37   Sciatic nerve of 45-g rat (*Experiment VII*) observed at 20 mm from the junction of the $L_5$ and $L_6$ branches of the lumbar plexus ("distal" region, at about 26–28 mm from the spinal cord). The axons are unreactive at 1 day (fig. 36), but strongly reactive at 16 days (fig. 37). (Reactions are seen at both times over Schwann cell cytoplasm, s).

# PROXIMO–DISTAL TRANSPORT OF [¹⁴C]NOR-ADRENALINE AND PROTEIN IN SYMPATHETIC NERVES

B. G. LIVETT, L. B. GEFFEN and L. AUSTIN

Departments of Biochemistry and Physiology, Monash University, Clayton, Victoria, Australia

(*Received 6 February* 1968)

**Abstract**—Both [¹⁴C]noradrenaline and [¹⁴C]leucine were injected into the coeliac ganglia of cats in an attempt to label the noradrenaline and protein of the granular vesicles, so that their movement in the splenic nerves could be followed.

When a constriction was placed on the nerves, labelled noradrenaline and protein accumulated just proximal to it, but there was no such accumulation below it, nor above a second, more distal constriction placed on the same nerve. This indicated that a neural transport mechanism, rather than uptake from the circulation, was responsible for the accumulation.

Peaks of labelled noradrenaline and protein were observed to move down the axon at about 5 mm/hr. In addition a slow moving component of axonal protein, advancing at about 1 mm/day, was detected.

The results demonstrate a rapid proximo–distal movement of noradrenaline and protein which could represent the transport of granular synaptic vesicles from their site of manufacture in the cell body to their site of storage in the nerve terminals within the spleen.

MOST of the noradrenaline in sympathetic nerves is bound within granular vesicles (WOLFE, POTTER, RICHARDSON and AXELROD, 1962; POTTER, 1966; RICHARDSON, 1966; VAN ORDEN, BLOOM, BARRNETT and GIARMAN, 1966), which are concentrated in the axon terminals. VON EULER (1959) and DAHLSTRÖM (1965) have postulated that the granular vesicles are synthesized in the neuronal soma and transported down the axon by the process of axoplasmic flow, first demonstrated by WEISS and HISCOE (1948). Evidence in favour of this hypothesis is that an accumulation of noradrenaline above a nerve ligature can be detected by fluorescence microscopy (DAHLSTRÖM, 1965; KAPELLER and MAYOR, 1967), and by biochemical extraction (DAHLSTRÖM and HÄGGENDAL, 1967; GEFFEN and RUSH, 1968). The electron microscope demonstration of an accumulation of a variety of granular vesicles above a constriction on splenic nerves (KAPELLER and MAYOR, 1966; 1967) and the presence of similar structures near the Golgi apparatus of the perikaryon, provide additional morphological support.

Since the granular vesicles in sympathetic terminals contain, in addition to noradrenaline, small quantities of proteins (AUSTIN, CHUBB and LIVETT, 1967), it should be possible to demonstrate that protein flows along the axon at the same rate as noradrenaline. In the previous paper (GEFFEN and RUSH, 1968), the rate of flow of noradrenaline in the cat splenic nerve was calculated as 1·4–3·3 mm/hr. This rate, though of the same order as that found by DAHLSTRÖM and HÄGGENDAL (1966, 1967) for noradrenaline in sympathetic fibres within sciatic nerves, (3–10 mm/hr), is much faster than that commonly found for protein movement in somatic nerves (1–5 mm/day) (see LUBIŃSKA, 1964).

In the present experiments, radioactive isotopes have been injected into the coeliac ganglion of the cat in an attempt to preferentially label both the noradrenaline and the protein of the granular vesicles, and to follow their movement in the splenic nerves. A preliminary account of this work has been reported elsewhere (Livett, Geffen and Austin, 1968).

METHODS

The experimental procedure is shown schematically in Fig. 1.

*Operative procedures.* Adult cats weighing 3–4·5 kg were anaesthetized with ethylchloride and ether, 12 hrs after being given intraperitoneal injections of iproniazid (50 mg/kg) to minimize metabolic oxidation of the injected [¹⁴C]noradrenaline. The abdomen was opened by a midline incision and

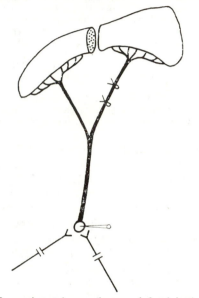

Fig. 1.—Diagram of experimental procedure used for injecting isotopes, showing sites of constriction of the nerves to the cat spleen. The splanchnic nerves, which supply the coeliac ganglion with its afferent supply were sectioned, as shown, and ligatures were placed on the major branch of the splenic nerves. Isotopes were injected directly into the coeliac ganglion with a microsyringe.

the left and right splanchnic nerves were divided close to the coeliac ganglion to prevent possible release of the isotopes by nerve impulses. The ganglion was then coated with silicone grease and, either [¹⁴C]noradrenaline (5–10 μC; 17·2 mc/m-mole), or [¹⁴C]leucine (5 μC; 305 mc/m-mole) (The Radiochemical Centre, Amersham) was injected beneath the capsule, using a microsyringe with an electrolytically polished steel needle of tip diameter 200 μ (Scientific-Glass Engineering, Melbourne). The isotope was injected in a total volume of 10–20 μl by two or three punctures of the ganglionic capsule through the silicone grease seal.

The splenic nerve fibres were dissected from the media of the main branch of the splenic artery, 4–8 cm from the coeliac ganglion and 2–4 cm from the hilum of the spleen. The major branch of the nerve was constricted at two points 1 cm apart, with fine silk thread against a glass rod, which was then removed and the tie on the nerves completed (Lubińska, 1959). The abdomen was then closed.

Six hours to 25 days later the abdomen was again opened under ether anaesthesia, and the splenic artery and nerves were dissected free by cutting all branches other than those going to the spleen. The artery was stripped of its adventitia and surrounding nerves at its bifurcation and cut. The cut ends of the vessel were retracted back through their sheaths by pulling on the intact proximal and distal ends of the artery. In this way, an artery free bundle of splenic nerves could be obtained for analysis, passing from the coeliac ganglion almost to the hilum of the spleen, a distance of up to 10 cm. The minor branch was combined with the corresponding portions of the major branch.

*Extraction and assay.* The excised nerves and ganglion were washed with saline, blotted, and placed on microscope slides chilled to 4°. The nerves were cut into 5 mm pieces and each weighed before either catecholamines or protein were extracted as follows (see Fig. 2)—

(a) *Catecholamines.* The tissue from animals injected with [$^{14}$C]noradrenaline was homogenized in 1 ml of ice cold 0·4 M-perchloric acid containing ethylenediamine tetraacetic acid (EDTA), 10 mg/ml., in a teflon-glass homogenizer, (AUSTIN, CHUBB and LIVETT, 1967). The homogenate was then transferred to a centrifuge tube, and the precipitated protein spun down and washed once with 0·5 ml

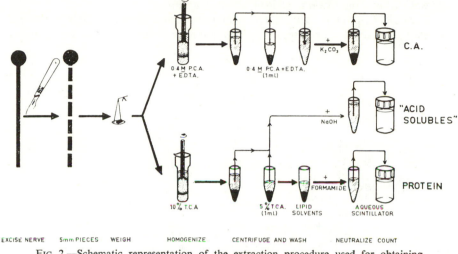

EXCISE NERVE   5mm PIECES   WEIGH        HOMOGENIZE     CENTRIFUGE AND WASH      NEUTRALIZE COUNT

FIG. 2.—Schematic representation of the extraction procedure used for obtaining noradrenaline, protein and acid solubles.

of 0·4 M-perchloric acid. The supernatants were combined, neutralized with 5 M-K$_2$ CO$_3$, the potassium perchlorate which formed was removed by centrifugation, and a portion of the supernatant containing the catecholamines counted in 10 ml of scintillator fluid (BRUNO and CHRISTIAN, 1961), using a Packard Scintillation spectrometer.

(b) *Protein.* Ganglia and portions of nerve taken from cats injected with [$^{14}$C]leucine were homogenized in 10% trichloracetic acid (TCA). The precipitate obtained after centrifuging the homogenate was washed once with 5% TCA, twice in ethanol–ether (1:2, v/v), twice in chloroform–methanol–water (38:19:3, by vol.), and then once with ether to remove lipids. The TCA extracts were combined, neutralized with 5 M-K$_2$ CO$_3$ and counted for free leucine and any other acid soluble metabolites. The lipid free proteins were dissolved in formamide and a portion counted, as above, for incorporation of [$^{14}$C]leucine. A portion was also taken for protein estimation by the method of LOWRY, ROSEBROUGH, FARR and RANDALL (1951).

Tissue from the spleen was treated in a similar manner except that it was homogenized in ice cold 1 M-K$_3$ PO$_4$ buffer, pH 6·5 before addition of TCA or perchloric acid–EDTA to make final concentrations of 10% and 0·4 M, respectively.

*Chromatography.* In some experiments samples of nerve and spleen were analysed to determine the distribution of tissue radioactivity amongst noradrenaline and its various metabolites (SJÖQVIST, TAYLOR and TITUS, 1967). After chromatography of extracts on Whatman P20 cellulose phosphate paper, the catecholamines were detected by the use of either potassium ferricyanide or ethylenediamine-NH$_3$ stains (UDENFRIEND, 1962). Strips were cut 0·9 cm wide, and counted in 5 ml of scintillator fluid.

*Quenching.* All samples were corrected for quenching by adding [$^{14}$C]acetate of known activity to the vials. The counting efficiency in this system was within the range 59–72 per cent, depending on the amount of protein present and the pH of the supernatants.

*Measurement of nerve lengths.* Calculation of the flow rate is subject to errors in measurement as follows. The distance of the site of constriction from the ganglion is subject to an error of up to 5 mm due both to difficulty in determining precisely the point of exit of the splenic nerves from the ganglion and to stretching of the nerves during their measurement. The distances given in the figures are measured *in situ*, and are the minimum distances travelled by the isotope.

RESULTS

(a) *Noradrenaline.* In some experiments, the tissues were removed from the animals 16–24 hr after injection of the isotopes, and the spleen was cut into two pieces. The portion of spleen supplied by the untied branch of the nerve contained 3–4 times as much [¹⁴C]noradrenaline as that supplied by the constricted branch (Table 1). The ganglion still contained large amounts of radioactivity (91·3 dis./min/ mg wet wt.) and the blood contained 380 dis./min/ml.

Chromatography of extracts containing the catecholamines from the coeliac ganglion, splenic nerves and spleen showed that noradrenaline was the main source of

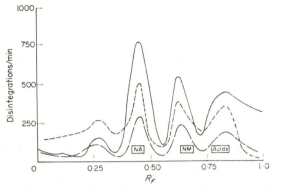

FIG. 3.—Distribution of radioactivity among noradrenaline and its metabolites. Extracts containing the catecholamines from the coeliac ganglion (—), splenic nerve (– – – – –) and spleen (— —) were chromatographed together with 0·5 μmoles each of carrier noradrenaline, (NA); normetanephrine, (NM); and 3,4 dihydroxy mandelic acid and 3-methoxy, 4-hydroxy mandelic acid (acids).
The chromatogram was developed in a solvent containing a mixture of 2 parts of 0·2 M-ammonium acetate pH 6·5 and one part of *n*-propanol for 20 hr at 20° (see Sjöqvist *et al.*, 1967).

the radioactivity, the rest being mostly normetanephrine and acid metabolites (Fig. 3). The splenic nerves were also removed after 16 hr, and when analysed for catecholamines it was found that [¹⁴C]noradrenaline accumulated just proximal to the upper constriction, a distance of 8 cm from the coeliac ganglion. However, there was no such accumulation above the lower constriction (Fig. 4a). Similar results were obtained from the nerves taken out after 24 hr (Fig. 4b).

When the nerves were taken out after a shorter period of time, 6 hr, it was possible to locate a peak of [¹⁴C]noradrenaline before it reached the constriction (Fig. 5). The peak of radioactivity, at a distance of approximately 3 cm away from the ganglion, indicates that the labelled noradrenaline has been transported down the nerve at a rate of about 5 mm/hr. The results obtained for the content of [¹⁴C]noradrenaline in the two portions of spleen removed after 6 hr, show no difference between the constricted and the normally innervated portions (Table 1).

(b) *Protein.* If [¹⁴C]leucine was injected into the ganglion, and time was allowed for the labelled protein to reach the nerve constriction, accumulation of [¹⁴C]protein could be observed above the upper but not the lower constriction (Fig. 6a).

In short term experiments (6 hr) a peak of labelled protein, moving at about 5 mm/hr was observed before it reached the constriction (Fig. 6b). There was no

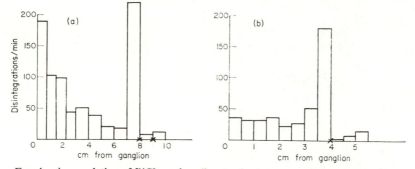

FIG. 4.—Accumulation of [¹⁴C]noradrenaline proximal to a constriction on the splenic nerves. The distribution of radioactivity in the splenic nerves 16 hr (a) and 24 hr (b) after injection of the isotope into the coeliac ganglion. The positions of the ligatures are shown (X).

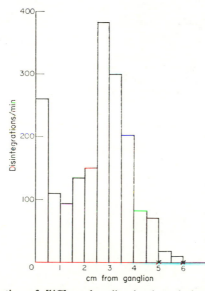

FIG. 5.—Distribution of [¹⁴C]noradrenaline in the splenic nerves after 6 hr. The positions of the nerve ligatures are marked (X).

TABLE 1.—CONTENT OF [¹⁴C]NORADRENALINE IN THE CAT SPLEEN

| Time (hr) | Portion of spleen | dis./min | Mass of tissue (g) | dis./min |
|---|---|---|---|---|
| 6 | Supplied by constricted nerves | 1820 | 10·83 | 169 |
| | Supplied by unconstricted nerves | 1057 | 6·44 | 164 |
| 16 | Supplied by constricted nerves | 2100 | 11·52 | 183 |
| | Supplied by unconstricted nerves | 5820 | 9·82 | 641 |
| 24 | Supplied by constricted nerves | 10920 | 11·94 | 916 |
| | Supplied by unconstricted nerves | 9350 | 3·62 | 2660 |

[¹⁴C]noradrenaline was injected into the coeliac ganglion, the major branch of the splenic nerves was constricted and, at the time specified, the spleen was removed in two portions.

461

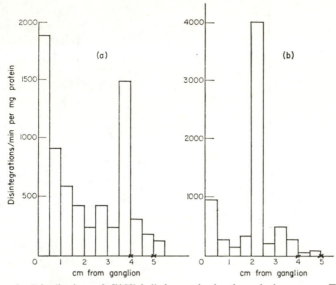

FIG. 6.—Distribution of [¹⁴C]labelled protein in the splenic nerves. The radio-activity in nerve proteins 6·5 hr (a) and 6 hr (b) after the injection of [¹⁴C]leucine into the coeliac ganglion is shown in two separate experiments. The positions of the nerve ligatures are marked (X).

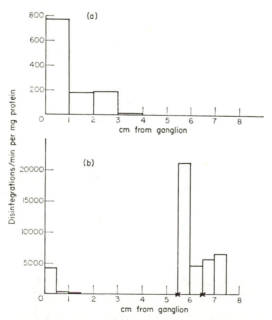

FIG. 7.—Distribution of protein labelled by injection of [¹⁴C]leucine in (a) unconstricted splenic nerves after 25 days, and (b), in the presence of nerve ligatures (X) after 15 days. In (b) regenerated nerve tissue had bypassed the constrictions.

significant accumulation of free leucine at the constriction and, except for the first half cm of nerve and the ganglion (5000 dis./min/mg protein), the concentration of free leucine in the splenic nerves (50–190 dis./min/mg protein) was less than 10 per cent of that incorporated into protein.

When animals had been injected with [$^{14}$C]leucine 15–25 days previously, and the splenic nerves had not been constricted, the pattern of incorporation was that shown in Fig. 7a. Since the counts were significant only in the first 3 cm of nerve, this suggests that some of the amino acid was incorporated into a slow moving protein component, which advanced as a front at a rate of about 1 mm/day. The specific activity of this slow moving protein was less than one-tenth of that found for the fast moving peak, being of the same order as the counts in the acid soluble fraction. For these long term experiments the splanchnic input to the coeliac ganglion was left intact in order not to interfere with the innervation of other viscera.

In another experiment in which the nerves had been ligated 15 days previously, it was observed that nerves had regenerated beyond the constricting ligatures, and that [$^{14}$C]leucine had been incorporated into this newly formed protein as well as into that of the slow moving fraction (Fig. 7b).

## DISCUSSION

The results demonstrate a rapid proximo–distal transport of noradrenaline and protein in the splenic nerves of the cat, supporting the hypothesis that granular vesicles containing noradrenaline are transported from the ganglion, along the post-ganglionic sympathetic axons to their terminals within the spleen.

Isotopically labelled noradrenaline and leucine were injected into the coeliac ganglion in an attempt to label both the noradrenaline and the protein of the granular vesicles, so that their movement in the splenic nerves could be followed. One of the assumptions that is made in calculating the flow rate for noradrenaline in experiments where the accumulation of fluorescence above a nerve constriction is measured (DAHLSTRÖM and HÄGGENDAL, 1966), is that no noradrenaline is synthesized by the granular vesicles in their movement down the axon. However, previous work in this and other laboratories, (AUSTIN, LIVETT and CHUBB, 1967; STJÄRNE, ROTH and LISHAJKO, 1967) has shown that the granular vesicles contain, as one of their proteins dopamine-$\beta$-hydroxylase. It is conceivable that some of the noradrenaline which accumulates above a nerve constriction is synthesized by the granular vesicles as they pass down the axon. The use of [$^{14}$C]noradrenaline in the present experiments overcomes this difficulty, while the injection of [$^{14}$C]leucine permitted the measurement of the rate of protein movement in the same system.

Both [$^{14}$C]noradrenaline and [$^{14}$C]protein accumulated above a constriction on the nerves but not below it, nor around a second, more distal tie placed at the same time as the first. This suggests that the accumulation was due to a peripherally directed neural transport of labelled isotope, rather than uptake at the constriction of isotope which had escaped into the circulation. The finding in short term experiments that peaks of radioactive noradrenaline and protein could be detected before they reached the constriction reinforces this conclusion. In the more chronic experiments, [$^{14}$C]-leucine was incorporated both into a slow moving protein component, which advanced distally from the ganglion at a rate of about 1 mm/day, and into newly formed regenerating nerve tissue, which grew peripherally from the site of a constriction.

When time was allowed for the [$^{14}$C]noradrenaline to reach the terminals in the spleen, the portion of spleen innervated by the constricted branch of the nerves contained much less [$^{14}$C]noradrenaline than the normally innervated portion. Nevertheless, the quantitative contribution of the labelled noradrenaline to the stores in the normal portion of the spleen was very low, which confirms the evidence of Geffen and Rush (1968).

The possibility that the isotopes diffused down endoneural spaces or blood vessels between the axons is made unlikely both by the distribution of radioactivity along the nerves, which is not an exponential decline from the ganglion, but is peaked, and by the failure to detect significant amounts of free [$^{14}$C]leucine in the nerves. In support of this, experiments aimed at the localization within nerves of labelled noradrenaline given intravenously, using electron microscopic autoradiography (Taxi and Droz, 1967), did not detect significant amounts of noradrenaline accumulating outside of the axons, unlike compounds for which no such selective uptake mechanism by nerve tissue exists, such as $^{24}$NaCl, $^{64}$CuCl$_2$ and various coloured dyes, which flow along a diffusion gradient in the endoneural fluid (Weiss, Wang, Taylor and Edds, 1945).

The rate of flow for [$^{14}$C]noradrenaline and [$^{14}$C]protein in the splenic nerves of 5 mm/hr, obtained in the present experiments is slightly greater than that calculated by Geffen and Rush (1968), for the movement of noradrenaline in the decentralized splenic nerves in the cat. This difference could be ascribed to our use of a monoamine oxidase inhibitor to reduce metabolic oxidation of noradrenaline. On the other hand, it is considerably in excess of the rate commonly found for protein movement in somatic nerves of 1–5 mm/day (Lubińska, 1964). Our finding of a second component of protein movement, advancing as a front at a similar rate of 1 mm/day probably reflects the outgrowth of structural proteins, such as those comprising the neurofilaments and axolemma, while the faster rate we report of 5 mm/hr could be that of the transport of soluble proteins and cytoplasmic structures, such as the granular vesicles, to the nerve terminals. Recently Grafstein (1967) has reported two different rates of protein transport in goldfish optic nerves.

Noradrenaline occurs throughout the whole neuron and its synthesis takes place both within ganglia and nerve fibres (Goodall and Kirshner, 1958; Stjärne et al., 1967) and within the nerve terminals (see Udenfriend, 1966). Recently evidence from fluorescence microscopy of cultures of fetal sympathetic neurons indicates that noradrenaline appears in the nerve terminals before it can be detected in the cell bodies (Sano, Odake and Yonezawa, 1967). Noradrenaline synthesis in the nerve terminals depends upon a continual supply both of the enzymes involved in its synthesis, and the proteins which bind and sequestrate the transmitter. These enzymes and proteins are probably synthesized in the cell body, where large amounts of RNA exist (Hydén, 1960), although the possibility that some may be made by a separate protein synthesizing system within the axon (Koenig, 1967; Morgan and Austin, 1968) cannot be discounted. The fast flow of protein which we report could function to provide the nerve terminals with the enzymes and other proteins required for the local synthesis and storage of the transmitter.

The question arises concerning the fate of the granular vesicles once they have reached the nerve terminals. The calculations of Dahlström and Häggendal (1967) and Geffen and Rush (1968), suggest they have a life of up to 100 days, and that they exchange their noradrenaline content repeatedly. In the adrenal medulla, release of the protein that binds catecholamine within the storage granules has been demonstrated to accompany the release of catecholamines (BLASCHKO, COMLINE, SCHNEIDER, SILVER and SMITH, 1967) and it remains to be shown whether a similar process, possibly of reverse pinocytosis of the contents of the granular vesicles, accompanies the release of noradrenaline from sympathetic nerves. The method employed in the present experiments may label the vesicular protein in a sufficiently preferential manner to examine this problem.

*Acknowledgements*—We thank Mr. R. A. RUSH for his assistance and Miss D. HARRISON for the preparation of the figures.
This work was supported by grants from the National Heart Foundation of Australia.

## REFERENCES

AUSTIN L., CHUBB I. W. and LIVETT B. G. (1967) *J. Neurochem.* **14**, 473.
AUSTIN L., LIVETT B. G. and CHUBB I. W. (1967) *Circulat. Res.* (11, Suppl III, 111.).
BLASCHKO H., COMLINE R. S., SCHNEIDER F. H., SILVER M. and SMITH A. D. (1967) *Nature (Lond.)* **215**, 58.
BRUNO G. A. and CHRISTIAN J. E. (1961) *Analyt. Chem.* **33**, 1216.
DAHLSTRÖM A. (1965) *J. Anat. (Lond.)* **99**, 4.
DAHLSTRÖM A. and HÄGGENDAL J. (1966) *Acta physiol. scand.* **67**, 278.
DAHLSTRÖM A. and HÄGGENDAL J. (1967) *Acta physiol. scand.* **69**, 153.
EULER U. S. VON (1959) In *Handbook of Physiology*, Section I, Neurophysiology (Edited by FIELD J.) Vol. 1, p. 222. Waverley Press, Baltimore.
GEFFEN L. B. and RUSH R. A. (1968) *J. Neurochem* **15**, 925.
GOODALL MC. C. and KIRSHNER N. (1958) *Circulation* **17**, 366.
GRAFSTEIN B. (1967) *Science* **157**, 196.
HYDÉN H. (1960) The neuron, In *The Cell*, Vol. IV (Edited by BRACHET J. and MIRSKY A.) p. 215. Academic Press, New York–London.
KAPELLER K. and MAYOR D. (1966) *J. Anat. (Lond.)* **100**, 439.
KAPELLER K. and MAYOR D. (1967) *Proc. roy. Soc. B* **167**, 282.
KOENIG E. (1967) *J. Neurochem.* **14**, 437.
LIVETT B. G., GEFFEN L. B. and AUSTIN L. (1968) *Nature (Lond.)* **217**, 278.
LOWRY O. H., ROSEBROUGH N. J., FARR A. L. and RANDALL R. J. (1951) *J. biol. Chem.* **193**, 265.
LUBIŃSKA L. (1959) *J. comp. Neurol.* **113**, 315.
LUBIŃSKA L. (1964) *Progr. Brain. Res.* **13**, 1.
MORGAN I. G. and AUSTIN L. (1968) *J. Neurochem.* **15**, 41.
POTTER L T. (1966) *Pharmacol. Rev.* **18**, 439.
RICHARDSON K. C. (1966) *Nature (Lond.)* **210**, 756.
SANO Y., ODAKE G. and YONEZAWA T. (1967) *Z. Zellforsch.* **80**, 345.
SJÖQVIST F., TAYLOR P. W. and TITUS E. (1967) *Acta physiol. scand.* **69**, 13.
STJÄRNE L., ROTH R. H. and LISHAJKO F. (1967) *Biochem. Pharmacol* **16**, 1729.
TAXI J. and DROZ B. (1967) *C.R. Acad. Sci. (Paris)* Série D. **263**, 1237.
UDENFRIEND S. (1962) *Fluorescence Assay in Biology and Medicine*. Academic Press, New York.
UDENFRIEND S. (1966) *Harvey Lect.* Series 60, p. 57. Academic Press, New York.
VAN ORDEN III L. S., BLOOM F. E., BARRNETT R. J. and GIARMAN N. J. (1966) *J. Pharmacol. exp. Ther.* **154**, 185.
WEISS P. and HISCOE H. (1948) *J. exp. Zool.* **107**, 315.
WEISS P., WANG H., TAYLOR C. A. and EDDS M. V. (1945) *Amer. J. Physiol.* **143**, 521.
WOLFE D., POTTER L. T., RICHARDSON K. C. AXELROD J. (1962) *Science.* **138**, 440.

STUDIES ON
THE TRANSLOCATION OF NORADRENALINE-CONTAINING
VESICLES IN POST-GANGLIONIC SYMPATHETIC NEURONES
*IN VITRO.* INHIBITION OF MOVEMENT BY COLCHICINE
AND VINBLASTINE AND EVIDENCE FOR THE
INVOLVEMENT OF AXONAL MICROTUBULES

BY P. BANKS, D. MAYOR, MARY MITCHELL AND
D. TOMLINSON

*From the Department of Biochemistry and Department of
Human Biology and Anatomy, Sheffield University,
Sheffield S10 2TN*

(*Received 12 March 1971*)

SUMMARY

1. Methods are presented for studying axonal transport mechanisms in preparations of constricted hypogastric nerve/inferior mesenteric ganglia maintained *in vitro* for periods up to 48 hr. Under these conditions the ultrastructure of the tissue is excellently preserved.

2. The proximo-distal movement of noradrenaline and noradrenaline storage vesicles in the non-myelinated axons of these preparations is inhibited by both colchicine (10 $\mu$g/ml.) and vinblastine sulphate (1 $\mu$g/ml.) whilst the movement of mitochondria appears to be unaffected.

3. Neither colchicine nor vinblastine sulphate depletes accumulated dense-cored vesicles of their stores of noradrenaline.

4. These drugs reduce the accumulation of noradrenaline and dense-cored vesicles against a constriction when they are in contact with the nerve trunks only, and are denied direct access to the nerve cell bodies in the ganglion.

5. The only other morphological change that can be attributed to the action of colchicine and vinblastine is a marked reduction in the number of axonal microtubules.

6. The experiments provide strong support for the view that the axonal system of microtubules is closely involved in the proximo-distal movement of noradrenaline storage vesicles within noradrenergic neurones. The microtubular system does not appear to be involved in mitochondrial movement.

Reprinted from *The Journal of Physiology* 216: 625–639 (1971) by permission of the publisher.

## INTRODUCTION

In recent years it has become evident that dense-cored vesicles containing noradrenaline are formed in the cell bodies of noradrenergic neurones and are then transported along the axons towards the sites of transmitter release in the terminal autonomic network (Banks, Mangnall & Mayor, 1969; Dahlström, 1969). This paper describes methods that allow the proximo-distal movement of noradrenaline storage vesicles (dense-cored vesicles) along post-ganglionic sympathetic axons to be studied *in vitro*. Besides enabling the effects of various metabolic inhibitors on the translocation process to be examined in the absence of more generalized side effects encountered *in vivo*, these preparations also make possible experiments that could not be performed with living animals. The problem investigated in the present series of experiments concerns the role of the axonal microtubules (neurotubules) in the translocation of dense-cored vesicles and the site of action of the antimitotic drugs colchicine and vinblastine, which are known to inhibit the movement of these visicles *in vivo* (Dahlström, 1970; Hökfelt & Dahlström, 1971).

## METHODS

*Ganglion/nerve preparation.* The two hypogastric nerves from sixty cats of both sexes weighing 1·0–2·5 kg were used. Under intraperitoneal Nembutal anaesthesia, the hypogastric nerves were constricted 1·5–2·5 cm distal to the inferior mesenteric ganglion with fine silk ligatures; these were used to suspend the preparation *in vitro*. A similar ligature was placed on a group of preganglionic nerves. In some cases the colonic nerves were ligated 1–1·5 cm from the inferior mesenteric ganglion. The mesenteric and connective tissue was then dissected from the nerves and ganglion. The latter was frequently in several parts on either side of the inferior mesenteric artery. The ligated preganglionic nerves were cut proximal to their ligature, other preganglionic fibres were cut and the ganglion/ligated hypogastric nerve preparation was excised *en bloc*. In those cases in which the ganglion was astride the artery, part of the vessel was included in the ganglionic mass. The preparation was then either suspended in a test-tube or placed in a specially designed two compartment Perspex box.

In all the experiments the ganglion/nerve preparations were maintained in Eagles Minimal Essential Medium (Eagle's Medium MEM, Wellcome Research Laboratories, Beckenham, Kent) without added calf serum and containing the following antibiotics: penicillin (100 u./ml.); streptomycin (100 $\mu$g/ml.); polymixin (100 u./ml.) and nystatin (25 u./ml.).

*Incubation in test-tubes.* In these experiments the ganglion/nerve preparations were maintained at 37° C in large test-tubes (Text-fig. 1) containing Eagle's medium and gassed with 95% $O_2 + 5\%$ $CO_2$ saturated with $H_2O$ by passage through Krebs bicarbonate saline at 37° C. In some experiments, after a 24 hr period of incubation, a second ligature was placed on the nerve trunks 0·5–1 cm proximal to the first ligature. The incubation was then continued for a further 24 hr.

*Incubations in two compartment boxes.* In some experiments it was desired to study the effects of colchicine and vinblastine on the axonal transport of noradrenaline when the drugs were in contact with the nerve trunks but were denied access to the neuronal cell bodies in the ganglion. For this purpose a two compartment box was designed which allowed the ganglion to be isolated from a substantial length of post-ganglionic nerve trunk by a water-tight partition (Text-fig. 2). In setting up the preparation, the lower half of the partition was placed in position after applying silicone grease (M 494 I.C.I. Ltd.) to the narrow surfaces. The upper partition was similarly greased and the 'half' holes on both partitions were filled with grease. The nerve trunks were then laid upon the grease in the lower 'half' hole and the upper part of the partition was placed in position on top of the lower part; the threads were then secured to the Perspex posts at each end of the box. The nerve trunk thus passed through a grease seal in the Perspex barrier. In all experiments 1 $\mu$c of [$^{14}$C]sodium acetate or [$^{14}$C]valine was added to the Eagle's medium on the ligated nerve trunk side of the preparation so that any leakage through

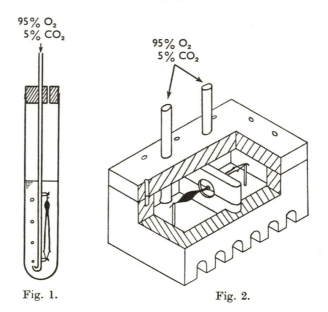

Fig. 1.                                        Fig. 2.

Text-fig. 1. Diagram of incubation test-tube. A single ganglion/nerve preparation was supported by silk threads tied to hooks attached to the gassing tube. The vessel contained 30 ml. Eagle's medium gassed with $O_2 + CO_2$ (95:5) and was maintained at 37° C in a water-bath. The thread tied to the post-ganglionic nerve trunk also provided the distal constricting ligature.

Text-fig. 2. Diagram of two-compartment Perspex box showing the positioning of the nerve/ganglion preparation. The preparation was mounted in the box with the nerve trunks passing through the silicone grease seal in the Perspex barrier as described in the text. The two compartments were then filled with Eagle's medium and 1 $\mu$C [$^{14}$C]valine or [$^{14}$C]acetate was added to the compartment containing the distal portion of the nerve trunk. Where appropriate colchicine or vinblastine sulphate was also added to that compartment. The lid was then screwed on and the box was submerged in a water-bath at 37° C and each compartment was gassed with 95% $O_2$ + 5% $CO_2$.

The dimensions of the box were $8.7 \times 6.3 \times 3.7$ cm and each of the two compartments had a volume of 35 ml.

the barrier could be detected by the appearance of radioactivity in the compartment containing the ganglion. Each compartment of the box was gassed with 95% $O_2 + 5\%$ $CO_2$ saturated with $H_2O$ by passage through Krebs bicarbonate saline at 37° C.

*Segmentation of the nerves.* After 24 or 48 hr incubation the nerves were placed on a dry postcard. The regions proximal to the ligature (and, where appropriate, adjacent to the situation of the water-tight partition) were cut into small segments 0·8 mm long (see Text-fig. 3 a, b).

*Electron microscopy.* In some of the incubation experiments in test-tubes, the colonic nerves were included in the ganglion/constricted nerve preparations. These colonic and/or the hypogastric nerves were used for electron microscopy. At the end

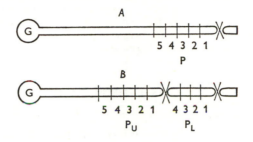

Text-fig. 3. Diagrams indicating the segmentation of the constricted nerves for chemical analysis and electron microscopy. G, inferior mesenteric ganglion. X, sites of constriction. A, Segments 1–5: proximal to single constriction from either test-tube or divided box experiments. B. Segments $P_L$1–4: above lower constriction applied when preparation excised from animal. Segments $P_U$ 1–5: above second or upper constriction applied after initial 24 hr incubation.

of the incubation period the nerves were placed in a pool of ice-cold fixative and segments P1 to P3 proximal to the constriction were cut as indicated in Text-fig. 3a. A 1 cm piece of nerve, situated about halfway between the ganglion and segment P3, and the ganglia were also cut into small pieces for electron microscopy. Two methods of fixation were used: (1) 1% osmium tetroxide adjusted to pH 7·3–7·4 with veronal acetate buffer for $1\frac{1}{2}$–2 hr, or (2) 3% glutaraldehyde in phosphate buffer at pH 7·3 for 4 hr. The tissue was then washed in frequent changes of the buffer for 24–48 hr and post-fixed in 1% aqueous osmium tetroxide for 2 hr. Following fixation by either method, the specimens were dehydrated in graded ethanols passed through epoxy propane and embedded in epoxy resin (Araldite, Ciba, England). The segments of nerve near to the site of constriction were orientated and cut longitudinally. The portions of the nerve remote from the site of constriction were cut transversely so that the number of microtubules in transverse or short oblique sections of non-myelinated axons could be counted. Ultra-thin sections were stained with lead citrate (Reynolds, 1963) and examined in either a Philips EM 200 or an A.E.I. 6B electron microscope. For quantitative studies on the microtubules, random fields were photographed at a primary magnification of 20,550 × . From these standard prints were produced to give a final magnification of 51,375 × . The number of microtubules cut either transversely or in short oblique section were counted in each non-myelinated axon. The axonal area was estimated by tracing their outline on to constant weight paper, cutting out the profiles and weighing the paper.

*Noradrenaline* present in corresponding segments from both hypogastric nerves of a single preparation was measured by the fluorimetric method of Häggendal (1963). The two segments were homogenized in 0·1 ml. ice-cold 1% perchloric acid and centrifuged. The supernatant was retained and the sediment was extracted with a further 0·1 ml. ice-cold 1% perchloric acid, before being recentrifuged. The two supernatants were pooled, diluted with 1 ml. $H_2O$, neutralized to pH 6·5 with 0·1M $K_2CO_3$ and then diluted to 2 ml. with $H_2O$. The $KClO_4$ was allowed to precipitate and a 1 ml. sample of the solution was used for the noradrenaline estimation without any further purification. In order to characterize the fluorescent material present after oxidation with $K_3Fe(CN)_6$ and subsequent treatment with 2,3-dimercapto-propanol (BAL) and NaOH, the emission spectrum of each sample was measured over the range 450–600 m$\mu$ using an excitation wave-length of 400 m$\mu$. In all instances the spectra corresponded with those given by similarly treated samples of noradrenaline. The difference in intensity of the fluorescence at 515 m$\mu$ between samples and their faded blanks (see Häggendal, 1963) was directly proportional to the noradrenaline content of the samples. A standard curve was prepared for each set of noradrenaline determinations.

## RESULTS

### Single ligation experiments in test-tubes

The ultrastructure of the ligated non-myelinated axons and the neuronal cell bodies in the ganglion was well preserved despite 48 hr incubation *in vitro*. The changes immediately above the constriction and at more proximal levels in the nerve were identical with those seen in similar situations in ligated cat hypogastric nerves *in vivo*, and the variation between adjacent axons was equally evident (see Kapeller & Mayor, 1969; Banks *et al.* 1969). Large numbers of granular vesicles, mitochondria and myelin figures accumulated in non-myelinated axons, many of which were extremely swollen and distorted (Pl. 1, fig. 1). There was also an increase in the tubulovesicular components of the axonal endoplasmic reticulum and microtubules were considerably more prominent than usual, especially in the less swollen and in the more normal looking axons some distance from the constriction (see Pl. 1, fig. 2). The cytology of the neuronal cell bodies was similar to that seen in both normal ganglia and in ganglia where the hypogastric and colonic nerves had been ligated for 2 days *in vivo* (Tomlinson, Mayor, Mitchell & Banks, 1971).

In ganglion/nerve preparations where the hypogastric nerves had been ligated at one point, the amount of noradrenaline accumulating in Segments P1 + P2 + P3 (see Text-fig. 3a) increased linearly during the first 48 hr of incubation in the test-tubes (Text-fig. 4). The amount of noradrenaline accumulating in this part of the nerve was approximately half the amount found in a similar region in previous experiments on ligated hypogastric nerves *in vivo* (Banks *et al.* 1969). This may be related to the smaller size of the cats used in the present series of experiments or to the fact that the preganglionic input to the ganglion had been severed. The method of least squares was used to calculate the best straight line fitting the experimental points (correlation coefficient 0·97). These data indicated that the noradrenaline accumulated proximal to the constriction at the rate of 0·007 mμ-mole/hr) and that the noradrenaline content of an 0·8 mm segment of nerve at zero time was 0·003 mμ-mole. Assuming that

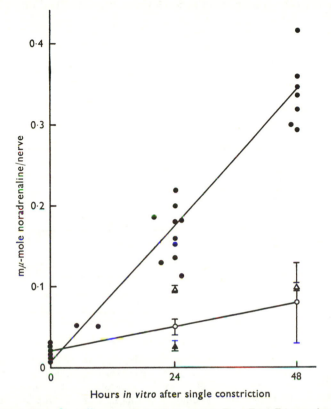

Text-fig. 4. Noradrenaline content of segments P1 + P2 + P3 proximal to a single constriction at different time intervals after incubation of a ganglion/ligated hypogastric nerve preparation in a test-tube. ●, Control incubation; ○, with added colchicine 10 μg/ml; ▲, with added vinblastine sulphate 10 μg/ml.; △, with added vinblastine sulphate 1 μg/ml.

the noradrenaline passes proximo-distally along non-myelinated axons (Mayor & Kapeller 1967; Banks et al. 1969) within granular vesicles, the rate of movement of the vesicles can be calculated to be 1·9 mm/hr. Direct analysis of 0·8 mm lengths of hypogastric nerves well away from the site of constriction showed that they contained 0·006 ± 0·001 mμ noradrenaline after 24 hr incubation in vitro. Using this value the rate of movement of the vesicles was found to be 0·9 mm/hr. Despite the discrepancy in the two values they are both close to the value of approximately 2 mm/hr found in ligated cat hypogastric nerves in previous experiments *in vivo* (Banks *et al.* 1969).

Incubation of ganglion/hypogastric nerve preparations with colchicine (10 $\mu$g/ml.) caused a marked reduction in the accumulation of noradrenaline adjacent to the constriction at both time intervals studied (Table 1 and Text-fig. 5).

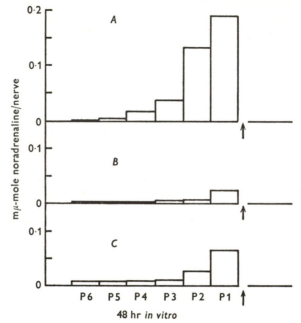

Text-fig. 5. Histograms illustrating the distribution of noradrenaline in constricted hypogastric nerve/inferior mesenteric ganglion preparations maintained for 48 hr *in vitro*. The site of constriction of the nerves is indicated by the vertical arrow. Segmentation as in Text-fig. 3*A*. *A*, Control incubation; *B*, with added colchicine 10 $\mu$g/ml.; *C*, with added vinblastine sulphate 1 $\mu$g/ml. Each of the histograms *A*, *B*, and *C* refers to a single experiment.

This was accompanied by a very obvious decrease in the number of dense-cored vesicles seen in axon profiles from segment P1 (Pl. 2). Furthermore the axons were frequently less swollen and appeared to contain fewer microtubules than those incubated without the drug. Mitochondria still accumulated in the axons close to the constriction despite the presence of colchicine. At a concentration of 1 $\mu$g/ml., colchicine showed only a slight tendency to inhibit noradrenaline accumulation.

Vinblastine sulphate (1 $\mu$g/ml.) was almost as potent in preventing the accumulation of noradrenaline and dense-cored vesicles as colchicine

(10 $\mu$g/ml.) and had similar effects upon the morphology of the axons close to the constriction (see Pl. 3). It did not prevent the accumulation of mitochondria immediately above the constriction.

These observations indicate that both colchicine and vinblastine inhibit the movement of noradrenaline in post-ganglionic noradrenergic nerves. However, they give no indication of the site of action of these drugs. They could, for example, inhibit the synthesis of dense-cored vesicles in the neuronal cell bodies, interfere with intra-axonal transport mechanisms or deplete dense-cored vesicles of their stored noradrenaline. Further experiments were designed to examine these possibilities.

TABLE 1. The effect of colchicine and vinblastine on the accumulation of noradrenaline in segments P1 + P2 + P3. Ganglion/hypogastric nerve preparations were incubated in test-tubes as described in the text for 24 or 48 hr in the presence or absence of drugs. Each hypogastric nerve carried a single ligature. Figures in parentheses indicate the number of observations

| | Noradrenaline accumulating (m$\mu$-mole/nerve ± s.e. of mean) | |
| --- | --- | --- |
| Drug added | 24 hr | 48 hr |
| None | 0·17 ± 0·01 (8) | 0·34 ± 0·02 (7) |
| Colchicine 1 $\mu$g/ml. | — | 0·22 ± 0·05 (4) |
| 10 $\mu$g/ml. | 0·06 ± 0·01 (4) | 0·08 ± 0·03 (3) |
| Vinblastine 1 $\mu$g/ml. | 0·10 ± 0·00 (2) | 0·10 ± 0·01 (2) |

*Asynchronous double ligation experiments in test-tubes*

In these experiments ganglion/ligated nerve preparations were incubated in test-tubes for 24 hr before a second ligature was placed on each nerve 0·5 cm proximal to the first ligature. Then, in all except the control experiments, either colchicine or vinblastine sulphate was added to the incubation medium and remained there throughout the second 24 hr period of incubation. In the control experiments, after a total period of 48 hr incubation, the amount of noradrenaline immediately proximal to the second or upper constriction did not differ significantly from the amount adjacent to the first or lower constriction (Table 2 and Text-fig. 6A).

The presence of colchicine (10 $\mu$g/ml.) or vinblastine sulphate (1 or 10 $\mu$g./ml.) in the incubation medium during the second 24 hr period greatly decreased the amount of noradrenaline accumulating close to the second or upper constriction. However, these drugs did not diminish the amount of noradrenaline found proximal to the first or lower constriction (Table 4 and Text-fig. 6B, C).

These experiments indicate that neither colchicine (10 $\mu$g/ml.) nor vinblastine sulphate (1 or 10 $\mu$g/ml.) deplete stores of noradrenaline accumulated against a ligature before their addition to the incubation medium. They also confirm the previous observations that incubation with colchicine (10 μg/ml.) or vinblastine (1 μg/ml.) prevents the accumulation of noradrenaline proximal to a ligature.

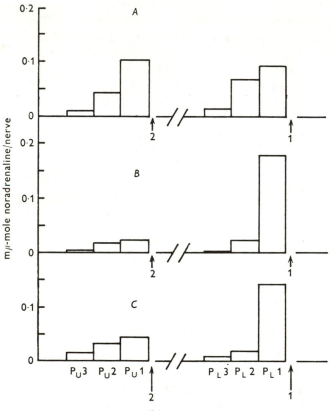

**48 hr** *in vitro*

Text-fig. 6. Histograms illustrating the distribution of noradrenaline in hypogastric nerve/inferior mesenteric ganglion preparations following asynchronous double ligation. Initially applied ligature indicated by vertical arrow 1. The second ligature (vertical arrow 2) was applied after 24 hr incubation. Drug was present only during the second 24 hr period of incubation. Total incubation period was 48 hr. Segmentation as in Text-fig. 3*B*. *A*, Control incubation; *B*, colchicine, 10 μg/ml., added after first 24 hr incubation; *C*, vinblastine sulphate, 1 μg/ml., added after first 24 hr incubation. Each of the histograms *A*, *B*, and *C* refers to a single experiment.

### Divided box experiments

In these experiments the ganglion/nerve preparations were set up as shown in Text-fig. 2. The grease seal in the Perspex barrier caused no obvious constriction of the nerve trunks but, as indicated by the lack of movement of radioactively labelled valine or acetate from one compartment to the other, it prevented any mixing of the Eagle's medium in the two compartments. The presence of colchicine (10 $\mu$g/ml.) or vinblastine (1 $\mu$g/ml.) in the compartment containing the ligated distal portion of the nerve trunks caused a considerable diminution in the amount of noradrenaline accumulating proximal to the constriction.

This reduction in the amount of noradrenaline close to the constriction was frequently associated with an accumulation of noradrenaline in the

TABLE 2. The lack of effect of colchicine and vinblastine on stores of noradrenaline accumulated proximal to a constriction before the addition of these drugs. Ganglion/ligated hypogastric nerve preparations were incubated *in vitro* for 24 hr. Then a second ligature was applied to each nerve proximal to the first and colchicine or vinblastine was added to the Eagle's medium for a further 24 hr incubation at 37° C. Segments $P_L1 + P_L2 + P_L3$ were immediately proximal to the first or lower constriction and segments $P_U1 + P_U2 + P_U3$ were proximal to the second or upper constriction. Figures in parentheses indicate number of observations

|  | Noradrenaline accumulating (m$\mu$-mole/nerve $\pm$ s.e. of mean) | |
|---|---|---|
|  | Segments | Segments |
| Drug | $P_U1 + P_U2 + P_U3$ | $P_L1 + P_L2 + P_L3$ |
| None | 0·16 ± 0·02 (4) | 0·18 ± 0·02 (4) |
| Colchicine 10 $\mu$g/ml. | 0·06 ± 0·01 (2) | 0·18 ± 0·03 (2) |
| Vinblastine 10 $\mu$g/ml. | 0·03 ± 0·00 (2) | 0·19 ± 0·06 (2) |
| 1 $\mu$g/ml. | 0·10 ± 0·00 (2) | 0·16 ± 0·01 (2) |

TABLE 3. Effect of colchicine and vinblastine on the movement of noradrenaline in nerve trunks isolated from the inferior mesenteric ganglion by a grease barrier (see text for arrangement of experimental box). Colchicine and vinblastine were present only in the compartment containing the distal ligated portion of the nerve trunks. Figures in parentheses indicate the number of observations

| Drug in nerve trunk compartment | Noradrenaline accumulating (m$\mu$-mole/nerve $\pm$ s.e. of mean) | |
|---|---|---|
|  | 24 hr | 48 hr |
| None | 0·23 ± 0·04 (3) | 0·29 ± 0·02 (3) |
| Colchicine 10 $\mu$g/ml. | 0·10 ± 0·02 (3) | 0·10 ± 0·04 (3) |
| Vinblastine 1 $\mu$g/ml. | — | 0·12 ± 0·02 (3) |

region of the nerve trunk either within or just proximal to the grease barrier. Such accumulations of noradrenaline in the vicinity of the barrier did not occur in control experiments.

These experiments indicate that when colchicine or vinblastine are in contact with the nerve trunk, but have no direct access to the neuronal cell bodies they are still able to inhibit the proximo-distal movement of noradrenaline and dense-cored vesicles.

### Effect of colchicine and vinblastine sulphate on axonal microtubules

Electron microscopic examination of P1 segments (compare Pl. 1 with Pls. 2, 3) led to the subjective impression that colchicine (10 $\mu$g/ml.) and vinblastine sulphate (1 $\mu$g/ml.) caused a reduction in the number of axonal microtubules. To carry out a quantitative assessment, the number of microtubules in transverse sections of non-myelinated axons midway between the ganglion and constriction were counted in control and drug-treated ganglion/nerve preparations incubated in test-tubes for 48 hr. This region was chosen because, although the axons were not entirely normal, they showed no gross distortion characteristic of the region immediately adjacent to the ligation (Pls. 4–6).

TABLE 4. The effect of colchicine and vinblastine sulphate on the number of microtubules in non-myelinated axons from transverse sections of ligated hypogastric nerve attached to the inferior mesenteric ganglion and maintained for 48 hr *in vitro*. The figures in parentheses indicate the number of axonal profiles counted

| Drug | Microtubules/axon $\pm$ s.e. of mean | Microtubules/$\mu^2$ of axon $\pm$ s.e. of mean |
|---|---|---|
| None | $16 \cdot 5 \pm 0 \cdot 5$ (91) | $75 \cdot 5 \pm 3 \cdot 1$ (91) |
| Colchicine 10 $\mu$g/ml. | $1 \cdot 1 \pm 0 \cdot 05$ (105) | $5 \cdot 3 \pm 0 \cdot 3$ (105) |
| Percentage reduction | $93 \cdot 3$ | $93 \cdot 0$ |
| Vinblastine sulphate 1 $\mu$g/ml. | $8 \cdot 4 \pm 0 \cdot 15$ (123) | $29 \cdot 0 \pm 1 \cdot 5$ (123) |
| Percentage reduction | $49 \cdot 1$ | $61 \cdot 5$ |

Data obtained from a total of 91 axons indicated that control axons incubated for 48 hr contained $16 \cdot 5 \pm 0 \cdot 5$ microtubules per axon. Axons from preparations incubated with colchicine (10 $\mu$g/ml.) or vinblastine sulphate (1 $\mu$g/ml.) for 48 hr contained only $1 \cdot 1 \pm 0 \cdot 05$ or $8 \cdot 4 \pm 0 \cdot 15$ microtubules per axon respectively (Table 4). The data in this Table suggest that the axons in control and colchicine-treated nerves were of a similar size whilst after treatment with vinblastine sulphate some axons were swollen.

The abundance and ultrastructural appearances of fine filamentous structures (neurofilaments) in both transverse and longitudinal sections of non-myelinated axons were not obviously changed by treatment with either colchicine or vinblastine sulphate. Furthermore no significant changes in the tubulo-vesicular components of the axonal endoplasmic reticulum were detected following treatment with either drug.

DISCUSSION

It is clear from these results that the production and transport of granular vesicles and noradrenaline can continue for up to 48 hr in constricted sympathetic neurones isolated from the body and maintained in an artificial environment. The preparations described have the advantage of eliminating many of the uncontrollable factors which arise in studying the effects of drugs on noradrenergic neurones in intact animals. This type of preparation should prove valuable for investigating various aspects of the cellular dynamics of the noradrenergic neurone. Furthermore, the double ligation experiments provide a novel method for studying the influence of drugs on noradrenaline storage granules in an intra-axonal environment which is more physiological than any that can be provided for granules isolated by traditional methods of tissue homogenization and centrifugation.

The present experiments suggest that colchicine and vinblastine prevent the accumulation of noradrenaline storage vesicles above a constriction by interacting with components of the post-ganglionic nerve trunk rather than by inhibiting the formation of the granular vesicles in the neuronal cell bodies, or by depleting the accumulated granular vesicles of their store of noradrenaline.

Since both colchicine and vinblastine are known to interact with the protein subunits of microtubules (Schmitt, 1969) it has been suggested that these fibrous protein elements are in some way involved in the rapid proximo-distal movement of granular vesicles within non-myelinated noradrenergic axons (Dahlström, 1970; Hökfelt & Dahlström, 1971). This view is supported by the present findings that low concentrations of colchicine or vinblastine, which greatly reduce the proximo-distal movement of granular vesicles and noradrenaline, also cause marked reductions in the number of microtubules present in the non-myelinated axons of constricted hypogastric nerves. The latter was the only ultrastructural change that could be unequivocally attributed to the action of colchicine and vinblastine, apart from the reduction in the number of granular vesicles accumulating against the constriction. There was no evidence to suggest that the microtubules were converted into neurofilaments (Hökfelt & Dahlström, 1971). Indeed such a conversion of microtubules to 'neurofilaments' is unlikely to occur in view of the very different amino acid compositions of their component proteins (Davison, 1970; Davison & Huneeus, 1970; Huneeus & Davison, 1970).

These results are consistent with the view that there is a close relationship between the structural integrity of the microtubules and the ability of noradrenergic axons to maintain the proximo-distal movement of granular vesicles.

Although a quantitative determination of the amount of cytochrome oxidase accumulating above a ligature has not been made in the present series of experiments, a subjective assessment of the number of mitochondria present in electron micrographs of segments P 1 to P 3 (Pls. 2, 3) suggests that colchicine and vinblastine have little, if any, effect upon the movement of mitochondria. This agrees with the observations of Kreutzberg (1969) on rat sciatic nerve and leads to the conclusion that microtubules are not involved in the movement of mitochondria. These findings support previous observations indicating that the mechanism responsible for the transport of granular vesicles differed from that involved in mitochondrial movement in constricted non-myelinated axons *in vivo* (Banks *et al.* 1969).

Although the experiments described in this paper are suggestive of a role for microtubules in the axonal transport of noradrenaline storage vesicles, the nature of the relationship between these two structural elements remains to be discovered. At the present time no close association between microtubules and vesicles, such as that observed by Smith, Järlfors & Beránek (1970) in lamprey nerves, has been found in noradrenergic neurones.

Financial support for this work from the Wellcome Trust, The Smith, Kline and French Foundation, the M.R.C. and the S.R.C. is acknowledged with gratitude. We are grateful to Miss R. Grigas, Mrs M. M. Hollingsworth, Mr T. Owen and Mr G. Bottomley for their assistance.

D.R.T. and M.M. are in receipt of Postgraduate Research Studentships from the Wellcome Foundation.

We thank Dr C. W. Potter for supplying us with Eagle's Medium.

### REFERENCES

BANKS, P., MANGNALL, D. & MAYOR, D. (1969). The redistribution of cytochrome oxidase, noradrenaline and adenosine triphosphate in adrenergic nerves constricted at two points. *J. Physiol.* **200**, 745–762.

DAHLSTRÖM, A. (1969). Synthesis, transport and life span of amine storage granules in sympathetic adrenergic neurones. In *Cellular Dynamics of the Neurone*, pp. 153–174, ed. BARONDES, S. H. New York and London: Academic Press.

DAHLSTRÖM, A. (1970). The effects of drugs on axonal transport of amine storage granules. In *New Aspects of Storage and Release Mechanisms of Catecholamines. Bayer Symposium II*, ed. SCHÜMANN, H. S. & KRONEBERG, G. Berlin, Heidelberg, New York: Springer-Verlag.

DAVISON, P. F. (1970). Microtubules and neurofilaments: possible implications in axoplasmic transport. In *Biochemistry of Simple Neuronal Modes. Advances in Biochemical Psychopharmacology*, vol. 2, pp. 289–302, ed. COSTA, E. & GIACOBINI, E. New York and London: Raven Press.

DAVISON, P. F. & HUNEEUS, F. C. (1970). Fibrillar proteins from Squid axons. II. Microtubule protein. *J. molec. Biol.* **52**, 429–439.

HÄGGENDAL, J. (1963). An improved method for fluorimetric determination of small amounts of adrenaline and noradrenaline in plasma and tissues. *Acta physiol. scand.* **59**, 242–254.

HÖKFELT, T. & DAHLSTRÖM, A. (1971). Electron microscopic observations on the distribution and transport of noradrenaline storage particles after local treatment with mitosis inhibitors. *Acta physiol. scand.* (in the Press).

HUNEEUS, F. C. & DAVISON, P. F. (1970). Fibrillar proteins from Squid axons. I. Neurofilament protein. *J. molec. Biol.* **52**, 415–428.

KAPELLER, K. & MAYOR, D. (1969). An electron microscopic study of the early changes proximal to a constriction in sympathetic nerves. *Proc. R. Soc.* B **172**, 39–51.

KREUTZBERG, G. (1969). Neuronal dynamics and axonal flow. IV. Blockage of intraaxonal enzyme transport by colchicine. *Proc. natn. Acad. Sci. U.S.A.* **62**, 722–728.

MAYOR, D. & KAPELLER, K. (1967). Fluorescence microscopy and electron microscopy of adrenergic nerves after constriction at two points. *Jl R. microsc. Soc.* **87**, 277–294.

REYNOLDS, E. S. (1963). The use of lead citrate at high pH as an electron-opaque stain in electron microscopy. *J. cell Biol.* **17**, 208–212.

SCHMITT, F. O. (1969). Fibrous proteins and neuronal dynamics. In *Cellular Dynamics of the Neuron*, Symposium of the International Society for Cell Biology, vol. 8, ed. by BARONDES, S. H. New York and London: Academic Press.

SMITH, D. S., JÄRLFORS, U. & BERÁNEK, R. (1970). The organization of synaptic axoplasm in the Lamprey (*Petromyzon marinus*) central nervous system. *J. cell Biol.* **46**, 199–219.

TOMLINSON, D. R., MAYOR, D., MITCHELL, M. & BANKS, P. (1971). Ultrastructural changes in constricted sympathetic nerves maintained *in vitro. J. Anat.* **108**, 612.

### EXPLANATION OF PLATES

#### PLATES 1–3

All electron micrographs are from nerves fixed in osmium tetroxide. The sections were stained with lead citrate. The magnification markers represent $1 \mu$. A indicates non-myelinated axons, S indicates Schwann cell cytoplasm.

#### PLATE 1

Electron micrographs from the middle of segment P1 (Text-fig. 3A) after 48 hr incubation in Eagle's medium only. Fig. 1 illustrates the accumulation of granular or dense-cored vesicles (g), agranular vesicles (a) in slightly swollen and deformed axons. Microtubules (arrowed) can be seen in the narrower axons. The mitochondria (m) are swollen.

Fig. 2 illustrates typical microtubules (arrowed) in a longitudinal section of a slightly swollen axon at higher magnification.

#### PLATE 2

Electron micrograph from the middle of segment P1 after 48 hr incubation in Eagle's medium with added colchicine (10 $\mu$g/ml). Several axons are swollen, mitochondria (m) have accumulated in several axons. Granular or dense-cored vesicles (g) are exceptionally rare and microtubules cannot be identified. The axoplasm has an amorphous appearance.

P. BANKS AND OTHERS

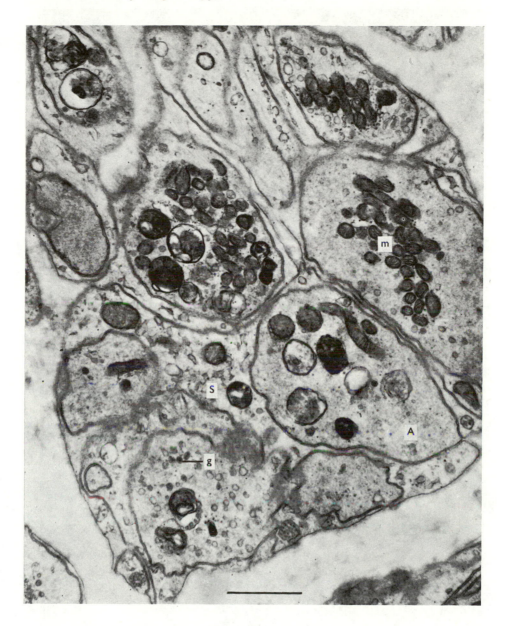

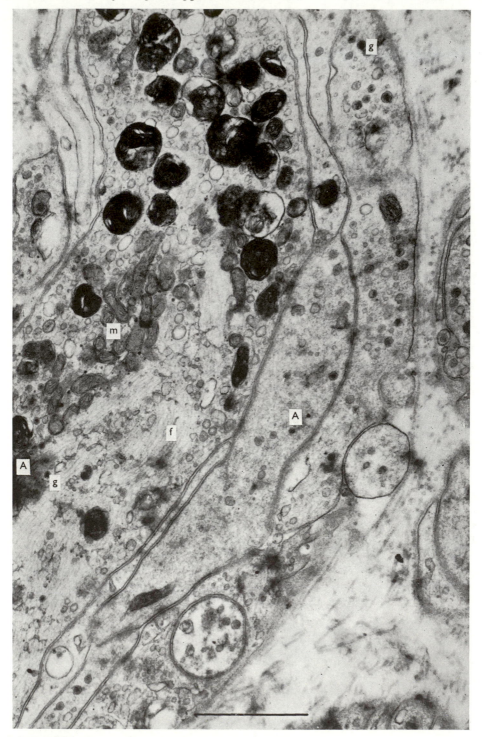

P. BANKS AND OTHERS

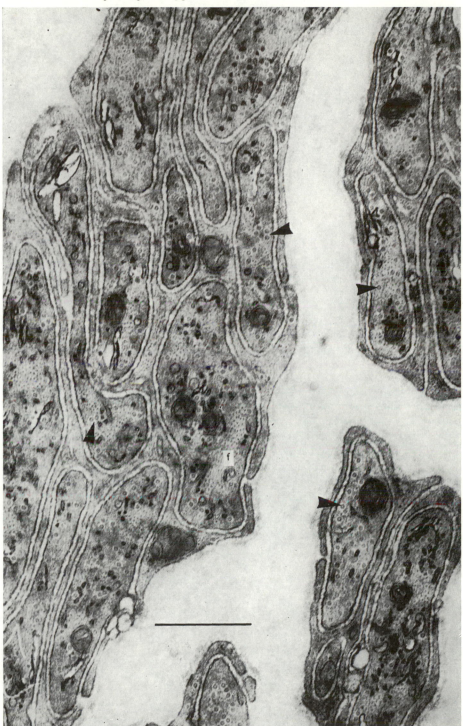

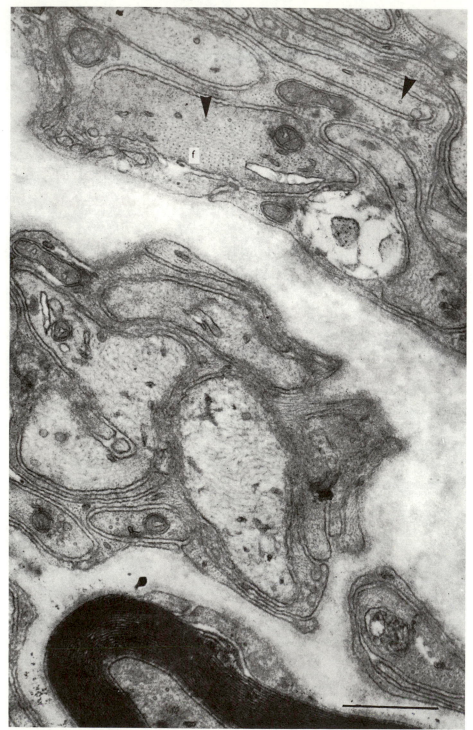

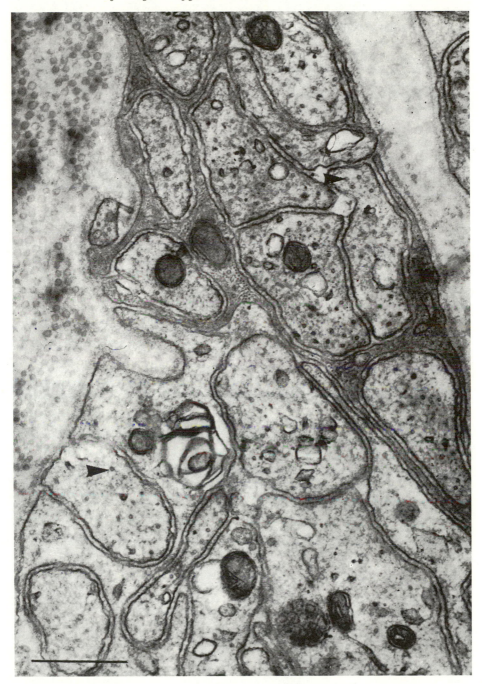

P. BANKS AND OTHERS

## PLATE 3

Electron micrograph from middle of segment P1 after 48 hr incubation in Eagle's medium with added vinblastine sulphate (1 $\mu$g/ml). The more swollen non-myelinated axon contains several mitochondria (m) and a few granular vesicles (g). Microtubules cannot be identified but fine filaments (f) are present.

## PLATES 4–6

In these electron micrographs from transverse sections of hypogastric nerves mid-way between segment P3 (see Text-fig. 3A) and the ganglion there is a considerable widening of the interstitial spaces and distortion of the non-myelinated axons cut in transverse or short oblique section due to the incubation for 48 hr in Eagle's medium *in vitro*. Glutaraldehyde followed by osmium tetroxide fixation. Magnification markers equal 0·5$\mu$.

## PLATE 4

From a control incubation, illustrates the abundance of microtubules (arrowed) with their typical clear halo when cut transversely. Fine filamentous structures (f) seen as dark gray or black dots in transvere sections are very common.

## PLATE 5

From an experiment with colchicine 10 $\mu$g/ml. added to the incubation medium. Note the paucity of microtubules (arrowed). Fine filaments (f) are just as common as in control incubation

## PLATE 6

From an experiment with vinblastine sulphate 1 $\mu$g/ml. added to incubation medium. The non-myelinated axons contain fewer microtubules (arrowed) than control axons (Pl. 4). The amorphous nature of the axoplasm obscures the fine filaments in this micrograph.

*Chapter 9*

# TRANSMITTERS IN THE CENTRAL NERVOUS SYSTEM

Transmitter identification in the mammalian central nervous system (CNS) presents a dilemma. On the one hand, all of the known or suspected transmitter compounds are found in the CNS, in which they probably actually serve as transmitters. On the other hand, it is extraordinarily difficult in the CNS to meet the rigorous standards of transmitter identification that have been established for peripheral synapses (Chapter 1). The major complication is anatomical: the extremely dense packing of neurons, glia, and their processes, and the large number of terminals that come from different sources and impinge on any particular neuron, make experimental isolation of a given synapse difficult. Faced with this difficulty, one may reasonably relax the rigid standards used to characterize peripheral transmitter systems and impose simplified, but not uncritical, criteria for CNS transmitters.

Most of the known transmitter substances are selectively concentrated in neurons that secrete them. Accordingly, a useful first indication of transmitter identity is the demonstration that a neuron, particularly within its terminals, accumulates high levels of the suspected transmitter or of a key enzyme of its biosynthesis. Concentrations of substances in various regions of the CNS are only marginally informative; it is their accumulation within particular cells that is important. An exception to this general rule arises in the case of transmitter candidates such as glycine and glutamate, which are common metabolites and are present in all cells.

A variety of methods serves to assign suspected transmitters to particular cells. For catecholamines and 5-hydroxytryptamine (5-HT), a fluorescence histochemical procedure has proved extremely valuable (Falck, 1962). In this technique CNS tissue slices are freeze-dried and exposed to formaldehyde vapor, whereupon cells with high amine concentrations fluoresce brightly. Catecholamines and 5-HT give

487

characteristic fluorescence spectra, allowing them to be assigned to specific cells. For several transmitter substances, including ACh (Goldberg and McCaman, 1973; Hanin and Jenden, 1969), GABA (Otsuka, Obata, Miyata, and Tanaka, 1971), and amines (Cattabini, Koslow, and Costa, 1972), there are also microchemical assay procedures sufficiently sensitive for quantification of the transmitter in single neurons, although only a few CNS cell types have been examined with these methods.

Less work has been done on location of specific proteins required for transmitter synthesis or storage. A number of investigators have reported progress in developing a histochemical method for the enzyme choline acetyltransferase (Burt, 1971). This procedure detects—as an insoluble, electron-dense precipitate—the sulfhydryl group that is freed when acetyl coenzyme A transfers its acetyl group to choline. Another method of great future promise is immunochemical labeling of specific cellular proteins. Chromogranin A and dopamine β-hydroxylase have been detected in noradrenergic neurons by this method (Geffen, Livett, and Rush, 1969, 1970). In principle, any protein that can be highly purified and is antigenic can be located by antibodies against it.

The efforts to assign transmitters to cells by pinpointing transmitter-synthesizing enzymes are predicated on the specific and exclusive association of those enzymes with neurons that use the biosynthetic products of the enzymes as transmitters. Another approach that has enjoyed greater development and application is location of transmitter-degrading enzymes, such as acetylcholinesterase (Karnovsky, 1964). Although the procedures for locating these enzymes are effective, this approach is less useful for establishing cellular transmitter chemistry, particularly at unstudied synapses, because the degradative enzymes are not confined to neurons that employ their substrates as transmitters.

Yet another way to locate cells of a particular transmitter chemistry may be to search for cells with an uptake system with high affinity for the transmitter candidate in question. Essentially all of the transmitter candidates can be located in tissues with the use of radioactive materials and autoradiographic techniques. Thus, for norepinephrine, a high-affinity uptake mechanism exists in noradrenergic nerve terminals while low-affinity systems operate in surrounding cell types (see Chapter 6). Similarly, high-affinity systems may transport glycine and glutamate into neurons that use them as transmitters, allowing autoradiographic detection of amino acid-releasing cells (Iversen and Bloom, 1972). But these autoradiographic results must be interpreted with caution. For example, in the lobster, Schwann and connective tissue cells vigorously take up GABA, but inhibitory nerve terminals that release GABA take it up only slightly or not at all (see Chapter 4).

A second indication that a substance may be a transmitter in the CNS is that its application to a postsynaptic cell evokes the same electrophysiological response (recorded intracellularly) as does stimulation of the presynaptic nerve innervating the test cell. Ideally, the suspected transmitter should be applied as closely as possible to the synapse, and should produce the same ionic conductance changes and have the same pharmacology as does the transmitter that is released by nerve stimulation. A good example of this type of investigation is the study by R. Werman, R.A. Davidoff, and M.H. Aprison (1968) of the iontophoretic application of glycine onto spinal cord motor neurons. GABA and glycine produce nearly identical responses in this system, but the pharmacological properties of the glycine response more closely resemble those of a natural inhibitory input (Curtis, Duggan, and Johnston, 1971). These studies raise the possibility that glycine may function as the inhibitory transmitter.

The papers we have selected for reprinting in this chapter describe the most complete attempt (prior to 1973; see Chapter 11) to demonstrate a transmitter system in the CNS. These studies take advantage of the highly stereotyped organization of the mammalian cerebellum and provide evidence that GABA may function as the neurotransmitter released at the terminals of Purkinje cell axons. The experimental approach was (a) to attempt to localize GABA in Purkinje cell bodies and their terminals; (b) to compare the physiological and pharmacological effects of GABA and of Purkinje cell stimulation; (c) to demonstrate directly that GABA is released into the fourth ventricle during cerebellar stimulation.

Before this work was begun, physiological studies had shown that the total output of the cerebellum (through the axons of Purkinje cells) is inhibitory. Recordings from neurons receiving monosynaptic input from Purkinje cells (*e.g.*, cells in Deiters' nucleus) showed that activation of Purkinje cells caused an inhibitory postsynaptic potential. K. Obata and coworkers reported on the physiological properties and pharmacology of this response in two papers (1967, 1970), the second of which is reprinted here. Their results show that both externally applied GABA and Purkinje cell stimulation produce a hyperpolarizing inhibitory response in Deiters' neurons; that the equilibrium potential for the two is the same; and that picrotoxin blocks both. The responses of the postsynaptic cell to GABA and to natural stimulation appear, therefore, to be identical.

M. Otsuka and coworkers (Otsuka, *et al.,* 1971, reprinted here) compared the GABA content of single cell bodies isolated from various kinds of neurons by manual microdissection. Because the isolated cell bodies carried adhering nerve terminals, the cellular content of GABA could not be unequivocally determined. The results were consistent, however, with the idea that Purkinje cell bodies contain high levels of GABA. In addition, cells from the dorsal part of Deiters' nucleus, receiving Purkinje cell input, had higher GABA levels than cells from the ventral part. After surgical removal of the cerebellar vermis and degeneration of Purkinje cell terminals, the GABA level fell only in the cells from the dorsal portion of the nucleus. This suggested that much of the GABA measured in these cells was actually in Purkinje terminals ending on the cells.

K. Obata and K. Takeda (1969, reprinted here) took advantage of the location of the cerebellar subcortical nucleii of the cat (which receive input from the cerebellum) immediately adjacent to the fourth ventricle. The cerebellum was massively stimulated during ventricular perfusion, and the GABA content of the perfusate was measured. Although the efflux of GABA showed large variations, more GABA was released with stimulation than at rest in all but one experiment, and the average GABA output was increased about two-fold with stimulation.

The three papers reprinted in this section strongly support the proposal that GABA may be the transmitter compound liberated by Purkinje cell terminals. Although the experiments discussed are a technical *tour de force,* the localization of GABA in Purkinje cells and their terminals still is not absolutely certain. Moreover, a quantitative comparison between the amount of GABA released and the amount required to elicit a response is not possible with the techniques used. The difficulties of rigorous transmitter identification in the CNS are thus well illustrated in the papers reprinted here. Nonetheless, the extreme interest of this important area of investigation and the continuing development and application of new technology, ensure rapid progress in the essential task of mapping the transmitter chemistry of the mammalian CNS.

## READING LIST

*Reprinted Papers*

1. Obata, K. and K. Takeda (1969). Release of $\gamma$-aminobutyric acid into the fourth ventricle induced by stimulation of the cat's cerebellum. *J. Neurochem.* 16: 1043–1047.

2. Obata, K., K. Takeda, and H. Shinozaki (1970). Further study on pharmacological properties of the cerebellar-induced inhibition of Deiters neurons. *Exp. Brain Res.* 11: 327–342.

3. Otsuka, M., K. Obata, Y. Miyata, and Y. Tanaka (1971). Measurement of γ-aminobutyric acid in isolated nerve cells of cat central nervous system. *J. Neurochem.* 18: 287–295.

*Other Selected Papers*

4. Falck, B. (1962). Observations on the possibilities of the cellular localization of monoamines by a fluorescence method. *Acta Physiol. Scand.* 56: Suppl. 197.

5. Karnovsky, M. (1964). The localization of cholinesterase activity in rat cardiac muscle by electron microscopy. *J. Cell Biol.* 23: 217–232.

6. Dahlström, A. and K. Fuxe (1965). Evidence for the existence of monoamine containing neurons in the central nervous system. I. Demonstration of monoamines in the cell bodies of brain stem neurons. *Acta Physiol. Scand.* 62: Suppl. 232.

7. Obata, K., M. Ito, R. Ochi, and N. Sato (1967). Pharmacological properties of the postsynaptic inhibition by Purkinje cell axons and the action of γ-aminobutyric acid on Deiters neurons. *Exp. Brain Res.* 4: 43–57.

8. Werman, R., R.A. Davidoff, and M.H. Aprison (1968). Inhibitory action of glycine on spinal neurons in the cat. *J. Neurophysiol.* 31: 81–95.

9. Geffen, L.B., B.G. Livett, and R.A. Rush (1969). Immunohistochemical localization of protein components of catecholamine storage vesicles. *J. Physiol.* 204: 593–605.

10. Hanin, I. and D.J. Jenden (1969). Estimation of choline esters in brain by a new gas chromatographic procedure. *Biochem. Pharmacol.* 18: 834–837.

11. Geffen, L.B., B.G. Livett, and R.A. Rush (1970). "Immunohistochemical localization of chromogranins in sheep sympathetic neurons and their release by nerve impulses," *in* H.G. Kroneberg and H.J. Schümann (Eds.), *New Aspects of Storage and Release Mechanisms of Catecholamines* (Bayer Symposium II), pp. 55–72. Berlin: Springer-Verlag.

12. Burt, A.M. (1971). The histochemical localization of choline acetyltransferase. *Progr. in Brain Res.* 34: 327–335.

13. Curtis, D.R., A.W. Duggan, and G.A.R. Johnston (1971). The specificity of strychnine as a glycine antagonist in the mammalian spinal cord. *Exp. Brain Res.* 12: 547–565.

14. Cattabini, F., S.H. Koslow, and E. Costa (1972). Gas chromato-graphy—mass fragmentography: a new approach to the estima-tion of amines and amine turnover. *Adv. Biochem. Psycho-pharm.* 6: 37–59.

15. Iversen, L.L. and F.E. Bloom (1972). Studies of the uptake of $^3$H-GABA and $^3$H-glycine in slices and homogenates of rat brain and spinal cord by electron microscopic autoradiography. *Brain Res.* 41: 131–143.

16. Otsuka, M., S. Konishi, and T. Takahashi (1972). A further study of the motoneuron-depolarizing peptide extracted from dorsal roots of bovine spinal nerves. *Proc. Japan Acad.* 48: 747–752.

17. Goldberg, A.M. and R.E. McCaman (1973). The determination of picomole amounts of acetylcholine in mammalian brain. *J. Neurochem.* 20: 1–8.

*Recent books describing methods of detecting neurotransmitters and their synthetic enzymes*

18. Costa, E., L. Iversen, and R. Paoletti (Eds.) (1972). *Studies of Neurotransmitters at the Synaptic Level. Adv. in Biochem. Psychopharmacol.,* Vol. 6. New York: Raven Press.

19. Eranko, O. (Ed.). *The Histochemistry of Nervous Transmission. Progr. in Brain Res.,* Vol. 34. Amsterdam: Elsevier.

# RELEASE OF γ-AMINOBUTYRIC ACID INTO THE FOURTH VENTRICLE INDUCED BY STIMULATION OF THE CAT'S CEREBELLUM

K. OBATA and K. TAKEDA

Department of Pharmacology, Faculty of Medicine, Tokyo Medical and Denta
University, Tokyo, Japan

(*Received* 6 *February* 1969. *Accepted* 14 *February* 1969)

**Abstract**—The fourth ventricle of the cat was perfused and the release of γ-aminobutyric acid (GABA) into the perfusate was measured. GABA was released at a rate of $6.69 \times 10^{-10}$ moles/min and increased about three times during cerebellar cortical stimulation at 200/sec. It is suggested that GABA is released from axon terminals of Purkinje cells in cerebellar subcortical nuclei.

THE CEREBELLAR corticofugal impulses along Purkinje cell axons produce the inhibitory postsynaptic potentials (IPSPs) monosynaptically in their target neurones of the cerebellar subcortical nuclei, as examined in the intracerebellar (ITO, YOSHIDA and OBATA, 1964) and Deiters' nuclei (ITO and YOSHIDA, 1966; ITO, OBATA and OCHI, 1966). When applied micro-iontophoretically, γ-aminobutyric acid (GABA) induces IPSP-like changes in Deiters neurones, i.e. a membrane hyperpolarization with concomitant increase of the membrane conductance and so mimics the action of the inhibitory transmitter substance released from axon terminals of Purkinje cells (OBATA, ITO, OCHI and SATO, 1967). In a further attempt to identify GABA as the natural transmitter, it is important to show that activation of Purkinje cell axons liberates GABA from their terminals in the cerebellar subcortical nuclei. In the cat, these nuclei are adjacent, and in some parts even exposed, to the fourth ventricle (see SNIDER and NIEMER, 1961). It may therefore be expected that GABA liberated in those nuclei would pass into the fourth ventricle. In the present study, the fourth ventricle was perfused and it was shown that the amount of GABA in the perfusates increased significantly during stimulation of the cerebellar cortex.

## METHODS

The experiments were carried out on adult cats anaesthetized with pentobarbitone sodium (30 mg/kg). In most cats (see Results) three to four hours before the beginning of the perfusion, amino-oxyacetic acid (AOAA) was injected subcutaneously (30 mg/kg) to try to prevent the enzymic destruction of the released GABA. Also, VAN GELDER (1965) suggested that AOAA impairs the blood–brain barrier and presumably also the cerebrospinal fluid–brain barrier for GABA by inhibiting GABA metabolism in the wall of blood vessels and ventricular systems. It was therefore expected that AOAA might facilitate the passage of released GABA through these barriers. After mounting on a stereotaxic frame, the animals were immobilized with gallamine triethiodide, while respiration was maintained artificially. Blood pressure was monitored continuously from the femoral artery. If the blood pressure rose markedly during cerebellar stimulation, as occurred occasionally, hexamethonium bromide (2–10 mg/kg, i.v.) was administered so that the blood pressure increase was confined within 30 mmHg.

Six needle electrodes, each of which had four or five uninsulated spots at 2 mm intervals along its shaft, were inserted into the posterior and anterior lobe cortices of the cerebellum (two into the vermis and four into the hemisphere on both sides; see Fig. 1). All the electrodes were used at the same time as the cathode for electrical stimulation against an anode formed by a silver plate placed on the temporal muscle. Stimuli were provided with pulses of 30–60 v amplitude and 0.2 msec duration repeated for 5 min at frequencies of up to 200/sec.

---

*Abbreviations used:* AOAA, amino-oxyacetic acid; IPSP, inhibitory postsynaptic potential.

Reprinted from the *Journal of Neurochemistry* 16: 1043–1047 (1969) by permission of the publisher.

The foramen of Magendie was opened and the nearby choroid plexus was dissected. A thin vinyl tubing (1–1·5 mm external diameter) was inserted into the fourth ventricle to a depth of 1·5–2 cm (Fig. 1). Perfusion fluid containing NaCl (9·0 g/l.) and CaCl$_2$ (0·2 g/l.) was oxygenated and warmed to 35–38° and was delivered into the fourth ventricle through the tubing at a constant rate of 1·0–1·5 ml/min. The effluent was collected by suction through a small wad of cotton wool placed on the caudal part of the medulla. The infused solution could thus be recovered with little loss. The perfusate was collected over a period of 5 min just before, during and after cerebellar stimulation. Gradual swelling of the cerebellum and the brain stem was considered to indicate an alteration in the experimental conditions and, as soon as it appeared, the perfusion was discontinued. The experiments were also discontinued if the perfusates became contaminated with blood that arose from

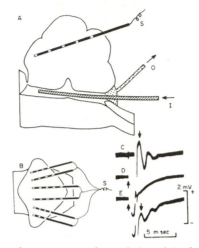

Fig. 1. A and B show the arrangement for perfusion of the fourth ventricle and for stimulation of the cerebellar cortex on the mid-sagittal and horizontal planes, respectively.
I: inlet and O: outlet tubings. Stimulating needle electrodes (S) were lacquered except at several spots marked with white. C–E were recorded extracellularly within Deiters' nucleus. C, antidromic field potentials induced by the stimulation of ipsilateral C$_3$ spinal segment. The initial positivity is marked by a downward arrow. D, single shock of cerebellar stimulation through the electrodes S. The moment of stimulation is indicated by an upward arrow. E, combined cerebellar and spinal stimulations at a brief interval. Note that the antidromic fields are depressed markedly in comparison with the control in C.

a lesion of the choroid plexus. In several cases, about 1 cm$^2$ of cortical surface on the vermis of the posterior lobe was enclosed with a wall of agar and was superfused continuously at a rate of 1·0–1·5 ml/min.

In some experiments, a needle electrode was inserted into Deiters' nucleus to record the antidromic field potentials that were induced by stimulation of the ipsilateral ventral surface of the C$_3$ spinal segment (Ito, Hongo, Yoshida, Okada and Obata, 1964). Following cerebellar stimulation there was a marked inhibition of the antidromic field potentials, indicating that Purkinje cell axons were excited effectively by that stimulation (Fig. 1 C–E).

GABA in the perfusates was isolated and assayed by the method developed by Otsuka, Iversen, Hall and Kravitz (1966), with minor modifications. To each sample, $5 \times 10^{-12}$ moles of [$^3$H]-GABA (specific activity, 5 c/m-mole, New England Nuclear Corp.) were added as an internal standard to estimate the overall recovery. Each sample was passed through a column (0·8 × 15 cm) of Dowex-50-H$^+$ resin and amino acids were eluted with pyridine or ammonia solution. After evaporation the concentrated eluate was passed through a column (0·4 × 5 cm) of Dowex-1-acetate resin to remove acidic amino acids. The effluent solution was taken to dryness and the residue was dissolved in 50 $\mu$l water. [$^3$H]GABA was measured in 5 $\mu$l portions and GABA was assayed enzymically in 10 $\mu$l portions (Jakoby and Scott, 1959); for each analysis a blank and two assay samples were run and an internal standard of $2·5 \times 10^{-10}$ moles of GABA was added to a fourth sample.

Amino acid analysis was carried out in the laboratory of Prof. Y. NAGAI (Institute for Hard Tissue Research), using an amino acid analyser (Mitamura Riken Co., Tokyo), following the procedures developed by SPACKMAN, STEIN and MOORE (1958).

## RESULTS

The total amount of free amino acids in the perfusate was 0·02–0·1 $\mu$moles/min without cerebellar stimulation and its change during the cerebellar stimulation did not exceed 10 per cent of each control. According to the amino acid analysis, glutamine formed about 60 per cent of the free amino acids and glutamic acid, glycine, alanine and valine showed separate peaks. The amount of GABA, however, was below the limit of sensitivity of the analysis (about $10^{-8}$ moles). The cerebellar stimulation did not produce any detectable change in the chromatographic pattern of the released amino acids. Enzymic assay revealed that the amount of GABA in the perfusates was much higher in cats which were treated with AOAA than in non-treated ones; the average spontaneous release was about $6 \times 10^{-10}$ moles/min in the former and about $1 \times 10^{-10}$ moles/min in the latter. The effects of cerebellar stimulation were studied only in the cats which received AOAA beforehand. Table 1 compares the amount of GABA measured in 5 min perfusates during the resting

TABLE 1.—GABA RELEASE INTO THE FOURTH VENTRICLE OF THE CAT

| Cat No. | Trial No. | Resting period before stimulation (A) ($\times 10^{-10}$ moles/min) | During 200/sec cerebellar stimulation (B) ($\times 10^{-10}$ moles/min) | B/A |
|---|---|---|---|---|
| 1 | 1 | 5·85 | 20·4 | 3·49 |
|  | 2 | 5·12 | 5·50 | 1·09 |
|  | 3 | 9·62 | 32·0 | 3·33 |
| 2 | 4 | 18·6 | 41·6 | 2·24 |
|  | 5 | 12·8 | 15·5 | 1·21 |
| 3 | 6 | 3·56 | 8·54 | 2·40 |
|  | 7 | 2·22 | 1·75 | 0·79 |
|  | 8 | 0·68 | 3·47 | 5·10 |
| 4 | 9 | 4·78 | 24·7 | 5·17 |
|  | 10 | 12·3 | 29·8 | 2·42 |
|  | 11 | 9·38 | 10·4 | 1·11 |
| 5 | 12 | 0·75 | 2·81 | 3·75 |
|  | 13 | 0·33 | 2·36 | 7·15 |
| Mean ± S.E.M. |  | 6·69 ± 1·55 | 15·45 ± 3·67* | 3·02 ± 0·53† |

\* $P < 0.05$ when compared with A.
† $P \blacktriangleleft 0.005$ when compared with unity.

periods just before the stimulation (A) and those during cerebellar stimulation at 200/sec (B). In the same cats stimulations were repeated at intervals of 15 min. Although both the spontaneous and evoked release of GABA varied over a fairly wide range, the ratio of GABA release during 200/sec stimulation to that released just before stimulation was significantly higher than unity, being three on average (Table 1). In some cases GABA release during the resting periods immediately following stimulation was measured and was similar to that before the stimulation. Stimulation at lower frequencies (20 and 50/sec) produced no detectable increase in GABA release.

Although any marked change in blood pressure was suppressed by an administration of hexamethonium (see Methods), a rise of up to 30 mmHg was sometimes observed during cerebellar stimulation. However, this was induced to the same extent by stimulation at various rates between 20 and 200/sec. and was not correlated to the amount of GABA in the perfusates. Concurrent perfusion of the cortical surface on the vermis of the posterior lobe revealed that GABA release from the cortex was $1-3 \times 10^{-11}$ moles/cm$^2$/min, either during the cerebellar stimulation or during the resting period.

## DISCUSSION

Spontaneous release of GABA into the fourth ventricle showed rather a wide variation in each experiment. This might be ascribable to fluctuation of experimental conditions such as the depth of anaesthesia, the stage of AOAA action or beginning of brain oedema. However, GABA release during 200/sec stimulation was significantly higher than just before the stimulation. Since the amount of GABA output had no correlation with systemic blood pressure, it is unlikely that the change in GABA release during stimulation arose from alterations in the brain circulation, but it does appear to have a causal relationship with neuronal activities evoked in the structures enclosing the fourth ventricle. The cerebellar cortex at the lingula, nodulus and uvula forms the roof of the fourth ventricle. These regions might be activated by cerebellar stimulation, either directly or indirectly through collaterals of cerebellar afferents (see ECCLES, ITO and SZENTÁGOTHAI, 1967). However, the release of GABA from the cortical surface in the proximity of the stimulating electrodes was relatively low and did not increase appreciably during cerebellar stimulation. This suggests that the cortical release of GABA contributes little, if at all, to the increase in GABA content shown for the perfusates of the fourth ventricle. Therefore, it appears likely that GABA in the perfusates is derived from the cerebellar subcortical nuclei which occupy a large part of tissues facing the fourth ventricle and where abundant Purkinje cell axons terminate forming inhibitory synapses.

It may be worth noting that some unusual features in the present results can also be interpreted satisfactorily on the basis of the electrophysiological findings on Purkinje cell activity (see ECCLES et al., 1967). It was reported that Purkinje cells discharge spontaneously at rates of 30–60 impulses/sec. This would account for the relatively large rate of the background GABA release (Table 1). It was further shown that electrical stimulation of the cerebellar cortex not only excites Purkinje cells, but also depresses them as a result of activation of the intracortical inhibitory neurones (ITO, KAWAI, UDO and SATO, 1968). The latter depressant effect lasts much longer than the former excitation and, under certain circumstances, the frequency of the impulses firing down Purkinje cell axons could be depressed in spite of their stimulation. This might be the reason why there was no significant increase in GABA release during stimulation at relatively low frequency (20—50/sec, see Results) and in some cases even at 200/sec stimulation.

The present results favour the previous postulate that GABA is the inhibitory transmitter liberated from axon terminals of Purkinje cells (OBATA et al., 1967). In order to confirm that the GABA released into the fourth ventricle actually originates from the cerebellar subcortical nuclei, a further investigation is now in progress with the direct perfusion of these nuclei.

*Acknowledgements*—The authors wish to express their thanks to Prof. M. OTSUKA and Dr. M. ITO for their constant interest and advice. They are also indebted to Dr. E. A. KRAVITZ for his comments on this manuscript.

## REFERENCES

ECCLES J. C., ITO M. and SZENTÁGOTHAI J. (1967) *The Cerebellum as a Neuronal Machine*. Springer-Verlag, New York.
ITO M., HONGO T., YOSHIDA M., OKADA M. and OBATA K. (1964) *Jap. J. Physiol.* **14**, 638.
ITO M., KAWAI N., UDO M. and SATO N. (1968) *Exp. Brain Res.* **6**, 247.
ITO M., OBATA K. and OCHI R. (1966) *Exp. Brain Res.* **2**, 350.
ITO M. and YOSHIDA M. (1966) *Exp. Brain Res.* **2**, 330.
ITO M., YOSHIDA M. and OBATA K. (1964) *Experientia (Basel)* **20**, 575.
JAKOBY W. B. and SCOTT E. M. (1959) *J. biol. Chem.* **234**, 937.
OBATA K., ITO M., OCHI R. and SATO N. (1967) *Exp. Brain Res.* **4**, 43.
OTSUKA M., IVERSEN L. L., HALL Z. W. and KRAVITZ E. A. (1966) *Proc. nat. Acad. Sci. (Wash.)* **56**, 1110.
SNIDER R. S. and NIEMER W. T. (1961) *A Stereotaxic Atlas of the Cat Brain*. The University of Chicago Press, Chicago.
SPACKMAN D. H., STEIN W. H. and MOORE S. (1958) *Analyt. Chem.* **30**, 1190.
VAN GELDER N. M. (1965) *J. Neurochem.* **12**, 239.

# Further Study on Pharmacological Properties of the Cerebellar-Induced Inhibition of Deiters Neurones

K. Obata, K. Takeda and H. Shinozaki

Department of Pharmacology, Faculty of Medicine,
Tokyo Medical and Dental University, Tokyo (Japan)

Received May 29, 1970

**Summary.** The pharmacological properties of Deiters neurones were studied in anaesthetized cats, together with their inhibition by cerebellar Purkinje cells. Purkinje cell inhibition, as detected by depression of antidromic field potentials of Deiters neurones, was blocked by relatively large doses of picrotoxin administered intravenously (5—10 mg/kg). The cerebellar inhibition was also detected as a depression of the discharge of Deiters neurones excited by electrophoretic administration of DL-homocysteic acid. This inhibition was abolished or reduced by picrotoxin, but was not altered by strychnine, administered either systemically or electrophoretically. $\gamma$-Aminobutyric acid (GABA), glycine, $\beta$-alanine and imidazole acetic acid, when administered electrophoretically, also depressed the antidromic field potentials and the spike discharges of Deiters neurones. Picrotoxin antagonized the effect of GABA but not of glycine, while strychnine blocked only the action of glycine. Intracellular recording from Deiters neurones revealed that both GABA and glycine, ejected extracellularly, hyperpolarized the membrane and increased the membrane conductance. The reversal of the GABA-induced hyperpolarization was at the same potential level as that of the inhibitory postsynaptic potentials induced by cerebellar stimulation. These results are consistent with the hypothesis that the inhibitory transmitter released from Purkinje cell axons is GABA or a related substance.

**Key Words:** Deiters neurones — Cerebellar inhibition — GABA — Glycine — Picrotoxin — Strychnine

Purkinje cells of the mammalian cerebellum project to the cerebellar nuclei and to some parts of the vestibular nuclear complex, including the dorsal portion of the nucleus of Deiters (Jansen and Brodal, 1954; Walberg and Jansen, 1961). The synaptic action of these Purkinje cell axons has been shown to be inhibitory (Ito and Yoshida, 1966; Ito, Obata and Ochi, 1966; Ito, Kawai and Udo, 1968a; Ito, Yoshida, Obata, Kawai and Udo, 1970e; Ito, Udo, Mano and Kawai, 1970d), and there is accumulating evidence which suggests that the inhibitory transmitter substance is $\gamma$-aminobutyric acid (GABA) or a related compound. GABA has been shown to hyperpolarize and increase the membrane conductance of Deiters neurones, as does the natural transmitter released from Purkinje cell axons (Obata, Ito, Ochi and Sato, 1967). This effect of GABA accounts for the depression of the discharges of impulses by Deiters neurones during administration of this amino acid (Bruggencate and Engberg, 1969a). Strychnine influences neither the cerebellar inhibition (Obata *et al.*, 1967) nor the action of GABA (Bruggencate and Engberg, 1969b) upon Deiters neurones.

The concentration of GABA in isolated Purkinje cells is high relative to that of spinal motoneurones (Obata, 1969; Obata, Otsuka and Tanaka, 1970a), and the release of GABA into the fourth ventricle, presumably from Purkinje cell axons, increases during stimulation of the cerebellar cortex (Obata and Takeda, 1969). A similar increased release has also been detected with local push-pull perfusion in the cerebellar nuclei, as well as in the nucleus of Deiters (K. Obata and H. Shinozaki, unpublished observations). More recently (Otsuka, Obata, Miyata and Tanaka, 1970), the GABA content of isolated dorsal Deiters neurones has been found to be high relative to that of ventral Deiters neurones which receive no Purkinje cell axons (Walberg and Jansen, 1961; Ito *et al.*, 1968a), and GABA levels in dorsal neurones are reduced significantly after chronic section of Purkinje cell axons. These results suggest that GABA is located in the axon terminals of Purkinje cells making contact with the dorsal Deiters neurones. Fonnum, Storm-Mathisen and Walberg (1970) demonstrated that the activity of glutamate decarboxylase, an enzyme associated with GABA synthesis (Kravitz, Molinoff and Hall, 1965), is high in the dorsal part of the nucleus of Deiters relative to its ventral part.

In efforts to identify GABA or a related substance as the natural inhibitory transmitter liberated from Purkinje cell axons, three major problems have been left unsolved. First, in previous experiments (Obata *et al.*, 1967), Purkinje cell inhibition of Deiters neurones could not be reduced by picrotoxin, a specific antagonist of the crustacean inhibitory neuromuscular junction (Robbins and van der Kloot, 1958; Grundfest, Reuben and Rickles, 1959) that is presumed to be operated by GABA (Kuffler, 1960; Takeuchi and Takeuchi, 1965). However, the effectiveness of picrotoxin in blocking postsynaptic inhibition has been reported recently in several regions of the mammalian CNS. A relatively large dose of picrotoxin given intravenously blocks the postsynaptic inhibition of oculomotor neurones by stimulating vestibular nuclei cells (Ito, Highstein and Tsuchiya, 1970a), as well as the inhibition of vestibular nuclei cells evoked from the cerebellar flocculus, an inhibition presumably involving Purkinje cell axons (Ito, Highstein and Fukuda, 1970b). Picrotoxin, ejected through micropipettes, reduces the depressant action of GABA on cuneate neurones (Galindo, 1969), and on spinal and Deiters neurones (Bruggencate and Engberg, 1969c; Engberg and Thaller, 1970), and also blocks both postsynaptic inhibition and GABA action on oculomotor neurones (Obata and Highstein, 1970). The present experiments confirmed that picrotoxin administered systemically or electrophoretically effectively blocks both Purkinje cell inhibition and GABA action upon Deiters neurones.

Secondly, glycine as well as GABA, has been postulated as a natural inhibitory transmitter substance, particularly in the spinal cord (Werman, Davidoff and Aprison, 1968; Curtis, Hösli, Johnston and Johnston, 1968a; Curtis, Hösli and Johnston, 1968b; Bruggencate and Engberg, 1968). In order to show that action of glycine is irrelevant to Purkinje cell inhibition of Deiters neurones, the differential blocking actions of strychnine on glycine, and of picrotoxin on GABA (Galindo, 1969; Bruggencate and Engberg, 1969c; Obata and Highstein, 1970), were tested in the present experiments. Finally, the similarity of the GABA-induced hyperpolarization of Deiters neurones to the inhibitory postsynaptic potentials (IPSPs) evoked by Purkinje cell impulses was indicated by demonstrating that both reach an equilibrium at the same level of membrane potential.

## Methods

Experiments were performed on 31 cats anaesthetized with pentobarbitone sodium (Nembutal, Abbott or Mintal, Tanabe; 35 mg/kg intraperitoneally initially, supplemented intravenously when necessary), immobilized with gallamine triethiodide (Gallamine, Teisan; 20 mg intravenously on occasion), and artificially respired. The dissection and experimental arrangements were as described previously (Ito, Hongo, Yoshida, Okada and Obata, 1964; Ito and Yoshida, 1966; Obata et al., 1967).

For electrophoretic drug administration, three types of micropipettes were used: coaxial, parallel, and five- or six-barrel. The inner recording barrel of the coaxial micropipettes was filled with 2M K-citrate solution, and the tip protruded from the orifice of the drug-containing outer barrel by 30—50 μm (cf. Obata et al., 1967). For the parallel micropipettes, a double-barrel intracellular microelectrode with a fine tip (see below) was glued to a single- or a double-barrel micropipette, used for electrophoretic administration and having a relatively coarse tip of 2—5 μm, the former extending 30—50 μm beyond the orifice of the latter. The double-barrel intracellular micropipette was filled with 2M K-citrate solution, each barrel having a resistance of 7—15 MΩ. The coupling resistance between the two barrels (cf. Coombs, Eccles and Fatt, 1955) was 50—100 kΩ. The voltage drop across this coupling resistance during passage of current through one barrel was detected by the other barrel, and was virtually cancelled by a bridge device (cf. Araki and Otani, 1955). The multi-barrel pipettes had tip diameters of 3—8 μm. The central barrel was filled with 5M NaCl solution and was used for recording (Curtis, 1964).

The following solutions were used in the micropipettes; 0.2M DL-homocysteic acid (DLH, Tokyo Kasei, pH 7.5 adjusted with NaOH), 1M GABA (Tokyo Kasei, pH 7 in most experiments and pH 2.5 with HCl, only when described), 1M glycine (Koso Chemicals, pH 7 usually and pH 2.5 with HCl when described), 1M β-alanine (Dai-ichi Pure Chemicals, pH 7), 1M imidazole acetic acid (Takeda, pH 2), 30mM strychnine nitrate (Sankodo, pH 5.5), 4.5 mM picrotoxin in 30mM NaCl (Tokyo Kasei, pH 7.5 with NaOH). All barrels of the pipettes were first filled with distilled water, which was replaced with NaCl or the drug solutions about 24 hrs before they were used. As reported by Davidoff and Aprison (1969), the pH of picrotoxin solutions decreases spontaneously, and picrotoxin becomes inactive in solutions of acidic or alkaline pH. In each of the present experiments picrotoxin solutions were freshly prepared and the pH was adjusted to 7.5 repeatedly over a 30 min period. After standing within micropipettes for a day, however, some changes may have occurred in the pH, and correspondingly in the activity of picrotoxin. Electro-osmotic outflow from glass micropipettes has been demonstrated to be a very effective method for ejecting substances without net electric charge (Krnjević and Whittaker, 1965; Obata, Takeda and Shinozaki, 1970b). Thus, in the present experiments, GABA, glycine and β-alanine in solutions of pH 7, and picrotoxin, were presumed to be ejected effectively by electro-osmosis. In this paper, the term "electrophoretic administration" is used to represent ejection both by iontophoresis and by electro-osmosis, as proposed by Curtis (1964). For intravenous injection, 3 mg/ml picrotoxin and 1 mg/ml strychnine nitrate solutions were prepared. Picrotoxin was dissolved just before each experiment (cf. Robbins and van der Kloot, 1958).

## Results

Location of micropipettes within the nucleus of Deiters was indicated by the fast negative field potentials induced antidromically by stimulation of the lateral vestibulospinal tract at the ipsilateral third cervical (C3) spinal level (Ito et al., 1964). These potentials were taken as an index of the activity of a population of Deiters neurones in the proximity of the micropipette. In this region, unitary spikes, recorded extracellularly, often discharged in response to electrophoretic administration of DLH with anionic currents of 5—200 nA (cf. Fig. 3C). These action potentials were diphasic, being initially negative and followed by a small positivity, and the discharge frequency was influenced very effectively by electrophoretic administration of GABA, glycine and $\beta$-alanine (cf. Curtis and Crawford, 1969). These extracellular units were identified as Deiters neurones by their activation with brief latencies (about 1 msec), presumably antidromically, following spinal cord stimulation (Ito et al., 1964). Impalement of individual Deiters neurones was indicated by a sudden appearance of a resting membrane potential of —40 to —70 mV, and the recording of antidromic action potentials (Ito et al., 1964).

Cerebellar inhibition of Deiters neurones was initiated by stimulating the vermal cortex of the culmen with concentric electrodes (cf. Ito and Yoshida, 1966), and was indicated by the following four types of events; a) reduction in amplitude of antidromic field potentials (cf. Obata and Takeda, 1969); b) depression of spontaneous or DLH-induced extracellular unit spike discharges; c) recording of small positive field potentials within the nucleus of Deiters, presumably caused by inhibitory postsynaptic currents flowing outwardly across activated inhibitory subsynaptic membrane (cf. Obata et al., 1967); d) recording of IPSPs from impaled Deiters neurones. All of the 120 neurones examined (74 extracellularly and 46 intracellularly) exhibited cerebellar inhibition in the form of (b) or (d), and were therefore considered to be dorsal Deiters neurones which receive Purkinje cell inhibition (Ito et al., 1968a).

*Action of Picrotoxin and Strychnine on Purkinje Cell Inhibition*
*Systemic Administration of Picrotoxin*

Figures 1 A—D illustrate that electrical stimulation of the cerebellum (3 stimuli) effectively depressed antidromic field potentials recorded in the nucleus of

---

Fig. 1. *The effect of picrotoxin upon field potentials associated with the cerebellar inhibition of Deiters neurones.* A, antidromic field potentials recorded within the nucleus of Deiters in response to stimulation of the third cervical (C3) spinal segment (downward arrow). B, C3 stimulation was preceded by a triple shock stimulation of the ipsilateral anterior vermis (300/sec). C, D, similar to A, B but recorded at a slower sweep velocity. E—H, as for A—D but after intravenous administration of picrotoxin, 3 mg/kg and 20 min later another 3 mg/kg were injected and 5—10 min thereafter E—H were recorded. Upward arrows in D and H point to the positive field potentials produced by the cerebellar stimulation. Each record in A—H consists of 3 superposed sweeps at a repetition rate of 5/sec. All fields were recorded with a 2M NaCl single microelectrode and the recording time constant was 0.3 sec. I, the relative amplitude of the antidromic field potentials (ordinate) (100% without conditioning by the cerebellar stimulation) as a function of the time interval between cerebellar stimulation and the testing C3 stimulation (abscissa). O, before; X, 7—9 min after injection of 3 mg/kg of picrotoxin; ●, 5—10 min after a further 3 mg/kg of picrotoxin (25—30 min after the first injection). Zero time (vertical solid line) represents the occurrence of the third cerebellar stimulus. Field potential amplitudes plotted to the left of the vertical line were not conditioned by cerebellar stimulation and the mean of these values was taken as 100% (horizontal dotted line). Note that the scaling of the abscissa is altered at 50 msec (vertical dotted line). J—M, positive field potentials recorded within the nucleus of Deiters following stimulation of the ipsilateral anterior vermis in another experiment. DC recording, single sweep. J. control; K, 3 min after intravenous injection of 3 mg/kg of picrotoxin; L, 3 min after another 3 mg/kg; M, 5 min after a further 3 mg/kg (total 9 mg/kg). The injections were given at intervals of 7 min. Arrows in J point to two peaks of the positivity (see text). Voltage calibrations: 1 mV for A—H, 0.5 mV for J—M. Time calibrations: 5 msec for A, B, E, F, 50 msec for C, D, G, H, 10 msec for J—M

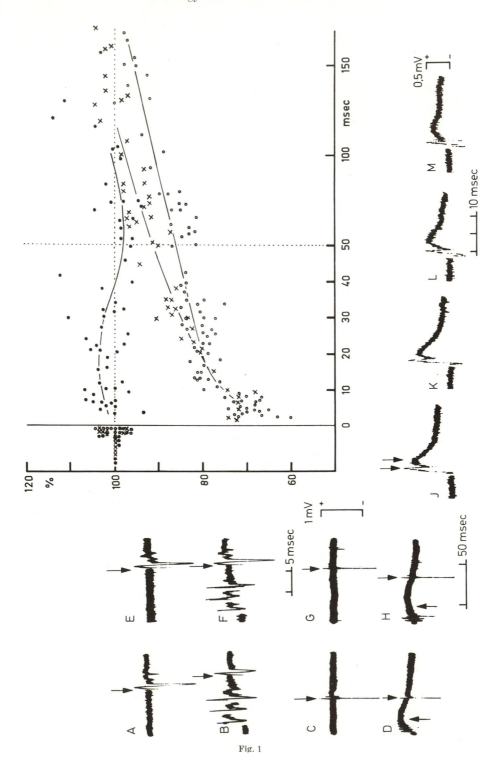

Fig. 1

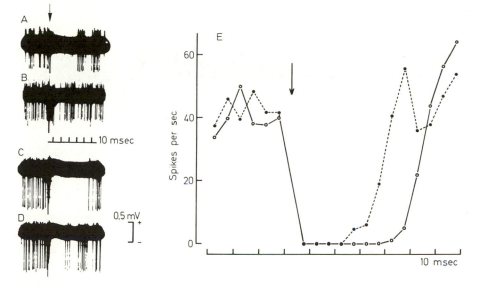

Fig. 2. *The effect of picrotoxin on the cerebellar inhibition of unit spike discharges of Deiters neurones.* A, spike discharges of a Deiters neurone induced by continuous administration of DLH (10 nA) from one barrel of a six-barrel pipette. The anterior vermis of the cerebellum was stimulated with a single pulse at the time indicated by the arrow. Ten sweeps superposed at a repetition rate of 5/sec. B, as in A, but 30 min after 10 mg/kg of picrotoxin injected intravenously. C, similar to A but another Deiters neurone. D, as in C, but during electrophoretic administration of picrotoxin (70 nA). E, the rate of DLH-induced spike discharges of the cell of C, D (ordinate) as a function of the time during each sweep (abscissa), the time of the cerebellar stimulus being indicated by a downward arrow. Each point represents the instantaneous frequency of firing, counted at 5 msec successive intervals in 500 sweeps: ○, before and ●, during the administration of picrotoxin. Voltage calibration, 0.5 mV. Time calibration, 10 msec

Deiters. The time course of this depression is plotted in Fig. 1 I (open circles). The intravenous administration of 3 mg/kg of picrotoxin reduced this inhibition only slightly (Fig. 1 I crosses), but the additional administration of 3 mg/kg abolished it, as shown in E—H, and plotted by closed circles in Fig. 1 I. In Fig. 1 D, a relatively slow inhibitory positivity followed the cerebellar stimulus. Intravenous administration of 6 mg/kg of picrotoxin reduced this positivity (H). Figures 1 J—M also show the effect of intravenously injected picrotoxin on positive field potentials evoked by a single cerebellar stimulus. In this experiment, these potentials had double peaks (arrows in J), probably corresponding to the mono- and polysynaptic components of the intracellularly recorded IPSPs (Ito and Yoshida, 1966; Ito *et al.*, 1966). This field was not affected by 3 mg/kg of picrotoxin (K), but was depressed by further administration of two additional similar doses (Figs. 1 L, M). In contrast, picrotoxin did not reduce, or even increased slightly, the spiky field potentials that preceded these positivities, representing the presynaptic volley in Purkinje cell axons (Ito and Yoshida, 1966) (not illustrated).

In Fig. 2A, spike discharges of a Deiters neurone were evoked by continuous administration of DLH from one barrel of a multi-barrel micropipette, and cerebellar stimulation depressed these discharges very effectively for a period of

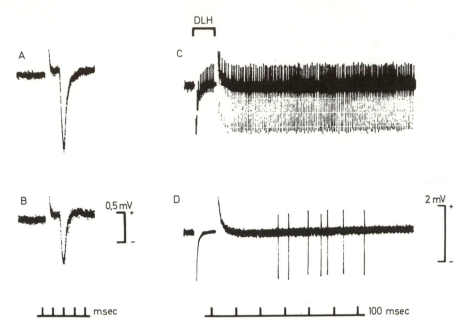

Fig. 3. *Depressant action of GABA on Deiters neurones. A*, antidromic field potential evoked within the nucleus of Deiters by stimulation of the vestibulospinal tract. *B*, as in *A*, but during administration of GABA (15 nA). Twenty sweeps superposed at a rate of 20/sec. *C*, unit spike discharges from a Deiters neurone produced by administering DLH with a pulse of 150 nA for 90 msec. The discharges ceased about 1 sec after the pulse. *D*, as in *C*, but during administration of GABA (12 nA). Calibrations, 0.5 mV for *A, B*; 2 mV for *C, D*. Time calibrations, msec for *A, B*; 100 msec for *C, D*

about 40 msec. Systemic administration of pictrotoxin (5—10 mg/kg) often caused an increase in the discharge frequency of Deiters neurones. This could, however, be prevented by administering pentobarbitone sodium (5—10 mg/kg, i. v.) beforehand. The records of Fig. 2 B, photographed after picrotoxin (10 mg/kg), demonstrates that picrotoxin greatly reduced cerebellar inhibition, there being only an incomplete depression of DLH-evoked spikes during a period of about 20 msec.

*Electrophoretic Picrotoxin*

In Fig. 2 D, cationic currents of 70 nA were passed through one barrel of a multi-barrel pipette which contained picrotoxin. The cerebellar inhibition of the DLH-induced spike discharges of a Deiters neurone (Fig. 2 C) was reduced, though to a lesser degree than after intravenous injection of picrotoxin (Fig. 2 B). The time course of the inhibition is compared in Fig. 2 E before (open circles) and during (closed circles) the passage of current through the picrotoxin-containing pipette.

The effect of picrotoxin increased to a maximum 2—3 min after the onset of its ejection, and diminished 1—2 min after the ejection ceased. In the present study picrotoxin was administered with currents less than 100 nA, and only partially blocked cerebellar inhibition of Deiters neurones (Fig. 2 E). With larger currents, the antidromic field potentials and spike discharges of Deiters neurones

504

were depressed, probably by anodal polarization of the neuronal membrane and/or a side effect of picrotoxin, as assumed by Galindo (1969).

*Strychnine*

Intravenous administration of a relatively large dose of strychnine nitrate, up to 0.7 mg/kg, did not change the cerebellar inhibition of DLH-induced firing of Deiters neurones. Electrophoretically administered strychnine (with cationic currents of up to 100 nA) was also ineffective in modifying this inhibition.

### Action of Depressants

The records of Figs. 3A and B show that GABA, electrophoretically administered, reduces the antidromic field potentials of Deiters neurones (Obata *et al.*, 1967). Furthermore, Figs. 3C and D demonstrate that GABA depresses the DLH-evoked unit discharges from a Deiters neurone, as reported by Bruggencate and Engberg (1969b). The degree of this depression increased as a function of the current ejecting GABA, as shown in Figs. 7A, B.

GABA, glycine, β-alanine and imidazole acetic acid all depressed spike discharges of Deiters neurones. To compare the potency of these substances, all were ejected from multi-barrel micropipettes filled with solutions of the same concentration and of similar pH. The currents required to just suppress the DLH-induced firing was taken to be reciprocally proportional to the potency of the ejected substance (cf. Curtis, 1964). The potency thus measured was highest for GABA, and on the basis of a GABA potency equal to 1, that of glycine was 0.3 (mean of 19 cells tested with 11 pipettes), β-alanine 0.4 (3 cells, 2 pipettes) and imidazole acetic acid 0.25 (18 cells, 8 pipettes).

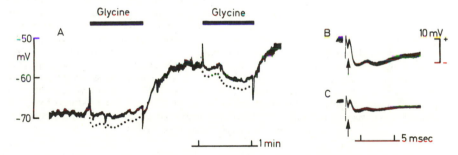

Fig. 4. *Action of glycine on intracellularly recorded potentials.* Coaxial electrodes with an outer barrel containing 1M glycine (pH 2.5). *A*, DC recording of the membrane potential of a Deiters neurone. During the periods indicated by bars, glycine was ejected from the outer barrel with cationic currents of 500 nA. Dotted lines indicate the net trans-membrane potential derived by correcting for the coupling artifact of 2.5 mV that was estimated just after withdrawal of the intracellular microelectrode. *B*, IPSPs induced by the cerebellar stimulation. *C*, as in *B* but during administration of glycine with a cationic current of 300 nA. Upward arrows indicate the "spiky" field potentials of the presynaptic velley

### Hyperpolarization by GABA and Glycine

The action of GABA and glycine was studied further by recording intracellularly from Deiters neurones. GABA, administered electrophoretically, hyperpolarized these cells as described previously (Obata *et al.*, 1967). Glycine also hyperpolarized Deiters neurones; in the cell of Fig. 4A, hyperpolarization of

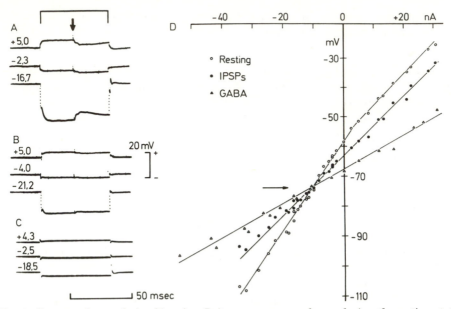

Fig. 5. *Current-voltage relationship of a Deiters neurone membrane during the resting state, cerebellar IPSPs and administration of GABA.* Parallel pipette. *A*, specimen records obtained with an intracellular double-barrel electrode. During the period shown by the uppermost horizontal bar (56 msec duration), polarizing currents (intensity indicated on each record, nA) were passed through one barrel. Plus sign (+) represents outward currents through the membrane, and minus (—) inward currents. The cerebellum was stimulated at the time indicated by the downward arrow. *B*, similar to *A*, but during electrophoretic administration of GABA (1M, pH 7, 270 nA) through the single extracellular pipette which was glued to the recording electrode. *C*, artifacts due to coupling resistance between the two barrels, recorded in the extracellular position by passing currents similar to those in *A* and *B*. *D*, current-voltage relationship derived from the series of records partly shown in *A*—*C*. *Ordinate*, membrane potential level. *Abscissa*, depolarizing (+) and hyperpolarizing (—) currents (nA) passed through the membrane. ○, measured just before cerebellar stimulation; ●, at the peak of the IPSPs; △, similar to ○ but during GABA administration (270 nA). Coupling artifacts (as shown in *C*) were corrected in plotting each point of *D*. The artifact produced by GABA-ejecting currents was so small (0.6 mV) that it was neglected in plotting *D*. Horizontal arrow marks the crossing point of three curves

5—6 mV (relative to the pre-ejection level) was produced by two administrations of glycine and depolarization followed the glycine ejections. The depolarization may have been due to either continuous deterioration of the cell, a change in the condition of impalement by the passage of current or a pharmacological effect of glycine. The IPSPs induced by cerebellar stimulation were reduced during the administration of glycine (Figs. 4 B, C), as has been observed during that of GABA (Obata *et al.*, 1967), presumably because the glycine-induced membrane hyper-polarization approached the equilibrium potential of the IPSPs. Since the spiky field potentials preceding the IPSPs were not influenced significantly (arrows in Figs. 4 B, C), glycine appeared to have no influence upon the impulse conduction along Purkinje cell axons.

In the experiment of Fig. 5, a double-barrel microelectrode was inserted into a Deiters neurone, whilst a GABA-containing pipette was located extracellularly.

One of the intracellular barrels was used for passing current pulses of about 50 msec duration across the membrane (marked by horizontal bar on the top of Fig. 5A), and the other for recording intracellular potentials. The cerebellum was stimulated to induce IPSPs during the passage of current (downward arrow in Fig. 5A). Figure 5D illustrates the current-voltage relationship of the membrane before (open circles) and during (closed circles) the cerebellar stimulation. These two lines crossed each other at —73 mV, indicating that the reversal potential of the IPSPs for this neurone was at this level (horizontal arrow), 15 mV below the resting potential.

During the administration of GABA, as shown in Fig. 5B, the IPSPs were greatly diminished in amplitude and the potential changes evoked by currents similar to those of Fig. 5A were reduced. The current-voltage curve during GABA (triangles in Fig. 5D) crossed the control curve (open circles) at the same level of membrane potential as the reversal potential for the IPSPs. Thus IPSPs and the GABA-induced hyperpolarization of this neurone had the same reversal potential.

The membrane conductance of Deiters neurones was measured from the current-voltage relationship. In Fig. 5D the increase in the membrane conductance during GABA was 78%. The average increase for 10 cells was 173% (range 25—600%) during the administration of GABA with currents of 100—500 nA from parallel micropipettes. The reversal potential for the glycine-induced hyperpolarization was also similar to that for the cerebellar-induced IPSPs. A large increase in the membrane conductance was also observed during the ejection of glycine (not illustrated).

### The Effect of Picrotoxin on Depression by GABA and Glycine

In the experiment which produced the records of Fig. 6, the currents ejecting GABA and glycine from a multi-barrel pipette were each adjusted to a level just adequate to abolish the spike discharges of a Deiters neurone (A). Two minutes after the beginning of the administration of picrotoxin from another barrel, the depression by GABA was reduced (B), and 2 min later, GABA was virtually ineffective, while the action of glycine remained unchanged (C). The effect of picrotoxin disappeared completely within 2 min of terminating the picrotoxin ejection (Fig. 6D).

Dose-response curves for GABA, before and during the administration of picrotoxin, are illustrated in Fig. 7A for DLH-induced firing of a Deiters neurone, and in Fig. 7B for the antidromic field potentials recorded within the nucleus of Deiters. Picrotoxin shifted both dose-response curves to the right (see Discussion). The blocking action of picrotoxin, administered electrophoretically, on depression by GABA was confirmed in all 9 cells and 2 foci of antidromic field potentials tested with 5 pipettes. No distinct action of picrotoxin could be detected in 6 cells examined with another 6 pipettes; this may be explained by a failure to eject picrotoxin from these pipettes, as suggested by Engberg and Thaller (1970) and/or by a degradative change in picrotoxin which occurred before ejection (see Methods).

On the other hand, administration of picrotoxin intravenously appeared to be not so effective against GABA depression as electrophoretic administration. In two cats, when Purkinje cell inhibition was almost abolished after intravenous

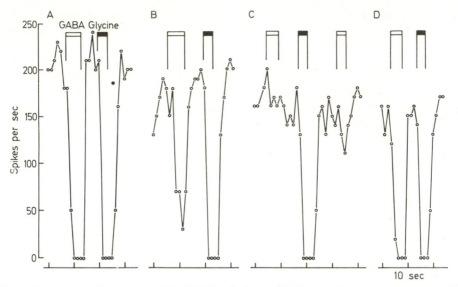

Fig. 6. *Interaction of picrotoxin with GABA and glycine.* DLH was administered continuously with a current of 30 nA and the cerebellar cortex was stimulated at a rate of 0.8/sec. The firing of a Deiters neurone was inhibited just after the cerebellar stimulation and then facilitated for a period of 100 msec or so due to disinhibitory mechanism (Ito, Kawai, Udo and Sato, 1968b). The frequency of firing was measured during 50 msec at the peak of this disinhibitory phase, and plotted as the ordinate. Hollow horizontal bars indicate the administration of GABA (17 nA), and filled bars that of glycine (71 nA). *A*, before; *B*, 2 min after; *C*, 4 min after onset of a picrotoxin-ejecting current (18 nA). *D*, 2 min after termination of a picrotoxin ejection that lasted for 5 min. *Abscissa*, time, 10 sec

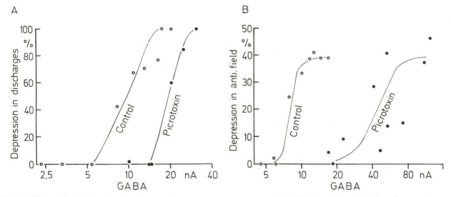

Fig. 7. *The effect of picrotoxin on dose-response curves of GABA action. A*, the depression of DLH-induced firing of a Deiters neurone by GABA. 100% represents complete suppression. *Abscissa*, currents used to eject GABA, logarithmic scale. ○, before; ●, during ejection of picrotoxin (33 nA). *B*, the percentage reduction in amplitude of antidromic field potentials recorded within Deiters nucleus. *Abscissa*, GABA currents, logarithmic scale. ○, before; ●, during ejection of picrotoxin (28 nA)

administration of 10 mg/kg of picrotoxin, 5 cells were sampled within the nucleus of Deiters. The firing of these cells by DLH could still be depressed by electrophoretic administration of GABA with relatively small currents of 10—20 nA.

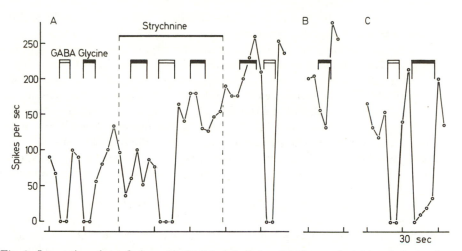

Fig. 8. *Interaction of strychnine with GABA and glycine.* DLH was administered electrophoretically with current pulses of 200 nA and 100 msec duration, repeated at a frequency of 0.2/sec. *Ordinate:* The frequency of firing induced in each trial measured at 300—400 msec after the onset of DLH-ejecting pulses. Hollow horizontal bars indicate the administration of GABA (15 nA) and filled bars that of glycine (85 nA). *A,* before, during and immediately after administration of strychnine with a cationic current of 100 nA. *B,* 5 min after; *C,* 20 min after the end of *A. Abscissa,* time, 30 sec

Although the sensitivity of these neurones to GABA was not measured before the injection of picrotoxin, these currents were of the same order of magnitude as found in many other experiments in the absence of picrotoxin.

### The Effect of Strychnine on Depression by GABA and Glycine

In the experiment of Fig. 8 A, GABA and glycine were administered from two barrels of a multi-barrel pipette upon a Deiters neurone with currents which were adjusted to levels just sufficient to stop the DLH-induced firing. Shortly after the onset of the ejection of strychnine from another barrel, the action of glycine was abolished, but that of GABA was unaffected. Figure 8C shows that the glycine action recovered after the termination of the strychnine current. Strychnine, ejected with currents up to 100 nA, produced no effect on the action of GABA.

Strychnine administered intravenously (up to 0.7 mg/kg) had no noticeable influence on the depressant action of either glycine or GABA (see Discussion). For example, for 40 min after the intravenous injection of 0.7 mg/kg of strychnine nitrate, the DLH-induced firing of a Deiters neurone was suppressed immediately by the electrophoretic administration of either glycine or GABA, using currents which were just-threshold for complete depression of the firing before the strychnine injection.

### Discussion

In a previous study (Obata *et al.,* 1967), intravenously administered picrotoxin did not block cerebellar inhibition of Deiters neurones, presumably because of the relatively small dose administered (up to 5 mg/kg, usually 2 mg/kg). In the present experiments, the dose of picrotoxin effective in blocking cerebellar inhibition ranged from 5—10 mg/kg. Similarly, a large dose of 5—10 mg/kg was required to block the inhibition of oculomotor neurones by secondary vestibular neurones (Ito et al., 1970a), and that of the vestibular nuclei cells by stimulating the flocculus (Ito et al., 1970b). A relatively small dose of 0.2—2 mg/kg of picrotoxin reduces presynaptic inhibition (Eccles, Schmidt and Willis, 1963), and "strychnine-resistant postsynaptic" inhibition, in the feline spinal cord (Kellerth and Szumski, 1966). Presynaptic inhibition in both the trigeminal nucleus (Shende and King, 1967) and the cuneate nucleus (Banna and Jabbur, 1969) is also affected by a relatively small dose of picrotoxin (0.2—1 mg/kg i. v.). At present it is not clear why such a wide range of picrotoxin doses are required for blocking these various central inhibitions.

The present experiments demonstrated that both GABA and glycine mimic the actions of natural inhibitory transmitter substances in hyperpolarizing the membrane of Deiters neurones toward the same equilibrium potential, and in increasing the membrane conductance. Antagonism by picrotoxin and strychnine, however, discriminates distinctively the action of GABA from that of glycine, as shown previously (Curtis et al., 1968a, b; Galindo, 1969; Bruggencate and Engberg, 1969c), and relates inhibition by Purkinje cells to GABA. A complication was introduced by the difference in the effects between systemically and electrophoretically administered picrotoxin or strychnine.

Cerebellar inhibition could be abolished by the intravenous injection of picrotoxin, but was only reduced moderately by the electrophoretic administration of picrotoxin. On the contrary, the depressant action of electrophoretically administered GABA was antagonized effectively by similarly given picrotoxin, but not influenced consistently by picrotoxin injected intravenously. Antagonism between glycine and strychnine was also distinct when both substances were administered electrophoretically. These apparently conflicting findings may be explained by assuming that intravenously administered substances, and the synaptically released transmitters, would affect the dendrosomatic membrane of Deiters neurones in a fairly uniform manner, while electrophoretically administered substances would be concentrated in close proximity of the orifice of the micropipette (cf. Curtis et al., 1968a; Curtis, Duggan and Johnston, 1969). Purkinje axon terminals are indeed distributed widely over the dendrosomatic membrane of Deiters neurones (Mugnaini and Walberg, 1967).

Recently Takeuchi and Takeuchi (1969) demonstrated at the crayfish neuromuscular junction that antagonism between GABA and picrotoxin is non-competitive. In Figs. 8A and B, the maximum effects of GABA were apparently the same before and during the action of picrotoxin, as might be expected if the antagonism was competitive. However, the mechanism of picrotoxin action cannot be concluded from this experiment; if picrotoxin ejected through a micropipette reached and affected only a relatively small area around the tip of the pipette, GABA administered with stronger currents would reach and be effective upon a larger area, and therefore would exert a depressant action without interference by picrotoxin (cf. Curtis et al., 1969).

The action of glycine, not blocked by picrotoxin, should have no relevance to the inhibitory synaptic action of Purkinje cell axons. Glycine may act as a transmitter of inhibitory fibres from other sources onto Deiters neurones. In fact, IPSPs could be induced in Deiters neurones during stimulation of the vestibular nerve (Ito, Hongo and Okada, 1969), and of the midbrain and the spinal cord (Ito, Udo and Mano, 1970c). Pharmacological properties of these inhibitions have yet to be investigated.

*Acknowledgement:* The authors wish to express their thanks to Prof. M. Ito for helpful advice and criticism. This work was supported in part by a grant from U.S. Public Health Service (NB-07440).

# References

Araki, T., Otani, T.: Response of single motoneurons to direct stimulation in toad's spinal cord. J. Neurophysiol. **18**, 472—485 (1955).

Banna, N.R., Jabbur, S.J.: Pharmacological studies on inhibition in the cuneate nucleus of the cat. Int. J. Neuropharmacol. **8**, 299—307 (1969).

Bruggencate, G. Ten, Engberg, I.: Analysis of glycine actions on spinal interneurones by intracellular recording. Brain Res. **11**, 446—450 (1968).

— — Effects of GABA and related amino acids on neurones in Deiters' nucleus. Brain Res. **14**, 533—536 (1969a).

— — The effect of strychnine on inhibition in Deiters' nucleus induced by GABA and glycine. Brain Res. **14**, 536—539 (1969b).

— — Is picrotoxin a blocker of the postsynaptic inhibition induced by GABA ($\gamma$-amino-butyric acid) ? Pflügers Arch. **312**, 121 (1969c).

Coombs, J.S., Eccles, J.C., Fatt, P.: The electrical properties of the motoneurone membrane. J. Physiol. (Lond.) **130**, 291—325 (1955).

Curtis, D.R.: Microelectrophoresis. In: Physical Techniques in Biological Research, vol. 5, pp. 144—190. Ed. by W.L. Nastuk. New York: Academic Press 1964.

— Crawford, J.M.: Central synaptic transmission — Microelectrophoretic studies. Ann. Rev. Pharmacol. **9**, 209—240 (1969).

— Hösli, L., Johnston, G.A.R., Johnston, I.H.: The hyperpolarization of spinal motoneurones by glycine and related amino acids. Exp. Brain Res. **5**, 235—258 (1968a).

— — — A pharmacological study of the depression of spinal neurones by glycine and related amino acids. Exp. Brain Res. **6**, 1—18 (1968b).

— Duggan, A.W., Johnston, G.A.R.: Glycine, strychnine, picrotoxin and spinal inhibition. Brain Res. **14**, 759—762 (1969).

Davidoff, R.A., Aprison, M.H.: Picrotoxin antagonism of the inhibition of interneurons by glycine. Life Sci. (Oxford) **8**, 107—112 (1969).

Eccles, J.C., Schmidt, R.F., Willis, W.D.: Pharmacological studies on presynaptic inhibition. J. Physiol. (Lond.) **168**, 500—530 (1963).

Engberg, I., Thaller, S.: On the interaction of picrotoxin with GABA and glycine in the spinal cord. Brain Res. **19**, 151—154 (1970).

Fonnum, F., Storm-Mathisen, J., Walberg, F.: Glutamate decarboxylase in inhibitory neurons. A study of the enzyme in Purkinje cell axons and boutons in the cat. Brain Res. **20**, 259—275 (1970).

Galindo, A.: GABA-picrotoxin interaction in the mammalian central nervous system. Brain Res. **14**, 763—767 (1969).

Grundfest, H., Reuben, J.P., Rickles, Jr., W.H.: The electrophysiology and pharmacology of lobster neuromuscular synapses. J. gen. Physiol. **42**, 1301—1323 (1959).

Ito, M., Highstein, S.M., Tsuchiya, T.: The postsynaptic inhibition of rabbit oculomotor neurones by secondary vestibular impulses and its blockage by picrotoxin. Brain Res. **17** 520—523 (1970a).

— — Fukuda, J.: Cerebellar inhibition of the vestibulo-ocular reflex in rabbit and cat and its blockage by picrotoxin. Brain Res. **17**, 524—526 (1970b).

— Hongo, T., Okada, Y.: Vestibular-evoked postsynaptic potentials in Deiters neurones. Exp. Brain Res. **7**, 214—230 (1969).

Ito, M., Hongo, T., Yoshida, M., Okada, Y., Obata, K.: Antidromic and trans-synaptic activation of Deiters' neurones induced from the spinal cord. Jap. J. Physiol. **14**, 638—658 (1964).

— Kawai, N., Udo, M.: The origin of cerebellar-induced inhibition of Deiters neurones. III. Localization of the inhibitory zone. Exp. Brain Res. **4**, 310—320 (1968a).

— — — Sato, N.: Cerebellar-evoked disinhibition in dorsal Deiters neurones. Exp. Brain Res. **6**, 247—264 (1968b).

— Obata, K., Ochi, R.: The origin of cerebellar-induced inhibition of Deiters neurones. II. Temporal correlation between the trans-synaptic activation of Purkinje cells and the inhibition of Deiters neurones. Exp. Brain Res. **2**, 350—364 (1966).

— Udo, M., Mano, N.: Long inhibitory and excitatory pathways converging onto cat's reticular and Deiters neurons and their relevance to the reticulofugal axons. J. Neurophysiol. **33**, 210—226 (1970c).

— — — Kawai, N.: Synaptic action of the fastigiobulber impulses upon neurones in the medullary reticular formation and vestibular nuclei. Exp. Brain Res. **11**, 29—47 (1970d).

— Yoshida, M.: The origin of cerebellar-induced inhibition of Deiters neurones. I. Monosynaptic initiation of the inhibitory postsynaptic potentials. Exp. Brain Res. **2**, 330—349 (1966).

— — Obata, K., Kawai, N., Udo, M.: Inhibitory control of intracerebellar nuclei by the Purkinje cell axons. Exp. Brain Res. **10**, 64—80 (1970e).

Jansen, J., Brodal, A.: Aspects of Cerebellar Anatomy. Oslo: Johan Grundt Tanum Forlag 1954.

Kellerth, J.-O., Szumski, A.J.: Effects of picrotoxin on stretch-activated post-synaptic inhibitions in spinal motoneurones. Acta physiol. scand. **66**, 146—156 (1966).

Krnjević, K., Whittaker, V.P.: Excitation and depression of cortical neurones by brain fractions released from micropipettes. J. Physiol. (Lond.) **179**, 298—322 (1965).

Kuffler, S.W.: Excitation and inhibition in single nerve cells. Harvey Lect. **54**, 176—218 (1960).

Kravitz, E.A., Molinoff, P.B., Hall, Z.W.: A comparison of the enzymes and substrates of gamma-aminobutyric acid metabolism in lobster excitatory and inhibitory axons. Proc. nat. Acad. Sci. (Wash.) **54**, 778—782 (1965).

Mugnaini, E., Walberg, F.: An experimental electron microscopical study on the mode of termination of cerebellar corticovestibular fibres in the cat lateral vestibular nucleus (Deiters' nucleus). Exp. Brain Res. **4**, 212—236 (1967).

Obata, K.: Gamma-aminobutyric acid in Purkinje cells and motoneurones. Experientia (Basel) **25**, 1283 (1969).

— Highstein, S.M.: Blocking by picrotoxin of both vestibular inhibition and GABA action on rabbit oculomotor neurones. Brain Res. **18**, 538—541 (1970).

— Ito, M., Ochi, R., Sato, N.: Pharmacological properties of the postsynaptic inhibition by Purkinje cell axons and the action of $\gamma$-aminobutyric acid on Deiters neurones. Exp. Brain Res. **4**, 43—57 (1967).

— Otsuka, M., Tanaka, Y.: Determination of gamma-aminobutyric acid in single nerve cells of cat central nervous system. J. Neurochem. **17**, 697—698 (1970a).

— Takeda, K.: Release of $\gamma$-aminobutyric acid into the fourth ventricle induced by stimulation of the cat's cerebellum. J. Neurochem. **16**, 1043—1047 (1969).

— — Shinozaki, H.: Electrophoretic release of $\gamma$-aminobutyric acid and glutamic acid from micropipettes. Neuropharmacol. **9**, 191—194 (1970b).

Otsuka, M., Obata, K., Miyata, Y., Tanaka, Y.: Measurement of $\gamma$-aminobutyric acid in isolated nerve cells of cat central nervous system. J. Neurochem. (1970) (in press).

Robbins, J., van der Kloot, W.G.: The effect of picrotoxin on peripheral inhibition in the crayfish. J. Physiol. (Lond.) **143**, 541—552 (1958).

Shende, M.C., King, R.B.: Excitability changes of trigeminal primary afferent preterminals in brain-stem nuclear complex of squirrel monkey (*Saimiri sciureus*). J. Neurophysiol. **30**, 949—963 (1967).

512

Takeuchi, A., Takeuchi, N.: Localized action of gamma-aminobutyric acid on the crayfish muscle. J. Physiol. (Lond.) **177**, 225—238 (1965).

— — A study of the action of picrotoxin on the inhibitory neuromuscular junction of the crayfish. J. Physiol. (Lond.) **205**, 377—391 (1969).

Walberg, F., Jansen, J.: Cerebellar corticovestibular fibers in the cat. Exp. Neurol. **3**, 32—52 (1961).

Werman, R., Davidoff, R.A., Aprison, M.H.: Inhibitory action of glycine on spinal neurons in the cat. J. Neurophysiol. **31**, 81—95 (1968).

Dr. K. Obata
Department of Pharmacology
Faculty of Medicine
Tokyo Medical and Dental University
Tokyo (Japan)

Dr. K. Takeda
Institute for Cardiovascular Diseases
Tokyo Medical and Dental University
Tokyo (Japan)

Dr. H. Shinozaki
Research Laboratory
Nippon Kayaku Co.
Tokyo (Japan)

# MEASUREMENT OF γ-AMINOBUTYRIC ACID IN ISOLATED NERVE CELLS OF CAT CENTRAL NERVOUS SYSTEM

M. Otsuka, K. Obata, Y. Miyata and Yuriko Tanaka

Department of Pharmacology, Faculty of Medicine, Tokyo Medical and Dental University, Bunkyo-ku, Tokyo, Japan

(Received 14 July 1970. Accepted 17 July 1970)

Abstract—A sensitive method for measuring γ-aminobutyric acid (GABA) has been developed. This method consists of a combination of the enzymic GABA assay of Jakoby and Scott (1959) with the enzymic cycling technique of Lowry, Passonneau, Schulz and Rock (1961) and permits the measurement of as little as $2 \times 10^{-14}$ mol of GABA. Using this method, GABA analyses were made on single isolated nerve cell bodies of different types from the CNS of the cat. Average GABA concentrations in these cell bodies were: spinal ganglion cells, 0·2 mM; spinal motoneurons, 0·9 mM; large cells of the ventral part of Deiters' nucleus, 2·7 mM; large cells of the dorsal part of Deiters' nucleus, 6·3 mM; cerebellar nuclei cells, 6·0 mM; cerebellar Purkinje cells, 6·6 mM; cerebral Betz cells, 2·5 mM.

The GABA concentrations in the isolated dorsal Deiters' cells were greatly reduced (1·7 mM) after the removal of the cerebellar vermis while those of the ventral Deiters' cells were unaffected by the denervation. These results suggest that GABA is concentrated within axon terminals, probably of Purkinje neurons, synapsing with the dorsal Deiters' cells. The results of GABA analyses on isolated nerve cells are discussed in relation to the relevant neuronal functions and the possible role of GABA as an inhibitory transmitter.

γ-Aminobutyric acid (GABA) has been shown to be an inhibitory transmitter in the crustacean nervous system (Kravitz, Kuffler and Potter, 1963; Takeuchi and Takeuchi, 1965; Otsuka, Iversen, Hall and Kravitz, 1966). Inhibitory neurons of the lobster contain GABA in much higher concentrations than the excitatory neurons (Kravitz et al., 1963; Otsuka, Kravitz and Potter, 1967). Conversely, if a neuron with an unknown function is shown to contain GABA in a high concentration, this suggests that the neuron is an inhibitory one with GABA as the transmitter. This suggestion has so far been confirmed in the chemical studies of single neurons of the lobster (Kravitz and Potter, 1965; Otsuka et al., 1967).

In the mammalian CNS it is also probable that GABA serves as a neuronal index with regard to the transmitter and function. There is an accumulating evidence which suggests that GABA functions as an inhibitory transmitter in the mammalian CNS (Obata, Ito, Ochi and Sato, 1967; Obata and Takeda, 1969; Krnjević and Schwartz, 1967). Here, however, the analysis of the GABA in single neurons is limited by the sensitivity of chemical assay. Since the sizes of mammalian neurons are in general smaller than those of Crustacea, it is to be expected that nerve cells of the mammalian CNS will contain much smaller amounts of GABA than the large crustacean neurons analysed in previous work. In the present study, we have, therefore, developed a method for microdetermination of GABA which, by combining the enzymic GABA analysis (Jakoby and Scott, 1959) and the enzymic cycling method (Lowry et al., 1961), permits the measurement of as little as $2 \times 10^{-14}$ mol of material, and using this method GABA analyses were made on several types of isolated nerve cells of cat CNS. Preliminary reports of this work have been published (Obata, Otsuka and Tanaka, 1970; Miyata, Obata, Tanaka and Otsuka, 1970).

## METHODS

*Macro-analysis of GABA in tissue slices*

Spinal cords and brain slices were removed from cats anaesthetized with pentobarbitone sodium. From these slices selected areas were dissected out with the aid of a dissecting microscope. For the dissection of vestibular and cerebellar nuclei, slices were stained with 0·1% methylene blue–Locke solution, but other tissues were dissected out without staining. After weighing the tissues, 1 ml of 0·1 N-HCl was added per 4–25 mg of fresh tissue. The above procedures were performed at room temperature (about 23°C) and the time taken from removing the tissues from the animal until they were placed in 0·1 N-HCl was less than 30 min, usually 4–10 min. Preliminary experiments showed that the post mortem increase in GABA concentration of the nervous tissues was about 20 per cent in 30 min (cf. Elliott, Tariq Kahn, Bilodeau and Lovell, 1965). Tissues in 0·1 N-HCl were homogenized and the GABA contents of the extracts were measured by enzymic assay (Hirsch and Robins, 1962; Kravitz *et al.*, 1963). When the tissues were stained with methylene blue, the dye slightly inhibited the NADPH production by GABA conversion. Therefore, the values of GABA contents obtained were corrected using standard curves obtained in the presence of methylene blue.

*Micro-analysis of GABA by the enzymic cycling method*

*Biochemicals.* GABA–glutamate transaminase and succinate semialdehyde dehydrogenase were extracted from *Pseudomonas fluorescens* ATCC-13430 following the method of Scott and Jakoby (1959) through the first part of step 4. The specificity of the enzyme preparation was checked for glycine, $\beta$-alanine, DL-$\beta$-hydroxy-$\gamma$-aminobutyric acid, L-ornithine, L-lysine, L-glutamic acid and L-glutamine. In the presence of the enzyme preparation, these compounds did not produce any detectable amount of NADPH under the condition used in the present study (see below). Glucose-6-P dehydrogenase, glutamate dehydrogenase and 6-P-gluconate dehydrogenase were obtained from Boehringer and Sons, Mannheim, Germany. Sulphate was removed by centrifugation from the suspensions of glucose-6-P dehydrogenase and glutamate dehydrogenase before they were added to the cycling reagent.

*Constriction pipettes.* Constriction pipettes of 0·1 to 0·2 $\mu$l (Fig. 1A) were constructed from commercially available 1 $\mu$l Lang–Levy pipettes. The pipettes were calibrated as described by Lowry, Roberts, Leiner, Wu and Farr (1954).

*Principle of method.* GABA–glutamate transaminase and succinate semialdehyde dehydrogenase carry out the following successive reactions (Jakoby and Scott, 1959):
(1) GABA + $\alpha$-ketoglutarate $\rightarrow$ succinate semialdehyde + glutamate
(2) succinate semialdehyde + NADP$^+$ + H$_2$O $\rightarrow$ succinate + NADPH + H$^+$.

Excess NADP$^+$ is destroyed by heating in weak NaOH. NADPH then catalyses the following cycling reactions in the presence of glutamate dehydrogenase and glucose-6-P dehydrogenase (Lowry *et al.*, 1961):
(3) NADPH + $\alpha$-ketoglutarate + NH$_4$$^+$ $\rightarrow$ NADP$^+$ + glutamate
(4) NADP$^+$ + glucose-6-P $\rightarrow$ NADPH + 6-P-gluconate + H$^+$.

The formed 6-P-gluconate reduces NADP$^+$ under the action of 6-P-gluconate dehydrogenase:
(5) 6-P-gluconate + NADP$^+$ $\rightarrow$ ribose-5-P + NADPH + H$^+$ + CO$_2$.

The native fluorescence of NADPH is then measured.

*Analytical procedure.* A 0·13 $\mu$l volume of reaction mixture containing 0·22 M-tris–HCl buffer (pH 8·0), 2·2 mM-$\alpha$-ketoglutarate, 30 $\mu$M-NADP$^+$, 8 mM-$\beta$-mercaptoethanol, 0–6 $\mu$M-GABA and 0·2–0·3 mg protein/ml bacterial enzymes (GABA–glutamate transminase and succinate semialdehyde dehydrogenase) was placed in a 0·1 ml tube, whose lower part of about 5 $\mu$l in volume was separated from the upper part by a stopper as shown in Fig. 1B. This type of stopper was simple and quite efficient in preventing evaporation. The reaction mixture was incubated at 38°C for 30 min, and then 1 $\mu$l of 0·17 N-NaOH was added. Tubes were again capped as shown in Fig. 1C and heated to 60°C for 15 min.

To each sample in a 0·1 ml tube in ice was added 20 $\mu$l of the cycling reagent containing 0·2 M-tris–HCl buffer (pH 7·8), 1 mM-glucose-6-P, 10 mM-$\alpha$-ketoglutarate, 0·03 M-ammonium acetate, 0·5 mg/ml bovine plasma albumin, 0·2 mM-EDTA, 0·2 mM-ADP, 0·3 mg/ml glutamate dehydrogenase and 0·06 mg/ml glucose-6-P dehydrogenase. The tubes were capped with Parafilm and incubated at 38°C in a water bath for 90 min, and thereafter heated to 100°C for 5 min. Each sample was transferred quantitatively to a 1 ml fluorometer tube containing 1 ml of 0·02 M-tris–HCl buffer (pH 8·0), 0·02 mM-NADP$^+$ and 0·1 mM-EDTA. The fluorescence of each sample was read in Farrand fluorometer, Model A-3, with a Corning 5860 primary filter (365 nm) and a Farrand interference filter (460 nm) as the secondary filter. To each tube, 5 $\mu$l of 6-P-gluconate dehydrogenase suspension (2 mg/ml in 2·8 M-ammonium sulphate) was added and, after 30 min at room temperature, the fluorescence of each sample was again measured. The NADPH produced was determined by the difference between the reading of fluorescence before adding 6-P-gluconate dehydrogenase and that 30 min after

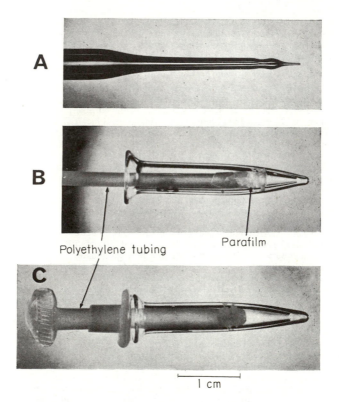

Polyethylene tubing          Parafilm

1 cm

Fig. 1.—Constriction pipette of 0·13 $\mu$l (A) and stoppers for microtubes (B and C). Microtubes contained 0·13 $\mu$l (B) and 1 $\mu$l (C) of water. For the use of these stoppers see text.

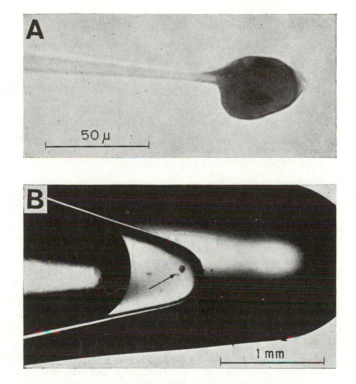

Fig. 3.—A: single Deiters' cell body attached to the tip of a dissecting glass needle and placed in xylene. B: a single Deiters' cell (arrow) was transferred into 0·13 $\mu$l of 0·1 N-HCl at the bottom of a microtube.

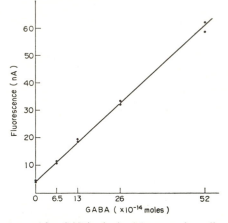

FIG. 2.—Standard curve for GABA obtained by enzymic cycling method. Ordinate records the difference between the fluorescence reading before adding 6-P-gluconate dehydrogenase and the reading 30 min after the addition of the enzyme. For details see text. Fluorescence units are galvanometer readings of the fluorometer and duplicates are recorded individually.

addition of the enzyme. An example of the standard curve is shown in Fig. 2. Reproducible measurements were obtained with samples ranging from $2-60 \times 10^{-14}$ mol. Overall amplification, i.e., the molar ratio of added GABA to 6-P-gluconate produced, was 5000–10,000.

*GABA analyses of isolated nerve cell bodies*

Tissue slices were stained with 0·1% brilliant blue 6B–Locke solution. For staining nerve cells, methylene blue is more satisfactory than brilliant blue, but methylene blue was unsuitable for the present purpose because the dye prevented the formation of NADPH by GABA conversion in the reaction mixture. Types of nerve cells were identified by their characteristic size and location. Deiters' nucleus was located according to the atlas of BERMAN (1968) with the aid of a stereotaxically placed needle. Under a dissecting microscope, a single nerve cell body was lifted out from the surface of the slice with a hand-held glass needle with a tip diameter of about 1 $\mu$m (HYDÉN, 1959; OBATA, 1969). The isolated nerve cell attached to the tip of a glass needle was soaked in xylene (Fig. 3A) and examined under a compound microscope ($\times 200$). When the cell was markedly contaminated by the surrounding tissues, it was discarded. The isolated cell body was photographed in xylene and its volume was calculated assuming the cell to be a prolate spheroid. The obtained value was used for the estimation of GABA concentration. Xylene was used during the microscopic observation because GABA is virtually insoluble in it (OTSUKA *et al.*, 1967). The shrinkage of isolated cells in xylene was found to be negligible. The isolated cells were placed in a desiccator and dried *in vacuo*. The collection of cells, usually 10–20 at a time, was performed at room temperature, and it usually took less than 30 min from the time the tissue was removed from the animal until the isolated cells were placed *in vacuo*. In some experiments on Deiters' cells, parts of brain stem, after being removed from the cat, were kept in a cold room (3°C) for less than 2 hr before collection of the cells was started. Preliminary experiments showed that keeping the brain in a cold room did not significantly influence the values of GABA concentration in tissue slices or in isolated nerve cells.

A glass needle with a dried cell at the tip was held in a micromanipulator and under a dissecting microscope the dried cell was transferred into 0·13 $\mu$l of 0·1 N-HCl at the bottom of a 0·1 ml microtube (Fig. 3B; LOWRY, ROBERTS and CHANG, 1956). To each microtube with 0·13 $\mu$l of 0·1 N-HCl, 1–5 cells were taken, and the sample was kept in a desiccator at 3°C to remove water and HCl. Just before assay, samples were further treated *in vacuo* for 10 min. To each sample, 0·13 $\mu$l of enzyme reagent containing GABA–glutamate transaminase and succinate semialdehyde dehydrogenase was added. Samples were incubated at 38°C and the assay was completed as described in the previous section. Blanks and GABA standards were run at the same time. A 0·13 $\mu$l volume of 0·1 N-HCl used for the extraction occasionally caused a slight increase in the blank value (corresponding to $0·5-1·0 \times 10^{-14}$ mol of GABA). In such a case, the obtained values of GABA analysis were corrected. The amount of tissue contained in 0·13 $\mu$l of reaction mixture with the bacterial enzymes was $3-500 \times 10^{-12}$ l. (see Tables 2 and 3). Preliminary experiments showed that brain tissue in an amount of

500 × 10⁻¹² l. per 0·13 $\mu$l of the reaction mixture gives a negligible tissue blank reading (amino-oxyacetic acid was added to the enzyme reagent in a concentration of 5 mM) and that the internal standard is 97 per cent in the presence of the tissue.

## RESULTS

*GABA concentrations in different regions of CNS.* In order to compare the values of GABA concentration in isolated nerve cells with those in their background, average GABA concentrations of tissues in which the nerve cells were located, were assayed and the results are shown in Table 1. GABA concentrations in all tissues except spinal ganglia ranged between 1 and 2 $\mu$mol/g of fresh tissue. The GABA

TABLE 1.—GABA CONTENT IN REGIONS OF CAT CNS

| Region of CNS | GABA ($\mu$mol/g wet wt.) |
|---|---|
| Spinal ganglia (L$_6$–S$_1$) | less than 0·06(2) |
| Ventral grey matter of spinal cord (L$_7$–S$_1$) | 1·0 ± 0·1(6) |
| Vestibular nuclei | 1·8 ± 0·2(3) |
| Cerebellar nuclei (lateral, interpositus and medial nuclei) | 1·8 ± 0·2(5) |
| Cerebellar cortex | 1·0 ± 0·1(4) |
| Cerebral cortex (anterior and posterior sigmoid gyri) | 1·4 ± 0·1(5) |

Figures represent the mean values ±S.E.M. The figures in brackets indicate the number of determinations.

concentration in spinal ventral grey matter is close to the value obtained by GRAHAM, SHANK, WERMAN and APRISON (1967) in the cat. The values for cerebral and cerebellar cortices as well as cerebellar nuclei are lower than those obtained by LOVELL, ELLIOTT and ELLIOTT (1963) in beef brain.

*GABA concentrations in isolated nerve cell bodies.* Table 2 shows the results of GABA analyses on samples, each consisting of 3–5 isolated nerve cell bodies of the same type. Spinal ganglion cells and spinal motoneurons contained low concentrations of GABA while cerebral Betz cells contained intermediate and cerebellar Purkinje cells and cerebellar nuclei cells contained high concentrations of GABA. Table 3 shows the results of GABA analyses on single isolated nerve cell bodies. All

TABLE 2.—GABA ANALYSIS ON POOLED NERVE CELL BODIES*

| Type of nerve cells | GABA content (10⁻¹⁴ mol) | Volume (10⁻¹² l.) | GABA concentration (mM) |
|---|---|---|---|
| Spinal ganglion cells | 1·2 ± 0·1 | 83·5 ± 40·1 | 0·2 ± 0·1(2) |
| Spinal motoneurons | 2·4 ± 0·5 | 24·4 ± 2·9 | 0·9 ± 0·1(6) |
| Cerebellar nuclei cells | 6·0 ± 0·8 | 8·1 ± 1·8 | 8·0 ± 1·1(4) |
| Purkinje cells | 2·1 ± 0·3 | 4·1 ± 0·1 | 5·5 ± 1·1(5) |
| Betz cells | 1·6 ± 0·2 | 8·0 ± 0·4 | 2·0 ± 0·2(3) |

* GABA analyses were made on samples, each consisting of 3–5 isolated nerve cell bodies. Each type of cell was collected from the regions of CNS given in Table 1.

Each value is recorded for an isolated cell, and represents the mean ±S.E.M. The figures in brackets indicate the number of determinations.

10 spinal motoneurons contained low concentrations of GABA (0–1·5 mM). Large cells from the dorsal part of Deiters' nucleus, in contrast, showed rather high concentrations of GABA, while large cells from the ventral part of the nucleus showed intermediate levels. In agreement with the results on pooled cells given in Table 2, all Betz cells contained intermediate concentrations of GABA, and many Purkinje cells and cerebellar nuclei cells showed quite high levels. The reliability of GABA

TABLE 3.—GABA ANALYSIS ON SINGLE ISOLATED NERVE CELL BODIES

| Spinal motoneurons | | | Ventral Deiters' cells | | | Dorsal Deiters' cells | | |
|---|---|---|---|---|---|---|---|---|
| GABA content ($10^{-14}$ mol) | Volume ($10^{-12}$ l.) | GABA concentration (mM) | GABA content ($10^{-14}$ mol) | Volume ($10^{-12}$ l.) | GABA concentration (mM) | GABA content ($10^{-14}$ mol) | Volume ($10^{-12}$ l.) | GABA concentration (mM) |
| 0 | 32·4 | 0 | 15·2 | 42·4 | 3·6 | 45·2 | 60·6 | 7·5 |
| 1·1 | 38·4 | 0·3 | 18·1 | 51·7 | 3·5 | 16·7 | 24·4 | 6·9 |
| 1·6 | 16·3 | 1·0 | 5·8 | 22·2 | 2·6 | 45·7 | 67·8 | 6·7 |
| 4·8 | 33·6 | 1·4 | 6·4 | 34·8 | 1·8 | 63·5 | 60·8 | 10·4 |
| 3·6 | 24·6 | 1·5 | 12·6 | 38·4 | 3·3 | 7·6 | 22·2 | 3·4 |
| 6·8 | 50·8 | 1·3 | 13·0 | 51·6 | 2·5 | 70·0 | 88·0 | 8·0 |
| 2·5 | 36·8 | 0·7 | 12·0 | 48·9 | 2·5 | 15·2 | 49·6 | 3·1 |
| 1·8 | 19·8 | 0·9 | 22·5 | 102·5 | 2·2 | 20·9 | 77·1 | 2·7 |
| 0·6 | 26·9 | 0·2 | 11·8 | 57·1 | 2·1 | 46·0 | 64·7 | 7·1 |
| 5·1 | 35·3 | 1·4 | | | | 31·4 | 43·0 | 7·3 |
| Mean ±S.E.M. 2·8 ± 0·7 | 31·5 ± 3·2 | 0·9 ± 0·2 | 13·0 ± 1·7 | 50·0 ± 7·5 | 2·7 ± 0·2 | 36·2 ± 6·7 | 55·8 ± 6·7 | 6·3 ± 0·8 |

| Cerebellar nuclei cells | | | Purkinje cells | | | Betz cells | | |
|---|---|---|---|---|---|---|---|---|
| GABA content ($10^{-14}$ mol) | Volume ($10^{-12}$ l.) | GABA concentration (mM) | GABA content ($10^{-14}$ mol) | Volume ($10^{-12}$ l.) | GABA concentration (mM) | GABA content ($10^{-14}$ mol) | Volume ($10^{-12}$ l.) | GABA concentration (mM) |
| 6·5 | 5·8 | 11·2 | 2·4 | 4·8 | 5·0 | 2·3 | 8·9 | 2·6 |
| 6·7 | 11·2 | 6·0 | 2·2 | 6·0 | 3·7 | 2·1 | 10·4 | 2·0 |
| 1·8 | 4·3 | 4·2 | 5·5 | 5·7 | 9·6 | 2·7 | 7·2 | 3·8 |
| 7·8 | 8·2 | 9·5 | 4·5 | 6·0 | 7·5 | 1·1 | 5·8 | 1·9 |
| 1·3 | 4·9 | 2·7 | 3·5 | 4·4 | 8·0 | 1·5 | 9·2 | 1·6 |
| 8·7 | 13·9 | 6·3 | 1·7 | 2·9 | 5·9 | 2·1 | 10·0 | 2·1 |
| 2·4 | 5·1 | 4·7 | 4·3 | 4·1 | 10·5 | 3·5 | 11·2 | 3·1 |
| 4·8 | 14·2 | 3·4 | 0·9 | 3·9 | 2·3 | 2·9 | 10·9 | 2·7 |
| Mean ±S.E.M. 5·0 ± 1·0 | 8·5 ± 1·5 | 6·0 ± 1·1 | 3·1 ± 0·6 | 4·7 ± 0·4 | 6·6 ± 1·0 | 2·3 ± 0·3 | 9·2 ± 0·7 | 2·5 ± 0·3 |

Each type of cell was collected from the regions of CNS given in Table 1.

analyses on single Betz cells and single Purkinje cells is rather low because the GABA content of a single cell was close to the lower limit of the assay. It is to be noted, however, that for each type of neurons the average value of GABA concentration obtained for individual cells (Table 3) is close to the mean value for pooled cells (Table 2).

*Effect of denervation on GABA contents of Deiters' cells.* Isolated nerve cell preparations assayed in the present study were very probably contaminated by presynaptic nerve terminals attached to the cell bodies. High GABA values in Tables 2 and 3, therefore, may be due to GABA being present at high concentrations in nerve terminals. This possibility was examined in the following experiments. Histological studies of WALBERG and JANSEN (1961) have shown that Purkinje neurons of the cerebellar vermis send their axons to the dorsal part of Deiters' nucleus but they do not send their fibres to the ventral part of the nucleus. Physiological studies showed that these Purkinje axons form inhibitory synapses with the dorsal Deiters' cells (ITO, KAWAI and UDO, 1968; OBATA *et al.*, 1967). On the basis of this information, an attempt was made to eliminate these Purkinje axon terminals from the dorsal Deiters' cells by denervation. In two cats the cerebellar vermis was totally removed (for the procedures of operation, see DUSSER DE BARENNE, 1924) and the animals were kept alive for 9 and 40 days respectively, after which they were killed and Deiters' cells were collected as described in Methods.

GABA concentrations in isolated Deiters' cells from the normal and operated cats are compared in Fig. 4. In normal cats, only one out of 10 dorsal Deiters' cells showed a value lower than 3 mM and the mean was 6·3 mM (see also Table 3). In the operated cats, by contrast, 10 out of 11 dorsal Deiters' cells showed values lower than 3 mM and the mean was 1·7 mM. Removal of the cerebellar vermis did not influence the GABA concentration in isolated Deiters' cells of the ventral part. These results suggest that GABA is present in a quite high concentration within presynaptic terminals attached to the dorsal Deiters' cell bodies. It is probable that these presynaptic terminals originate from Purkinje cells in the cerebellar vermis (see Discussion).

## DISCUSSION

The importance of chemical studies of single neurons has been emphasized by many authors (LOWRY *et al.*, 1956; GIACOBINI, 1968; KRAVITZ *et al.*, 1963; KUFFLER and NICHOLLS, 1966). Transmitter substances are certainly among the first substances worth measuring in individual neurons. In the crustacean nervous system, a good correlation was found between the GABA contents of single neurons and their physiological functions, so that a high content of GABA has always designated a cell as inhibitory (KRAVITZ and POTTER, 1965; OTSUKA *et al.*, 1967). In the present study in the mammalian CNS, however, the interpretation of the results of GABA analyses on isolated nerve cells is more complicated. A single cell preparation in the present study contained not only the desired cell body but also presynaptic terminals attached to the cell body and possibly glial cells, small nerve cells and nerve fibres in the immediate vicinity of the cell. So far by light microscopy the amount of contaminating tissues was estimated to be rather small (cf. Fig. 3A). However, an electron-microscopic examination will be needed to further clarify the fine structure of the isolated nerve cells and the adhering tissues (BONDAREFF and HYDÉN, 1969).

The GABA concentrations in isolated dorsal Deiters' cells showed high values, and they were markedly reduced after the removal of cerebellar vermis. It may be argued that the reduction of GABA levels in dorsal Deiters' cells after denervation was brought about by a general deterioration of the tissue caused by the operation procedures. However, 9 and 40 days after the operation the regions of Deiters' nucleus from which the cells were collected seemed apparently normal and no sign of circulatory disturbances was seen in these regions. Furthermore, the GABA

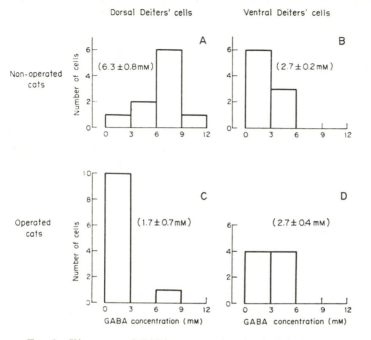

FIG. 4.—Histograms of GABA concentrations in single isolated Deiters' cell bodies from normal and operated (cerebellar vermis removed) cats. A: dorsal Deiters' cells and B: ventral Deiters' cells from normal cats (same experiments as in Table 3). C: dorsal and D: ventral Deiters' cells from operated cats. In each histogram, numbers in brackets represent a mean value of GABA concentration and s.e.m. Average volume of an isolated cell body was $34\cdot6 \pm 6\cdot0 \times 10^{-12}$ l. and $50\cdot6 \pm 10\cdot0 \times 10^{-12}$ l. for dorsal and ventral Deiters' cells, respectively, in operated cats. Those in normal cats are given in Table 3.

concentrations in isolated ventral Deiters' cells, collected from the regions neighbouring the dorsal Deiters' nucleus, were not influenced by the removal of the cerebellar vermis (Fig. 4). The most probable explanation for the reduction of GABA concentrations in isolated dorsal Deiters' cells after denervation is that GABA is concentrated in presynaptic terminals attached to the dorsal Deiters' cell bodies. Since the volume occupied by the inhibitory terminals is probably a minor portion of the total volume of an isolated cell preparation, GABA concentration in the nerve terminals may be considerably higher than 6·3 mM assessed for the GABA level of dorsal Deiters' cells in the normal cat.

In the present study each type of nerve cell was identified on the basis of its characteristic size and location. Individual nerve cells were arbitrarily sampled among hundreds of neurons of the same type. It is by no means assured that morphologically similar neurons in a given region of CNS are also alike with regard to the transmitter chemistry in their cell bodies and in presynaptic terminals attached to the cells (cf. Otsuka et al., 1967). So far in the present study, however, GABA contents of isolated cells of each type showed a certain common tendency for low, intermediate or high levels.

It is interesting to correlate the present results of GABA analyses with the relevant neuronal functions on the basis of the hypothesis that GABA is specifically concentrated in some inhibitory neurons. Low values of GABA concentrations were obtained for the isolated cell bodies of spinal motoneurons and spinal ganglion cells. These results indicate that the GABA concentrations in the cell bodies of these neurons are low, and further suggest that there are not abundant presynaptic terminals with a high GABA content in the close vicinity of these cell bodies. Spinal motoneurons are excitatory, and it has been suggested that the principal transmitter of the postsynaptic inhibition of motoneurons is not GABA but possibly glycine (Werman, Davidoff and Aprison, 1968; Curtis, Hösli, Johnston and Johnston, 1968). Spinal ganglion cells are also excitatory and histological observations have shown that their cell bodies are mostly free from synaptic contacts (Rosenbluth and Palay, 1960).

The present results of GABA analyses on Deiters' cells before and after the removal of cerebellar vermis (Fig. 4) may satisfactorily be explained by assuming that GABA is concentrated in Purkinje axon terminals originating from cerebellar vermis and synapsing with dorsal Deiters' cells (see Results). There is a considerable evidence suggesting that GABA is the inhibitory transmitter of Purkinje neurons (Obata et al., 1967; Obata and Takeda, 1969). The present findings on Deiters' cells are consistent with, and therefore give an additional evidence to, this hypothesis. Deiters' neurons, on the other hand, are known to be excitatory (Grillner, Hongo and Lund, 1970) and they may not contain a high concentration of GABA. Studies on the metabolism of GABA in the crustacean nervous system have shown that the activity of glutamate decarboxylase, the enzyme synthesizing GABA, is about 11 times higher in inhibitory axons than in excitatory ones (Kravitz, Molinoff and Hall, 1965). In this connection the recent observations of Fonnum, Storm-Mathisen and Walberg (1970) on this enzyme are quite in parallel with our findings. Fonnum et al. (1970) assayed the activity of glutamate decarboxylase in tissue sections from the dorsal and ventral parts of Deiters' nucleus of the cat and found that the activity of the enzyme is 2–3 times higher in the dorsal part than in the ventral part, and further that the enzyme activity in the dorsal part is greatly reduced while that in the ventral part is unaffected by the removal of cerebellar vermis.

GABA concentrations in isolated cerebellar nuclei cells and Purkinje cells also showed high levels, which are considerably higher than their background concentrations determined in tissue slices. Cerebellar nuclei cells are known to be excitatory (Eccles, Ito and Szentágothai, 1967). Purkinje neurons form inhibitory synapses with cerebellar nuclei cells (Ito, Yoshida, Obata, Kawai and Udo, 1970). Therefore, as in the case of dorsal Deiters' cells, GABA may be concentrated in Purkinje axon terminals attached to the cell bodies of cerebellar nuclei. As mentioned above, there is evidence to suggest that Purkinje neurons are inhibitory, with GABA as the transmitter (Ito and Yoshida, 1966; Obata et al., 1967). Therefore, the cell bodies of Purkinje neurons may contain a high concentration of GABA. However, cerebellar basket cells, which form synapses with Purkinje cell bodies, are also known to be inhibitory (ECCLES et al., 1967). High GABA values obtained for Purkinje cell bodies, therefore, might be due to GABA being concentrated in the axon terminals of basket neurons (KURIYAMA, HABER, SISKEN and ROBERTS, 1966).

Intermediate values of GABA concentration were obtained for cerebral Betz cells, which are known to be excitatory. KRNJEVIĆ and SCHWARTZ (1967) suggested that the inhibitory transmitter of the presynaptic terminals synapsing with cortical pericruciate neurons is probably GABA. The results presented in this paper are altogether consistent with the hypothesis that GABA is specificially concentrated in certain inhibitory neurons of the mammalian CNS. If this is proved, studies of GABA distribution at cellular level will afford a valuable means of mapping certain inhibitory pathways in the mamalian CNS.

*Acknowledgements*—We wish to thank Professor H. MANNEN, Department of Anatomy, Tokyo Medical and Dental University, for much helpful advice. This investigation was supported in part by a Research Grant from the United States Public Health Service (NB-07440).

## REFERENCES

BERMAN A. L. (1968) *The Brain Stem of the Cat.* University of Wisconsin Press, Madison.
BONDAREFF W. and HYDÉN H. (1969) *J. Ultrastruct. Res.* **26**, 399.
CURTIS D. R., HÖSLI L., JOHNSTON G. A. R. and JOHNSTON I. H. (1968) *Exp. Brain Res.* **5**, 235.
DUSSER DE BARENNE J. G. (1924) In *Handbuch der Neurologie des Ohres.* Band I, p. 589. Urban & Schwarzenberg, Berlin.
ECCLES J. C., ITO M. and SZENTÁGOTHAI J. (1967) *The Cerebellum as a Neuronal Machine.* Springer-Verlag, Berlin.
ELLIOTT K. A. C., TARIQ KHAN R., BILODEAU F. and LOVELL R. A. (1965) *Can. J. Biochem.* **43**, 407.
FONNUM F., STORM-MATHISEN J. and WALBERG F. (1970) *Brain Res.* **20**, 259.
GIACOBINI E. (1968) In *Neurosciences Research* (Edited by EHRENPREIS S. and SOLNITZKY O. C.) Vol. I., p. 1. Academic Press, New York.
GRAHAM L. T., SHANK R. P., WERMAN R. and APRISON M. H. (1967) *J. Neurochem.* **14**, 465.
GRILLNER S., HONGO T. and LUND S. (1970) *Exp. Brain Res.* **10**, 94.
HIRSCH H. E. and ROBINS E. (1962) *J. Neurochem.* **9**, 63.
HYDÉN H. (1959) *Nature, Lond.* **184**, 433.
ITO M., KAWAI N. and UDO M. (1968) *Exp. Brain Res.* **4**, 310.
ITO M. and YOSHIDA M. (1966) *Exp. Brain Res.* **2**, 330.
ITO M., YOSHIDA M., OBATA K., KAWAI N. and UDO M. (1970) *Exp. Brain Res.* **10**, 64.
JAKOBY W. B. and SCOTT E. M. (1959) *J. biol. Chem.* **234**, 937.
KRAVITZ E. A., KUFFLER S. W. and POTTER D. D. (1963) *J. Neurophysiol.* **26**, 739.
KRAVITZ E. A., MOLINOFF P. B. and HALL Z. W. (1965) *Proc. natn. Acad. Sci. U.S.A.* **54**, 778.
KRAVITZ E. A. and POTTER D. D. (1965) *J. Neurochem.* **12**, 323.
KRNJEVIĆ K. and SCHWARTZ S. (1967) *Exp. Brain Res.* **3**, 320.
KUFFLER S. W. and NICHOLLS J. G. (1966) *Ergebn. Physiol.* **57**, 1.
KURIYAMA K., HABER B., SISKEN B. and ROBERTS E. (1966) *Proc. natn. Acad. Sci. U.S.A.* **55**, 846.
LOVELL R. A., ELLIOTT S. J. and ELLIOTT K. A. C. (1963) *J. Neurochem.* **10**, 479.
LOWRY O. H., PASSONNEAU J. V., SCHULZ D. W. and ROCK M. K. (1961) *J. biol. Chem.* **236**, 2746.
LOWRY O. H., ROBERTS N. R. and CHANG M. W. (1956) *J. biol. Chem.* **222**, 97.
LOWRY O. H., ROBERTS N. R., LEINER K. Y., WU M. and FARR A. L. (1954) *J. biol. Chem.* **207**, 1.
MIYATA Y., OBATA K., TANAKA Y. and OTSUKA M. (1970) *J. Physiol. Soc. Japan.* In press.
OBATA K. (1969) *Experientia* **25**, 1283.
OBATA K., ITO M., OCHI R. and SATO N. (1967) *Exp. Brain Res.* **4**, 43.
OBATA K., OTSUKA M. and TANAKA Y. (1970) *J. Neurochem.* **17**, 697.
OBATA K. and TAKEDA K. (1969) *J. Neurochem.* **16**, 1043.
OTSUKA M., IVERSEN L. L., HALL Z. W. and KRAVITZ E. A. (1966) *Proc. natn. Acad. Sci. U.S.A.* **56**, 1110.
OTSUKA M., KRAVITZ E. A. and POTTER D. D. (1967) *J. Neurophysiol.* **30**, 725.
ROSENBLUTH J. and PALAY S. L. (1960) *Anat. Rec.* **136**, 268.
SCOTT E. M. and JAKOBY W. B. (1959) *J. biol. Chem.* **234**, 932.
TAKEUCHI A. and TAKEUCHI N. (1965) *J. Physiol., Lond.* **177**, 225.
WALBERG F. and JANSEN J. (1961) *Exp. Neurol.* **3**, 32.
WERMAN R., DAVIDOFF R. A. and APRISON M. H. (1968) *J. Neurophysiol.* **31**, 81.

*Chapter 10*
# NEURONS *IN VITRO*

Cultivation of cells and tissues *in vitro* allows the investigation of biological phenomena in an environment that can be controlled and manipulated. Culture techniques have been of major importance for studies of animal viruses, of mechanisms of cell growth, and of cell and tissue differentiation. Although investigations *in vitro* have been less prominent in neurobiology and have been concerned mainly with establishing that nerve cells in culture retain their distinctive neuronal properties, recent advances in the field have made clear the potential power of the technique for research on fundamental neurobiological problems. While cell culture has barely begun to contribute to our understanding of synaptic chemistry, its unmistakable promise recommends its inclusion here.

*In vitro* work on nervous tissue dates from the inception of tissue culture itself. In the first decade of this century, R.G. Harrison (1907) reported maintenance of neural tissue from embryonic frogs in sterile lymph. He was able to demonstrate conclusively that axons are not formed by the fusion of chains of Schwann cells, and he inferred that they arise from neurons. These observations provided strong support for the concept of the neuron that had been proposed by Ramon y Cajal and others in the late 1800's.

Following Harrison's pioneering work, techniques were developed for the culture of avian and mammalian nervous tissue. The first major phase of *in vitro* investigation involved the study of "explant" cultures, prepared from slices or chunks of embryonic nervous tissue. The basic architecture of these tissue fragments is preserved, though cellular migrations and the development of necrotic zones often occur. Earlier investigations emphasized morphology and demonstrated a variety of developmental processes in cultured tissue, including formation of synaptic contacts, outgrowth of neurites, myelination of axons, stimulation of growth of neurons by specific biological factors (*e.g.,* the well-known nerve growth factor), and migration of neurons and glia *in vitro.* Electrophysiological studies, moreover, have shown that cells in such explant cultures can generate action potentials and form functioning synapses (Crain, 1956; 1970).

Studies of explant cultures have been very important in demonstrating that complex nervous tissue can survive, mature, and remain active for long periods of time *in vitro.* Attempts to investigate particular neuron-neuron interactions or other events at the cellular level in these cultures are frustrated, however, by the heterogeneity, high density, and complex interrelationships of cells in the explants. Use of monolayer cultures, in which the numbers of cells and cell types are reduced, has overcome many of these problems. Such simplification allows direct morphological and physiological examination of individual neurons and permits experimental study *in vitro* of processes such as synapse formation. Neurons can be challenged with their target cells or with foreign cells, and the results directly monitored. For biochemical studies, large numbers of reproducible cultures can be prepared in which the environment around the cells can be controlled.

Primary monolayer cultures are generally prepared from embryonic or neonatal nervous tissue that is dissociated, by treatment with proteolytic enzymes or by simple mechanical agitation, into single cells or small groups of cells. The cells are then plated at low numerical density on collagen-coated glass or plastic surfaces in culture dishes containing a complex nutrient medium. Two major problems must be confronted in establishing good cultures: one is prevention of overgrowth of neuronal cultures with various non-neural, dividing cell types such as fibroblasts (mature neurons do not divide); the other is separation of different neuronal cell types from a complex population. Several satisfactory solutions to the first problem are now known, such as use of inhibitors of DNA synthesis or choice of a medium that suppresses the dividing cells (for examples, see Bray, 1970; Okun, 1972; and the reprinted article by Fischbach, 1972). The second problem, the sorting of various cell types, remains formidable, with only the barest advances toward solution.

Low-density monolayer cultures, from which essentially all non-neuronal cells have been eliminated, have been prepared from spinal cord, sympathetic ganglia, and dorsal root ganglia. Heart and skeletal muscle cells also have been grown; the skeletal myoblasts fuse *in vitro* to form myotubes and subsequently differentiate into mature striated muscle. The potentialities of these cultures are well illustrated in the reprinted paper (Fischbach, 1972) on formation of neuromuscular synapses. After myotubes had formed from myoblasts *in vitro,* Fischbach added dispersed spinal cord cells to the cultures. He selected as likely synapses points of contact between nerve and muscle cells by visual inspection and examined them with electrophysiological techniques. The neuromuscular junctions formed in these cultures resembled adult junctions *in vivo,* but the two differed in interesting ways. For example, no acetylcholinesterase was found at the junctions formed *in vitro.* Moreover Fischbach obtained possible clues about the early stages of synapse formation, such as a suggestion of early electrical coupling between cells. Clearly these studies set the stage for more extensive investigations.

Despite their promise, primary cultures have obvious limitations. For a variety of purposes it is desirable to have cells that can divide and mature into neurons in culture. For biochemical analysis greater amounts of material may be needed than what is readily available from primary cultures. Also, dividing cells should allow the establishment of genetically pure, *in vitro* lines from which mutants could be derived. One could then use the techniques of animal cell genetics to study the mechanisms by which neurons develop a characteristic form, electrical excitability, and the capacity to make and secrete neurotransmitters.

To date, no one has induced mature neurons to divide, or adapted isolated neuroblasts from embryos to culture. The only existing solution to the problem has been the development of cell lines derived from tumors. G. Augusti-Tocco and G. Sato (1969, reprinted here) established clonal cell lines that displayed neuronal morphology and contained the neuronal enzymes, choline acetyltransferase and tyrosine hydroxylase. They derived these lines from a transplantable mouse neuroblastoma, which was first described at the Jackson Laboratories in 1940, and was maintained by passage from animal to animal. The cellular origin of the tumor has not been firmly established, but it is thought to have derived from the neural crest tissue that forms adrenal medullary cells and postganglionic sympathetic neurons. Augusti-Tocco and Sato "adapted" the tumor cells by alternate passage through culture and animal hosts. This procedure was developed by V. Buonassisi, G. Sato, and A. Cohen (1962) and selects for actively dividing cells in culture, but discriminates, in the animal host phase, against the stromal cells that usually predominate in such cultures.

The availability of the neuroblastoma cells has stimulated an enormous amount of investigation into their properties. Various cell lines have been shown to conduct action potentials, to respond to neurotransmitters, and to contain specific enzymes for the synthesis of transmitters. Although it has been difficult to obtain stable neuroblastoma cell lines, certain clones have been isolated that have especially high levels of choline acetyltransferase or tyrosine hydroxylase. In addition, attempts are in progress to produce and isolate other types of tumors, from which cells with different characteristics can be obtained. One major reservation remains. The derivation of cell lines from tumors, to obtain dividing and therefore pathological neuron-like cells, may yield cells that are unlike neurons in other important respects as well. Before the full potential of these tumor cells is realized, the extent of such deviations must be carefully determined.

## READING LIST

### Reprinted Papers

1. Augusti-Tocco, G. and G. Sato (1969). Establishment of functional clonal lines of neurons from mouse neuroblastoma. *Proc. Nat. Acad. Sci.* 64: 311–315.
2. Fischbach, G.D. (1972). Synapse formation between dissociated nerve and muscle cells in low density cell cultures. *Devel. Biol.* 28: 407–429.

### Historical Paper

3. Harrison, R.G. (1907). Observations on living, developing nerve fibers. *Proc. Soc. Exp. Biol. Med.* 4: 140–143.

### Neuronal Culture

4. Crain, S.M. (1956). Resting and action potentials of cultured chick embryo spinal ganglion cells. *J. Comp. Neurol.* 104: 285–330.
5. Varon, S. and C.W. Raiborn (1969). Dissociation, fractionation, and culture of embryonic brain cells. *Brain Res.* 12: 180–199.
6. Bray, D. (1970). Surface movements during the growth of single explanted neurons. *Proc. Nat. Acad. Sci.* 65: 905–910.
7. Crain, S.M. (1970). Bioelectric interactions between cultured fetal rodent spinal cord and skeletal muscle after innervation *in vitro. J. Exp. Zool.* 173: 353–370.
8. Okun, L.M. (1972). Isolated dorsal root ganglion neurons in culture: cytological maturation and extension of electrically active processes. *J. Neurobiol.* 3: 111–151.
9. Fischbach, G.D. and S.A. Cohen (1973). The distribution of acetylcholine sensitivity over uninnervated and innervated

muscle fibers grown in cell culture. *Devel. Biol.* 31: 147–162.

10. Mains, R.E. and P.H. Patterson (1973a). Primary cultures of dissociated sympathetic neurons. I. Establishment of long-term growth in culture and studies of differentiated properties. *J. Cell Biol.* 59: 329–345.

11. Mains, R.E. and P.H. Patterson (1973b). Primary cultures of dissociated sympathetic neurons. II. Initial studies on catecholamine metabolism. *J. Cell Biol.* 59: 346–360.

12. Mains, R.E. and P.H. Patterson (1973c). Primary cultures of dissociated sympathetic neurons. III. Changes in metabolism with age in culture. *J. Cell Biol.* 59: 361–366.

*Neuroblastoma*

13. Buonassisi, V., G. Sato, and A.I. Cohen (1962). Hormone-producing cultures of adrenal and pituitary tumor origin. *Proc. Nat. Acad. Sci.* 48: 1184–1190.

14. Nelson, P., W. Ruffner, and M. Nirenberg (1969). Neuronal tumor cells with excitable membranes grown *in vitro. Proc. Nat. Acad. Sci.* 64: 1004–1010.

15. Schubert, D., S. Humphreys, C. Boroni, and M. Cohn (1969). *In vitro* differentiation of a mouse neuroblastoma. *Proc. Nat. Acad. Sci.* 64: 316–323.

16. Blume, A., F. Gilbert, S. Wilson, J. Farber, R. Rosenberg, and M. Nirenberg (1970). Regulation of acetylcholinesterase in neuroblastoma cells. *Proc. Nat. Acad. Sci.* 67: 786–792.

17. Seeds, N.W., A.G. Gilman, T. Amano, and M. Nirenberg (1970). Regulation of axon formation by clonal lines of a neural tumor. *Proc. Nat. Acad. Sci.* 66: 160–167.

18. Harris, A.J., S. Heinemann, D. Schubert, and H. Tarakis (1971). Trophic interaction between cloned tissue culture lines of nerve and muscle. *Nature* 231: 296–301.

19. Harris, A.J. and M.J. Dennis (1970). Acetylcholine sensitivity and distribution on mouse neuroblastoma cells. *Science* 167: 1253–1255.

20. Minna, J., P. Nelson, J. Peacock, D. Glazer, and M. Nirenberg (1971). Genes for neuronal properties expressed in neuroblastoma X L cell hybrids. *Proc. Nat. Acad. Sci.* 68: 234–239.

21. Amano, T., E. Richelson, and M. Nirenberg (1972). Neurotransmitter synthesis by neuroblastoma clones. *Proc. Nat. Acad. Sci.* 69: 258–263.

# ESTABLISHMENT OF FUNCTIONAL CLONAL LINES
# OF NEURONS FROM MOUSE NEUROBLASTOMA*

By Gabriella Augusti-Tocco† and Gordon Sato

GRADUATE DEPARTMENT OF BIOCHEMISTRY, BRANDEIS UNIVERSITY,
WALTHAM, MASSACHUSETTS

Communicated by Marshall Nirenberg, June 27, 1969

*Abstract.*—Clonal lines of neurons were obtained in culture from a mouse neuroblastoma. The neuroblastoma cells were adapted to culture growth by the animal-culture alternate passage technique and cloned after single-cell plating. The clonal lines retained the ability to form tumors when injected back into mice. A striking morphological change was observed in the cells adapted to culture growth; they appeared as mature neurons, while the cells of the tumor appeared as immature neuroblasts.

Acetylcholinesterase and the enzymes for the synthesis of neurotransmitters, cholineacetylase and tyrosine hydroxylase were assayed in the tumor and compared with brain levels; tyrosine hydroxylase was found to be particularly high, as described previously in human neuroblastomas. The three enzymes were found in the clonal cultures at levels comparable to those found in the tumors. Similarly, there were no remarkable differences between the three clones examined.

---

The difficulty in separating glial cells and neurons has proved to be a major obstacle in the biochemical characterization of the components of the nervous system. Methods of separation, which yield homogeneous populations of cells, are limited by the low amount of cells obtainable.[1, 2] On the other hand, the methods described for large scale preparation[3-5] give highly heterogeneous fractions and produce a large amount of cell damage.[6] Clonal cell lines of the components of nervous tissue would, therefore, provide a useful tool for the study of neurobiology. Recently, a glial cell line which retains in culture the ability to synthesize the brain specific protein S-100 has been developed from a rat brain tumor.[7] This cell line was obtained using the technique of alternate animal-culture passage described by Buonassisi *et al.*[8] to obtain in culture functional cell lines from functional tumors.

Previous work on human neuroblastomas indicates that this is a functional tumor and can adapt to growth in culture. Short-term cultures of human neuroblastoma explants have been reported to metabolize norepinephrine as *"in vivo";*[9] also long-term cultures of human neuroblastoma have been described to be able to rapidly metabolize norepinephrine.[10] Fast degradation of norepinephrine[11-12] and high tyrosine hydroxylase content[13] have been reported as biochemical features of neuroblastoma.

The availability of a transplantable mouse neuroblastoma offered the opportunity to apply the alternate animal-culture passages technique to select clonal lines which are more adaptable to the culture conditions and at the same time maintain their function. Choline acetylase, acetylcholinesterase, and tyrosine

Reprinted from *Proceedings of the National Academy of Sciences* 64: 311–315
(1969) by permission of the publisher.

hydroxylase activities were measured as a test of the functional capacity of the derived cell cultures.

*Materials and Methods.*—The mouse neuroblastoma, C 1300, was obtained from Jackson Laboratory, Bar Harbor, Maine. C-14 acetyl CoA, spec. act. 60 mc/mM, was obtained from New England Nuclear Corp., Boston, Mass.; 3,5 H-3 L-tyrosine, 36 c/mM, from Amersham/Searle Corp., Des Plaines, Ill.; Triton X-100, L-tyrosine and butyrylthiocholine from Mann Research Laboratories, New York, N.Y.; acetyl CoA, choline iodide, acetylthiocholine iodide, neostigmine methyl sulfate, 5,5'-dithio-bis-(2-nitrobenzoic acid) (DTNB), 6-7-dimethyl-5,6,7,8-tetrahydropterine hydrochloride from Calbiochem, Los Angeles, Calif.; Dowex 50 X8, 100–200 mesh, and Dowex 1 X10, 200–400 mesh from Baker, Phillipsburg, N.J.

*Tissue culture methods:* The technique of alternate passage animal-culture[8] was followed to adapt the neuroblastoma cells to growth in monolayer culture. The tumor tissue was dissociated by viokase treatment and the single cells plated in Falcon plastic plates or flasks pretreated with 5% gelatin solution. The medium used was Ham's F 10[14] supplemented with 15% horse serum and 2.5% fetal calf serum.

Clonal lines were isolated following the single-cell plating technique described by Puck *et al.*[15] from cultures at the second or third passage *in vitro*. Tumors grown from clonal cultures injected into host animal will be referred to as clonal tumors and designated with the lettering of the clone of origin.

*Enzyme assays:* Tyrosine hydroxylase and choline acetylase were assayed as described by Wilson *et al.*[16] Acetylcholinesterase was assayed according to the method of Ellman,[17] with 1 ml as final volume of the reaction mixture. The assays were run using as substrate both acetylthiocholine ($0.5 \times 10^{-3} M$) and butyrylthiocholine ($1 \times 10^{-3} M$) to ascertain that true acetylcholinesterase activity was measured. Cholinesterases nonspecific for acetylcholine hydrolyze butyrylcholine at a faster rate than acetylcholine.[18, 19] The tumors were finely minced with scissors and then homogenized in the appropriate buffer in a glass homogenizer with a motor-driven Teflon pestle. Cultures were washed twice with phosphate buffered saline solution (PBS: NaCl 8 gm, KCl 0.2 gm, $Na_2HPO_4$ 1.15 gm, $KH_2PO_4$ 0.2 gm, $MgCl_2$ 0.1 gm, $CaCl_2$ 0.1 gm per liter at pH 7) and scraped with a rubber policeman directly in the required volume of buffer for homogenization. Alternatively, the cells were scraped in 2–3 ml of PBS, centrifuged down at low speed, and then homogenized in the required volume of buffer; this procedure was followed when several flasks were needed for an assay.

Proteins were determined by the Lowry method,[20] and all enzyme activities expressed as $\mu$mole or m$\mu$moles of substrate converted in 10 min per milligram protein.

*Results.—Morphology:* Neuroblastomas have been described as highly undifferentiated tumors. The C 1300 Jackson tumor, described as a spontaneous tumor of the region of spinal cord, showed the usual morphology of neuroblastomas. Histological section of the tumor revealed the presence of only round cells. Fibers were absent.

When placed into culture, the cells undergo a striking change in morphology. The most striking characteristic of these cells is the large number of elongated processes which emanate from the cell body. These processes begin development soon after subculture or the initiation of primary culture, and within a few days form a complex network. A typical colony of a clonal line is shown in Figure 1. In each colony the cells remain rather sparse. After a few days in culture, round cells appear on the colonies (Fig. 2). They pile up on the colonies and form clumps, which tend to float away, while the cells with long processes remain attached to the plates.

*Enzyme assay:* The clonal line NB42B and the cultures obtained from the

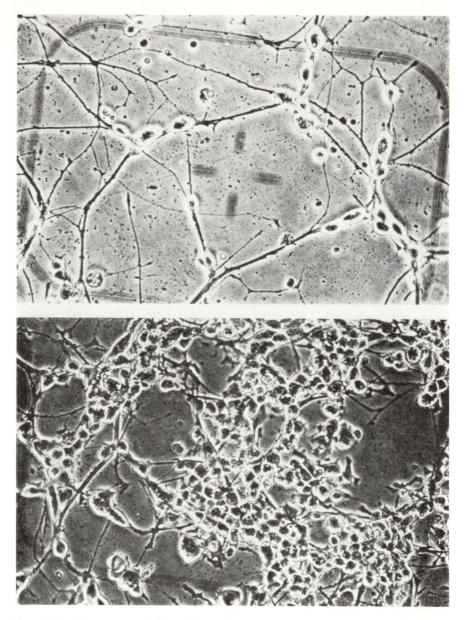

FIGS. 1-2.—Phase contrast photomicrograph (×370).  4-month-old continuous culture of clone NB42B.

clonal tumor NB41A and NB41B were assayed for acetylcholinesterase, choline acetylase, and tyrosine hydroxylase activities.   These results are reported in Table 1.   The three enzymes were present in the original tumor.   As compared with the brain, the tumor showed a higher content of tyrosine hydroxylase and a lower content of choline acetylase and acetylcholinesterase. The three clones studied, both as tumors and in culture, did not show striking differences in their enzyme contents. The differences observed between tumor and brain were much greater. Some variations, however, seem to occur going from tumor to culture. Choline acetylase activity is lower and possibly tyrosine hydroxylase activity is higher in culture than in the tumor (NB41A and NB41B). Similarly, the clonal tumors NB41A and NB41B seem to have higher choline acetylase activity and lower tyrosine hydroxylase activity than the original tumor. Acetylcholinesterase content appears to be more constant in all the conditions.

Choline acetylase, tyrosine hydroxylase, and specific acetylcholinesterase were not detected in control culture of mouse fibroblasts (AF1—Table 1).

*Discussion.*—Morphological observations indicate that the neuroblastoma cells can adapt to culture conditions and, moreover, that the culture conditions stimulate the immature neuroblasts present in the tumor to complete (or at least to proceed further in) their maturation. The same observations had been described a few years ago by Goldstein,[21-22] culturing explants of human neuroblastoma.

TABLE 1.    *Enzyme activities of neuroblastoma cell lines and tumors.*

| | Choline Acetylase | | Tyrosine Hydroxylase | | Acetylcholinesterase | | | |
| | | | | | Acetyl | | Butyryl | |
| | Tumor | Culture | Tumor | Culture | Tumor | Culture | Tumor | Culture |
|---|---|---|---|---|---|---|---|---|
| Brain | 8.1 | | 0.003 | | 1.16 | | 0.031 | |
| Neuroblastoma | 0.206 | ... | 0.0541 | ... | 0.125 | ... | 0.045 | ... |
| NB41A | 0.790 | 0.126 | 0.0041 | ... | 0.107 | 0.144 | 0.024 | ... |
| NB41B | 0.840 | 0.275 | 0.0082 | 0.0140 | 0.340 | 0.192 | 0.026 | ... |
| NB42B | ... | 0.210 | ... | 0.0145 | ... | 0.247 | ... | n.d. |
| AF 1 | ... | n.d. | ... | n.d. | ... | 0.034 | ... | 0.066 |

Choline acetylase and tyrosine hydroxylase activities are expressed in m$\mu$moles/10 min/mg protein; acetylcholinesterase in $\mu$moles/10 min/mg protein; n.d. indicates that enzyme activity was not detectable at homogenate concentration at least as high as that of neuroblastoma cells. NB41A and NB41B, cultures obtained from clonal tumors of mouse neuroblastoma; NB42B, clonal line of mouse neuroblastoma; AF1, clonal line of mouse fibroblast.

The data reported in Table 1 show that the neuroblastoma cells, adapted to growth in monolayer, keep the ability of the tumor of origin to synthesize the key enzymes for the transmission of the nerve impulse. At present, it is not possible to evaluate the significance of the observed variations of enzyme activities. In fact, specific activity of enzymes in the various tumors could be affected by the variable extent of necrotic areas; on the other hand, it has not yet been determined whether the enzyme activity of the cultured cells may vary during the growth cycle and therefore, whether the measured enzyme activity is the maximal one the cells can reach under the conditions of culture. Further work is in progress to ascertain this.

Our findings of the enzymes for the synthesis of norepinephrine and acetylcholine and acetylcholinesterase in clonal cell lines is in agreement with the Burn and Rand hypothesis for the transmission of impulse in adrenergic fibers[23] and demonstrate that the two neurotransmitters are present in the same neurons.

*Summary.*—Clonal lines of neurons were obtained from a mouse neuroblastoma by alternate animal-culture passage technique. Choline acetylase, acetylcholinesterase, and tyrosine hydroxylase activities were assayed.    Enzyme activities of cultures and tumors were of the same order of magnitude.

The authors acknowledge the expert technical assistance of Mrs. Maria Brasats.

* This is publication no. 667 of the Graduate Department of Biochemistry, Brandeis University, Waltham, Massachusetts 02154.    Supported by grants from the National Science Foundation (GB 7104) and the National Institutes of Health (CA 4123).

† On leave of absence from International Laboratory of Genetics and Biophysics (CNR), Naples, Italy.

[1] Hyden, H., *Nature*, **184**, 433 (1959).

[2] Roots, B. I., and P. V. Johnston, *J. Ultrastruct. Res.*, **10**, 350 (1964).

[3] Rose, S. P. R., *Biochem. J.*, **102**, 33 (1967).

[4] Satake, M., and S. Abe, *J. Biochem.*, **59**, 72 (1966).

[5] Bocci, V., *Nature*, **212**, 826 (1964).

[6] Cremer, J. E., P. V. Johnston, B. I. Roots, and A. J. Trevor, *J. Neurochem.*, **15**, 1361 (1968).

[7] Benda, P., J. Lightbody, G. Sato, L. Levine, and W. Sweet, *Science*, **161**, 370 (1968).

[8] Buonassisi, V., G. Sato, and A. I. Cohen, these PROCEEDINGS, **48**, 1184 (1962).

[9] La Brosse, E. H., J. Belehradek, G. Barski, C. Bohuon, and O. Schweisguth, *Nature*, **203**, 195 (1964).

[10] Goldstein, M., B. Anagnoste, and M. N. Goldstein, *Science*, **160**, 768 (1968).

[11] Robinson, R., in *Neuroblastomas Biochemical Studies*, ed. C. Bohuon (New York: Springer-Verlag, 1966), p. 37.

[12] Bohuon, C., E. H. La Brosse, M. Assicot, and A. Amar-Costesec, in *Neuroblastomas Biochemical Studies*, ed. C. Bohuon (New York: Springer-Verlag, 1966), p. 16.

[13] Goldstein, M., in *Neuroblastomas Biochemical Studies*, ed. C. Bohuon (New York: Springer-Verlag, 1966), p. 66.

[14] Ham, R. G., *Exptl. Cell Res.*, **29**, 515 (1963).

[15] Puck, T. T., P. I. Marcus, and S. J. Cieciura, *J. Exptl. Med.*, **103**, 273 (1956).

[16] Wilson, S., J. Farber, and M. Nirenberg, personal communication.

[17] Ellman, J. L., K. D. Courtney, V. Andres, Jr., and R. M. Featherstone, *Biochem. Pharmacol.*, **1**, 88 (1961).

[18] Augustinsson, K.-B., *Arch. Biochem.*, **23**, 111 (1969).

[19] Nachmansohn, D., and M. A. Rothenberg, *J. Biol. Chem.*, **158**, 653 (1945).

[20] Lowry, O. H., N. F. Rosebrough, A. L. Farr, and R. J. Randall, *J. Biol. Chem.*, **193**, 265 (1951).

[21] Goldstein, M. N., and D. Pinkel, *J. Natl. Canc. Inst.*, **20**, 675 (1958).

[22] Goldstein, M. N., J. A. Burdman, and L. J. Journey, *J. Natl. Canc. Inst.*, **32**, 165 (1964).

[23] Burn, J. H., and M. J. Rand, *Ann. Rev. Pharmacol.*, **5**, 163 (1965).

# Synapse Formation between Dissociated Nerve and Muscle Cells in Low Density Cell Cultures

GERALD D. FISCHBACH

*Behavioral Biology Branch, National Institute of Child Health and Human Development, National Institutes of Health, Bethesda, Maryland 20014*

*Accepted February 14, 1972*

Some of the neurons dissociated from embryonic chick spinal cord and maintained in low density cell cultures establish functional contacts with muscle fibers that had formed *in vitro* from previously plated myoblasts. Exposure of young muscle cultures to D-arabinofuranosylcytosine and subsequent maintenance of combined neuron–muscle cultures in low embryo extract media eliminated most of the peripheral and central supporting cells. The synapses are cholinergic, and transmitter release which, even in the youngest cultures is quantal, is regulated by $Ca^{2+}$ and $Mg^{2+}$. The major functional differences from adult vertebrate neuromuscular junctions are: slow synaptic potential time course, low end-plate potential quantum content and miniature end-plate potential frequency, occurrence of spontaneous end-plate potentials, and lack of functional acetylcholinesterase. In addition, direct electrical coupling between nerve and muscle has been observed in four cases.

## INTRODUCTION

Physiological data have been presented for the formation *in vitro* of functional neuromuscular junctions between explants of spinal cord and connected or separate but adjacent explants of muscle (Crain, 1970; Robbins and Yonezawa, 1971), between explants of spinal cord and myotubes formed from dissociated mononucleated myoblasts (Kano and Shimada, 1971), and between isolated neurons and muscle cells maintained in low-density cell cultures (Fischbach, 1970).

In addition to the precise, long-term control of the environment offered by all these tissue culture systems, the low density cell culture system offers the advantage that both the neuron cell body and muscle fiber of each synaptic pair can be identified, and, in most cases, the entire extent of each cell can be visualized in unstained cultures. Another advantage is that after dissociation into separate elements the potential exists for isolation and selective plating of different classes of neurons (Varon and Raiborn, 1969).

The architecture of the nerve terminal arbor as revealed by silver impregnation and cholinesterase stains and the ultrastructure of nerve-muscle contacts in the highly organized "organotypic" explants are nearly identical to adult neuromuscular junctions (Bornstein *et al.*, 1968; Veneroni and Murray, 1969; Nakai, 1969; Peterson and Crain, 1970). In comparison, nerve-muscle contacts in cell cultures are rather primitive. After 10–14 days fine neurites which terminate over muscle cells in one or a few simple swellings or boutons, are not covered by Schwann cells, there are no postsynaptic gutters or folds or membrane thickenings and the muscle fibers are not covered by a basal lamina (Shimada, 1968; Shimada *et al.*, 1969a). Rather simple *en plaque* endings and nonmuscle nuclei, possibly Schwann cells, have been observed in older cultures (Shimada *et al.*, 1969b; Shimada and Kano, 1971).

One purpose of this study, therefore, was to determine the extent to which the function of nerve-muscle synapses that form in cell culture resembles that of adult neuromuscular junctions. In addition, attempts were made to even further simplify the cultures by eliminating connective tissue cells with drugs that kill dividing cells.

## METHODS

Cultures were prepared under sterile conditions in a manner similar to that of Shimada *et al.* (1969a). Dissections, performed in Earle's balanced salt solution (BSS) under a dissecting microscope with transmitted bright field illumination, were completed within 10–15 min.

Pectoral muscles were removed from 11-day embryos and minced into small pieces (ca. 1 mm²). The fragments were sucked into a Pasteur pipette (ca. 5 cc), transferred to 2.5 cc of a 0.25% solution of recrystalized trypsin (GIBCO) in BSS prepared without added $Ca^{2+}$ or $Mg^{2+}$ and incubated at 37°C for 30 min in a stoppered test tube. The tissue fragments were then pelleted (1000 rpm), resuspended in complete media (see below) and trituated with a Pasteur pipette. The final yield could be significantly increased by narrowing the tip of the Pasteur pipette in a flame. The suspension was then filtered through a double layer of lens paper held in Swinnex filter holder and a sample of the isolated, mononucleated cells that passed through were counted in a hemacytometer. One pectoral muscle (one-half of the breast plate) yielded about $3 \times 10^6$ mononucleated cells. The lens paper removed large clumps of tissue, but, occasionally, aggregates of 2–4 cells appeared in the filtrate.

The aim of the present experiments was to obtain relatively pure cultures of muscle fibers free of connective tissue cells so that neurons could be easily located and fine neurites tracked in combined cultures. This was achieved by a combination of three techniques. (1) The percentage of fibroblasts in the suspension was reduced by the selective plating procedure described by Yaffe (1968). Approximately $10^6$ cells were plated in a final volume of 3 cc of complete media (see below) in 60-mm Falcon tissue culture dishes (Falcon Plastics) and kept at 37°C for 30–45 min, after which time the media was gently removed and the cells remaining in suspension (unattached) counted. The recovered cells (usually 50–75% of the initial innoculum) were then plated in collagen coated (Bornstein, 1958) 60 mm tissue culture dishes at a density of 100,000 cells/cc (3 cc total). The plating medium was composed of Eagle's Minimum Essential Medium in Earle's Salt Solution (80% by volume), horse serum (10%), chick embryo extract (CEE) (10%), glutamine 2 m$M$, penicillin (50 $\mu$/cc), and streptomycin (50 $\mu$g/cc). The glucose concentration of Earle's salt solution is 100 mg/100 ml. Fresh complete media was prepared each week and stored at 4°C. Horse serum (Microbiological Associates) was heat inactivated at 56°C for 30 min, stored at $-20$°C and thawed immediately prior to use. Serum was discarded after the second thaw. (2) Many of the mononucleated stellate cells, presumably fibroblasts, that escaped the preliminary incubation were eliminated by exposure to $10^{-5}$ $M$ D-arabinofuranosylcytosine (ara-C), a drug which inhibits DNA synthesis and also reduces the viability of dividing cells (Graham and Whitmore, 1970). The drug was added in fresh plating medium after 2–3 days—a time when myotubes were beginning to form but background stellate cells were still isolated and few in number—and was removed after 24–48 hr. The use of this inhibitor was suggested by W. Dryden. (3) The rate of division of fibroblasts that "escaped" both the preincubation and drug treatment was slowed by maintenance of the cultures in medium containing only 2% CEE.

Spinal cord cells were dissociated from the brachial enlargement and immediately adjacent cervical and thoracic segments of cords from 7-day embryos in the same manner described for myoblasts. The cord was approached from the ventral aspect and dissected free of attached dorsal root ganglia and connective tissue. Each cord fragment yielded about 0.6 × $10^6$ cells. Although freshly isolated cells possessed only one truncated process, or none at all, more than 95% were viable as judged by the exclusion of basic dyes; 0.1 × $10^6$–0.2 × $10^6$ spinal cord cells were added to muscle cultures in 3 cc of fresh 2% CEE media within 3 days of removing the ara-C, usually within 1 day. In addition, spinal cord cells were plated alone (0.05 × $10^6$ to 0.5 × $10^6$ cells/dish) in 10% CEE or 2% CEE medium. In several experiments, spinal cord cells were plated in 10% CEE medium, exposed to D-arabinofuranocylcytosine ($10^{-5}$ $M$) for 2 days and were subsequently maintained in 2% CEE medium. A collagen substrate was essential for the prolonged survival of neurons, especially when they were plated at less than 0.1 × $10^6$ cells/dish.

All cultures were maintained at 37°C in an atmosphere of 5% $CO_2$ and 95% air saturated with water vapor. The medium was changed every 2–3 days.

For electrophysiological measurements, the lid of the culture dish was removed and the dish was placed in a well of a Perspex slab mounted on the fixed stage of an inverted phase contrast microscope. Recording and stimulating microelectrodes, mounted on Leitz micromanipulators were introduced from above through a slit in a covering lid. A long working distance (80 mm) condenser allowed easy manipulation of the electrodes. The entire stage was heated and warm, moist $CO_2$ was introduced over the lip of the culture dish through a port in the side of the Perspex slab. The current through the heating coil and the flow of $CO_2$ were adjusted to maintain the bath temperature between 35–37°C and the pH at 7.4. During recording sessions, the cells were kept in either 5 cc of complete medium or, when ion concentrations were varied, in 5 cc of Earle's salt solution. No deterioration in morphology or electrical activity occurred

even after 8 hr under these conditions. In fact, many cultures were returned to the incubator and restudied at a later date.

Intracellular records were obtained with 3 $M$ KCl filled glass (0.012 inch wall thickness) microelectrodes. Signals were led via chlorided silver wires to unity gain cathode follower amplifiers and after further dc amplification were displayed on ac and dc coupled traces of a Tektronix 565 oscilloscope. Directly coupled potentials were also monitored on a penwriter. Each microelectrode was connected in a bridge circuit so that it could be used simultaneously for intracellular recording and stimulation (Araki and Otani, 1955); the stimulus was applied through a $10^9$ Ω resistor connected in series with the microelectrode. The indifferent electrode, a chlorided silver wire connected to ground, was immersed in a well of 3 $M$ KCl that contacted the bath through an agar–saline bridge. Best results were obtained with electrodes that measured between 30 and 50 MΩ when filled with 3 $M$ KCl. Stable recordings could not be reliably obtained from small (less than 15 $\mu$ diameter) muscle cells with lower resistance (larger tip) electrodes. Higher resistance electrodes did not improve recording stability, and they usually introduced several problems such as change in resistance (and hence bridge balance) during current flow, marked rectification of outward currents greater than ca 0.5 nA and significant increase in baseline noise.

Focal extracellular stimulation was achieved through a microelectrode filled with 4 $M$ NaCl. The return lead, a platinum wire immersed in the bath, was isolated from ground. The tips of stimulating electrodes were ground to about 2 $\mu$ diameter by repeated bumping on the edge of a microscope slide, and, when filled with 4 $M$ NaCl, they measured 5–10 MΩ.

Mechanical vibrations were minimized by mounting the microscope and manipulators on a heavy steel plate which, in turn, rested on a heavy marble table. The plate was decoupled from the table with sheets of foam rubber and the table from the floor with hard, corrugated rubber slabs.

## RESULTS

A brief description of separate muscle and nerve cell cultures precedes the electrophysiological findings in combined cultures.

### Muscle Cultures

A profound and prolonged reduction in numbers of fibroblasts in cultures derived from pectoral muscles of 11-day embryos was achieved by the protocol described in Methods: (1) preincubation of the initial cell suspension in uncoated tissue culture dishes, (2) exposure of young cultures to D-arabinofuranosylcytosine (ara-C) for 1–2 days, and (3) subsequent maintenance of cultures in a medium containing only 2% embryo extract. Figure 1 shows typical fields of 10-day cultures treated with $10^{-7}$ $M$ (B), $10^{-6}$ $M$ (C) or $10^{-5}$ $M$ (D) for 48 hr beginning on the second day after plating (300,000 cells/60-mm plate). Cultures treated with $10^{-5}$ $M$ resembled clones of muscle cells: they were virtually devoid of fibroblasts. Like fibers in isolated muscle clones (Hauschka and Konigsburg, 1966), muscle cells in drug-treated cultures did not differentiate and could not be maintained without a collagen substrate. The few fibroblasts that remained were extended ($>150$ $\mu$), contained clusters of refractile bodies, and either divided very slowly or not at all because the plates did not become confluent even after 2 months *in vitro*. Timing was critical at the plating density employed. If the drug was added on day 0 or 1, the cultures remained

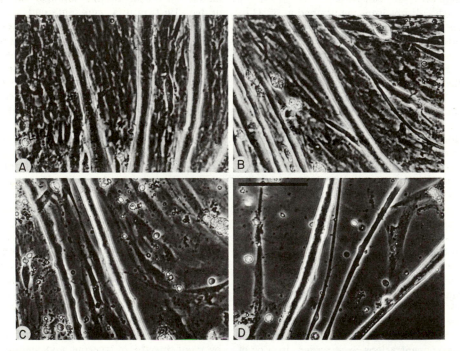

FIG. 1. Reduction in fibroblast number by ara-C. Ten-day muscle cultures. (A) Control. (B, C, and D) Representative fields in cultures treated with $10^{-7}$ $M$ (B), $10^{-6}$ $M$ (C), and $10^{-5}$ $M$ (D) ara-C for 2 days beginning on the second day after plating. Bar = 100 $\mu$.

sparse and the individual myofibers thin. If added after day 4 when fibroblasts were more numerous and many contacted young myotubes and each other, the drug was less effective. The effect of $10^{-6}$ $M$ (Fig. 1C) was variable. The initial decrease in fibroblast number was never as great as after treatment with $10^{-5}$ $M$, and the reduction was not maintained. The plates were usually confluent after only 2 weeks. Cultures exposed to $10^{-7}$ $M$ (Fig. 1B) were indistinguishable from controls (Fig. 1A). This dose-response relation is remarkably similar to that found by Graham and Whitmore (1970) in a study of L-cell viability.

Muscle differentiation was not prevented by drug treatment and subsequent reduction in embryo extract. On the contrary, cross striations were usually evident earlier and hypolemmal nuclei were more obvious in treated cultures (Fig. 1). Some fibers rounded up into multinucleated sacs, but the same phenomenon occurred in control plates. Nor did the drug affect the electrical properties or chemosensitivity (Fischbach *et al.*, 1971; Fischbach and Cohen, 1972) of the muscle membrane or prevent synapse formation.

Aminopterin, another drug which inhibits DNA synthesis, was also effective in eliminating fibroblasts. The effect of $10^{-6}$ $M$ aminopterin was indistinguishable from that of ara-C at $10^{-5}$ $M$. Coleman and Coleman (1968) obtained a significant "purification" of chick limb muscle cell cultures after addition of 5-fluorodeoxyuridine.

*Spinal Cord Cultures*

Spinal cord cells dissociated from 7-day embryos plated at densities ranging between $1.0 \times 10^4$ and $5.0 \times 10^5$ cells/dish and maintained in 10% CEE media survived for as long as 2 months in culture. Many of the cells, presumably neuroblasts, extended processes as long as 100 $\mu$ within 24 hr after plating (Fig. 2A). Unipolar and bipolar forms predominated,

but many multiprocessed cells were evident at this time. After 7–14 days, several cell types could be distinguished. Nonneuronal, polygonal, phase light cells that grew in sheets (Fig. 2B) and small, rounded, phase dark cells that grew in clusters (Fig. 2C) increased in number with time and eventually formed a confluent, multilayered mat. Neurons (Fig. 2D), those cells capable of generating action potentials, varied widely in perikaryon size and shape and in neurite length and pattern. They were usually situated on top of the nonneuronal background cells. All of the spinal cord neurons were easily distinguished from dorsal root ganglion (DRG) cells cultured under the same conditions (Fig. 2E). Thus, the morphological variety among the spinal cord cells is probably not an artifact of the two-dimensional culture system, but reflects real differences between cell types.

The pale, polygonal and dark, round background cells could be virtually eliminated from the cultures by treatment with ara-C ($10^{-5}$ $M$) or aminopterin ($10^{-6}$ $M$) for 48 hr beginning on the second day after plating and subsequent maintenance in 2% CEE media. A smaller but definite reduction in background cells could be achieved simply by maintenance in 2% CEE media beginning on the second day. Apparently healthy neurons—nonvacuolated cells with central nuclei, extensive processes and normal electrical properties —survived on the collagen substrate in complete isolation from other cell bodies for as long as 2 months (Fig. 3A).

In older drug-treated cultures (more than 3 weeks) many of the cell bodies were found in small aggregates of 3–6 cells and which were usually connected to nearby clusters by thick fascicles composed of several processes (Fig. 3B). The cells in each aggregate were enmeshed in a dense network of fine neurites (Fig. 3C). Similar aggregation occurred, but was less common, in untreated cultures and the

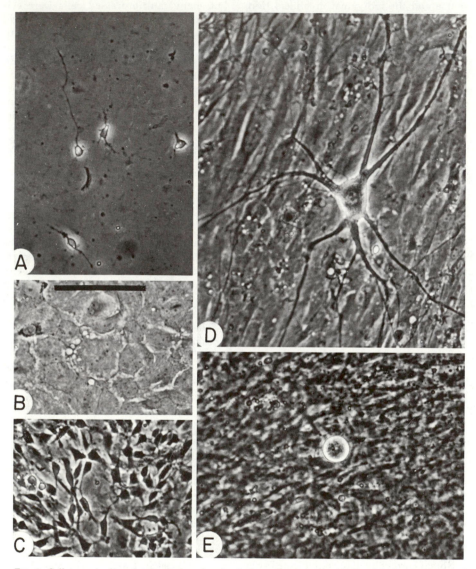

FIG. 2. Cell types in dissociated spinal cord and spinal ganglion cultures. (A) Small isolated, spinal cord cells with long processes 24 hr after plating. (B and C) Nonneuronal cells in an 11-day culture. (D) A large, multiprocessed spinal cord neuron, 14-day culture. (E) A typical, round dorsal root ganglion cell, 23-day culture. The thin process exits below the cell body and is not visible. Bar = 100 μ.

FIG. 3. Neurons in a 33-day culture that was treated with ara-C from day 2 through 4. (A) An isolated neuron. (B) Low-power dark-field view showing small aggregates of cells connected by relatively large nerve fascicles. (C) One of the clusters shown in (B). Note the dense neuropil. Bar = 100 μ in A and C; 640 μ in B.

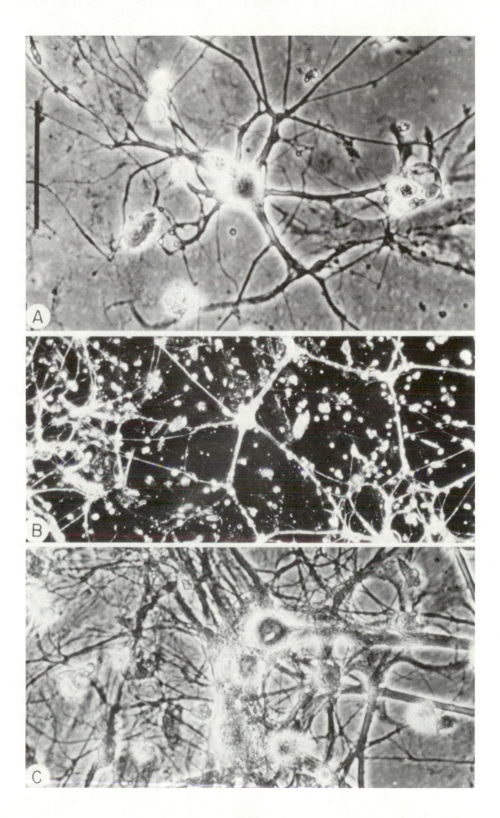

density of the neurites within each cluster was never as great as in drug-treated cultures. It is not clear whether these effects are directly related to the drugs or are secondary to the depletion of background cells.

A description of the morphological and electrical properties of the neurons will be presented in a separate publication.

*Combined Cultures*

At the time of addition of neurons, most of the muscle cells were elongated (>500 $\mu$) multinucleated, branched myotubes. Although striations and hypolemmal nuclei were apparent in several fibers, spontaneous contractions were rare. Spinal cord cells distributed evenly among the muscle fibers after addition to the "purified" cultures: no segregation according to cell type was noted. Small cells extended processes that contacted muscle fibers within 24–48 hr, and after 1–2 weeks, many mature neurons were located directly over or immediately adjacent to muscle cells (Fig. 4). In some cases, neurites coursed along a muscle fiber for several hundred microns (Fig. 4A). Nonneuronal spinal cord cells initially "filled in" areas bounded by muscle fibers, but after 4–5 weeks, despite maintenance in 2% CEE media, they overgrew some of the muscle cells.

*Stimulus-Evoked Potentials*

Evidence of functional synapses was sought by intracellular microelectrode recording from muscle cells and electrical stimulation of nearby neurons in cultures that ranged in age from 8 to 30 days (4–25 days after addition of spinal cord cells). When the neuron cell body was within the field of view (ca. 1 mm), the stimulus was usually applied through an intracellular electrode. Figure 5A shows recordings from a synaptically connected nerve-muscle pair. A brief depolarizing potential in the muscle ($m$ trace) followed an action potential evoked in the neuron ($n$ trace) shortly after the onset of a pulse of outward (depolarizing) current ($i$ trace). The neuronal membrane potential changes were recorded by the same electrode used to inject the stimulating current (see Methods). Even though end plates have not been described in dissociated cell cultures, the muscle response following nerve cell stimulation will be described as an end-plate potential (epp). The resting membrane potentials of muscle cells varied between 30 and 70 mV (see Fischbach *et al.*, 1971) and those of the neurons between 30 and 60 mV. In the best experiments, the cells could be held for more than 30 min.

In other cases, epps were detected after stimulation of nerve processes through an extracellular electrode (Fig. 5B, C). The stimulus was extremely focal; the muscle response was lost following movements of the extracellular electrode of less than 5 $\mu$. Thus, fine neurites could be stimulated selectively.

Synapses were not ubiquitous. On the contrary, epps were detected in only 5–10% of the muscles upon which a nerve process appeared to end, or over which a fine process coursed for more than 100 $\mu$. Although motoneurons—those neurons that innervated muscle fibers—were relatively large and multipolar, the occurrence of functional contacts could not, invariably, be predicted from the size or form of the neuron. For example, epps were recorded from the muscle cell shown in Fig. 4C but not from those shown in Fig. 4A or B after stimulation of the respective neurons.

Evidence was sought, but not found, for synaptic transmission from cells dissociated from lumbar and thoracic dorsal root ganglia to muscle. DRG cells added to muscle cultures exactly as described for spinal cord cells (1 × 10$^5$ cells/dish) were readily identified by their characteristic round shape, thin processes and distinc-

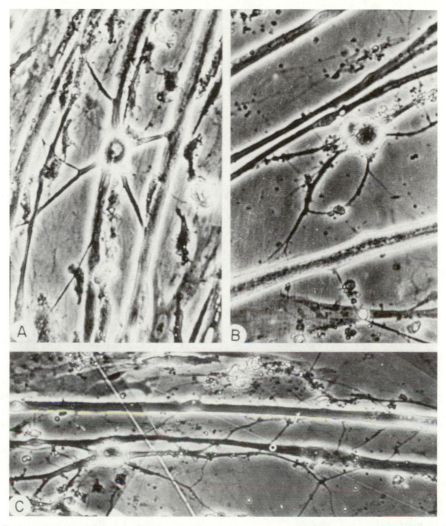

FIG. 4. Neuron-muscle pairs in combined spinal cord-muscle cultures. (A, B, and C) 25-day, 19-day, and 15-day cultures, respectively. See text. Bar = 50 $\mu$.

tive, prolonged action potential (Crain, 1956; Scott *et al.*, 1969).

The detailed arrangement of nerve endings could not be visualized with the phase contrast optics employed, but one or a few fine nerve processes appeared to terminate on the muscle cell at most functional contacts. However, in a few cases epps were recorded in muscle cells after focal stimulation of relatively large neurites that crossed the fibers and clearly continued beyond. On two occasions, mechanical prodding of the neurite directly over the muscle cell resulted in bursts of small (miniature) synaptic potentials (see below).

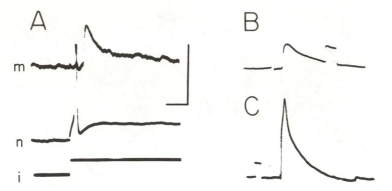

FIG. 5. Stimulus evoked synaptic potentials. (A) Intracellular stimulation. *m*, muscle; *n*, neuron; *i*, current traces (see text). Bars = 50 mV, *n* trace; 3.5 mV, *m* trace, and 10 msec. (B and C) Extracellular stimulation. Note partial spike in (C). Calibration pulse 5 mV, 5 msec in both.

Schwann cells have not been detected at functional nerve-muscle contacts. Nuclei in the region of functional endings examined in enlarged micrographs of living tissue observed under phase contrast optics and of fixed preparations impregnated with silver or stained for cholinesterase (Karnovsky and Roots, 1964) did not differ in any detail from other nuclei distributed throughout the muscle cell.

In a sample of 30 functional contacts the size of evoked epps ranged widely between 1.7 mV and 32.7 mV (Table 1). Some of the largest triggered partial (Fig. 5C) or full spikes. The mean time to peak and time to ½ decay, 2.86 msec and 11.2 msec, are slow compared to values obtained at amphibian (Fatt and Katz, 1951) and mammalian (Boyd and Martin, 1956) adult neuromuscular junctions.

The latency between the maximum rate of rise of the nerve spike and the onset of the epp fell between 2 and 5 msec in different nerve muscle pairs. Most of this delay probably reflects the conduction time of the presynaptic neurite because when the stimulus was applied near the nerve ending with an extracellular electrode, the latency was usually less than 1 msec. In one experiment in which the neuron cell body was 460 $\mu$ from the

TABLE 1

END-PLATE POTENTIAL (epp) SIZE AND TIME COURSE[a]

|  | $N$ | Amplitude (mv) | TTP (msec) | $T_{1/2}$ (msec) |
|---|---|---|---|---|
| Mean | 30 | 9.63 | 2.86 | 11.2 |
| Range |  | 1.7–32.7 | 1.3–5.0 | 5.2–21.4 |

[a] TTP is the time to peak and $T_{1/2}$ is the time at which the epp declined to ½ of the peak value. $N$ is the number of nerve-muscle pairs.

muscle fiber, the latency was 4.2 msec. Allowing 1 msec for synaptic delay, the estimated axon conduction velocity is ca. 0.1 meter/sec. This slow rate is consistent with the electron microscopic finding that the nerve processes are not myelinated (J. Heuser, personal communication).

*Spontaneous Potentials*

Small, potential fluctuations that resemble miniature end-plate potentials (mepps) of adult neuromuscular junctions were detected at most functional contacts in the absence of imposed stimulation. They usually occurred at a low rate, ca. 1–10 per minute, but in a few cases they appeared more frequently and were analyzed in more detail (Fig. 6, inset). In addition to their small size, they are analogous to adult mepps because waiting times between potentials were exponen-

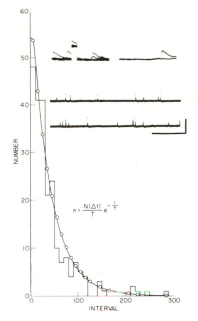

FIG. 6. Miniature end-plate potentials. In set: upper traces are superimposed sweeps. Calibration pulse = 5 mV and 5 msec; lower traces are contiguous segments of a moving film record. Bars = 5 mV, 2 sec. The continuous line superimposed on the interval histogram represents the theoretical exponential distribution of intervals between randomly occurring events.

tially distributed (Fig. 6), because their size was not greatly altered by reduction in $Ca^{2+}$ or increase in $Mg^{2+}$ concentration (del Castillo and Katz, 1956a: review) and because they persisted in the presence of tetrodotoxin ($10^{-7}$ gm/ml) (Fig. 7), a drug that blocks nerve and muscle action potentials but does not affect the spontaneous leak of transmitter (Katz and Miledi, 1967). The mean amplitudes of samples of 30–200 mepps ranged between 0.36 mV and 3.25 mV. Amplitude histograms were approximately bell-shaped but, in every case, were clearly skewed to the right (Fig. 8).

A striking interaction between stimulus evoked and spontaneous transmitter release was observed at most functional contacts. Mepps usually appeared on the

falling phase of evoked epps (Fig. 9) and, in several cases, the increase in frequency was more than 100-fold and persisted for several seconds. In some instances, mepps were detected for the first time only after one or two epps were elicited.

On occasion, a group of muscle fibers were observed to twitch in a characteristic patterned—either regular or bursting— manner. Penetration of such active fibers invariably revealed large as well as small spontaneous depolarizing potentials (Fig. 10). The rates of rise of the large and small potentials were usually identical, which indicates that they arose at the same synaptic locus. Evidence that the small potentials are mepps was presented above. The large potentials probably result from spontaneous impulse activity in the innervating neuron because they recurred in a distinctly nonrandom manner (Fig. 10A; see Fischbach, 1970; Fig. 3), there was little or no overlap between their amplitude distributions and those of the mepps (Fig. 10C), they were abolished by TTX ($10^{-7}$ gm/ml), and, finally, identical potentials could usually be elicited

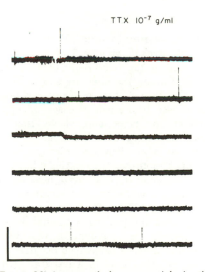

FIG. 7. Miniature end-plate potentials in the presence of tetrodotoxin ($10^{-7}$ gm/ml). Bars = 2 mV and 10 sec.

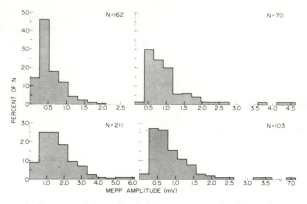

FIG. 8. Miniature end-plate potential amplitude histograms. The baseline noise was ca. 0.1 mV in each case. *N* is the number of observations (mepps). Note that each histogram is skewed to the right.

by extracellular stimulation of a nearby nerve process.

Intracellular records have not been obtained from neurons responsible for spontaneous epps, but many other neurons in culture are spontaneously active (Fig. 11). It is not yet clear, however, whether spontaneously occurring epps are due to impulses conducted from the neuron soma or to local activity restricted to the nerve terminals.

### Multiple Innervation

Samples from a series of synaptic potentials evoked at a rate of 0.5/sec and recorded at the same point (near a nerve ending) along the fiber are shown in Fig. 12. The falling phase of every epp in the series was prolonged. The second epp is smaller and rises more slowly than the first suggesting that the fiber is innervated at more than one point. According to this hypothesis, the relatively large and rapidly rising epp occurred near the recording electrode and the smaller slower epp originated at a more distant site. It is likely that the prolonged falling phase of the rapidly rising potentials was due to the simultaneous or delayed occurrence of a second, slow epp. In a few trials (third trace) the onset of the slow preceded that of the fast and superimposition was clear.

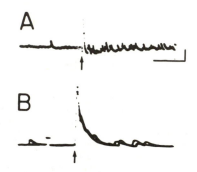

FIG. 9. Increase in mepp frequency following single evoked epps. (A) and (B) are different nerve-muscle junctions. Two traces are superimposed in (B). Epps were evoked by extracellular stimulation superimposed in B. Epps were evoked by extracellular stimulation at the arrows. Calibration pulse = 5 mV, 5 msec in (B). Bars = 5 mV and 0.2 sec in (A).

Another class of still smaller and slower epps recorded at the same point (fourth trace) suggests a third even more distant source.

In all, only 6 fibers were found in which spontaneous or evoked epps similar to those of Fig. 12 suggested electrotonically distinct sites of multiple innervation.

### Equilibrium Potential

Potentials recorded at chemical synapses result from a transient increase in permeability of the postsynaptic mem-

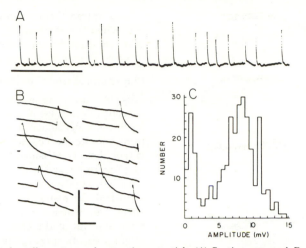

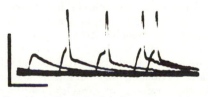

FIG. 10. Large and small spontaneously occurring potentials. (A) Continuous record. Bar = 1 sec. (B) Potentials recorded at the same point as in (A) displayed on repetitive sweeps with a faster time base Bars = 10 mV (applies to A as well) and 20 msec. (C) Bimodal amplitude histogram.

FIG. 11. Action potentials in a neuron triggered by large, spontaneously occurring excitatory synaptic potentials. Superimposed sweeps. Bars = 50 mV and 10 msec.

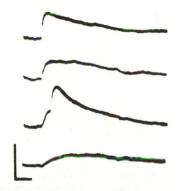

FIG. 12. Samples from a series of epps recorded at the same point elicited by stimulating a single neuron at a rate of 1/sec. The different rates of rise suggest that the neuron innervates the muscle fiber at more than one point (see text). Calibration = 5 mV and 5 msec.

brane. The size of the synaptic potential depends on the net current flow through the activated membrane which, in turn, depends on the transmembrane potential gradient. At the adult neuromuscular junction, the membrane potential at which the net current flow is zero, the equilibrium potential, is about −15 mV (Fatt and Katz, 1951; Takeuchi and Takeuchi, 1959). Thus, if the epps are chemically mediated and if the permeability change involves the same ions as at adult junctions, then epp amplitude should increase when the muscle membrane is hyperpolarized and decrease when it is depolarized. This, in fact, occurred in each of the 7 cases tested.

Figure 13 shows epps superimposed on hyperpolarizing and depolarizing electrotonic potentials which were established by current pulses delivered through the recording electrode. Successive epps varied in amplitude (see below), so the average response at each membrane potential was displayed by superimposing several traces. A plot of mean epp size vs mem-

547

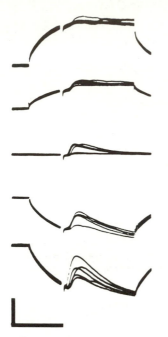

FIG. 13. Epps superimposed on electrotonic potentials. The membrane was hyperpolarized (lower two traces) and depolarized (upper two traces) by inward and outward current pulses (not shown), respectively—delivered through the recording electrode. Each record is several superimposed traces. The gap in each record marks the time of neurite stimulation. Bars = 20 mV and 20 msec.

brane potential was linear and the equilibrium potential, determined by extrapolation, was −8 mV.[1] Equilibrium potentials, determined in the same manner in 3 other fibers, ranged between −15 and −5 mV. These estimates were confirmed by interpolation in three other experiments in which it was possible to displace the membrane potential over a wider range with steady currents delivered through a

[1] Epp amplitude would vary if the membrane conductance changed as a function of membrane potential. However, the conductance of all muscle cells tested in a normal ionic environment remained constant over a range of 25–30 mV in the hyperpolarizing direction to 10–15 mV in the depolarizing direction. In a few cases, the current–voltage relation remained linear over a much wider range.

second intracellular microelectrode (Fig. 14). When the membrane was depolarized past the equilibrium potential, the epps reversed in polarity.

## Curare and Anticholinesterases

$d$-Tubocurare added to the bath in a concentration range of $10^{-7}$ gm/ml to $10^{-6}$ gm/ml rapidly blocked the abrupt, patterned twitches characteristic of innervated fibers (see below) and in every one of 10 trials in which mepps or epps were recorded, curare ($10^{-7}$ gm/ml) reduced or abolished the response (Fig. 15A, B). The effect was reversed usually within 15 min after removal of the drug. Curare did not affect neuron spike generation, muscle membrane potential, or muscle twitches evoked by direct stimulation.

The action of curare, together with the sensitivity of the muscle membrane to iontophoretically applied acetylcholine (ACh) (Fischbach, 1970) suggest that nerve-muscle transmission, in this culture system, is mediated by ACh. No physiological evidence was obtained, however, for the presence of acetylcholinesterase, another feature of adult cholinergic syn-

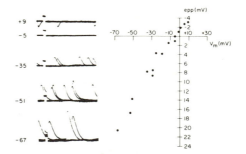

FIG. 14. The superimposed traces show the change in amplitude of spontaneously occurring epps as the membrane potential ($V_m$) was shifted by steady currents injected through a second intracellular electrode to the values indicated at the left of each record. No deflection was observed at −5 mV of $V_m$ and at +9 mV (inside positive) the potentials were inverted. Calibration = 5 mV and 5 msec. Each point in the graph represents the mean amplitude of 5–10 epps.

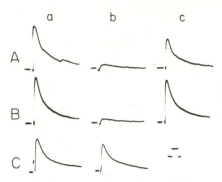

FIG. 15. A and B: The effect of *d*-tubocurare ($10^{-7}$ gm/ml) on epps recorded in 2 different fibers. *a*, control; *b*, 30 min after addition of the drug; *c*, 30 min after removal of drug. C: Lack of effect of physostigmine ($10^{-6}$ gm/ml). *a*, control; *b*, ca. 30 min after addition of the anticholinesterase. Calibration = 5 mV and 5 msec.

apses. Neither physostigmine or neostigmine, inhibitors of the enzyme, affected the size or time course of spontaneous or evoked synaptic potentials (Fig. 15C) in a dose range of $10^{-7}$ gm/ml to $10^{-4}$ gm/ml. Attempts to demonstrate the enzyme in the region of nerve endings by the histochemical method of Karnofsky and Roots (1964) have been negative. Suggestive densities appeared in the region of only one of many functional endings examined.

## Quantum Content

At junctions which exhibited epps or relatively rapid and constant rise times, i.e., which were innervated at one point or a few "electrotonically identical" points, successive responses varied markedly in amplitude, and in some series, many stimuli failed to evoke a response. Neither phenomenon can be attributed to inadequate stimulation because both occurred with stimulation through an intracellular electrode that produced a constant spike in the neuron (Fig. 16).

Such amplitude variation and the occurrence of true mepps is *prima facie* evidence that synaptic transmission is quantal: that each epp is due to the action of an integral number of units or quanta

of transmitter (del Castillo and Katz, 1956a). In fact, amplitude histograms of epps evoked at 0.5/sec or 1.0/sec were multimodal. Figure 17 shows four repre-

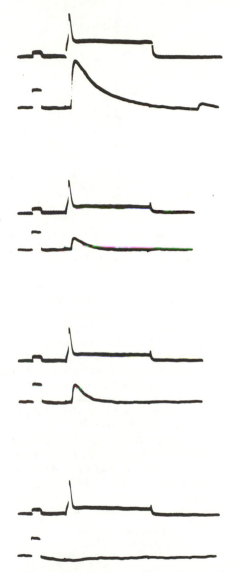

FIG. 16. Variation in amplitude of successive epps (lower traces of each pair) during repetitive stimulation at 1.0/sec despite constant action potential size in the innervating neuron (upper traces). Calibration = 5 mV, 5 msec.

549

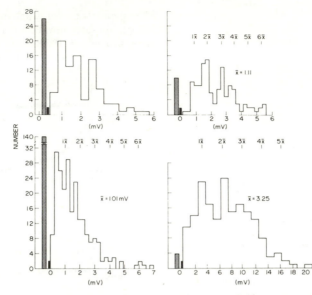

FIG. 17. Stimulus evoked epp amplitude histograms. Width of the solid bar indicates the size of the baseline noise. Hatched bar shows the number of failures. Multiples of $\overline{X}$, the mean amplitude of mepps recorded at the same point are indicated above three of the histograms.

sentative histograms in which the amplitudes cluster about certain "preferred" values which fall at multiples of the smallest class. Mepps, thought to result from the spontaneous discharge of single transmitter units provide an estimate of quantum size. Mepps were recorded in three of the experiments shown in Fig. 17 and, as indicated, the relative peaks in the epp histogram coincide with multiples of the mean quantum size ($\overline{X}$).

If epp amplitude is linearly proportional to quantum content, then the mean quantum content of a series of epps, $M$, can be estimated from the ratio $m = $ epp/mepp where bars indicate average values (del Castillo and Katz, 1956a).[2]

[2] When the epp size is a significant fraction of the resting membrane potential, the postsynaptic conductance increment is not linearly related to transmitter release (del Castillo and Katz, 1956a). Therefore, the amplitude of all epps larger than 3 mV was corrected by the factor suggested by Martin (1955): epp $= 1/(1\text{-epp}/V_0)$ where $V_0$ is the difference between the membrane potential and the epp equilib-

Such estimates obtained from junctions bathed in Earle's balanced salt solution ranged between about 1 and 30 (Table 2). These values are low compared with estimates of 200–400 obtained at adult neuromuscular junctions in a normal ionic environment (Martin, 1955). In one series, epps which, on occasion, were large enough to trigger muscle action potentials, were composed, on the average, of only 10 quanta.

Transmitter release from adult vertebrate motor nerve terminals can be described by the Poisson probability law (del Castillo and Katz, 1956a). This implies that the probability, $p$, of release of an individual quantum following a nerve impulse is small and that the total number of quanta available for release, $n$, is large. If the same law holds at nervemuscle junctions formed in culture then

rium potential. The latter was assumed equal to $-10$ mV (see above).

$M = np$, the parameter of the Poisson density function can be estimated in two additional ways: (1) $m' = ln\ (N/N_o)$, where $N$ is the number of stimuli or "trials" in a given series and $N_o$ is the number of trials in which a stimulus failed to evoke an epp; (2) $m'' = (1 + cv^2)CV^2$ where CV is the coefficient of variation (standard deviation/mean) of the series of evoked epps and cv is the coefficient of variation of the mepps recorded at the same point (del Castillo and Katz, 1956a; Brown, 1962). Agreement between $m'$, $m''$, and $n$ was fairly good (Table 2).

The general correspondence between $m'$ and $m''$ and $m$ is not strong evidence for the Poisson law. It is possible that $n$ is small and $p$ relatively large so that the release of transmitter would be more accurately predicted by the binomial probability law. In this case

$$(1 + cv^2)/CV^2 = m/(1 + m/n)$$

and

$$ln\ (N/N_o) = ln\ (1 - p)^{-n}$$
$$= m(1 + (1p/2) + (1/3)p^2 + \ldots)$$

If $n$ is greater than 20, $m$ less than 10, and $p$ less than 0.4, $m'$ and $m''$ would still fall within 50% of $m$. Moreover, estimates of $m$ and $m''$ are only approximate because the amplitude distribution of the basic random variable is apparently skewed (Fig. 8) (see Soucek, 1971).

No attempt has been made to relate changes in $M$ to time after synapse formation, but no obvious correlation of $m$ with culture age was observed. For example, $m$ at one junction in a 9-day culture (6 days after addition of neurons) was 9.53 and at another junction, and in a 32-day culture (23 days after addition of neurons) was 1.19.

## Effect of $Ca^{2+}$ and $Mg^{2+}$

Transmitter release at adult neuromuscular junctions depends on the relative concentrations of $Ca^{2+}$ and $Mg^{2+}$ ions in the bathing medium (del Castillo and Katz, 1956a); epp quantum content is reduced following decrease in $Ca^{2+}$ or increase in $Mg^{2+}$. The same ions controlled

stimulus-evoked transmitter release at each of 6 synapses tested *in vitro*. Figure 18 shows the effect of reducing $Ca^{2+}$ from 2.0 mM to 0.5 mM (a) or increasing $Mg^{2+}$ from 1.0 to 11.0 mM (B) at two different synapses. In both cases, the epp amplitude is reduced and the relative variation of successive responses is increased. In these and in other experiments, the quantum size was unchanged within the accuracy of the measurements. That is,

TABLE 2

The Quantum Content of Junctions at Which More Than One Estimate Was Obtained Expressed as Mean ± Standard Error[a]

| $N$ | $\overline{epp}/\overline{mepp}$ | $ln\ (N/N_o)$ | $\dfrac{1 + cv^2}{CV^2}$ |
|---|---|---|---|
| 376 | 1.04 ± 0.08 | 0.93 ± 0.06 | 0.98 ± 0.12 |
| 63 | 1.22 ± 0.14 | — | 2.76 ± 0.65 |
| 67 | — | 1.31 ± 0.20 | 1.19 ± 0.34 |
| 133 | 2.49 ± 0.17 | 2.59 ± 0.30 | 2.24 ± 0.37 |
| 50 | — | 2.53 ± 0.48 | 2.64 ± 0.70 |
| 100 | 2.73 ± 0.44 | 3.22 ± 0.49 | 1.76 ± 0.32 |
| 211[S] | 5.21 ± 0.14 | — | 8.14 ± 0.86 |
| 132 | 6.07 ± 0.35 | — | 6.54 ± 0.85 |
| 147 | 7.76 ± 0.38 | — | 6.51 ± 0.21 |
| 56 | 8.05 ± 0.62 | — | 3.82 ± 0.88 |
| 252[S] | 8.86 ± 0.32 | — | 10.5 ± 0.94 |
| 75 | 9.53 ± 0.62 | — | 11.72 ± 1.91 |
| 149 | 9.67 ± 0.62 | — | 18.8 ± 1.89 |
| 103[S] | 29.88 ± 2.79 | — | 21.70 ± 2.42 |

[a] $N$ is either the number of stimuli in each series or, in samples of spontaneously occurring epps (indicated by superscript S), the number of epps.

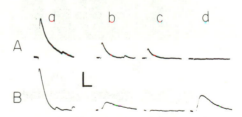

Fig. 18. The effect of reduction in $Ca^{2+}$ from 2.0 mM to 0.5 mM (A) or increase in $Mg^{2+}$ from 1.0 mM to 11.0 mM (B). a, control; b, c, and d, successive epps evoked after the indicated concentration changes. A and B are from different muscle fibers (see text). Bars = 5 mV and 10 msec for A and B$a$; 2.5 mV and 5 msec for B$b$, c and d.

the mean mepp size was not decreased by more than 20% following the same changes in $Ca^{2+}$ and $Mg^{2+}$ concentration.

### Electrical Coupling

Evidence for direct electrical coupling between spinal cord and muscle cells has been obtained on four occasions. Mepps (Fig. 19B) were recorded on penetration of the muscle fiber shown in Fig. 19A. Depolarization of the nearby neuron through an intracellular electrode produced a spike that was followed after about 2 msec by a typical epp (Fig. 19C). In this case, the epp was superimposed on a small, steady depolarization of the muscle membrane that began with the onset of the stimulating current and persisted until the

pulse was terminated. Reversal of the current polarity produced hyperpolarizing potentials in the nerve and muscle (Fig. 19D); the coupling element did not rectify. The coupling potential was not due to the potential field created in the bath by the stimulating current because identical pulses produced no visible deflection in the muscle trace after the recording electrode was withdrawn to a position immediately outside of the fiber (Fig. 19E). Rather, it suggests the presence of a relatively low resistance path between the interiors of the two cells that is insulated from the extracellular medium (Bennett, 1966).

Electrotonic spread of current between nerve and muscle was observed in two

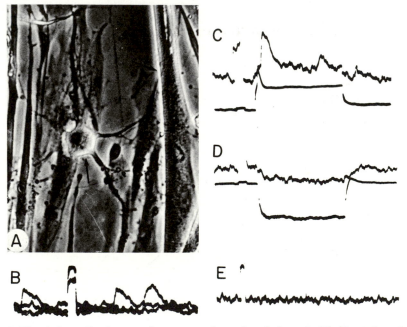

FIG. 19. Electrical coupling between the neuron and muscle cell shown in (A). Mepps (superimposed traces in B) were recorded on penetration of the muscle fiber at the point marked by the arrow. Outward and inward current pulses (ca. 5 nanoamperes) injected into the neuron depolarized and hyperpolarized the muscle membrane (upper traces in C and D, respectively). The voltage response of the neuron is shown in the lower trace of each pair. Current pulses are not shown. Note the epp superimposed on the electrotonic potential in (C). Two mepps appear on the same trace. (D) Absence of a potential change to identical current pulses after the muscle electrode was withdrawn from the fiber. Calibration pulse = 2 mV and 5 msec in all traces. Bar in (A) = 50 $\mu$.

other cases in which the neuron cell bodies were separated from the muscle fibers by 50–100 $\mu$. In one pair, a synaptic potential followed some of the neuron spikes. In the other, the membrane potential of the neuron was low and a spike could not be elicited. Although this failure probably was due to injury on electrode penetration and although the cell had several long processes, it cannot unambiguously be identified as a neuron.

In the fourth instance, the neuron cell body partially overlay the muscle fiber. At first, stimulation of the neuron resulted only in a epp in the muscle but, after several minutes of repetitive stimulation at 0.5/sec, each current pulse produced a relatively large, steady depolarizing potential in the muscle, in addition to the epp, and reversal of the stimulus polarity at this time resulted in a hyperpolarizing potential in the muscle cell. Electrical coupling, in this case, probably occurred between the neuron perikaryon and contiguous muscle, rather than at the end of a neurite because the ratio of the pre- and postsynaptic electrotonic potentials was close to unity and because the neuron action potential appeared almost simultaneously in the nerve and muscle records. This site—near the stimulating electrode —together with the delay in onset of the coupling suggest that the low resistance path was somehow "caused" by the intracellular electrode. Nevertheless, it demonstrates clearly that nerve and muscle membranes can fuse to form an effective insulating sheath. The coupling persisted after relocation of the stimulating electrode in the neuron at a point clearly removed from the underlying muscle, and it remained unchanged for 3 days, after which time the culture was discarded.

## DISCUSSION

The function of chick nerve-muscle synapses that form in low density cell cultures is, in broad outline, identical to that of adult vertebrate neuromuscular junctions. The major discrepancies—low mepp frequency and epp quantum content, slow rise and fall of synaptic potentials, and the occurrence of spontaneous epps correspond rather precisely to certain features of embryonic neuromuscular junctions.

Diamond and Miledi (1962) found that the mepp frequency at neuromuscular junctions of 17-day mouse embryos was 1/100 of the adult rate and did not attain adult values until 3 weeks after birth. The epp quantum content was not measured. The mepp time course was slow and unaffected by cholinesterase inhibitors. Occasional spontaneously occurring "giant" postsynaptic potentials similar to those shown in Fig. 10 triggered muscle action potentials and twitches. They related the low mepp frequency to the relatively simple structure of the embryonic nerve terminal arbor and, by inference, to the paucity of "active spots" of transmitter release (del Castillo and Katz, 1956b). In adult frogs, both mepp frequency and epp quantum content depend on end-plate size as measured by the histochemical localization of acetylcholinesterase (Kuno et al., 1971). The same explanation probably accounts for the low transmitter output observed *in vitro*. In a cell culture system similar to the one employed in the present experiments, silver-impregnated neurites terminate over muscle cells in a few bulbous swellings or boutons or simple arbors (see Introduction for references). It must be remembered, however, no evidence that the terminal specializations are indeed functional endings has as yet been presented. A comparison of simultaneous intracellular and extracellular recordings with silver strains of the same nerve terminals would settle the question.

The slow time course of the synaptic potentials might, as suggested by Diamond and Miledi (1962), be explained by prolonged transmitter action which, in turn, is due to the lack of surface or active acetylcholinesterase at functional nerve-muscle junctions. Inhibitors of the enzyme do not further prolong the epps in cell cultures (Fig. 15) or in cultures of explanted spinal cord fragments and dissociated muscle (Kano and Shimada, 1971). In addition, a prolonged postsynaptic conductance change would result if the transmitter were released from a relatively distant source (del Castillo and Katz, 1955). Hirano (1964) found postsynaptic membrane thickening in embryonic chick muscle fibers when the ingrowing neurite was still about 2000 Å away. The fact that the mean amplitudes of mepps, which should be more critically dependent on diffusion distance, were similar to adult values, does not argue against this interpretation because larger values are expected considering the relatively high input resistance (2–10 MΩ; see Fischbach et al., 1971) of the muscle cells (Katz and Thesleff, 1957).

The occasional large spontaneous synaptic potentials observed at the embryonic mouse junctions were described as "giant mepps" but, the large spontaneous potentials observed in this study clearly resulted from impulse activity in the innervating neuron. Patterned spontaneous twitches and bursts of electrical activity have been observed in combined spinal cord-muscle explants (Szepsenwohl, 1947; Crain, 1970). Spontaneous movements that must arise from nerve impulses and that do not depend on peripheral or suprasegmental input have been described in young chick embryos (Hamburger and Balaban, 1963). Such discharges in vivo and in vitro might be due to a relative decrease in inhibitory synaptic input, to a spatial reorganization of synaptic input, or to change in membrane properties of the motoneuron.

The number of presumptive nerve-muscle synapses which, in fact, were functional, i.e., at which stimulus evoked or spontaneous depolarizing potentials greater than 0.1 mV were detected in the muscle fiber, was low. Most of the neurons in the brachial cord segments of 7- to 7.5-day embryos are probably already specified as to future function because, at this age, mitotic activity has fallen to less than 25% and 50% of the peak values in the basal and alar plates, respectively (Hamburger, 1948; Fig. 8). The mutually exclusive relation between DNA synthesis and cell differentiation postulated in other tissues (Holtzer, 1968) seems to apply to the nervous system: retinal ganglion cells are "instructed" about future synapse formation in the tectum within 10 hr after cessation of DNA synthesis (Jacobsen, 1968). Thus, although the spinal cord cells are small and round immediately after plating, the great majority of those destined to form neurons are probably not multipotent, and one explanation for the low incidence of functional nerve-muscle contacts is simply that only a few cholinergic motor neuroblasts were added to the muscle cultures.

Alternative explanations, that actual or potential functional contacts are common, but that they rapidly degenerate or do not form because of mechanical, osmotic, or metabolic factors, must be investigated.

Description of the precise sequence of events during nerve-muscle synapse formation will probably depend on development of a system in which prospective motoneurons can be identified with high reliability prior to their contacting muscle cells. Nevertheless, the present results raise some interesting questions.

Is electrical coupling between nerve and muscle an early stage in chemical synapse formation? Coupling is not a general characteristic of contacting cells in the monolayer culture system employed in the present study; current did not pass between the great majority of nerve-muscle or nerve-nerve pairs tested. The fact that typical epps were recorded in the muscle cell after stimulation of the neuron in three of the four electrically coupled pairs (the fourth was not adequately tested) suggests that coupling is, somehow related to chemical synapse formation. The low incidence would be expected if the specialized contacts that provide the low resistance intercellular path were restricted to a brief period of time. Other interpretations are certainly possible. Although coupling is not an artifact due to extracellular current flow (Fig. 19), the possibility that, in each case, current passed between nerve and muscle through a third, intervening cell has not been ruled out. This indirect path is not unlikely as electrical coupling has observed between a variety of cell types in culture (Hyde *et al.*, 1969; Walker and Hild, 1969; Furshpan and Potter, 1970; Michalke and Lowenstein, 1971) and between cells from the same and from different germ cell layers in early squid (Potter *et al.*, 1966) and chick (Sheridan, 1968) embryos. The low incidence may, in part, be due to the unfavorable recording situation imposed by the high axoplasmic resistance of the fine neurite and the low input resistance of the muscle fiber (Bennett, 1966).

Gap or tight junctions (Brightman and Reese, 1969) have not been described at nerve-muscle contacts in embryos or *in vitro*. But Kelly and Zacks (1970) found regions of close apposition and increased membrane density between embryonic rat muscle cells and in growing neurites, and James and Tresman (1969) found that neurites growing out of explants of chick spinal cord extended long cytoplasmic fingers that deeply indented previously plated muscle fibers.

Is multiple innervation an early stage in synapse formation? Does it reflect differences in fully differentiated nerve and or muscle cells? Is it simply an artifact of the culture technique? The membranes of multiply innervated adult muscle fibers are distinguished by a relatively high resistivity (Fedde, 1969; Stefani and Steinbach, 1969) and absence of inward (hyperpolarizing) rectification when bathed in isotonic $K_2SO_4$ (Stefani and Steinbach, 1969). Comparison of these properties in multiply and singly innervated and in uninnervated fibers might answer these questions.

Is the availability of ACh a determinant of neuromuscular junction formation? If low transmitter output is, as suggested, due to a dearth of points of transmitter release, then existing active spots must be quite mature in terms of transmitter synthesis and storage, and it seems unlikely that these processes are rate limiting in the formation of functional contacts.

As judged by light microscopy and preliminary electron microscopy, neurons in these relatively "clean" cell cultures are not surrounded by glia or satellite cells; muscle fibers are not invested in a basal lamina, and contacting nerve terminals are not covered by Schwann cells. Thus, none of these factors are necessary for synapse formation *in vitro*. Perhaps they play a role in the maintenance or further maturation of the synapse such as organization of a complex terminal arbor, development of postsynaptic structural specialization, localization of acetylcholinesterase (see Hall and Kelly, 1971; Betz and Sackmann, 1971) or modulation of postsynaptic acetylcholine receptors (see Fischbach and Cohen, 1972). Their absence is not a drawback but, rather, points to a great advantage of dissociated cell cultures, because it might be possible to isolate the missing elements from another source and assay their effect on individual neurons and synapses.

I would like to express my gratitude to Mrs. Marie Neal for expert technical assistance in preparing and maintaining the cultures and to Dr. Phillip G. Nelson for many critical discussions. Stephen Cohen participated in some of the experiments.

## REFERENCES

ARAKI, T., and OTANI, T. (1955). Response of single motoneurons to direct stimulation in toads spinal cord. *J. Physiol. (London)* **190**, 123–137.

BENNETT, M. V. L. (1966). Physiology of electrotonic junctions. *Ann. N. Y. Acad. Sci.* **137**, 509–539.

BETZ, W., and SACKMANN, B. (1971). Disjunction of frog neuromuscular synapses by treatment with proteolytic enzymes. *Nature (London)* **232**, 94–95.

BORNSTEIN, M. B. (1958). Reconstituted rat-tail collagen used as a substrate for tissue culture on coverslips on Maximow slides and roller tubes. *Lab. Invest.* **7**, 134–140.

BORNSTEIN, M. B., IWANAMI, H., LEHRER, G. M., and BRIETBART, L. (1968). Observations on the appearance of neuromuscular relationships in cultured mouse tissues. *Z. Zellforsch. Nikrosk. Anat.* **92**, 197–206.

BOYD, I. A., and MARTIN, A. R. (1956). The end-plate potential in mammalian muscle. *J. Physiol. (London)* **132**, 74–91.

BRIGHTMAN, M. W., and REESE, T. A. (1969). Junctions between intimately opposed cell membranes in the vertebrate brain. *J. Cell Biol.* **40**, 648–677.

BROWN, W., JR. (1962). Appendix to: EDWARDS, C., and IKEDA, K. Effects of 2-PAM and succinylcholine on neuromuscular transmission in the frog. *J. Pharmacol. Exp. Ther.* **138**, 322–328.

COLEMAN, J. R., and COLEMAN, A. W. (1968). Muscle differentiation and macromolecular synthesis. *J. Cell Physiol.* **72**, Suppl. 1, 19–34.

CRAIN, S. (1956). Resting and action potentials of cultured chick embryo spinal ganglion cells. *J. Comp. Neurol.* **104**, 285–330.

CRAIN, S. (1970). Bioelectric interactions between cultured fetal rodent spinal cord and skeletal muscle after innervation *in vitro*. *J. Exp. Zool.* **173**, 353–370.

DEL CASTILLO, J., and KATZ, B. (1955). On the localization of acetylcholine receptors. *J. Physiol. (London)* **128**, 157–181.

DEL CASTILLO, J., and KATZ, B. (1956a). Biophysical aspects of neuromuscular transmission. *Progr. Biophys. Biophys. Chem.* **6**, 121–170.

DEL CASTILLO, J., and KATZ, B. (1956b). Localization of active spots within the neuromuscular junction of the frog. *J. Physiol. (London)* **132**, 630–649.

DIAMOND, J., and MILEDI, R. (1962). A study of fetal and newborn rat muscle fibers. *J. Physiol. (London)* **162**, 393–408.

FATT, P., and KATZ, B. (1951). An analysis of the endplate potential recorded with an intracellular electrode. *J. Physiol. (London)* **115**, 320–370.

FEDDE, M. R. (1969). Electrical properties and acetylcholine sensitivity of singly and multiply innervated avian muscle fibers. *J. Gen. Physiol.* **53**, 624–637.

FISCHBACH, G. D. (1970). Synaptic potentials recorded in cell cultures of nerve and muscle. *Science* **169**, 1331–1333.

FISCHBACH, G. D., and COHEN, S. (1972). The acetyl-

choline sensitivity of uninnervated and innervated muscle fibers in cell culture. In preparation.

FISCHBACH, G. D., NAMEROFF, M., and NELSON, P. G. (1971). Electrical properties of chick skeletal muscle fibers developing in cell culture. *J. Cell Physiol.* **78**, 289–300.

FURSHPAN, E. J., and POTTER, D. D. (1968). Low-resistance junctions between cells in embryos and tissue culture. *Curr. Top. Develop. Biol.* **3**, 95–127.

GRAHAM, F. L., and WHITMORE, G. F. (1970). The effect of 1-β-D-arabinofuranosylcytosine on growth, viability and DNA synthesis of mouse L-cells. *Cancer Res.* **30**, 2627–2634.

HALL, Z. W., and KELLY, R. B. (1971). Enzymatic detachment of endplate acetylcholinesterase from muscle. *Nature (London)* **232**, 62–63.

HAMBURGER, V. (1948). The mitotic patterns in the spinal cord of the chick embryo and their relation to histogenetic processes. *J. Comp. Neurol.* **88**, 221–283.

HAMBURGER, V., and BALABAN, M. (1963). Observations and experiments on spontaneous rhythmical behavior in the chick embryo. *Develop. Biol.* **7**, 533–545.

HAUSCHUKA, S., and KONIGSBERG, I. (1966). The influence of collagen on the development of muscle clones. *Proc. Nat. Acad. Sci. U.S.A.* **55**, 119.

HIRANO, H. (1967). Ultrastructural study on the morphologenesis of the neuromuscular junction in the skeletal muscle of the chick. *Z. Zellforsch. Mikrosk. Anat.* **79**, 198–208.

HOLTZER, H. (1968). Induction of chondrogenesis: A concept in quest of mechanisms. *In* "Epithelial-Mesenchymal Interactions" (R. Fleischmajer, ed.), pp. 152–164. Williams & Wilkins, Baltimore, Maryland.

HYDE, A., BLONDEL, B., MATTER, A., CHENEVAL, S. P. FILLOUX, B., and GIRADIER, L. (1969). Homo- and heterocellular junctions in cell cultures: an electrophysiological and morphological study. *Progr. Brain Res.* **31**, 283.

JACOBSON, M. (1968). Cessation of DNA synthesis in retinal ganglion cells correlated with the time of specification of their central connections. *Develop. Biol.* **17**, 219–232.

JAMES, D. W., and TRESMAN, R. L. (1969). An electron-microscopic study of the de novo formation of neuromuscular junctions in tissue culture. *Z. Zellforsch. Mikrosk. Anat.* **100**, 126–140.

KARNOVSKY, M., and ROOTS, L. (1964). A "direct-coloring" thiocholine method for cholinesterases. *J. Histochem. Cytochem.* **12**, 219–221.

KATZ, B., and MILEDI, R. (1967). Tetrodotoxin and neuromuscular transmission. *Proc. Roy Soc. Ser. B* **167**, 8–22.

KATZ, B., and THESLEFF, S. (1957). On the factors which determine the amplitude of the "miniature endplate potential." *J. Physiol. (London)* **137**, 267–278.

KANO, M., and SHIMADA, Y. (1971). Innervation of skeletal muscle cells differentiated *in vitro* from chick embryo. *Brain Res.* **27**, 402–405.

KELLY, A. M., and ZACKS, S. J. (1969). The fine structure of motor endplate morphogenesis. *J. Cell Biol.* **42**, 154–169.

KUNO, M., TURKANIS, S., and WEAKLY, J. (1971). Correlation between nerve terminal size and transmitter release of the neuromuscular junction of the frog. *J. Physiol. (London)* **213**, 545–556.

MARTIN, A. R. (1955). A further study of the statistical composition of the end-plate potential. *J. Physiol. (London)* **130**, 114–122.

MICHALKE, W., and LOWENSTEIN, W. R. (1971). Communication between cells of different type. *Nature (London)* **232**, 121–122.

NAKAI, J. (1969). The development of neuromuscular junctions in cultures of chick embryo tissues. *J. Exp. Zool.* **170**, 85–106.

PETERSON, E. R., and CRAIN, S. M. (1970). Innervation in cultures of fetal rodent skeletal muscle by organotypic explants of spinal cord from different animals. *Z. Zellforsch. Mikrosk. Anat.* **106**, 1–21.

POTTER, D. D., FURSHPAN, E., and LENNOX, E. J. (1966). Connections between cells of the developing squid as revealed by electrophysiological methods. *Proc. Nat. Acad. Sci. U.S.A.* **55**, 328–335.

ROBBINS, N., and YONEZAWA, T. (1971). Developing neuromuscular junctions: first signs of chemical transmission during formation in tissue culture. *Science* **172**, 395–397.

SCOTT, B. S., ENGELBERT, W. E., and FISHER, K. C. (1969). Morphological and electrophysiological characteristics of dissociated chick embryonic spinal ganglion cells in culture. *Exp. Neurol.* **23**, 230–248.

SHERIDAN, J. D. (1968). Electrophysiological evidence for low-resistance intercellular junctions in the early chick embryo. *J. Cell Biol.* **38**, 650–659.

SHIMADA, Y. (1968). Suppression of myogenesis by heterotypic and heterospecific cells in monolayer cultures. *Exp. Cell Res.* **51**, 564–578.

SHIMADA, Y., and KANO, M. (1971). Formation of neuromuscular junctions in embryonic cultures. *Arch. Histol. Japan.* **33**, 95–114.

SHIMADA, Y., FISCHMAN, D. A., and MOSCONA, A. A. (1969a). Formation of neuromuscular junctions in embryonic cell cultures. *Proc. Nat. Acad. Sci. U.S.A.* **62**, 715–721.

SHIMADA, Y., FISCHMAN, D. A., and MOSCONA, A. A. (1969b). The development of nerve-muscle junctions in monolayer cultures of embryonic spinal cord and skeletal muscle cells. *J. Cell Biol.* **43**, 382–387.

SOUCEK, B. (1971). Influence of the latency fluctuations and the quantal process of transmitter release on the endplate potentials amplitude distribution. *Biophys. J.* **11**, 127–139.

STEFANI, E., and STEINBACH, A. B. (1969). Resting potential and electrical properties of frog slow muscle fibers. Effect of different external solutions. *J. Physiol. (London)* **203**, 383–401.

SZEPSENWOHL, J. (1947). Electrical excitability and spontaneous activity in explants of skeletal and heart muscle of chick muscle. *Anat. Rec.* **98**, 67.

TAKEUCHI, A., and TAKEUCHI, N. (1959). Active phase of frogs end-plate potential. *J. Neurophysiol.* **22**, 395–411.

VARON, S., and RAIBORN, C. W., JR. (1969). Dissociation, fractionation and culture of embryonic brain cells. *Brain Res.* **12**, 180–199.

VENERONI, C., and MURRAY, M. (1969). Formation *de novo* and development of neuromuscular junctions in vitro. *J. Embryol. Exp. Morphol.* **21**, 369–382.

WALKER, F., and HILD, W. (1969). Neuroglia electrically coupled to neurons. *Science* **165**, 602–604.

YAFFE, D. (1968). Retention of differentiation potentialities during prolonged cultivation of myogenic cells. *Proc. Nat. Acad. Sci. U.S.A.* **61**, 477–483.

*Chapter 11*

# CYCLIC AMP

The work of E.W. Sutherland and his colleagues and students over the last fifteen years has demonstrated that the effects of many hormones, including the catecholamine epinephrine, are mediated within cells by adenosine-3',5'-phosphate (cAMP). The primary action of these hormones is to increase the activity of adenyl cyclase, the enzyme that forms cAMP and is found in the surface membrane of target cells. Stimulation of adenyl cyclase causes an increase in intracellular cAMP that is responsible for the diverse effects of the hormones. The similarities and possible evolutionary relationships between systems of hormonal communication and those of synaptic transmission raise the possibility that cAMP plays a correspondingly important role in the nervous system. Indeed, this speculation is bolstered by the observation that brain levels of cAMP and adenyl cyclase are among the highest in the body. One of the most provocative areas of current neurochemical investigation lies in exploring and defining the role of cAMP in synaptic transmission.

The enzyme involved in the initial step of hormone action, adenyl cyclase, catalyzes the formation of cAMP and pyrophosphate from ATP in a reaction requiring magnesium ions. The enzyme exists in a wide variety of animal tissues; in each tissue, however, enzymic activity is increased only by appropriate hormones. For instance, adrenocorticotrophic hormone stimulates adenyl cyclase from the adrenal cortex, and epinephrine and glucagon stimulate the liver enzyme. No fewer than five different hormones influence enzyme activity in adipose tissue. L. Birnbaumer and M. Rodbell (1969), in studies on adenyl cyclase activity in membrane fragments from fat cells, showed that the hormones all affect the same cyclase catalytic site, although they apparently act through different receptor sites. These and other observations suggest that the hormone receptors are regulatory subunits overseeing a single catalytic subunit of adenyl cyclase.

The conversion of cAMP to 5'-AMP, catalyzed by a specific phosphodiesterase, renders it physiologically inactive. This phosphodiesterase is found in both particulate and soluble fractions after tissue homogenization and is inhibited by methylxanthine derivatives such as caffeine and theophylline (Butcher and Sutherland, 1962).

cAMP was originally discovered in studies of the stimulation by epinephrine and glucagon of glycogen breakdown in liver (Rall, Sutherland, and Berthet, 1957). Even now, the glycogenolysis caused by epinephrine administration to liver or skeletal muscle is probably the best understood cellular process in which cAMP participates. The initial effect of epinephrine is activation of adenyl cyclase to cause an increase in intracellular cAMP. Thereafter a cascading series of reactions leads to the ultimate increase in glycogen breakdown. In the first step cAMP activates a protein kinase that catalyzes a phosphoryl transfer from ATP to the enzyme phosphorylase kinase, changing the phosphorylase kinase to a more active species. This enzyme in turn catalyzes an ATP-dependent phosphorylation of phosphorylase $b$, converting it to phosphorylase $a$. Under physiological conditions, phosphorylase $b$ is less active than phosphorylase $a$ in gylcogenolysis. The result of the reaction is thus to activate phosphorylase and increase glycogen breakdown. The protein kinase that is stimulated by cAMP also catalyzes phosphorylation of the enzyme glycogen synthetase, in this case converting it to a less active species (Soderling, et al., 1970). Both phosphorylase $a$ and glycogen synthetase revert to their original forms when the phosphoryl-protein linkages are hydrolyzed by phosphatases.

In these two examples, the initial step in the action of cAMP is stimulation of a protein kinase. The wide-spread occurrence of such cAMP-sensitive protein kinases led P. Greengard to propose that cAMP generally affects cellular processes by activating protein kinases, which then modify enzymes or other proteins by catalyzing their phosphorylation. A protein kinase, requiring cAMP for full activity, has been partially purified from bovine brain and shown to catalyze the phosphorylation of several proteins, although its physiological substrates are unknown (Miyamoto, Kuo, and Greengard, 1969). A second enzyme, having a higher affinity for guanosine-3',5'-phosphate (cGMP) than for cAMP, has also been isolated from several sources. This finding and studies demonstrating the natural occurrence of cGMP suggest the existence of a parallel but separate intracellular signaling system, similar to the cAMP system but possibly leading to the phosphorylation of different proteins.

The similarity between the effects of epinephrine and of sympathetic nerve stimulation, documented so extensively by T. Elliot (see Chapter 1), suggests that the hormone and the sympathetic neurotransmitter may have a common mode of action. All of the effects of the hormone epinephrine that have been shown to be caused by cAMP can also be produced by exogenous norepinephrine, or, in the case of sympathetically innervated tissues, by nerve stimulation. Both epinephrine and norepinephrine stimulate adenyl cyclase, and drugs that antagonize the interactions of catecholamines with β-receptors also block the effects of the catecholamines on adenyl cyclase. These results suggest that the adrenergic receptor may be a regulatory subunit of adenyl cyclase, and that some of the effects of the neurotransmitter may be mediated by cAMP. The question arises whether cAMP is involved in the electrical as well as the metabolic actions of the neurotransmitter.

G. Siggins, B. Hoffer, and F. Bloom (1971, reprinted here) provided the first experimental demonstration that cAMP could affect electrical signaling in neurons. Their earlier experiments had shown that Purkinje cells in the cerebellum are contacted by afferent endings containing norepinephrine, that norepinephrine administered by iontophoresis reduces the rate of firing of Purkinje cells, and that the effects of norepinephrine are blocked by an antagonist of β-receptors. In the paper reprinted here, they reported that iontophoretically applied cAMP also reduced the firing rate of most Purkinje cells, but that adenosine mono- and triphosphates did not have this effect. The dibutyryl analogue of cAMP was somewhat less effective than cAMP itself. The effects of norepinephrine and cAMP were increased by administration of phosphodiesterase inhibitors. In later experiments Siggins, et al. (1971) made intracellular recordings during iontophoresis. Both norepinephrine and cAMP hyperpolarized the Purkinje cells, and in most cases caused a membrane conductance decrease.

The studies of P. Greengard and his colleagues on sympathetic ganglia have also implicated cAMP in synaptic transmission. They initially observed that stimulation of preganglionic axons caused an increase in the cAMP content of the superior cervical ganglion (McAfee, Shorderet, and Greengard, 1971, reprinted here). Because cAMP levels did not increase when the preganglionic axons (cholinergic) were stimulated in the presence of cholinergic blocking agents, or when the postganglionic axons were stimulated, these investigators concluded that the cAMP increase was associated with synaptic transmission. Sympathetic ganglia contain a class of small, intensely fluorescent (SIF) cells that may receive input from the preganglionic fibers and terminate on the large noradrenergic postganglionic cells of the ganglion, which are called principal cells. The SIF cells contain high concentrations of dopamine. It is thought that the slow inhibitory potentials observed in the principal cells after preganglionic stimulation result from secretion of dopamine from the SIF cells onto the principal cells. Because of the involvement of a catecholamine, Greengard and Kebabian (1971, reprinted here) focused their attention on this synapse. They showed that incubation of the ganglion with dopamine increased the ganglionic cAMP content; in addition, ganglionic homogenates contained adenyl cyclase activity that was stimulated by dopamine. Both the increase in cAMP and the slow potential change caused by dopamine were blocked by phentolamine, an $\alpha$-adrenergic blocking agent. Later, McAfee and Greengard (1972, reprinted here) found, by recording with sucrose-gap techniques from the ganglion, that both the neurally evoked slow inhibitory potential and the potential produced by dopamine were amplified in the presence of the phosphodiesterase inhibitor, theophylline. Furthermore, monobutyryl cAMP produced a potential change similar to that found with dopamine. Greengard and his colleagues favor the view that the slow inhibitory potential is mediated by an increase in cAMP that occurs in response to stimulation of adenyl cyclase by neurally released dopamine.

The studies of Greengard, Bloom, and their colleagues thus show that cAMP can change the potential across neuronal membranes. Unfortunately in neither system is the mechanism of the potential change caused by the transmitter well enough understood to make a detailed comparison with the effects of cAMP and its analogues possible. cAMP could act by altering the ionic conductance of the membrane or by activating an electrogenic pump, either directly or through an effect on energy metabolism.

In heart muscle, however, it has been possible to examine the effects of these substances on the passive ionic currents underlying the action potential. Experiments using voltage clamp techniques have shown that epinephrine, theophylline, and monobutyryl cAMP all have similar effects on both inward and outward currents during the plateau phase (Tsien, Giles, and Greengard, 1972).

In addition to the possibility that cAMP mediates the potential changes caused by catecholamines, the suggestion has recently been made that changes in cGMP levels may be related to the effects produced by parasympathetic (cholinergic) nerve stimulation in cardiac and smooth muscle. ACh increases the cGMP levels in these tissues, and the increase is blocked by parasympathetic blocking agents such as atropine (George, *et al.*, 1970; Lee, Kuo, and Greengard, 1972).

562

At the vertebrate neuromuscular junction cyclic nucleotides have also been implicated in cholinergic transmission. Here, however, the involvement is presynaptic. cAMP, dibutyryl cAMP, epinephrine, and inhibitors of cAMP hydrolysis, such as theophylline, all increase the quantal content of end-plate potentials and the frequency of miniature end-plate potentials at the neuromuscular junction (Goldberg and Singer, 1969). The exact role play by cAMP in transmitter secretion is obscure, but these findings are similar to those obtained in studies of secretion from pancreatic islet cells or from salivary glands, suggesting the possibility of a general role of cAMP in secretory processes.

## READING LIST

*Reprinted Papers*

1. Siggins, G.R., B.J. Hoffer, and F.E. Bloom (1971). Studies on norepinephrine-containing afferents to Purkinje cells of rat cerebellum. III. Evidence for mediation of norepinephrine effects by cyclic 3',5'-adenosine monophosphate. *Brain Res.* 25: 535–553.
2. McAfee, D.A., M. Schorderet, and P. Greengard (1971). Adenosine 3',5'-monophosphate in nervous tissue: Increase associated with synaptic transmission. *Science* 171: 1156–1158.
3. Kebabian, J.W. and P. Greengard (1971). Dopamine-sensitive adenyl cyclase: Possible role in synaptic transmission. *Science* 174: 1346–1349.
4. McAfee, D.A. and P. Greengard (1972). Adenosine 3',5'-monophosphate: Electrophysiological evidence for a role in synaptic transmission. *Science* 178: 310–312.

*Other Selected Papers*

5. Rall, T.W., E.W. Sutherland, and J. Berthet (1957). The relationship of epinephrine and glucagon to liver phosphorylase. IV. Effect of epinephrine and glucagon on the reactivation of phosphorylase in liver homogenates. *J. Biol. Chem.* 224: 463–475.
6. Butcher, R.W. and E.W. Sutherland (1962). Adenosine 3',5'-phosphate in biological materials. I. Purification and properties of cyclic 3',5'-nucleotide phosphodiesterase and use of this enzyme to characterize adenosine 3',5'-phosphate in human urine. *J. Biol. Chem.* 237: 1244–1250.
7. Birnbaumer, L. and M. Rodbell (1969). Adenyl cyclase in fat cells. II. Hormone receptors. *J. Biol. Chem.* 244: 3477–3482.

8. Goldberg, A.L. and J.J. Singer (1969). Evidence for a role of cyclic AMP in neuromuscular transmission. *Proc. Nat. Acad. Sci.* 64: 134–141.

9. Miyamoto, E., J.F. Kuo, and P. Greengard (1969). Cyclic nucleotide-dependent protein kinases. III. Purification and properties of adenosine 3′,5′-monophosphate-dependent protein kinase from bovine brain. *J. Biol. Chem.* 244: 6395–6402.

10. George, W.J., J.B. Polson, A.G. O'Toole, and N.D. Goldberg (1970). Elevation of guanosine 3′,5′-cyclic phosphate in rat heart after perfusion with acetylcholine. *Proc. Nat. Acad. Sci.* 66: 398–403.

11. Soderling, T.R., J.P. Hickenbottom, E.M. Reimann, F.L. Hunkeler, D.A. Walsh, and E.G. Krebs (1970). Inactivation of glycogen synthetase and activation of phosphorylase kinase by muscle adenosine 3′,5′-monophosphate-dependent protein kinases. *J. Biol. Chem.* 245: 6317–6328.

12. Levey, G.S. (1971). Restoration of norepinephrine responsiveness of solubilized myocardial adenylate cyclase by phosphatidylinositol. *J. Biol. Chem.* 246: 7405–7407.

13. Siggins, G.R., A.P. Oliver, B.J. Hoffer, and F.E. Bloom (1971). Cyclic adenosine monophosphate and norepinephrine: Effects on transmembrane properties of cerebellar Purkinje cells. *Science* 171: 192–194.

14. Lee, T.-P., J.F. Kuo, and P. Greengard (1972). Role of muscarinic cholinergic receptors in regulation of guanosine 3′,5′-cyclic monophosphate content in mammalian brain, heart muscle and intestinal smooth muscle. *Proc. Nat. Acad. Sci.* 69: 3287–3291.

15. Tsien, R.W., W. Giles, and P. Greengard (1972). Cyclic AMP mediates the effects of adrenaline on cardiac Purkinje fibers. *Nature New Biol.* 240: 181–183.

# STUDIES ON NOREPINEPHRINE-CONTAINING AFFERENTS TO PURKINJE CELLS OF RAT CEREBELLUM. III. EVIDENCE FOR MEDIATION OF NOREPINEPHRINE EFFECTS BY CYCLIC 3',5'-ADENOSINE MONOPHOSPHATE

G. R. SIGGINS, B. J. HOFFER AND F. E. BLOOM

*Laboratory of Neuropharmacology, Division of Special Mental Health Research, National Institute of Mental Health, Saint Elizabeths Hospital, Washington, D.C. 20032 (U.S.A.)*

(Accepted August 3rd, 1970)

## INTRODUCTION

The preceding papers in this series[7,33] have dealt with the cytochemical and microiontophoretic evidence for an inhibitory, norepinephrine-mediated afferent pathway to rat cerebellar Purkinje cells. Norepinephrine (NE) selectively depresses the spontaneous action potentials of virtually all Purkinje cells. This response is blocked by MJ-1999, a $\beta$ sympatholytic agent[43]. The mechanism of action of catecholamines on peripheral sympathetic end organs has been attributed to an increased formation of 3',5'-adenosine monophosphate (cyclic AMP) caused by stimulation of adenyl cyclase[67]. The rat cerebellum is one of the richest sources of both cyclic AMP (C-AMP) and adenyl cyclase[17,38,66,71,72], and the cyclase activity or the cyclic nucleotide can be even further increased *in vitro* by catecholamine[35,38,50,63]. Thus, it seemed appropriate to test whether these biochemical data might apply to the molecular mechanisms underlying responses of Purkinje cells to NE.

Preliminary studies[31,64] have indicated that cyclic AMP does indeed mimic the effects of NE on Purkinje cells, and that inhibition of phosphodiesterase (the enzyme which catabolizes cyclic AMP) by methyl xanthines[13] enhances the responses to both NE and cyclic AMP. Further support for the proposed cyclic AMP intermediation of cerebellar NE responses is derived from recent observations on the specific effects of prostaglandins[31,32]. These acidic lipids may occur naturally in cerebellum[14] and other central nervous structures[37,53,54], as well as in a variety of peripheral organs[2].

In this paper, detailed observations of the interactions between NE, cyclic AMP and prostaglandins are reported. Data on the microiontophoretic effects of additional endogenous brain amines, adenine nucleotides, and of calcium and metal chelators have been included to indicate the specificity of the NE–cyclic AMP relationship in the rat cerebellum, and the specific blocking effects of PGE$_1$ on this NE response[31,32]. The results further support the contention that NE transmission across cerebellar cortical synapses not only may be mediated by cyclic AMP but also may be modulated by endogenous prostaglandins.

METHODS

The adult rats used in this study were surgically prepared by the procedures outlined in the preceding paper[33]. Techniques for recording electrical activity of single Purkinje cells, evaluating mean spike frequency, computing interspike interval histograms, and ejecting drugs by microiontophoresis from 5-barrel micropipettes were as previously described[33]. All drug effects described in this report refer to iontophoretic administration, unless otherwise stated. The drugs used in iontophoresis experiments, and their concentrations in the micropipettes were: 0.5 $M$ D,L-norepinephrine HCl (Mann Chemical Laboratories); 0.5 $M$ adenosine 3′,5′-monophosphate (Calbiochem); 0.5 $M$ $N^6,O^{2'}$-dibutyryl adenosine 3′,5′-monophosphate (Calbiochem); 0.1 $M$ theophylline (Calbiochem); 0.2 $M$ aminophylline ((theophylline)$_2$ ethylenediamine, Sigma); 0.5 $M$ adenosine 5′-monophosphate (Calbiochem); 0.5 $M$ adenosine triphosphate (Calbiochem); 0.018 $M$ prostaglandin $E_1$ (Upjohn); 0.014–0.028 $M$ prostaglandin $E_2$ (Upjohn); 0.028 $M$ prostaglandin $F_{1a}$ and $F_{2a}$ (Upjohn); 0.03 $M$ sodium linoleate (Calbiochem); 0.03 $M$ sodium linolenate (Calbiochem); 0.5 $M$ gamma-aminobutyric acid HCl (Aldrich Chemical Co.); 0.1 $M$ disodium (ethylenedinitrilo) tetraacetic acid (EDTA) (J. T. Baker Co.); 0.1 $M$ sodium citrate (Allied Chemical Corp.); 0.2 $M$ calcium chloride (Allied Chemical Corp.); 0.5 $M$ sodium nicotinate (Fischer); 0.5 $M$ histamine dihydrochloride (Calbiochem).

The pH of these solutions was maintained between the limits of 3 and 8, in accordance with previously established limits of microiontophoresis controls[40,61]. The prostaglandin solutions were kept below pH 8.0 to avoid oxidation or polymerization. With poorly soluble substances such as cyclic AMP, dibutyryl cyclic AMP, and the prostaglandins, diluted NaOH was added to the solutions to permit adjustment of pH for maximum solubility and microiontophoretic mobility. In some cases this permitted the ejection of a weakly ionized agent by 'electroosmosis' (see Discussion, ref. 61). Maximum solubilization of substances was occasionally facilitated by sonication of the mixture for short (0.5–1 min) periods. To prevent the conversion of the relatively soluble aminophylline to the sparingly soluble theophylline in the presence of atmospheric carbon dioxide, fresh aminophylline solution was quickly placed in a barrel of the pipette assembly and the open top of the barrel sealed with plasticene.

For intravenous administration of drugs, the left jugular vein of the rat was cannulated with PE 50 tubing. In an effort to obtain a sufficiently concentrated solution of theophylline at 20–40 mg/ml Ringer's solution, warming to about 50°C was necessary. Aminophylline was adequately soluble for i.v. injection in a concentration of 250 mg/ml at room temperature. Aminophylline was injected in volumes of 0.10–0.20 ml, and the theophylline in 0.5–1.2 ml. After determining threshold responses (see Results) of Purkinje cells to iontophoretically applied NE and cyclic AMP, either aminophylline or theophylline was slowly infused over a period of 5–10 min, and the cannula then flushed with 0.2–0.3 ml of Ringer's solution. Threshold responses to NE and cyclic AMP were then redetermined. Electrocardiograms were recorded throughout these experiments.

In an effort to rule out possible presynaptic effects of cyclic AMP, methyl

TABLE I

DIRECT EFFFCTS OF IONTOPHORETICALLY APPLIED ADENINE NUCLEOTIDES ON SPONTANEOUS DISCHARGES
OF PURKINJE CELLS

| Agent | No. cells studied | Responsive | Slowed | Accelerated | Biphasic or reversible |
|---|---|---|---|---|---|
| Cyclic AMP | 110 | 92 | 67 | 16 | 9 |
| Dibutyryl cyclic AMP | 25 | 14 | 10 | 4 | 0 |
| ATP | 8 | 6 | 1 | 5 | 0 |
| 5'-AMP | 7 | 3 | 0 | 3 | 0 |

xanthine, and prostaglandin on adrenergic terminals, Purkinje cells were studied in several animals pretreated with 6-hydroxydopamine HBr (6-HODA; Aldrich Chemical Co.). These animals, taken from the same series of intracisternally injected rats described previously[6,7], show a complete depletion of endogenous norepinephrine from the cerebellum, lack of ability to take up $^3$H-NE, and extensive ultrastructural degeneration of nerve fibers terminating on Purkinje cells[6,7]. Such findings seem compatible with a loss of the presumed NE-containing input to the cerebellar cortex.

RESULTS

*Adenine nucleotides*

The effects of iontophoretically applied cyclic AMP have been studied in 110 Purkinje cells. Of these, 92 cells (84%) showed reproducible changes in spontaneous discharge frequency in response to the substance (Table I, Figs. 1–4). Responses to identical ejection currents of drugs were always of equivalent magnitude when drugs were ejected sequentially on a periodic basis, over short time periods (less than 1 min) and when spike size did not change. The great majority of cells (61%) displayed reductions in rate; firing rates of 15% were increased. A reversible or biphasic type of response was seen in 8% of all cells. In the 'reversible' case, the response to two different applications of cyclic AMP reversed direction spontaneously over a period of time or when the micropipette was moved slightly; biphasic responses were usually characterized by an initial speeding of rate during cyclic AMP application which was slowly succeeded by marked depression during or immediately after application.

In most respects, the depression of spontaneous rate by iontophoretically applied cyclic AMP resembled that of iontophoretic NE. For example, both agents were usually capable of abolishing ordinary spike activity[20] with sufficient ejection current. In contrast to the effects of GABA, which abolishes all spontaneous discharge, neither NE or cyclic AMP appeared to affect the high frequency 'climbing fiber' responses[20], even when ordinary single spikes were completely eliminated. Interspike interval histograms were computed from the activity which persisted during submaximal doses of NE or cyclic AMP. Most probable single interspike intervals were the

567

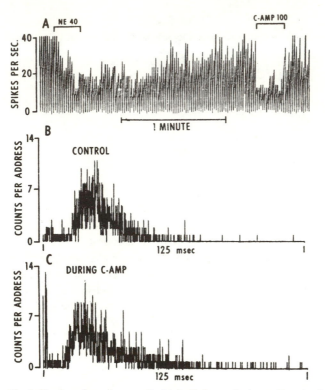

Fig. 1. Slowing of spontaneous Purkinje discharges by iontophoresis of 40 nA of norepinephrine and 100 nA of cyclic AMP (C-AMP). (Same cell illustrated for other purposes in ref. 33.) A, Polygraph record of mean discharge rate with time. Note more rapid onset and termination of depressant response with cyclic AMP than with NE. In this and subsequent polygraph records, brackets indicate duration of drug application and numbers following drugs show ejection currents (in nA). B and C, Interspike interval histograms of spontaneous activity during control periods and during several submaximal applications of cyclic AMP, respectively. The peak of the histograms demonstrate the modal (most probable )intervals to be nearly identical (about 16 msec) in both B and C. In each histogram 1000 spikes were deposited in 500 addresses, each of 0.25 msec interval.

same as those of control histograms (Fig. 1, see preceding report) but there were more frequent interspike intervals of long duration. The only consistent difference between responses to NE and cyclic AMP was the shorter response latency with cyclic AMP (Fig. 1).

The dibutyryl derivative of cyclic AMP depressed discharge rates in 8 of 20 cells and elevated rates in only 4 cells (Table I). In cases where cyclic AMP and dibutyryl cyclic AMP were applied onto the same cells from different barrels of the same 5-barrel pipette, ejection currents required to evoke threshold or maximal responses were similar for each drug. Although this equipotency is not supported by findings in some other tissues[12,30,52] we cannot presently eliminate the possibility of differences in electrophoretic mobility of the two substances. Other factors may also be operative (see Discussion).

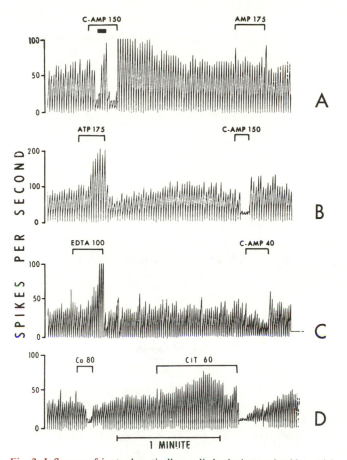

Fig. 2. Influence of iontophoretically applied adenine nucleotides, calcium chelators and $Ca^{2+}$ on spontaneous discharge of Purkinje cells. A and B taken from same cell. Heavy bar during cyclic AMP administration in A shows cathodal stimulation of the cell through another (NaCl) barrel of the 5-barrel pipette. Increased discharge during this stimulation suggests that the cyclic AMP depression is not the result of local anesthesia or hyperdepolarization. Note that while cyclic AMP only depresses activity in these cells, 5'-AMP does nothing (A), and ATP (B), EDTA (C), and citrate (D), all accelerate firing. Calcium always slowed activity (D). Often, supramaximal currents of ATP and the chelators accelerated discharge presumably to the point of 'depolarization block'.

In an effort to define the specificity of cyclic AMP effects, other adenine nucleotides were also tested. ATP was iontophoretically applied to 8 Purkinje cells and found to elevate the discharge rates in 5 cases (Table I, Fig. 2). Likewise, 5'-adenosine monophosphate accelerated firing in 3 of 7 Purkinje cells (Table I, Fig. 2). Clearly, these nucleotides have little or no ability to reproduce the depressant action of cyclic AMP.

*Calcium and metal chelators*

Adenine nucleotides can chelate divalent metals[5,15]. An attempt was made to

TABLE II

DIRECT ACTION OF IONTOPHORETICALLY APPLIED $Ca^{2+}$ AND CHELATORS ON SPONTANEOUS DISCHARGE OF SINGLE PURKINJE CELLS

| Agent | No. cells studied | Responsive | Slowed | Accelerated | Biphasic or reversible |
|---|---|---|---|---|---|
| $Ca^{2+}$ | 17 | 17 | 17 | 0 | 0 |
| EDTA | 9 | 8 | 0 | 8 | 0 |
| Na citrate | 9 | 9 | 0 | 9 | 0 |

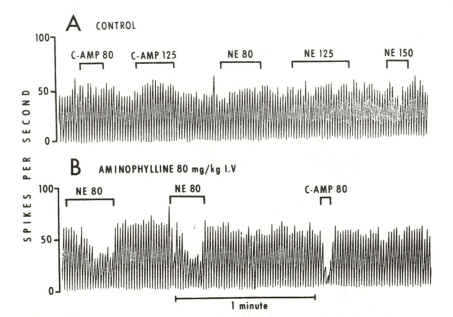

Fig. 3. Potentiation of Purkinje cell inhibitory responses to NE and cyclic AMP by intravenous aminophylline. Mean spontaneous discharge rate of same Purkinje cell before (A) and 10 min after (B) intravenous injection of aminophylline (80 mg/kg). This cell is one of few which showed accelerated firing with cyclic AMP in control conditions (A, see Fig. 4 also). However, after i.v. aminophylline, the response to cyclic AMP (note lower current required) is reversed to blockade of discharge (B). Note that after aminophylline injection a previously ineffective current (80 nA) of NE is sufficient to reduce mean discharge rate by about half.

control for this possible effect on Purkinje cells by changing extracellular calcium concentrations. The response of rat Purkinje cells to iontophoretically applied $Ca^{2+}$ was extraordinarily reproducible; in all 17 cells studied, $Ca^{2+}$ slowed the spontaneous discharge (Table II, Fig. 2). In contrast to $Ca^{2+}$, metal chelators always accelerated the firing rate of Purkinje cells. Thus, in 9 cells studied, 8 cells responded to iontophoretically administered Na EDTA with speeding (Fig. 2). Likewise, Na citrate accelerated the firing rates of all 9 cells examined (Fig. 2). Both EDTA and citrate were capable of elevating discharge rates to the point of 'depolarization block', whereupon spike size decreases, and discharge becomes rapid and abruptly stops. Under these circumstances, electrical stimulation of the cell via the 'salt' barrel was ineffective in eliciting discharges. Fig. 2 shows the striking similarity between this effect of $Ca^{2+}$-chelators and 5'-AMP and ATP.

*Phosphodiesterase inhibitors*

Parenterally administered theophylline (60–150 mg/kg, i.v.) and aminophylline (40–122 mg/kg, i.v.) usually accelerated firing or had little direct effect on Purkinje cell firing rate. Yet the agents greatly potentiated the response to given iontophoretic currents of NE within 25 min after injection. In addition, the duration of the NE response was often increased following theophylline (see ref. 64, Fig. 3).

Depressant responses to iontophoretic cyclic AMP were also potentiated by intravenous theophylline (4 of 4 cells) and aminophylline (4 of 4 cells). Significantly, the occasional elevations in firing rate encountered with cyclic AMP were reversed to depression by this treatment (Fig. 3).

Although analysis of spike size revealed little change during and after injection of theophylline or aminophylline, we could still not ensure that blood pressure changes and resultant cellular movement had not altered the position of the cell relative to the micropipette assembly. Such changes could alter local drug concentrations, and therefore disturb the response intensity to equal pulses of NE or cyclic AMP. In fact,

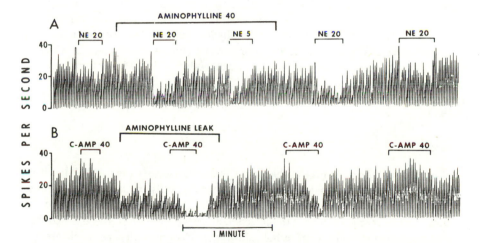

Fig. 4. Potentiation of the responses to NE and cyclic AMP by iontophoretically applied aminophylline. A, Slightly effective current of NE (20 nA) becomes almost maximally effective during and shortly after aminophylline (40 nA) is ejected. Previously subthreshold current (5 nA) of NE is now very effective during aminophylline administration. B, Same cell as in A, 20 min later. Leakage of aminophylline from micropipette is now sufficient to directly reduce discharge rate. Slight excitation of the unit is noted with 40 nA of cyclic AMP before aminophylline, although during and shortly after aminophylline application, only reduction in firing rate is seen with the same current of cyclic AMP. Recovery of the original excitatory response seen about 2 min after reinstituting aminophylline 'holding' current.

571

TABLE III

DIRECT EFFECT OF IONTOPHORETICALLY APPLIED METHYL XANTHINE ON SPONTANEOUS ACTIVITY OF SINGLE PURKINJE CELLS

| Agent | No. cells studied | Responsive | Slowed | Accelerated | Biphasic or reversible |
|---|---|---|---|---|---|
| Aminophylline | 39 | 39 | 38 | 0 | 1 |
| Theophylline | 19 | 18 | 12 | 4 | 2 |

analysis of EKGs often revealed alterations of cardiovascular activity, consistent with the literature on methyl xanthines[57]. Even though one would not expect random blood pressure changes to uniformly increase the intensity of response to NE and cyclic AMP as we have found, we nonetheless attempted microiontophoretic application of theophylline to eliminate tissue movement as a factor. Microiontophoresis of theophylline moderately potentiated the effects of NE or cyclic AMP in only 6 of 16 studied cells. However, the low solubility (about 0.1 $M$) of theophylline made its microiontophoresis difficult.

However, iontophoretically applied aminophylline which is more soluble (0.2 $M$) was decidedly more effective: in 10 Purkinje cells studied, leakage (no 'holding' current) or weak currents (10–40 nA) of aminophylline just before and during test pulses of NE or cyclic AMP markedly accentuated the depressant responses to NE (10 cells) and cyclic AMP (5 cells) (Fig. 4). These quantities of ejected aminophylline generally had only slight or no direct effect on tonic Purkinje firing rate. As with injected methyl xanthine, iontophoretic aminophylline reversed the occasional acceleratory responses of cyclic AMP to those of slowing (Fig. 4). In 3 cases in which a biphasic response (see above) was previously evoked by cyclic AMP, only the depressant action was potentiated. Larger currents (5–80 nA) of aminophylline and theophylline directly reduced discharge rate of the vast majority of Purkinje cells tested (Table III).

*Histamine*

In view of recent claims that histamine, like NE, elevates cyclic AMP levels in cerebellar slices[35,63], we applied histamine to Purkinje cells by microiontophoresis. Discharge rates were slowed in all 16 cells so studied. In this respect the constancy of histamine action resembles that of the catecholamines[33,64]. However, it was noted that ejection currents necessary for threshold slowing of Purkinje cells was much greater than with NE. The mean threshold current ($\pm$ S.E.) with histamine ($109 \pm 11$ nA) was significantly ($P < 0.001$) higher than that with NE ($61 \pm 3$ nA).

*Prostaglandins*

Members of the E and F families of prostaglandin were studied. The direct effects of these substances on Purkinje cells are shown in Table IV. It will be noted that

TABLE IV

EFFECTS OF PROSTAGLANDINS AND THEIR PRECURSORS ON SPONTANEOUS ACTIVITY OF PURKINJE CELLS
AND ON THE EFFECT OF NE

0 = no effect; E = elevated discharge rate; R = reduced; B or R = biphasic or reversible; A = slight or variable antagonism; PA = pronounced and repeatable antagonism.

| Agent | Direct action (no. cells) | | | | Antagonism of NE response (no. cells) | | |
|---|---|---|---|---|---|---|---|
| | O | E | R | B or R | O | A | PA |
| PGE$_1$ | 8 | 21 | 4 | 0 | 2 | 6 | 19 |
| PGE$_2$ | 5 | 9 | 10 | 0 | 2 | 3 | 8 |
| PGF$_{1a}$ | 6 | 9 | 3 | 5 | 14 | 0 | 1 |
| PGF$_{2a}$ | 3 | 10 | 5 | 3 | 14 | 2 | 1 |
| Linoleic | 11 | 1 | 0 | 0 | 9 | 0 | 0 |
| Linolenic | 7 | 3 | 3 | 0 | 11 | 0 | 0 |

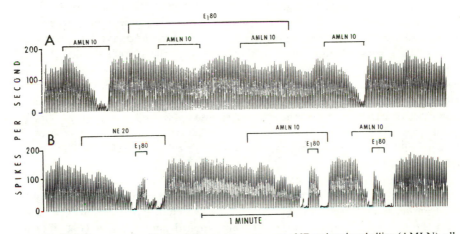

Fig. 5. Blockade by prostaglandin E$_1$ of depressant responses to NE and aminophylline (AMLN), all applied iontophoretically to a normal Purkinje cell. A, Nearly total inhibition of the effects of aminophylline (10 nA) by prior and concurrent application of PGE$_1$, 80 nA. B, Same cell, showing Purkinje cell depressant responses to NE 20 nA and aminophylline 10 nA; during the consequent responses, 80 nA of PGE$_1$ is ejected, restoring discharge rates to near normal.

a mixture of responses are obtained depending upon the prostaglandin tested. With PGE$_1$ a preponderance (64%) of cells responded with accelerated rate. By contrast, PGE$_2$ evoked slightly more depressant responses (42%) than acceleratory ones (38%). Although the majority of cells responding to PGF$_{1a}$ and PGF$_{2a}$ showed accelerated rates, more units showed biphasic or reversible responses with the F$_a$ series than the E series. Furthermore, tachyphylaxis of the type described by Avanzino et al.[1] was seen only with the F series of prostaglandins.

Although the direct responses to the E group of prostaglandins were mixed, reproducible blockade of NE depressant responses was usually found (Fig. 5). This antagonism of NE was manifested in two ways: (a) reduction or obliteration of the control NE response by the prior (about 0.5 min) and concurrent application of PGE from another barrel of the same pipette assembly, and (b) reversal of the maximal NE response when iontophoretic application of PGE was initiated after NE had already stopped cell firing (Fig. 5; see ref. 32, Fig. 2). In these tests control responses to NE or PGE alone were recorded several times before and after NE blockade was attempted. For those cells responding with elevated rates to prostaglandin alone, ejection currents of prostaglandin which had no direct effect were used to block NE action.

The great majority of cells exhibited antagonism of NE by $PGE_1$ or $E_2$ (Table IV). In a total of 40 cells tested with $PGE_1$ or $E_2$, 27 cells exhibited consistent reversals of the NE response by 40 % or more; another 9 cells showed occasional or only slight blockade of NE effects by $PGE_1$ or $E_2$. However, a clear-cut blockade of NE responses was seen only rarely with iontophoretic application of $PGF_{1\alpha}$ (3 of 17 cells, Table IV). Furthermore, one unit showed potentiation of NE responses with iontophoretic application of $PGF_{2\alpha}$. No potentiation was ever seen with $PGE_1$ or $E_2$.

Several lines of evidence suggest that the inhibition of NE response by $PGE_1$ or $PGE_2$ is a specific antagonism. First, the closely related $PGF_\alpha$ series is not particularly effective against NE. Further, neither linoleic nor linolenic acid, two fatty acid precursors of the prostaglandins, ever antagonized NE in the 13 cells studied (Fig. 7, Table IV), in spite of occasional direct excitatory effects. Additional evidence that the reversal of the NE response is not merely a result of a nonspecific elevation in discharge rate by PGE is found in the 15 cells where $PGE_1$ or $E_2$ had no direct effect, or actually suppressed discharges, yet still blocked the response to NE (Fig. 7; see ref. 32, Fig. 2). Finally, maximal doses of $PGE_1$ or $E_2$ had no effect on the depressant responses of Purkinje cells to iontophoretically applied GABA (7 cells), or cyclic AMP (10 cells) (ref. 32, Fig. 2).

Although the lack of prostaglandin effect on cyclic AMP responses would seem to point to an action of prostaglandin at some step at or before cyclic AMP formation (presumed adrenergic receptors, adenyl cyclase, etc.), $PGE_1$ curiously antagonized the slowing action of iontophoretically applied aminophylline (Fig. 5) (7 of 7 Purkinje cells). Evaluation of this unexpected effect will be presented in the Discussion.

*Nicotinate*

Nicotinic acid has been reported to reduce cyclic AMP levels of isolated fat cells in the presence of catecholamine[11], perhaps by stimulating phosphodiesterase[39]. Since high concentrations of this agent are sufficiently soluble and charged for iontophoretic administration, its effects on the NE responses of Purkinje cells were also tested. The reduction in firing rate produced by iontophoretically applied NE was markedly reduced in 5 of 5 cells by iontophoresis of nicotinate from another barrel of the same 5-barrel micropipette (Fig. 6). The antagonism by nicotinate had several characteristics similar to that of $PGE_1$ and $E_2$. For example, nicotinate reversed NE responses regardless of which of the two agents were first applied. Furthermore, pronounced

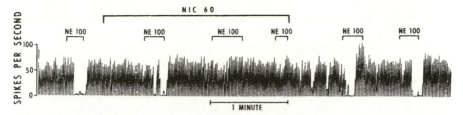

Fig. 6. Inhibitory action of iontophoretically applied nicotinate (NIC, 60 nA) on responses of Purkinje cells to periodic NE (100 nA) administration. Note the total blockade of maximal NE responses by a dose of nicotinate which has no direct action on the spontaneous discharge rate.

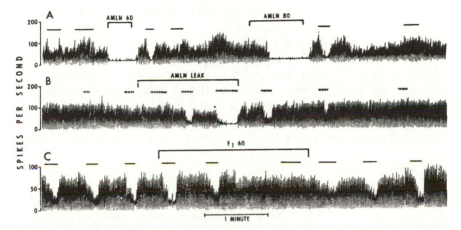

Fig. 7. Effects and interactions of iontophoretically applied NE, aminophylline, cyclic AMP and PGE₁ on Purkinje cells of 6-hydroxydopamine treated animals. A, The only Purkinje cell observed which showed a 'reversible' or 'biphasic' response to NE (solid bars above record indicate application of 80 nA NE). Aminophylline (AMLN) 60 nA abolishes action potentials. Within 1 min after recovery from direct effects of aminophylline, NE 80 nA now abolishes firing. B, Same cell as in A. Application of cyclic AMP 200 nA (dashed lines above record) has no effect on firing rate until aminophylline is allowed to leak out of the micropipette. During this time and for 1.5 min after 'holding' current is reinstated, cyclic AMP 200 nA now abolishes or slows discharges. C, Different cell. Near maximal, reproducible responses to application of NE 80 nA (indicated by solid bars above the record) are blocked by concomitant iontophoretic application of PGE₁ 60 nA. Note that the latter is in itself incapable of altering discharge rate.

antagonism was seen with ejection currents of nicotinate which had no observable direct effect on spontaneous Purkinje discharge rate (see Fig. 6).

*6-hydroxydopamine treated rats*

In an effort to determine whether some of the agents used in this study were exerting an indirect effect on Purkinje cells via a presynaptic action on adrenergic nerve terminals (see refs. 3, 23, 29, 73), the cerebellar cortices of several 6-hydroxydopamine (6-HODA) treated rats were studied. Purkinje cells of these rats have no functional adrenergic terminals (see Methods and refs. 6, 7).

575

When cyclic AMP was iontophoretically applied to 19 Purkinje cells of 3 different 6-HODA treated rats, 5 cells did not respond, 11 units displayed reduced firing rates and 3 increased their discharge activity. As in normal rats, depressant responses to NE and cyclic AMP were greatly enhanced in 6-HODA treated rats by i.v. aminophylline and by iontophoretically applied aminophylline (Fig. 7) (6 of 6 units examined). Two of the 3 cells excited by cyclic AMP were subjected to methyl xanthine, one iontophoretically and one parenterally. Both now were depressed by cyclic AMP. Furthermore, 2 of the 5 cells which did not initially respond to cyclic AMP (200 nA ejection current) exhibited reduced firing rates to cyclic AMP (125 nA) during iontophoretic application of aminophylline (Fig. 7).

Prostaglandin $E_1$ also showed similar effects in cerebella of 6-HODA treated and normal rats. Thus, $PGE_1$ (but not linolenic acid) showed marked antagonism of NE responses (Fig. 7) without affecting those to cyclic AMP (8 of 8 cells studied in two animals). Furthermore, $PGE_1$ was still capable of inhibiting the slowing of discharge rate in response to iontophoresis of aminophylline. The only pharmacological difference apparent between normal and 6-HODA treated rats was in the direct responses of Purkinje cells to $PGE_1$: only 2 of 28 cells studied showed elevations in rate, compared to 21 of 33 cells in normal rats. Such a disparity in the two groups may indicate tonic presynaptic release of NE in normal cerebella (see ref. 32).

DISCUSSION

The surprisingly reproducible effect of iontophoretically applied NE in inhibiting the spontaneous activity of rat Purkinje cells has led to attempts to uncover the mechanism of this response. Iontophoretically applied cyclic AMP nearly always mimicked the action of NE. Data from other experiments point toward intermediation of NE effects by cyclic AMP. Thus, inhibition of phosphodiesterase by theophylline[13] or aminophylline reproducibly potentiates the inhibitory actions of both NE and cyclic AMP. Furthermore, nicotinic acid and prostaglandins of the E group block the response of Purkinje cells to NE. Both these agents can antagonize the ability of catecholamines to elevate cyclic AMP levels in peripheral tissues[10,11,39].

Although an enhanced formation of cyclic AMP in response to NE cannot presently be measured directly in individual Purkinje cells, there have been biochemical findings of increased cyclic AMP production by particulate brain fractions[38,56] and slices of cerebellum[35,50,63] exposed to catecholamine. On the other hand, Weiss[69] has not observed an NE stimulation of the adenyl cyclase activity of cerebellar homogenates, suggesting that extraction or homogenization procedures may obscure physiological modulation of cyclase activity[72].

Biochemical studies on cerebellar slices showed that histamine also increases cyclic AMP levels[35,63]. In the present study all 16 cells examined responded to histamine in a manner analogous to NE and cyclic AMP. The apparent lesser potency of histamine compared to NE may arise from differences in iontophoretic mobility. However, histamine stimulates cyclic AMP accumulation less than NE in cerebellar slices[35,63]. The reverse is true in cerebral slices[36].

In spite of the predominant depressant responses of Purkinje cells to cyclic AMP, some attention should be given to those cells which either did not respond (16%), which displayed elevations in rate (15%) or which generated biphasic or reversible responses (8%). In an effort to improve the responsiveness of Purkinje cells, the dibutyryl derivative of cyclic AMP was administered by 5-barrel micropipette. Yet, in contrast to its greater effectiveness in several peripheral tissues[12,30,52], the dibutyryl derivative showed no greater potency either in terms of incidence or intensity of response than the parent compound.

In assessing the significance of this finding it is important to evaluate the mechanisms commonly advanced for the greater potency of the dibutyryl derivative. One advantage proposed is the greater ability of dibutyryl cyclic AMP to pass through barriers to diffusion in the tissue[52], since most other nucleotides are reputed not to traverse plasma membranes without dephosphorlylation[41,59]. In our iontophoresis experiments the increased diffusibility of dibutyryl cyclic AMP may be of no advantage since the micropipette may already have broken down the majority of diffusion barriers surrounding the Purkinje cells.

A second proposal for the greater efficacy of the dibutyryl derivative is its lower affinity as a substrate for phosphodiesterase, thus slowing its hydrolysis[52]. It may be relevant to the present study that the reported phosphodiesterase activity of the rat cerebellum is the lowest in the brain[71]. Thus, if the major advantage of the dibutyryl derivative resides in its inaccessibility to phosphodiesterase, one would expect the cerebellum to show the least difference between the potencies of cyclic AMP and the derivative. In fact, cyclic AMP and dibutyryl AMP are equipotent in producing behavioral effects in rats and cats when injected by microcannula into the cerebellar substance; in other brain areas only the dibutyryl derivative is effective[26]. Moreover, there are other tissues outside the brain which respond to cyclic AMP[24,28,45,49] and a few which are no more responsive to dibutyryl cyclic AMP than the parent compound[30,44,60].

The reported low activity of phosphodiesterase in the rat cerebellum may also account for the dramatic effectiveness of methyl xanthines in enhancing NE and cyclic AMP depressant effects. Hence, low quantities of the xanthine would abolish the already scant phosphodiesterase activity without overt toxicity.

In spite of its low activity, the presence, and especially the location, of phosphodiesterase may be of profound importance in determining the response of each Purkinje cell to cyclic AMP. There is biochemical evidence that brain phosphodiesterase is distributed in particulate and soluble fractions[17,71]; histochemical analysis has revealed neuronal and neuroglial localization of this enzyme[62]. It is thus conceivable that the unresponsiveness of some Purkinje cells to cyclic AMP resulted from the extraneuronal destruction of the substance before it could exert its intracellular action. In fact, all cells unresponsive to or accelerated by cyclic AMP in normal (5 cells) and 6-HODA treated (4 cells) rats showed exclusively depressant responses with cyclic AMP after methyl xanthine administration (Figs. 3, 4, and 7).

The cause of the occasional elevation in discharge rate with cyclic AMP is more puzzling. It was noted that ATP and 5'-AMP almost exclusively accelerated firing rates (Fig. 2). These adenine nucleotides have in common a metal chelating ability[5,15] which could account for the elevations in firing rate. This proposal is supported indirectly by the observations that $Ca^{2+}$ always slowed and chelators always accelerated Purkinje discharge rates (Fig. 2), in accord with the findings of Curtis *et al.*[16] and Galindo *et al.*[25]. One might conjecture, therefore, that cyclic AMP, acting either pre- or postsynaptically, speeds the activity of some Purkinje cells through calcium chelation. However, other mechanisms of action (such as indirect effects on presynaptic endings, blood vessels, etc.) cannot be excluded at present.

Indeed, the function of $Ca^{2+}$ in excitable membranes is complex, but it appears to be required for stabilization of the membrane at the 'resting' level[68]. Furthermore, it has been shown that adenyl cyclase itself is modulated by $Ca^{2+}$ (refs. 8, 70) and that some cyclic AMP membrane effects may be mediated by $Ca^{2+}$ (refs. 22, 55). Possibly, chelation of $Ca^{2+}$ or other divalent cations could influence adenyl cyclase activity or cyclic AMP effects.

In any event, the inhibitory action of cyclic AMP generally predominates over speeding effects, although occasionally the two effects may be balanced to some degree, as in the 'biphasic' or 'reversible' responses. The primary action of the cyclic AMP would appear to be a reduction in firing rate since the occasional excitatory responses produced by cyclic AMP are reversed to those of depression by methyl xanthines. Accordingly, the few excitatory responses to cyclic AMP may arise from secondary effects such as $Ca^{2+}$ chelation, while the principal intracellular, discharge-reducing effects are masked by the phosphodiesterase.

One may always question whether substances administered by iontophoresis affect presynaptic as well as postsynaptic elements. This question is especially important in the present study, since several investigators have reported presynaptic actions of cyclic AMP[27], methyl xanthines[3,27,73] and prostaglandins[23,29], the latter two substances on adrenergic terminals. For this reason, 6-HODA treated rats, lacking any significant NE-containing axons or terminals in the cerebellum[6,7] were tested. In all respects, responses of Purkinje cells to cyclic AMP and methyl xanthine in these animals were identical to those of normal animals. Furthermore, the NE and cyclic AMP potentiating action of methyl xanthine and the antagonism of NE effects by $PGE_1$ in 6-HODA animals were as pronounced as in normals (Fig. 7). Thus it does not seem likely that either cyclic AMP, methyl xanthine or prostaglandin act at adrenergic terminals on Purkinje cells. This finding is corroborated by recent research on neonatal rats[65]. At 1–4 days of age Purkinje cells do not have electrophysiologically or ultrastructurally demonstrable synaptic terminations of any type; still, inhibitory responses to NE are antagonized by iontophoretically applied prostaglandin $E_1$. Moreover, these immature, asynaptic Purkinje cells respond to cyclic AMP only by depression of spontaneous activity.

Turning now to the protaglandins, the specificity of $PGE_1$ and $E_2$ antagonism of NE has been evaluated in an earlier report[32]. These agents will not antagonize cyclic AMP or GABA inhibitory effects on Purkinje cells, nor will fatty acid precursors of the prostaglandins affect responses to NE. The present study shows that prostaglandins $F_{1a}$ and $F_{2a}$ are also not effective against NE. In fact, one cell showed an enhanced response to NE after $PGF_{2\alpha}$. Thus, $PGE_1$ and $PGE_2$ appear to be unique in their inhibition of NE response.

In most respects the influence of $PGE_1$ and $PGE_2$ on Purkinje cells resembles that of $PGE_1$ on isolated fat cells[2,10,46]. For example, responses to catecholamines are inhibited while those to cyclic AMP are not affected. Moreover, $PGE_1$ and $PGE_2$ were found to block the slowing action of iontophoretically applied aminophylline, much as $PGE_1$ inhibits the lipolytic effect of theophylline in fat cells[46]. These findings point to an action of prostaglandin at some point beyond the adenyl cyclase enzyme. It is possible that $PGE_1$ has a dual action, wherein adenyl cyclase activity is inhibited and phosphodiesterase is stimulated. However, a more plausible explanation may be a primary effect of prostaglandin on membrane permeability, thus changing the ionic environment of the enzymes[34] or allowing intracellular cyclic AMP to diffuse out of the cell. Such a mechanism, among others, has been proposed for the antilipolytic action of insulin on fat cells[58,70], and might account for the lack of $PGE_1$ effects on adenyl cyclase activity in homogenates of cerebellum, pineal gland (Weiss, personal communication) and fat pad[10], or on slices of brain[50]. However, the slowing action of methyl xanthine and its antagonism by prostaglandin may be unrelated to phosphodiesterase activity[2,4].

It is interesting to speculate as to the function of prostaglandins in the central nervous system. They are found in synaptosome fractions of cerebral cortex[37] and are released from the surface of cerebral cortex spontaneously and in response to stimulation of the spinal cord[53] and the reticular formation[9]. Moreover, prostaglandins are released spontaneously from superfused cerebellar cortex[14].

However, indications as to the function of prostaglandin in the central nervous system are scant. Thus, although prostaglandins have been shown to alter synaptic transmission in spinal cord[18,51], and to exert direct effects on the electrical activity of brain stem neurons[1], it is difficult to determine whether they function as local modulators of synaptic transmission, as neurotransmitters, or are merely some by-product of fatty acid metabolism. In the cerebellum, the highly variable direct action of each of the prostaglandins on the spontaneous activity of Purkinje cells, and the invariably potent antagonism of NE responses by $PGE_1$ and $E_2$, suggest they may act as modulators of adrenergic transmission rather than as neurotransmitters[32].

Finally, in view of the multiplicity of known inhibitory inputs to the Purkinje cell via interneurons[20], the question of the function of the newly described adrenergic pathway still remains. It is tempting to hypothesize that the adrenergic pathway introduces the potential for a slow, metabolically coupled change in excitability, distinct from the rapidly subsiding passive changes in ion conductance of classical inhibitory synapses[19]. Such a 'metabolic synaptic' mechanism has been proposed for the 'slow IPSP' of frog and rabbit sympathetic neurons[21,42,47] in which the neurotransmitter may also be a catecholamine[21,42]. An adrenergic system of this type in the cerebellum would provide considerably more plasticity in the time dimension. Recent electrophysiological studies with intracellular techniques appear to support the metabolic nature of this response to norepinephrine[48].

SUMMARY

The relationship between cerebellar adenyl cyclase and norepinephrine (NE) receptivity of cerebellar Purkinje cells was explored by recording their spontaneous discharge during microiontophoretic application of various substances. The depression in firing rate of single Purkinje cells produced by NE was usually mimicked by adenosine 3'5'-monophosphate (cyclic AMP). The synthetic dibutyryl derivative of cyclic AMP, however, was no more potent than the parent compound. Two other adenine nucleotides, adenosine triphosphate (ATP) and 5'-AMP generally accelerated discharge rate or had no effect. The excitatory effects of the nucleotides may be related to chelation of divalent cations, since EDTA and citrate were universally found to accelerate unit firing while calcium ions always slowed or blocked spontaneous activity.

Further evidence for a link between the effects of NE and cyclic AMP was seen with the administration of the methyl xanthines, which inhibit the enzymatic breakdown of cyclic AMP by phosphodiesterase. Theophylline and aminophylline, whether parenterally or iontophoretically administered, markedly potentiated the depressant effects of both NE and cyclic AMP on Purkinje cells. Methyl xanthines usually transformed the infrequent speeding effects of cyclic AMP to those of slowing, or brought about an inhibitory response in cells previously non-responsive to cyclic AMP. Furthermore, iontophoresis of prostaglandins $E_1$ and $E_2$ (but not $F_{1a}$, $F_{2a}$, linoleic or linolenic acids), and of nicotinate, reported to reduce cyclic AMP levels in peripheral neuro-effector systems, also block the action of iontophoretically applied NE in rat cerebellum.

To determine if the locus of the action of the various iontophoretically applied substances was exerted presynaptically on the proposed adrenergic terminals on Purkinje cells, 6-hydroxydopamine (6-HODA) treated animals were studied. Under these conditions the effects of all the drugs and their interactions appeared identical to those of normal cerebella, in spite of biochemical and histochemical evidence for complete degeneration of adrenergic nerve terminals.

These studies provide indirect evidence for mediation of NE effects by cyclic AMP in a living single cell system. Thus, they parallel *in vitro* studies with cerebellar slices which show an increase in cyclic AMP levels with NE, as well as histamine. Taken with the histochemical data for norepinephrine nerves terminating on Purkinje cells, the findings point to a possible transsynaptic modulation of adenyl cyclase activity.

ACKNOWLEDGEMENTS

We are greatly indebted to Dr. Benjamin Weiss for his advice during the course of these experiments and his comments in the preparation of this manuscript; we acknowledge the skillful technical assistance of A. Paul Oliver, Odessa Colvin and Hamilton Poole. We also thank Dr. John Pike of the Upjohn Company for the kind gift of the prostaglandins used in this study.

## REFERENCES

1 AVANZINO, G. L., BRADLEY, P. B., AND WOLSTENCROFT, J. H., Actions of prostaglandins $E_1$, $E_2$ and $F_{2a}$ on brain stem neurons, *Brit. J. Pharmacol.*, 27 (1966) 157–163.

2 BERGSTROM, S., CARLSON, L. A., AND WEEKS, J. R., The prostaglandins: A family of biologically active lipids, *Pharmacol. Rev.*, 20 (1968) 1–48.

3 BERKOWITZ, B. A., TARVER, J. H., AND SPECTOR, S., Norepinephrine release by theophylline and caffeine, *Fed. Proc.*, 28 (1969) 415.

4 BIANCHI, C. P., *Cell Calcium*, Appleton-Century-Crofts, New York, 1968.

5 BJERRUM, J., SCHWARZENBACH, G., AND SILLEN, L. G., Stability constants. Part I. Organic ligands, *Spec. Publ. Chem. Soc.*, 6 (1957).

6 BLOOM, F. E., ALGERI, S., GROPPETTI, A., REVUELTA, A., AND COSTA, E., Lesions of central norepinephrine terminals with 6-OH-dopamine: Biochemistry and fine structure, *Science*, 166 (1969) 1284–1286.

7 BLOOM, F. E., HOFFER, B. J., AND SIGGINS, G. R., Studies on norepinephrine-containing afferents to cerebellar Purkinje cells of rat cerebellum. I. Localization of the fibers and their synapses, *Brain Research*, 25 (1971) 501–521.

8 BRADHAM, L. S., HOLT, D. A., AND SIMS, M., The effect of $Ca^{2+}$ on the adenyl cyclase of calf brain, *Biochim. biophys. Acta (Amst.)*, 201 (1970) 250–260.

9 BRADLEY, P. B., GILLIAN, M. SAMUELS R., AND SHAW, J. E., Correlation of prostaglandin release from the cerebral cortex of cats with the electrocorticogram, following stimulation of the reticular formation, *Brit. J. Pharmacol.*, 37 (1969) 151–157.

10 BUTCHER, R. W., AND BAIRD, C. E., Effects of prostaglandins on adenosine 3′,5′-monophosphate levels in fat and other tissues, *J. biol. Chem.*, 243 (1968) 1713–1717.

11 BUTCHER, R. W., BAIRD, C. E., AND SUTHERLAND, E. W., Effects of lipolytic and antilipolytic substances on adenosine 3′,5′-monophosphate levels in isolated fat cells, *J. biol. Chem.*, 243 (1968) 1705–1712.

12 BUTCHER, R. W., HO, R. J., MENG, H. C., AND SUTHERLAND, E. W., Adenosine 3′,5′-monophosphate in biological materials. II. The measurement of adenosine 3′,5′-monophosphate in tissues and the role of the cyclic nucleotide in the lipolytic response of fat to epinephrine, *J. biol. Chem.*, 240 (1965) 4515–4523.

13 BUTCHER, R. W., AND SUTHERLAND, E. W., Adenosine 3′,5′-phosphate in biological materials. I. Purification and properties of cyclic 3′,5′-nucleotide phosphodiesterase and use of this enzyme to characterize adenosine 3′,5′-phosphate in human urine, *J. biol. Chem.*, 237 (1962) 1244–1250.

14 COCEANI, F., AND WOLFE, L. S., Prostaglandins in brain and the release of prostaglandin-like compounds from the cat cerebellar cortex, *Canad. J. Physiol. Pharmacol.*, 43 (1965) 445–450.

15 COHN, M., AND HUGHES, T. R., Nuclear magnetic resonance spectra of adenosine di- and triphosphate, *J. biol. Chem.*, 237 (1962) 176–181.

16 CURTIS, D. R., PERRIN, D. D., AND WATKINS, J. C., The excitation of spinal neurons by the iontophoretic application of agents which chelate calcium, *J. Neurochem.*, 6 (1960) 1–20.

17 DE ROBERTIS E., RODRIGUEZ DE LORES ARNAIZ, G., AND ALBERICI, M., Subcellular distribution of adenyl cyclase and cyclic phosphodiesterase in rat brain cortex, *J. biol. Chem.*, 242 (1967) 3487–3493.

18 DUDA, P., HORTON, E. W., AND MCPHERSON, A., The effects of prostaglandins $E_1$, $F_{1a}$ and $F_{2a}$ on monosynaptic reflexes, *J. Physiol. (Lond.)*, 196 (1968) 151–162.

19 ECCLES, J. C., *The Physiology of Synapses*, Academic Press, New York, 1964.

20 ECCLES, J. C., ITO, M., AND SZENTÁGOTHAI, J., *The Cerebellum as a Neuronal Machine*, Springer, Berlin, 1967.

21 ECCLES, R. M., AND LIBET, B., Origin and blockade of the synaptic responses of curarized sympathetic ganglia, *J. Physiol. (Lond.)*, 157 (1961) 484–503.

22 ENTMAN, M. L., LEVEY, G. S., AND EPSTEIN, S. E., Demonstration of adenyl cyclase activity in canine cardiac sarcoplasmic reticulum, *Biochem. biophys. Res. Commun.*, 35 (1969) 728–733.

23 EULER, U. S. VON, AND HEDQVIST, P., Inhibitory action of prostaglandins $E_1$ and $E_2$ on the neuromuscular transmission in the guinea pig vas deferens, *Acta physiol. scand.*, 77 (1969) 510–512.

24 EXTON, J. H., AND PARK, C. R., The stimulation of gluconeogenesis from lactate by epinephrine, glucagon, and cyclic 3′,5′-adenylate in the perfused rat liver, *Pharmacol. Rev.*, 18 (1966) 181–188.

25 GALINDO, A., KRNJEVIĆ, K., AND SCHWARTZ, S., Micro-iontophoretic studies on neurones on the cuneate nucleus, *J. Physiol. (Lond.)*, 192 (1967) 359–377.

26 GESSA, G. L., TAGLIAMONTE, A., AND KRISHNA, G., Behavioral and vegetative effects produced by dibutyryl cyclic AMP injected into different brain areas. In E. COSTA AND P. GREENGARD (Eds.) *Advances in Biochemical Psychopharmacology, Vol. 3,* Raven, New York, 1970, pp. 371–381.

27 GOLDBERG, A. L., AND SINGER, J. J., Evidence for a role of cyclic AMP in neuromuscular transmission, *Proc. nat. Acad. Sci. (Wash.),* 64 (1969) 134–141.

28 GRANTHAM, J. J., AND ORLOFF, J., Effect of prostaglandin E₁ on the permeability response of the isolated collecting tubule to vasopressin, adenosine 3′,5′-monophosphate, and theophylline, *J. clin. Invest.,* 47 (1968) 1154–1161.

29 HEDQVIST, P., AND BRUNDIN, J., Inhibition by prostaglandin E₁ of noradrenaline release and of effector response to nerve stimulation on the cat spleen, *Life Sci.,* 8 (1969) 389–395.

30 HENION, W. F., SUTHERLAND, E. W., AND POSTERNAK, TH., Effects of derivatives of adenosine 3′,5′-phosphate on liver slices and intact animals, *Biochim. biophys. Acta (Amst.),* 148 (1967) 106–113.

31 HOFFER, B. J., SIGGINS, G. R., AND BLOOM, F. E., Cyclic 3′,5′-adenosine monophosphate (C-AMP) mediation of the response of rat cerebellar Purkinje cells to norepinephrine (NE): Blockade with prostaglandins, *Pharmacologist,* 11 (1969) 238.

32 HOFFER, B. J., SIGGINS, G. R., AND BLOOM, F. E., Prostaglandins E₁ and E₂ antagonize norepinephrine effects on cerebellar Purkinje cells. Microelectrophoretic study, *Science,* 166 (1969) 1418–1420.

33 HOFFER, B. J., SIGGINS, G. R., AND BLOOM, F. E., Studies on norepinephrine-containing afferents to Purkinje cells of rat cerebellum. II. Sensitivity of Purkinje cells to norepinephrine and related substances administered by microiontophoresis, *Brain Research,* 25 (1971) 523–534.

34 JESSUP, S. J., McDONALD-GIBSON, W. J., RAMWELL, P. W., AND SHAW, J. E., Biosynthesis and release of prostaglandins on hormonal treatment of frog skin, and their effect on ion transport, *Fed. Proc.,* 29 (1970) 387.

35 KAKIUCHI, S., AND RALL, T. W., The influence of chemical agents on the accumulation of adenosine 3′,5′-phosphate in slices of rabbit cerebellum, *Mol. Pharmacol.,* 4 (1968) 367–378.

36 KAKIUCHI, S., AND RALL, T. W., Studies on adenosine 3′,5′-phosphate in rabbit cerebral cortex, *Molec. Pharmacol.,* 4 (1968) 379–388.

37 KATAOKA, K., RAMWELL, P. W., AND JESSUP, R., Prostaglandins: Localization in subcellular particles of rat cerebral cortex, *Science,* 157 (1967) 1187–1188.

38 KLAINER, L. M., CHI, Y.-M., FREIDBERG, S. L., RALL, T. W., AND SUTHERLAND, E. W., The effects of neurohormones on the formation of adenosine 3′,5′-phosphate by preparations of brain and other tissues, *J. biol. Chem.,* 237 (1962) 1239–1243.

39 KRISHNA, G., WEISS, B., DAVIES, J. L., AND HYNIE, S., Mechanism of nicotinic acid inhibition of hormone-induced lipolysis, *Fed. Proc.,* 25 (1966) 719.

40 KRNJEVIĆ, K., AND PHILLIS, J. W., Iontophoretic studies of cortical neurones in the mammalian cerebral cortex, *J. Physiol., (Lond.)* 165 (1963) 274–304.

41 LEIBMAN, K. C., AND HEIDELBERGER, C., The metabolism of ³²P labeled ribonucleotides in tissue slides and cell suspensions, *J. biol. Chem.,* 216 (1955) 823–830.

42 LIBET, B., Generation of slow inhibitory and excitatory postsynaptic potentials, *Fed. Proc.,* 29 (1970) in press.

43 LISH, P. M., WEIKEL, J. H., AND DUNGAN, K. W., Pharmacological and toxicological properties of two new beta adrenergic receptor antagonists, *J. Pharmacol. exp. Ther.,* 149 (1965) 161–173.

44 MacMANUS, J. P., AND WHITFIELD, J. F., Stimulation of DNA synthesis and mitotic activity of thymic lymphocytes by cyclic adenosine 3′,5′-monophosphate, *Exp. Cell Res.,* 58 (1970) 188–191.

45 MOSINGER, B., AND VAUGHAN, M., The action of cyclic 3′,5′-adenosine monophosphate on lipolysis in rat adipose tissue, *Biochim. biophys. Acta (Amst.),* 144 (1967) 569–582.

46 MÜHLBACHOVÀ, E., SOLYOM, A., AND PUGLISI, L., Investigations on the mechanism of the prostaglandin E₁ antagonism to norepinephrine and theophylline-induced lipolysis, *Europ. J. Pharmacol.,* 1 (1967) 321–325.

47 NISHI, S., AND KOKETSU, K., Origin of ganglionic inhibitory postsynaptic potential, *Life Sci.,* 6 (1967) 2049–2055.

48 OLIVER, A. P., SIGGINS, G. R., HOFFER, B. J., AND BLOOM, F. E., Changes in transmembrane potential of Purkinje cells of rat cerebellum during microelectrophoretic administration of norepinephrine (NE), *Fed. Proc.,* 29 (1970) 251.

49 ORLOFF, J., HANDLER, J. S., AND BERGSTROM, S., Effect of prostaglandin on the permeability response of the toad bladder to vasopressin, theophylline and adenosine 3′,5′-phosphate, *Nature (Lond.),* 205 (1965) 397–398.

50 PALMER, E. C., SULSER, F., AND ROBISON, G. A., The effects of neurohumoral agents on the level of cyclic AMP in different brain areas *in vitro, Pharmacologists*, 11 (1969) 157.

51 PHILLIS, J. W., AND TEBĒCIS. A. K., Prostaglandins and toad spinal cord responses, *Nature (Lond.)*, 217 (1968) 1076–1077.

52 POSTERNAK, TH., SUTHERLAND, E. W., AND HENION, W. F., Derivatives of cyclic 3',5'-adenosine monophosphate, *Biochim. biophys. Acta (Amst.)*, 65 (1962) 558–560.

53 RAMWELL, P. W., AND SHAW, J. E., The spontaneous and evoked release of non-cholinergic substances from the cerebral cortex of cats, *Life Sci.*, 2 (1963) 419–426.

54 RAMWELL, P. W., SHAW, J. E., AND JESSUP, R., Spontaneous and evoked release of prostaglandins from frog spinal cord, *Amer. J. Physiol.*, 211 (1966) 998–1004.

55 RASMUSSEN, H., AND TENENHOUSE, A., Cyclic adenosine monophosphate, $Ca^{2+}$ and membranes, *Proc. nat. Acad. Sci. (Wash.)*, 59 (1968) 1364–1370.

56 RIGBERG, M., VACIK, J. P., AND SHELVER, W. M., Utilization of radiometric analysis for measurement of activation of adenyl cyclase by sympathomimetic amines, *J. pharmacol. Sci.*, 58 (1969) 358–359.

57 RITCHIE, J. M., Central nervous system stimulants. II. The xanthines. In L. S. GOODMAN AND A. GILMAN (Eds.), *The Pharmacological Basis of Therapeutics*, Macmillan, New York, 1965, pp. 354–366.

58 RODBELL, M. J., AND JONES, A. B., Metabolism of isolated rat cells, *J. biol. Chem.*, 241 (1966) 140–142.

59 ROLL, P. M., WEINFIELD, H., CARROLL, E., AND BROWN, G., The utilization of nucleotides by the mammal. IV. Triply labeled purine nucleotides, *J. biol. Chem.*, 220 (1956) 439–465.

60 RYAN, W. L., AND HEIDRICK, M. L., Inhibition of cell growth *in vitro* by adenosine 3',5'-monophosphate, *Science*, 27 (1968) 1484–1485.

61 SALMOIRAGHI, G. C., AND WEIGHT, F., Micromethods in neuropharmacology: An approach to the study of anesthetics, *Anesthesiology*, 28 (1967) 54–64.

62 SHANTA, T. R., WOODS, W. D., WAITZMAN, M. B., AND BOURNE, G. H., Histochemical method for localization of cyclic 3',5'-nucleotide phosphodiesterase, *Histochemie*, 7 (1966) 177–191.

63 SHIMIZU, H., DALY, J. W., AND CREVELING, C. R., A radioisotopic method for measuring the formation of adenosine 3',5'-cyclic monophosphate in incubated slices of brain, *J. Neurochem.*, 16 (1969) 1609–1619.

64 SIGGINS, G. R., HOFFER, B. J., AND BLOOM, F. E., Cyclic adenosine monophosphate: Possible mediator for norepinephrine effects on cerebellar Purkinje cells, *Science*, 165 (1969) 1018–1020.

65 SIGGINS G. R., WOODWARD, D., HOFFER, B. J., AND BLOOM, F. E., Responsiveness of cerebellar Purkinje cells to norepinephrine (NE), cyclic AMP (C-AMP) and prostaglandin $E_1$ ($PGE_1$) during synaptic morphogenesis in neonatal rat, *Pharmacologist*, 12 (1970) 198.

66 SUTHERLAND, E. W., RALL, T. W., AND MENON, T., Adenyl cyclase. I. Distribution, preparation and properties, *J. biol. Chem.*, 237 (1962) 1220–1227.

67 SUTHERLAND, E. W., ROBISON, G. A., AND BUTCHER, R., Some aspects of the biological role of adenosine 3',5'-monophosphate, *Circulation*, 37 (1968) 279–306.

68 TASAKI, I., *Nerve Excitation, A Macromolecular Approach*, Thomas, Springfield, Ill., 1968.

69 WEISS, B., Differences in the stimulation effects of norepinephrine (NE) and sodium fluoride on adenyl cyclase (AC) of pineal gland and cerebellum, *Fed. Proc.*, 27 (1968) 752.

70 WEISS, B., Factors affecting adenyl cyclase activity and its sensitivity to biogenic amines. In J. J. BLUM (Ed.), *Biogenic Amines as Physiological Regulators*, Prentice Hall, Englewood Cliffs, N.J., 1970, in press.

71 WEISS, B., AND COSTA, E., Regional and subcellular distribution of adenyl cyclase and 3',5'-cyclic nucleotide phosphodiesterase in brain and pineal gland, *Biochem. Pharmacol.*, 17 (1968) 2107–2116.

72 WEISS, B., AND KIDMAN, A. D., Neurobiological significance of cyclic 3',5'-adenosine monophosphate. In E. COSTA AND P. GREENGARD (Eds.), *Advances in Biochemical Psychopharmacology*, Vol. 1, Raven, New York, 1969, pp. 131–164.

73 WESTFALL, D. P., AND FLEMING, W. W., Sensitivity changes in the dog heart to norepinephrine, calcium and aminophylline resulting from pretreatment with reserpine, *J. Pharmacol. exp. Ther.*, 159 (1968) 98–106.

# ADENOSINE 3',5'-MONOPHOSPHATE IN NERVOUS TISSUE: INCREASE ASSOCIATED WITH SYNAPTIC TRANSMISSION

*Donald A. McAfee,*
*Michel Schorderet and*
*Paul Greengard*
*Department of Pharmacology,*
*Yale University School of Medicine,*
*New Haven, Connecticut 06510*

*Brief periods of stimulation of the preganglionic nerve fibers produced a severalfold increase in the content of adenosine 3',5'-monophosphate in superior cervical sympathetic ganglia, whereas postganglionic stimulation did not. These and other experiments indicated that the increased concentrations of adenosine 3'5'-monophosphate were closely associated with the process of synaptic transmission. This increase occurred primarily in postsynaptic cells.*

There is considerable evidence which suggests that adenosine 3',5'-monophosphate (cyclic AMP) may be involved in regulation of metabolism and function in the nervous system. Several reviews of this subject have appeared recently (1). Included in the evidence is the finding that electrical stimulation of brain slices results in an increase in the concentration of cyclic AMP (2). However, it was not possible to conclude from those experiments whether the effect on the concentration of cyclic AMP reflected what might be seen under more physiological conditions of nervous activity, nor could it be ascertained at what level of cellular organization this biochemical effect had occurred. In the hope of answering these questions, we studied the effect of nervous activity on the concentration of cyclic AMP in various types of peripheral nervous tissue. Such tissues are amenable to experimental manipulation under relatively physiological conditions. We determined the cyclic AMP content of these small tissues by using a sensitive analytical method for cyclic AMP recently developed in our laboratory (3). Our experiments provide the first demonstration that the cyclic AMP content of nervous tissue can change in response to synaptic activity.

Superior cervical sympathetic ganglia were removed from New Zealand white rabbits (weight, 4 to 5 kg) which had been anesthetized with urethane (1000 mg per kilogram of body weight; administered intravenously). Ganglia were carefully decapsulated, mounted on stimulating and recording electrodes in an appropriate chamber, and continuously superfused with oxygenated Locke's solution (4). After the response to single shocks was monitored, the ganglia were stimulated through the preganglionic nerve trunk by means of supramaximum shocks at a frequency of 10 per second for various periods of time. Immediately following the stimulus period the ganglia were homogenized in ice-cold 6 percent trichloroacetic acid, and the precipitate was removed by low-speed centrifugation. For comparison, the contralateral ganglion of each pair served as an unstimulated control. The cyclic AMP in the trichloroacetic acid extract was isolated by minor modification of the procedure of Krishna et al. (5). The amount of cyclic AMP was determined according to its ability to activate a protein kinase purified from bovine heart, by means of the assay method described previously (3). Each extract was analyzed in duplicate at two different dilutions, in both the absence and the presence of authentic cyclic AMP added as an internal standard. The protein in the trichloroacetic acid precipitate was determined by the method of Lowry et al. (6). In some experiments, the cervical vagus, with or without the inclusion of the nodose ganglion, was prepared and studied in a similar manner. The nodose ganglion was studied because it contains nerve cell bodies but not synapses.

The mean concentration of cyclic AMP in a population of 29 unstimulated superior cervical sympathetic ganglia was $17.3 \pm 1.3$ pmole per milligram of protein. Stimulation of the preganglionic (cervical sympathetic) nerve trunk at a frequency of 10 per second for 30 seconds caused a considerable increase in the cyclic AMP

Table 1. Effect of preganglionic stimulation on the content of cyclic AMP in rabbit superior cervical sympathetic ganglia. One ganglion from each rabbit was stimulated at a frequency of 10 per second. The contralateral ganglion served as an unstimulated control. The data have been calculated as the mean $\pm$ standard error for the number ($N$) of rabbits indicated in the second column. In the last column, the concentration of cyclic AMP in the stimulated ganglia is expressed as the percentage of that in the unstimulated control ganglia. Temperature, 33°C.

| Duration of stimulation (min) | N | Cyclic AMP (picomoles per milligram of protein) | | | Percentage of control |
| --- | --- | --- | --- | --- | --- |
| | | Unstimulated ganglion | Stimulated ganglion | Absolute increase | |
| 0.5 | 5 | $23.2 \pm 5.5$ | $43.4 \pm 11.2$ | $20.3 \pm 13.0$ | $249 \pm 113$ |
| 1.0 | 5 | $13.1 \pm 1.3$ | $61.8 \pm 6.1$ | $48.7 \pm 5.2$ | $479 \pm 39$ |
| 2.0 | 11 | $18.0 \pm 1.7$ | $70.2 \pm 9.1$ | $52.1 \pm 8.2$ | $399 \pm 40$ |
| 4.0 | 4 | $14.2 \pm 2.9$ | $57.0 \pm 3.0$ | $43.5 \pm 4.3$ | $483 \pm 136$ |
| 8.0 | 4 | $16.4 \pm 1.0$ | $72.0 \pm 4.5$ | $55.7 \pm 4.6$ | $445 \pm 41$ |

content of the superior cervical ganglion. The concentration of cyclic AMP reached a maximum of about 450 percent of the unstimulated control value within 1 minute of stimulation and remained at this elevated level during the next several minutes of stimulation (Table 1). When experiments with the superior cervical ganglia were carried out at 26°C rather than 33°C, a smaller increase in cyclic AMP, to about 250 percent of control, was observed in response to 2 minutes of preganglionic stimulation (Table 2).

A number of experiments indicate that the increase in cyclic AMP, observed in the superior cervical ganglion as a result of stimulation of the preganglionic nerve trunk, is closely associated with the process of synaptic transmission. Thus, stimulation of these ganglia through the postganglionic (internal carotid) nerve trunk did not result in any significant change in the cyclic AMP content of the ganglia (Table 2). Stimulation of the vagus nerve did not cause any significant increase in the concentration of cyclic AMP either of the nerve itself or of the nodose ganglion (Table 2) under conditions of stimulation that caused a severalfold elevation of cyclic AMP in the superior cervical ganglia. Moreover, the concentration of cyclic AMP in the vagus nerve showed no measurable change even when the nerve was stimulated at a frequency of 50 per second for periods varying between 0.3 and 2.5 minutes. These are conditions that are known to cause large changes in the energy metabolism of the vagus nerve (7). The absence of any significant change in the concentration of cyclic AMP upon stimulation of the vagus nerve, stimulation of the nodose ganglion, or postganglionic stimulation of the superior cervical ganglion indicates that the increase in cyclic AMP observed upon preganglionic stimulation of the superior cervical ganglion is indeed associated with the process of synaptic transmission.

It is important to know whether this increase in cyclic AMP, associated with synaptic activity, occurs in the nerve endings of the preganglionic cholinergic nerve fibers or in cells innervated by these nerve endings. In order to distinguish between these two possibilities, we studied the effect of hexamethonium and atropine on the increase in cyclic AMP normally observed in response to preganglionic stimulation. Hexamethonium and atropine are competitive antagonists of the action of acetylcholine on the postsynaptic acetylcholine receptors. It is generally accepted that, in the presence of these antagonists, the preganglionic nerve endings secrete acetylcholine in a normal fashion, but the postsynaptic electrical response is inhibited. When isolated superior cervical ganglia were superfused for 30 minutes with Locke's solution containing 1 m$M$ hexamethonium chloride plus 0.1 m$M$ atropine sulfate, which nearly abolished the postsynaptic

Table 2. Effect of stimulation on the content of cyclic AMP in various preparations of isolated peripheral nervous tissue. Preparations were stimulated at a frequency of 10 per second. The contralateral tissue served as the unstimulated control in each experiment. The data have been calculated as the mean ± standard error for the number (N) of rabbits indicated in the fourth column.

| Nervous tissue | Temperature (°C) | Duration of stimulation (min) | N | Cyclic AMP (picomoles per milligram of protein) | | |
| --- | --- | --- | --- | --- | --- | --- |
| | | | | Unstimulated | Stimulated | Absolute increase |
| Superior cervical ganglion, preganglionic stimulation | 26 | 2 | 5 | 17.1 ± 2.5 | 40.9 ± 3.5 | 23.8 ± 1.9 |
| Superior cervical ganglion, postganglionic stimulation | 26 | 2 | 5 | 14.2 ± 1.4 | 13.7 ± 1.4 | −0.5 ± 0.4 |
| Nodose ganglion | 33 | 2 | 7 | 17.5 ± 5.3 | 21.2 ± 4.6 | 3.7 ± 5.8 |
| Cervical vagus | 33 | 2 | 5 | 23.4 ± 3.0 | 19.9 ± 3.2 | −3.9 ± 5.0 |
| Superior cervical ganglion, preganglionic stimulation | 33 | 1 | 5 | 13.1 ± 1.3 | 61.8 ± 6.1 | 48.7 ± 5.2 |
| Superior cervical ganglion, preganglionic stimulation, 1 mM hexamethonium chloride plus 0.1 mM atropine sulfate | 33 | 1 | 4 | 17.6 ± 1.4 | 22.0 ± 1.4 | 4.4 ± 1.6 |

587

electrical response, the increase in cyclic AMP was also almost abolished (Table 2). When lower doses of these antagonists and longer
durations of stimulation were used, so that there was less inhibition
of the postsynaptic electrical response, there was also a smaller degree
of inhibition of the increase in cyclic AMP that occurred in response
to preganglionic stimulation. These results indicate that the increase in
the concentration of cyclic AMP associated with synaptic transmission occurred in cells innervated by the preganglionic nerve endings. At most, only a small part of the increase in cyclic AMP could
have occurred in the presynaptic terminals themselves. This conclusion is consistent with denervation studies (8) which suggest that
adenyl cyclase and phosphodiesterase are located in postjunctional
cells and is also consistent with recent cytochemical studies (9) which
demonstrate the localization of phosphodiesterase activity post-
synaptically in the vicinity of the synaptic membrane.

It will be important to identify the postsynaptic cells responsible
for the increase in cyclic AMP. There are two types of cells in the
superior cervical ganglion which appear to be innervated by the preganglionic nerve fibers. Thus, besides the postganglionic neurons,
there are present small intensely fluorescent (SIF) cells that also
receive preganglionic innervation. There is evidence that these SIF
cells function as internuncials to produce the slow postsynaptic
potential changes observed in the postganglionic neurons following
synaptic transmission: the SIF cells are not only innervated by the
preganglionic nerve endings, but they also closely abut and synapse
with the soma and dendrites of postganglionic neurons (10); the
SIF cells contain high concentrations of dopamine (11); and exogenous dopamine is known to produce changes in postsynaptic potential
similar to those observed after synaptic activity in sympathetic ganglia
(12). Thus, the slow changes in postsynaptic potential observed after
synaptic activity may result from dopamine, released from the internuncial cell, acting upon the postganglionic neurons (12). It is well
established that concentrations of cyclic AMP in brain slices are
increased by certain biogenic amines (13). On the other hand, there
is no evidence that acetylcholine causes an increase in cyclic AMP
content of nervous tissue. It is, therefore, worth considering the
possibility that the increase in cyclic AMP, observed during synaptic
activity, occurs largely in the postganglionic neurons and is the result
of the action of dopamine, secreted from the internuncial cells, on
adenyl cyclase in the postganglionic neurons. Recent observations in
our laboratory are consistent with such a scheme. Thus, it has been
found that low concentrations of dopamine cause an increased accumulation of cyclic AMP in isolated slices of bovine superior cervical
ganglia (14). Moreover, it seems possible that the postsynaptic hyper-

polarization observed in sympathetic ganglia is caused by cyclic AMP which, as demonstrated in the present study, accumulates as a result of synaptic activity. In support of this notion, exogenous norepinephrine causes a hyperpolarization of the cerebellar Purkinje cell membrane, and this effect can be mimicked by cyclic AMP (15). It seems quite possible, as has been suggested previously (16), that cyclic AMP might produce long-lasting physiological effects on synaptic membranes through a mechanism comprised of the activation of a protein kinase (17) and the consequent catalysis of the phosphorylation of a protein constituent of the synaptic membrane. We have, in fact, been able to demonstrate high endogenous levels both of a cyclic AMP—dependent protein kinase (18) and of a substrate (19) for the protein kinase in fractions rich in synaptic membranes isolated from rat cerebral cortex.

In summary, our working hypothesis, which is consistent with the experimental data so far available, is that dopamine-containing internuncial cells, when activated by acetylcholine released from preganglionic nerve endings, secrete dopamine; the dopamine activates a dopamine-sensitive adenyl cyclase in the postganglionic neurons leading to the formation of cyclic AMP; and the newly formed cyclic AMP, in turn, causes the slow hyperpolarization of these ganglion cells, with consequent modification of their responsiveness to activity in the preganglionic nerve fibers. The present data indicate that adrenergic modulation of cholinergic transmission in sympathetic ganglia may occur through the mediation of cyclic AMP. Such an integrative role for cyclic AMP in ganglia suggests one important generalized function for this nucleotide in nervous tissue: cyclic AMP may provide a molecular basis for integrative actions within the nervous system.

## REFERENCES AND NOTES

1. P. Greengard and E. Costa, Eds., *Role of Cyclic AMP in Cell Function* (Raven, New York, 1970).
2. S. Kakiuchi, T.W. Rall, H. McIlwain, *J. Neurochem.* 16, 485 (1969).
3. J.F. Kuo and P. Greengard, *J. Biol. Chem.* 245, 4067 (1970).
4. The composition (in millimoles per liter) of Locke's solution was: NaCl, 136; KCl, 5.6; $NaHCO_3$, 20.0; $NaH_2PO_4$, 1.2; $CaCl_2$, 2.2; $MgCl_2$, 1.2; and glucose, 5.5. Solutions were equilibrated with a gas mixture of 95 percent $O_2$ and 5 percent $CO_2$ and had a $pH$ of 7.2 at 25°C.

5. G. Krishna, B. Weiss, B.B. Brodie, *J. Pharmacol. Exp. Ther.* 163, 379 (1968).

6. O.H. Lowry, N.J. Rosebrough, A.L. Farr, R.J. Randall, *J. Biol. Chem.* 193, 265 (1951).

7. P. Greengard and R.W. Straub, *J. Physiol. (London)* 148, 353 (1959); M. Chmouliovsky, M. Schorderet, R.W. Straub, *ibid.* 202, 90P (1969); P. Montant and M. Chmouliovsky, *Experientia* 24, 762 (1968).

8. B. Weiss and E. Costa, *Science* 156, 1750 (1967); B. McL. Breckenridge and R.E. Johnson, *J. Histochem. Cytochem.* 17, 505 (1969).

9. N.T. Florendo, P. Greengard, R.J. Barrnett, *J. Histochem. Cytochem.* 18, 682 (1970).

10. T.H. Williams and S.L. Palay, *Brain Res.* 15, 17 (1969); M.R. Matthews and G. Raisman, *J. Anat.* 105, 255 (1969); G. Siegrist, M. Dolivo, Y. Dunant, C. Foroglou-Kerameus, Fr. de Ribaupierre, Ch. Rouiller, *J. Ultrastruct. Res.* 25, 381 (1968).

11. A. Björklund, L. Cegrell, B. Falck, M. Ritzén, E. Rosengren, *Acta Physiol. Scand.* 78, 334 (1970).

12. B. Libet and T. Tosaka, *Proc. Nat. Acad. Sci. U.S.* 67, 667 (1970).

13. S. Kakiuchi and T.W. Rall, *Mol. Pharmacol.* 4, 367 (1968); T.W. Rall and A. Sattin, in *Role of Cyclic AMP in Cell Function,* P. Greengard and E. Costa, Eds. (Raven, New York, 1970), p. 113; H. Shimizu, C.R. Creveling, J.W. Daly, *ibid.,* p. 135; G. Krishna, J. Forn, K. Voigt, M. Paul, G.L. Gessa, *ibid.,* p. 155.

14. J. Kebabian and P. Greengard, in preparation.

15. B.J. Hoffer, G.R. Siggins, F.E. Bloom, in *Role of Cyclic AMP in Cell Function,* P. Greengard and E. Costa, Eds. (Raven, New York, 1970), p. 349; G.R. Siggins, A.P. Oliver, B.J. Hoffer, F.E. Bloom, *Science* 171, 192 (1971).

16. P. Greengard and J.F. Kuo, in *Role of Cyclic AMP in Cell Function,* P. Greengard and E. Costa, Eds. (Raven, New York, 1970), p. 287.

17. E. Miyamoto, J.F. Kuo, P. Greengard, *J. Biol. Chem.* 244, 6395 (1969).

18. H. Maeno, E.M. Johnson, P. Greengard, *ibid.* 246, 134 (1971).

19. E.M. Johnson, H. Maeno, P. Greengard, in preparation.

20. Supported by PHS grants NS08440 and MH17387, NSF grant GB-27510, and a Swiss Academy of Medical Sciences Fellowship to M.S.

# DOPAMINE-SENSITIVE ADENYL CYCLASE: POSSIBLE ROLE IN SYNAPTIC TRANSMISSION

*John W. Kebabian and Paul Greengard*
*Department of Pharmacology,*
*Yale University School of Medicine,*
*New Haven, Connecticut 06510*

*An adenyl cyclase activated by low concentrations of dopamine has been found in the mammalian superior cervical sympathetic ganglion. The existence of this enzyme may account for the increased amount of adenosine 3',5'-monophosphate associated with synaptic activity in the ganglion. The results suggest that the physiological effects of dopamine in the ganglion, and possibly elsewhere in the nervous system, may be mediated by stimulating the synthesis of adenosine 3',5'-monophosphate.*

Experiments in our laboratory (*1*) have demonstrated that preganglionic stimulation of the superior cervical sympathetic ganglion of the rabbit, under relatively physiological conditions, produced a severalfold increase in the content of adenosine 3',5'-monophosphate (cyclic AMP) in the ganglion. In contrast, postganglionic stimulation produced no increase in the cyclic AMP content of the ganglion. From these and other observations, it was concluded that the increased amount of cyclic AMP was associated with the process of synaptic transmission within the ganglion, and that the increase occurred primarily in postsynaptic cells. This and a variety of other evidence, summarized elsewhere (*2, 3*), suggests that the cyclic AMP system may be intimately associated with the physiology of synaptic transmission. It therefore seemed of considerable importance to clarify the mechanism responsible for the increase in cyclic AMP associated with synaptic transmission in the ganglion.

Catecholamines have been shown to increase the cyclic AMP content of many tissues, including brain. There is evidence that suggests adrenergic regulation of synaptic transmission in the superior cervical ganglion (*4–6*). Superior cervical ganglia from several species, including bovine and rabbit, contain two catecholamines, dopamine and norepinephrine, in comparable amounts (*7*); and we have, therefore, studied the ability of these two catecholamines to stimulate the formation of cyclic AMP. Our experiments, with blocks of tissue prepared from bovine ganglia, indicate that dopamine, in low concentrations, and norepinephrine, in higher concentrations, increase the amount of cyclic AMP in intact cells. In addition, in experiments with homogenates of bovine ganglia, it was found that dopamine stimulates adenyl cyclase activity, but does not significantly alter phosphodiesterase activity. These observations support the hypothesis that small chromaffin-like interneurons release dopamine in response to preganglionic stimulation, and that this catecholamine activates adenyl cyclase in postganglionic neurons, thereby mediating the increased amount of cyclic AMP that follows preganglionic stimulation (*1*). Our experiments provide experimental evidence for a new type of adenyl cyclase, one with apparent specificity for dopamine, and suggest a mechanism, at the cellular and molecular levels, for the action of dopamine in the ganglion and possibly in other regions of the nervous system.

The amount of cyclic AMP accumulation in blocks of ganglion tissue was determined by means of the prelabeling technique (*8*) in which the amount of radioactive cyclic AMP formed from prelabeled adenosine triphosphate is determined (*9*). The relative potencies of dopamine and norepinephrine in causing the accumulation of cyclic AMP in blocks of ganglion tissue were compared (Fig. 1). At low concentrations dopamine was more effective than norepinephrine in causing the accumulation of cyclic AMP. The maximum responses to the two catecholamines were approximately equal, although in some experiments the maximum response to norepinephrine was somewhat greater than to dopamine. In each of several experiments similar to that shown in Fig. 1, a half-maximum increase in cyclic AMP accumulation occurred in the presence of 6 to 10 $\mu M$ dopamine. Moreover, in those experiments, 42 $\mu M$ norepinephrine produced a response approximately equal to that seen with 7 $\mu M$ dopamine.

In some experiments, the absolute amount of cyclic AMP was also determined by means of the protein kinase assay method (*11*). The results obtained with the two methods were similar. For instance, in one experiment the absolute amount of cyclic AMP in prelabeled but nonincubated tissue was 14.5 pmole per milligram of protein. Incubation in the presence of 10 m$M$ theophylline alone caused a 2.6-fold increase in the absolute amount of cyclic AMP and a 3.2-fold increase in the amount of radioactive cyclic AMP. Incubation in the presence

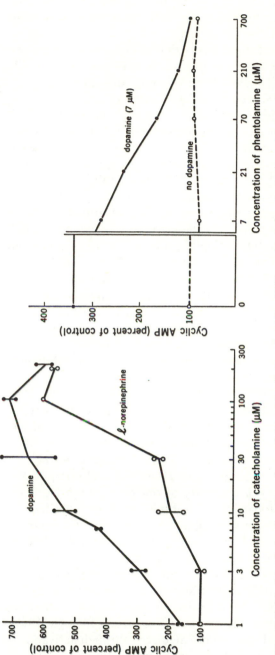

Fig. 1 (left). Stimulation by dopamine and *l*-norepinephrine of cyclic AMP accumulation in blocks of bovine superior cervical ganglion. Tissue was incubated for 5 minutes at 37°C in oxygenated Krebs-Ringer bicarbonate buffer, *p*H 7.4, containing 10 m*M* theophylline and the indicated amount of catecholamine. Cyclic AMP accumulation during incubation in the presence of catecholamine and theophylline is expressed as the percentage of that observed during incubation in the presence of theophylline alone. The curves are drawn through the average of two data points; each data point represents the mean of duplicate determinations on an individual sample.    Fig. 2 (right). Effect of the α-blocker, phentolamine, on cyclic AMP accumulation, in the presence and absence of 7 μ*M* dopamine, in blocks of bovine superior cervical ganglion. Tissue was incubated for 5 minutes at 37°C in oxygenated Krebs-Ringer bicarbonate buffer, *p*H 7.4, containing 10 m*M* theophylline and the indicated amounts of dopamine and phentolamine. Cyclic AMP accumulation is expressed as the percentage of that observed in the presence of theophylline alone. Each point represents the mean of determinations on two to four samples analyzed in duplicate.

593

of 30 $\mu M$ dopamine plus 10 m$M$ theophylline caused a 9.7-fold increase in the absolute amount of cyclic AMP and a 9.1-fold increase in the amount of radioactive cyclic AMP.

We have studied the effect of agents that antagonize the actions of catecholamines in other tissues on the accumulation of cyclic AMP in the superior cervical ganglion. Phentolamine, an $\alpha$-adrenergic antagonist, prevented the increase in cyclic AMP produced by 7$\mu M$ dopamine, whereas it did not appreciably alter the accumulation of cyclic AMP in the absence of added dopamine (Fig. 2). The response to 7 $\mu M$ dopamine was reduced by about 50 percent in the presence of 28 $\mu M$ phentolamine. Another $\alpha$-adrenergic antagonist, phenoxybenzamine, at a concentration of 70 $\mu M$, abolished the increase in cyclic AMP produced by 7 $\mu M$ dopamine. In contrast, propranolol, the $\beta$-adrenergic antagonist, was ineffective, at concentrations from 7$\mu M$ to as high as 210 $\mu M$, in preventing the increase in cyclic AMP mediated by 7 $\mu M$ dopamine. Interestingly, propranolol (120 $\mu M$) caused a substantial reduction of the increase in cyclic AMP mediated by 40 $\mu M$ norepinephrine. Two other $\beta$-adrenergic antagonists, dichloroisoproterenol and MJ 1999 [4'-(2-isopropylamino-l-hydroxyethyl) methanesulfonanilide], each tested at concentrations as high as 400 $\mu M$, were also ineffective in preventing the accumulation of cyclic AMP mediated by 7 $\mu M$ dopamine; in contrast, each of these agents, tested at a dose of 400 $\mu M$, reduced the increase in cyclic AMP mediated by 40 $\mu M$ norepinephrine.

It is important to know whether the accumulation of cyclic AMP observed in response to dopamine results from an increased synthesis or from a decreased degradation of the cyclic nucleotide. In order to distinguish between these two possibilities, we studied the effects of dopamine on the adenyl cyclase activity and phosphodiesterase activity of homegenates of ganglia (12). Dopamine and norepinephrine each stimulated adenyl cyclase activity of the ganglion homogenate (Table 1). In contrast, dopamine did not inhibit phosphodiesterase activity of the ganglion homogenate, nor did it increase the inhibition observed in the presence of theophylline. These observations indicate that catecholamine-sensitive adenyl cyclase activity exists within the superior cervical ganglion, and that the dopamine-mediated accumulation of cyclic AMP is the result of an increase of adenyl cyclase activity rather than an inhibition of phosphodiesterase activity.

The present data provide the first evidence, in any biological system, that the effects of dopamine are mediated through activation of adenyl cyclase (13). In previous studies, in which slices of intact mammalian nervous tissue were used, dopamine had little or no effect on the amount of cyclic AMP (14). Moreover, although dopamine was

Table 1. The effects of catecholamines and theophylline on adenyl cyclase activity and phosphodiesterase activity of homogenates of the bovine superior cervical ganglion. Activity is expressed as nanomoles per milligram of protein per minute. Each value represents the mean of determinations on two samples.

| Additions | Activity (nmole/min) | Percent of control |
|---|---|---|
| | *Adenyl cyclase* | |
| None | $33 \times 10^{-3}$ | 100 |
| Dopamine (7 $\mu M$) | $59 \times 10^{-3}$ | 179 |
| Norepinephrine (7 $\mu M$) | $56 \times 10^{-3}$ | 170 |
| | *Phosphodiesterase* | |
| None | 17.1 | 100 |
| Dopamine (7 $\mu M$) | 16.7 | 97 |
| Dopamine (30 $\mu M$) | 17.4 | 100 |
| Theophylline (10 m$M$) | 2.2 | 13 |
| Theophylline (10 m$M$) plus dopamine (30 $\mu M$) | 2.8 | 16 |

able to stimulate the adenyl cyclase activity of rat erythrocyte ghosts, the concentration of dopamine required for half-maximum activation of the enzyme was 17 to 350 times greater than that required for other catecholamines, and the maximum activation by dopamine was only 50 percent of the stimulation by other catecholamines (*15*). However, on the basis of our studies, we propose as a working hypothesis that the other biological actions of dopamine, including those within the basal ganglia, are also mediated by the activation of adenyl cyclase in the responsive tissues.

It is of interest to consider our results in relation to the increase in cyclic AMP that occurs in the superior cervical ganglion in association with the process of synaptic transmission (*1*). We have attempted (*1*) to account for this increase in cyclic AMP by the following schema: (i) physiological activity in the preganglionic neurons, in addition to directly activating the postganglionic neurons, also excites small dopamine-containing interneurons; (ii) the excitation of these interneurons causes them to secrete dopamine; and (iii) the dopamine thus released activates dopamine-sensitive adenyl cyclase in the postganglionic neurons. A variety of anatomical, pharmacological, and biochemical evidence supports this proposal concerning the cell types and neurotransmitter within the superior cervical ganglion that are responsible for the increased amount of cyclic AMP associated with synaptic activity. Although dopamine and norepinephrine, the two catecholamines found within the ganglion, can each cause an accumulation of cyclic AMP, these two substances are found in different cell types. Norepinephrine is found within the postganglionic neurons. Dopamine, on the other hand, is concentrated in small interneurons (16). These interneurons, which possess many of the morphological features of the chromaffin cells of the adrenal medulla, form synapses on the postganglionic neurons (17). Preganglionic, cholinergic fibers synapse on these interneurons as well as directly on the postganglionic neurons. Pharmacological evidence that the increase in cyclic AMP caused by preganglionic stimulation involves the dopamine-containing interneurons comes from studies with both adrenergic and cholinergic blocking agents. Recently, it has been found (18) that low concentrations of phentolamine blocked the increase in cyclic AMP associated with preganglionic stimulation, but MJ 1999, at concentrations up to 200 $\mu M$, did not. Thus, the increase in cyclic AMP caused by stimulation of preganglionic nerve fibers was antagonized by adrenergic blocking agents in a manner similar to the increase in cyclic AMP caused by exogenous dopamine. It has also been found that atropine, which appears to block the excitation of the interneurons (5), also prevents the increase in cyclic AMP that follows preganglionic stimulation (18). In contrast, hexamethonium, which blocks the action of acetylcholine on the postganglionic neurons but does not appear to affect the interneurons (5), does not prevent the increase in cyclic AMP that follows preganglionic stimulation (18). Finally, the biochemical data, which demonstrate the stimulation by dopamine of cyclic AMP synthesis in the ganglion, support the schema outlined above.

The physiological significance of the increase in cyclic AMP associated with synaptic activity in these ganglia is a matter of considerable interest. It is possible that this increase in cyclic AMP may be responsible for the slow hyperpolarization (slow inhibitory post-synaptic potential) of the ganglion that follows preganglionic stimulation. Recent observations support this idea. Exogenous dopamine (6, 18) is able to hyperpolarize the postganglionic neurons of the rabbit superior cervical ganglion. As described above, the increase in cyclic AMP seen in response either to preganglionic stimulation or to exogenous dopamine can be antagonized by $\alpha$-adrenergic blocking agents. The slow hyperpolarization that follows preganglionic stimulation (5), as well as that caused by exogenous dopamine (6), are also antagonized by $\alpha$-adrenergic blocking agents. Moreover, 1 m$M$ theophylline when added to the medium bathing the rabbit superior cervical ganglion causes a substantial increase in the magnitude of the slow hyperpolarization that follows preganglionic stimulation (18), implicating cyclic AMP in the production of this physiological response.

The biochemical events by which cyclic AMP might induce the hyperpolarization of the postganglionic cell membrane are not known. However, it has been suggested that the diverse effects of cyclic AMP in various tissues may be mediated through regulation of the activity of protein kinases (*2, 19*). A hypothesis worthy of consideration [compare (*1, 2*)] is that the ability of cyclic AMP to hyperpolarize the nerve cell membrane results from the activation of a protein kinase, with the consequent phosphorylation of a protein constituent of the nerve cell membrane, leading to a change in membrane properties concerned with ion movement.

The hyperpolarization of the membrane of the postganglionic neuron alters the responsiveness of the neuron to subsequent activity in the presynaptic fibers. Thus, the role of the increase in ganglionic cyclic AMP that follows preganglionic stimulation may be to mediate dopaminergic transmission and thereby to modulate cholinergic transmission. The extent to which cyclic AMP may also be involved in synaptic transmission elsewhere in the nervous system is an important area for future investigation.

## REFERENCES AND NOTES

1. D.A. McAfee, M. Schorderet, P. Greengard, *Science* 171, 1156 (1971).
2. P. Greengard and J.F. Kuo, in *Role of Cyclic AMP in Cell Function,* P. Greengard and E. Costa, Eds., (Raven, New York, 1970), p. 287.
3. B.J. Hoffer, G.R. Siggins, F.E. Bloom, in *ibid.,* p. 349.
4. E. Bulbring, *J. Physiol. London* 103, 55 (1944); M. Goffart, in *L'Adrénaline et la Noradrénaline dans la Regulation des Fonctions Homeostatasiques* (Centre National de la Recherche Scientifique, Paris, 1957), p. 213; E. Costa, A.M. Revzin, R. Kuntzman, S. Spector, B.B. Brodie, *Science* 133, 1822 (1961).
5. R.M. Eccles and B. Libet, *J. Physiol. London* 157, 484 (1961).
6. B. Libet and T. Tosaka, *Proc. Nat. Acad. Sci. U.S.* 67, 667 (1970).
7. R. Laverty and D. Sharman, *Brit. J. Pharmacol.* 24, 538 (1965); R.H. Roth, personal communication.
8. J.F. Kuo and E.C. DeRenzo, *J. Biol. Chem.* 244, 2252 (1969).
9. Superior cervical ganglia from young calves of both sexes were removed immediately after death, at a local abattoir, and

placed in ice-cold oxygenated Krebs-Ringer bicarbonate buffer that contained (in millimoles per liter): NaCl, 122; KCl, 3; $MgSO_4$, 1.2; $CaCl_2$, 1.3; $KH_2PO_4$, 0.4; $NaHCO_3$, 25; and D-glucose, 10. This buffer had been previously equilibrated with a gas mixture of 95 percent $O_2$ and 5 percent $CO_2$ and had a $p$H of 7.4 at 25°C. The ganglia were then desheathed, and were cut freehand with a razor blade into thin slices. These slices were rapidly brought back to the laboratory in oxygenated Krebs-Ringer bicarbonate buffer at 4°C and maintained at that temperature until they were cut into small blocks with a McIlwain tissue chopper (settings 0.52 mm by 0.26 mm). On sectioning, the blocks were placed in an oxygenated Krebs-Ringer bicarbonate buffer at 37°C. The blocks were then preincubated for 45 minutes in 32 ml of oxygenated Krebs-Ringer bicarbonate buffer at 37°C, containing 11.9 $\mu M$ [8-[14]C] adenine (specific activity 41.6 mc/mmole) and then washed extensively with oxygenated Krebs-Ringer bicarbonate buffer at 37°C, to remove extracellular adenine. For incubation, portions of tissue were transferred to homogenizers in which there were 5.0 ml of oxygenated Krebs-Ringer bicarbonate buffer (37°C), containing $10^{-2} M$ theophylline and appropriate concentrations of test agents. Unless otherwise stated incubation time was 5 minutes. Throughout the period of preincubation and incubation, blocks of tissue were prevented from settling by the gas mixture bubbling through the solution. At the end of the incubation, the Krebs-Ringer bicarbonate buffer was removed by aspiration, 1.5 ml of ice-cold 6 percent trichloroacetic acid was added, and the tissue was immediately homogenized. Tritiated carrier cyclic AMP (0.1 $\mu$mole) was added to each sample and the homogenate was centrifuged. The supernatant was decanted for cyclic AMP assay. The precipitate was suspended in 2.0 ml of 1.0$N$ NaOH and protein was determined by the method of O.H. Lowry, N.J. Rosebrough, A.L. Farr, R.J. Randall, *J. Biol. Chem.* 193, 265 (1951), with bovine serum albumin as the standard. The supernatant solution was extracted three times with 1.0 ml of diethyl ether. Cyclic AMP was isolated by minor modification of the method of Krishna *et al.* (*10*), and the amounts of [3]H and [14]C in the isolated sample were counted simultaneously in a Packard Tricarb liquid scintillation system. The amount of radioactivity present in the cyclic AMP of the original samples was calculated per milligram of protein with the use of the recovery of tritiated cyclic AMP to correct each sample for loss during the isolation procedure. The data were corrected by subtracting the amount of radioactive cyclic AMP present in prelabeled but nonincubated tissue.

10. G. Krishna, B. Weiss, B.B. Brodie, *J. Pharmacol. Exp. Ther.* 163, 379 (1968).

11. J.F. Kuo and P. Greengard, *J. Biol. Chem.* 245, 4067 (1970).

12. For studies of homogenates, ganglia were prepared by means of a McIlwain tissue chopper, in a manner similar to the procedure used for the prelabeling technique, and then homogenized manually for 60 seconds with 1.4 volumes of 6 m$M$ tris-(hydroxymethyl)-aminomethane-maleate buffer, $p$H 7.4. Adenyl cyclase activity of the homogenates was measured in the presence of 10 m$M$ theophylline, by a slight modification of the method of Krishna *et al.* (*10*). Phosphodiesterase activity of the homogenates was measured by minor modification of the procedure of J. Beavo, J. Hardman, E.W. Sutherland, *J. Biol. Chem.* 245, 5649 (1970).

13. The possibility exists that, in our experiments with intact ganglion cells, exogenous dopamine could become concentrated by postganglionic neurons and converted into norepinephrine, and that this newly synthesized norepinephrine, rather than the exogenous dopamine per se, would activate the adenyl cyclase. We consider this to be improbable for several reasons. (i) Low concentrations of dopamine were effective in stimulating the formation of cyclic AMP in homogenates of bovine ganglia; these homogenates were unfortified by the addition of cofactors necessary for the enzymatic conversion of dopamine to norepinephrine. (ii) As described above, experiments with the β-adrenergic antagonist, propranolol, have shown that this agent does not affect the dopamine-mediated increase in cyclic AMP, but does reduce the accumulation of cyclic AMP caused by norepinephrine. (iii) We have found that cocaine (210 $\mu M$), which has been shown to block the uptake of dopamine and norepinephrine by various tissues, caused a slight increase in the dopamine-mediated accumulation of cyclic AMP in blocks of bovine ganglia, whereas a decrease would be expected if the intracellular accumulation of dopamine and its conversion to norepinephrine were required. Thus, these data indicate that exogenous dopamine caused the accumulation of cyclic AMP in the ganglion by direct stimulation of an adenyl cyclase sensitive to low concentrations of dopamine.

14. S. Kakiuchi and T.W. Rall, *Mol. Pharmacol.* 4, 379 (1968); H.

Shimizu, C.R. Creveling, J.W. Daly, *Proc. Nat. Acad. Sci. U.S.* 65, 1033 (1970).

15. H. Sheppard and C.R. Burghardt, *Mol. Pharmacol.* 6, 425 (1970); *ibid.* 7, 1 (1971).

16. K.A. Norberg, M. Ritzen, U. Understedt, *Acta Physiol. Scand.* 67, 260 (1966); A. Björklund, L. Cergrell, B. Falck, M. Ritzen, E. Rosegren, *ibid.* 78, 334 (1970); F. Cattabeni, S.H. Koslow, E. Costa, *Pharmacologist* 13, 203 (1971).

17. T.H. Williams and S.L. Palay, *Brain Res.* 15, 17 (1969); M.R. Mathews and G. Raisman, *J. Anat.* 105, 255 (1969); G. Siegrist, M. Dolivo, Y. Dunant, C. Foroglou-Kermas, Fr. de Ribaupierre, Ch. Rouiller, *J. Ultrastruct. Res.* 25, 381 (1968).

18. P. Greengard, D.A. McAfee, M. Schorderet, J.W. Kebabian, in *Proceedings of the International Symposium on the Physiology and Pharmacology of Cyclic AMP,* P. Greengard, R. Paoletti, A.G. Robison, Eds. (Raven, New York, in press).

19. J.F. Kuo and P. Greengard, *J. Biol. Chem.* 244, 3417 (1969); *Proc. Nat. Acad. Sci. U.S.* 64, 1349 (1969); *J. Biol. Chem.* 245, 2493 (1970); P. Greengard, J.F. Kuo, E. Miyamoto, *Advan. Enzyme Regul.* 9, 113 (1971).

20. Supported by PHS grants NS 08440 and MH 17387 and NSF grant GB 27510. J.W.K. was supported by PHS training grant GM-00105.

# ADENOSINE 3',5'-MONOPHOSPHATE: ELECTROPHYSIOLOGICAL EVIDENCE FOR A ROLE IN SYNAPTIC TRANSMISSION

*Donald A. McAfee and Paul Greengard*
*Department of Pharmacology,*
*Yale University School of Medicine,*
*New Haven, Connecticut 06510*

*Synaptic potentials and changes in resting membrane potentials of superior cervical ganglia of the rabbit were measured in the presence of adenosine 3'5'-monophosphate and agents that affect its metabolism. Adenosine 3'5'-monophosphate and its mono- and dibutyryl derivatives caused a hyperpolarization of the postganglionic neurons. Theophylline potentiated the slow inhibitory postsynaptic potential that follows synaptic transmission, as well as the hyperpolarization of postganglionic neurons caused by exogenous dopamine. Conversely, prostaglandin $E_1$ inhibited both the slow inhibitory postsynaptic potential and the dopamine-induced hyperpolarization. We hypothesize that the slow inhibitory postsynaptic potential as well as the dopamine-induced hyperpolarization result from increased amounts of adenosine 3'5'-monophosphate in the postganglionic neurons. The dibutyryl derivative of guanosine 3'5'-monophosphate caused a depolarization of the postganglionic neurons, which is consistent with the possibility that guanosine 3'5'-monophosphate mediates synaptic transmission at muscarinic cholinergic synapses.*

Studies in our laboratory have implicated adenosine 3',5'-monophosphate (cyclic AMP) in the physiology of synaptic transmission in the mammalian superior cervical sympathetic ganglion (*1–4*). Stimulation of preganglionic fibers causes an increase in the amount of cyclic AMP in this ganglion (*1, 2*). In addition, dopamine, a putative neurotransmitter in the ganglion (*2–6*), increases the amount of ganglionic cyclic AMP (*3*) and causes a hyperpolarization of the postganglionic neurons (*5, 6*) (see Fig. 1). The effects of dopamine, both

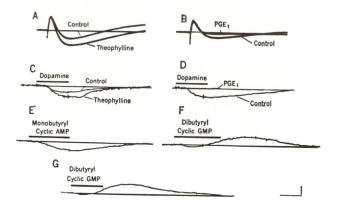

Fig. 1. (A to F) Effect of cyclic nucleotides, and of agents which affect cyclic AMP metabolism, on synaptic and resting membrane potentials recorded by means of the sucrose gap technique from postganglionic neurons of the superior cervical sympathetic ganglion of the rabbit. (A and B) Oscillographic traces of electrotonically conducted synaptic potentials elicited in response to a single supramaximum stimulus to the preganglionic nerve. Hexamethonium chloride (600 $\mu M$) was present to abolish propagated responses. (A) Responses obtained in Locke solution and after 30 minutes of superfusion with Locke solution containing 1.5 m$M$ theophylline are superimposed. (B) Responses obtained in normal Locke solution and after 15 minutes of superfusion with Locke solution containing $3 \times 10^{-7} M$ PGE$_1$ are superimposed. Results similar to those illustrated here were obtained when $d$-tubocurarine (125 $\mu M$) was used instead of hexamethonium chloride to abolish propagated responses. This dose of $d$-tubocurarine also abolished the initial EPSP. (C and D) Resting membrane potential changes in response to a brief period of superfusion with dopamine. (C) Responses to 50 $\mu M$ dopamine before (control) and 30 minutes after the start of superfusion with 2 m$M$ theophylline are superimposed. (D) Responses to 200 $\mu M$ dopamine before (control) and 20 minutes after the start of superfusion with $6 \times 10^{-7} M$ PGE$_1$ are superimposed. (E and F) Changes in membrane potential in response to a brief period of superfusion with 2.5 m$M$ monobutyryl cyclic AMP (E) or 25 $\mu M$ dibutyryl cyclic GMP (F). (G) Change in membrane potential of the cervical vagus nerve in response to a brief period of superfusion with 200 $\mu M$ dibutyryl cyclic GMP. The duration of superfusion with Locke solutions containing dopamine or cyclic nucleotides is indicated by the solid bars. All records are d-c recording, hyperpolarization downward. Calibration marks: (A and B) 1 second, 800 $\mu$v; (C to G) 2 minutes, 400 $\mu$v.

on cyclic AMP (*3*) and on postganglionic membrane potential (*5, 6*), are antagonized by $\alpha$-adrenergic blocking agents. To account for these and other results, we have suggested (*2–4*) that dopamine, released from interneurons during activity, causes an increase in the amount of cyclic AMP in the postganglionic neurons and that it is this increased cyclic AMP which is responsible for the slow inhibitory postsynaptic potential (slow-IPSP) that follows preganglionic stimulation. We now report the results of electrophysiological studies designed to test certain predictions made by this hypothesis, namely, (i) that cyclic AMP would hyperpolarize the postganglionic neurons; (ii) that theophylline, a phosphodiesterase inhibitor which potentiates the accumulation of cyclic AMP in the ganglion (7), would also potentiate the slow-IPSP as well as the hyperpolarization due to dopamine; and (iii) that prostaglandin $E_1$ (PGE$_1$), which has been shown to affect adenylate cyclase activity of almost all tissues studied, might alter the slow-IPSP as well as the hyperpolarization due to dopamine.

Changes in membrane potential of postganglionic neurons in superior cervical sympathetic ganglia of the rabbit were measured by the sucrose gap technique (8). Preganglionic stimulation of this ganglion results in the generation of an initial brief excitatory postsynaptic potential (initial EPSP), followed successively by a slow-IPSP that reaches a maximum within 600 msec, and a slow excitatory postsynaptic potential (slow-EPSP) lasting approximately 30 seconds. The slow-IPSP, but not the initial EPSP, was potentiated in amplitude and duration in the presence of theophylline (Fig. 1A). Theophylline did not inhibit either the amplitude or the duration of the slow-EPSP (not shown). The hyperpolarization of the postganglionic neurons induced by exogenous dopamine was also potentiated by theophylline (Fig. 1C). The response to dopamine was tested by switching for 3 minutes from a superfusate of normal Locke solution to one containing 50 $\mu M$ dopamine (prepared 2 to 5 minutes previously) and then by returning to the normal Locke solution. Theophylline (1 to 5 m$M$) in nine experiments caused an increase of $44 \pm 7$ percent (mean $\pm$ S.E.M.) in the amplitude of the slow-IPSP, and an increase of $54 \pm 9$ percent in the amplitude of the hyperpolarization induced by 50 to 200 $\mu M$ dopamine. The effect of the theophylline could be reversed by superfusion of the ganglion with normal Locke solution for 90 minutes.

In each of 15 ganglion preparations studied, $10^{-7} M$ to $10^{-6} M$ PGE$_1$ virtually abolished the slow-IPSP within 10 to 20 minutes and substantially reduced the slow-EPSP, but had no effect on the initial EPSP. (A transient hyperpolarization of the postganglionic neurons of 5 to 10 minutes duration, was usually observed on starting PGE$_1$ superfusion.) The effect of $3 \times 10^{-7} M$ PGE$_1$ on the slow-IPSP is illustrated in Fig. 1B. A concentration of PGE$_1$ of $1 \times 10^{-8} M$ caused a 50 percent decrease in the amplitude of the slow-IPSP. In nine ganglion preparations, the effect of PGE$_1$ was tested on the hyperpolarization induced by 50 to 200 $\mu M$ dopamine. It was found that PGE$_1$ abolished, or largely reduced, the dopamine-induced hyperpolarization at the same concentrations as were effective in abolishing the slow-IPSP (Fig. 1D). The effects of PGE$_1$ could be largely reversed on prolonged superfusion with normal Locke solution.

Monobutyryl cyclic AMP, applied in a concentration of 1 to 2.5 m$M$, hyperpolarized 8 of 11 ganglia tested (Fig. 1E). Qualitatively similar results were obtained with cyclic AMP and dibutyryl cyclic AMP, but not with adenosine 5'-monophosphate, adenosine, or butyric acid. Cyclic AMP and its derivatives were never observed to cause depolarization. The lack of any response, by some of the preparations, to the direct application of cyclic AMP or its derivatives may be due to a low permeability of neuronal membranes to cyclic AMP.

Studies have shown that acetylcholine can cause an increase in the amount of guanosine 3',5'-monophosphate (cyclic GMP) in heart and brain tissue (9). Moreover, available evidence indicates the existence, on postganglionic neurons of the superior cervical ganglion, of muscarinic-type receptors that respond to acetylcholine by causing a prolonged depolarization of the neurons (10). These same receptors are probably involved in the generation of the slow-EPSP (10). In view of the possibility that cyclic GMP might mediate this muscarinic depolarizing action of acetylcholine, we have studied the effect of cyclic GMP and dibutyryl cyclic GMP on the resting membrane potential of postganglionic neurons. Cyclic GMP itself did not cause a change in membrane potential. However, exposure of the ganglia to dibutyryl cyclic GMP, in low concentrations (2.5 to 5.0 × 10$^{-5}$$M$) for 4 minutes, caused a small, transient hyperpolarization followed by a depolarization of the postganglionic nerve cells in each of seven preparations tested (Fig. 1F). A depolarization of several millivolts could be achieved by maintaining the ganglion in solutions of dibutyryl cyclic GMP for longer periods of time (5 to 10 minutes). Higher doses (100 to 250 $\mu M$) of dibutyryl cyclic GMP greatly enhanced the rate of depolarization of the postganglionic neurons but either had no effect on, or decreased the size of, the transient hyperpolarization. These observations are in contrast to those made on liver slices where both cyclic AMP and cyclic GMP caused a hyperpolarization (11). Conceivably, cyclic GMP may mediate the slow-EPSP and, thereby, increase the responsiveness of the postganglionic neurons to subsequent excitatory input. If so, this would indicate that cyclic AMP and cyclic GMP function in opposite directions, that is, in a push-pull fashion to exert long-term control over neuronal excitability in the sympathetic ganglion.

Dopamine, theophylline, PGE$_1$, cyclic GMP, and cyclic AMP and its butyryl derivatives, when tested on axons of the cervical vagus nerve in the same concentrations that had been used on the ganglion, were found to cause little or no effect on the membrane potential. High concentrations of dibutyryl cyclic GMP (1 to 4 × $10^{-4}M$) had an effect on the vagus nerve (Fig. 1G) similar to that which had been observed on the ganglion with lower concentrations.

We have been able to demonstrate consistently and reproducibly, with each of 13 preparations, that the excitability of postganglionic neurons in the superior cervical ganglion was diminished during the period of the slow-IPSP and that this inhibition was markedly potentiated by theophylline. These effects are illustrated in Fig. 2 where the unconditioned response to a submaximum test stimulus is compared with the response to the same strength of stimulus applied 600 msec after a stronger conditioning stimulus, that is, at the time of maximum development of the slow-IPSP. The upper portion of Fig. 2 contains two superimposed oscillographic traces of compound action potentials derived from the postganglionic nerve with platinum bipolar recording electrodes. The test response in trace a was elicited without a prior conditioning stimulus and therefore did not occur during a slow-IPSP. The test response elicited 600 msec after a conditioning response (trace b) and, therefore, during the slow-IPSP, was reduced 24 percent in amplitude and 20 percent in area compared to the unconditioned test response. The lower portion of Fig. 2 con-

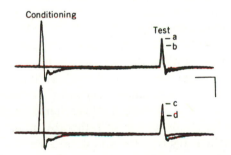

Fig. 2. Compound action potentials, elicited by submaximum stimulation of the preganglionic (cervical sympathetic) nerve, and recorded from platinum bipolar electrodes on the postganglionic (internal carotid) nerve 2 to 3 mm distant from the pole of the ganglion. Upper row, superimposed traces a and b recorded during superfusion of the ganglion with normal Locke solution. Lower row, superimposed traces c and d recorded 24 minutes after start of superfusion with Locke solution containing 5 mM theophylline. Traces a and c, response to a single test stimulus only. Traces b and d, response to a conditioning stimulus followed 600 msec later by response to a test stimulus. Conditioning stimuli were just maximum for the $S_a$ elevation [see (10)]; voltage of the test stimuli was one-half that of the conditioning stimuli; pulse width for both kinds of stimuli was 0.5 msec. Calibration mark: 200 μv, 100 msec. Bandwidth, 2 hz to 10 khz.

tains two superimposed oscillographic traces of compound action potentials obtained under experimental conditions identical to those of the upper portion of Fig. 2, except that the ganglion had been superfused for 24 minutes with 5 m$M$ theophylline. The unconditioned test response (trace c) and the conditioning response (early part of trace d) were unaffected by theophylline. In contrast, the conditioned test response (later part of trace d) was considerably more reduced in amplitude (46 percent) and area (44 percent) than prior to theophylline. This increased inhibition of synaptic transmission after a conditioning stimulus, observed in the presence of theophylline, can be attributed to the potentiation of the slow-IPSP achieved by this phosphodiesterase inhibitor (Fig. 1A).

Our results indicate that cyclic AMP can mimic the electrophysiologic effects of dopamine, a putative ganglionic neurotransmitter. Cyclic AMP has been found to mimic the hyperpolarizing action of β-adrenergic agonists on the Purkinje cells of the rat cerebellum (12) and on the smooth muscle cells of the rabbit pulmonary artery (13). In the case of the Purkinje cells, theophylline potentiated, and PGE$_1$ blocked the inhibition of spontaneous discharge caused by application of exogenous norepinephrine (12).

Our electrophysiological data support the hypothesis that cyclic AMP plays a role in synaptic transmission in sympathetic ganglia. There appear to be both direct excitatory and interneuron-mediated inhibitory input from the preganglionic fibers to the postganglionic neurons of the superior cervical ganglion (10, 14). Our evidence supports the idea (2–4) that the slow-IPSP is generated by an increase in the amount of cyclic AMP in the postganglionic neurons in response to dopamine released from the interneurons. The hyperpolarization of the postganglionic neurons makes them less responsive to subsequent excitatory input. According to this scheme, cyclic AMP mediates dopaminergic transmission and, thereby, modulates cholinergic transmission in the ganglion, the modulation being of an inhibitory type that produces a negative feedback and limits the effectiveness of subsequent excitation.

## REFERENCES AND NOTES

1. D.A. McAfee, M. Schorderet, P. Greengard, *Pharmacologist* 12, 488 (1970).
2. ——, *Science* 171, 1156 (1971).
3. J.W. Kebabian and P. Greengard, *ibid.* 174, 1346 (1971).
4. P. Greengard, D.A. McAfee, J. Kebabian, in *Advances in Cyclic*

*Nucleotide Research,* P. Greengard, R. Paoletti, G.A. Robison, Eds. (Raven, New York, in press), vol. 1.

5. B. Libet and T. Tosaka, *Proc. Nat. Acad. Sci. U.S.A.* 67, 667 (1970). B. Libet, *Fed. Proc.* 29, 1945 (1970).

6. P. Greengard and D.A. McAfee, *Biochem. Soc. Symp.,* in press.

7. D.A. McAfee, P. Kalix, M. Schorderet, P. Greengard, in preparation.

8. H.W. Kosterlitz, G.M. Lees, D.I. Wallis, *J. Physiol. London* 195, 39 (1968). Ganglia were removed from New Zealand white rabbits under urethane anesthesia (1 g/kg), were decapsulated, and were positioned in the sucrose gap apparatus. The preganglionic (cervical sympathetic) nerve was stimulated through platinum bipolar electrodes. Locke solution containing various agents superfused the ganglion at 1 to 2 ml/min. A short segment of the proximal portion of the postganglionic (internal carotid) nerve was superfused with 315 m$M$ sucrose, at 0.3 ml/min, and normal Locke solution superfused the distal end of the postganglionic nerve at 0.5 to 1 ml/min. Solution flow through the various chambers was monitored by precision flow meters. The d-c potential difference between the ganglion and the end of the postganglionic nerve (that is, across the sucrose gap) was amplified and displayed on an oscilloscope and on a strip-chart servo recorder. The potential difference across the sucrose gap with the ganglion in normal Locke solution was 5 mv or less, and the resistance was usually 0.4 to 0.8 megohm. The design of the sucrose gap apparatus and the precise control of flow rates reduced flow artifacts and eliminated associated problems. The composition of the Locke solution (in millimoles per liter) was: NaCl, 136; KCl, 5.6; $NaHCO_3$, 20.0; $NaH_2PO_4$, 1.2; $CaCl_2$, 2.2; $MgCl_2$, 1.2; and glucose, 5.5. The Locke solution was equilibrated with a gas mixture of 95 percent $O_3$ and 5 percent $CO_2$ and had a $p$H of 7.2 to 7.3 at the temperature of the experiments (23° to 25°C).

9. W.J. George, J.B. Polson, A.G. O'Toole. N.D. Goldberg, *Proc. Nat. Acad. Sci. U.S.A.* 66, 398 (1970); J.A. Ferrendelli, A.L. Steiner, D.R. McDougal, D.M. Kipnis, *Biochem. Biophys. Res. Commun.* 41, 1061 (1970); J. F. Kuo, T.-P. Lee, P.L. Reyes, K.G. Walton, T.E. Donnelly, P. Greengard, *J. Biol. Chem.* 247, 16 (1972).

10. R.M. Eccles and B. Libet, *J. Physiol. London* 157, 484 (1961).

11. A.P. Somlyo, A.V. Somlyo, N. Friedman, *Ann. N.Y. Acad. Sci.* 185, 108 (1971).

12. G.R. Siggins, B.J. Hoffer, F.E. Bloom, *Science* 165, 1018 (1969).

13. A.V. Somlyo, G. Haeusler, A.P. Somlyo, *ibid.* 169, 490 (1970).
14. T.H. Williams and S.L. Palay, *Brain Res.* 15, 17 (1969); A. Björk-lund, L. Cegrell, B. Falck, M. Ritzén, E. Rosengren, *Acta Physiol. Scand.* 78, 334 (1970).
15. Supported by PHS grants NS 08440 and MH 17387, NSF grant GB 27510, and a postdoctoral fellowship from the Connect-icut Heart Association to D.A.M.

Acetylcholine

$$CH_3\overset{\overset{\displaystyle O}{\|}}{C}-OCH_2CH_2\overset{+}{N}(CH_3)_3$$

Adenosine -3′, 5′ -phosphate (cAMP)
Monobutyryl-cAMP is butyrylated
at position *a*; dibutyryl-cAMP is
butyrylated at positions *a* and *b*.

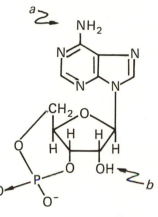

Atropine

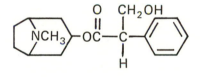

Caffein

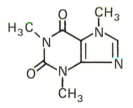

Carbamylcholine (carbachol)

$$H_2N\overset{\overset{\displaystyle O}{\|}}{C}-OCH_2CH_2\overset{+}{N}(CH_3)_3$$

Cocaine

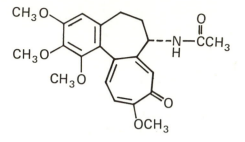

Colchicine

Curare (tubocurarine)

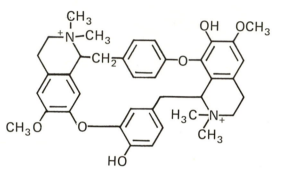

Cycloheximide

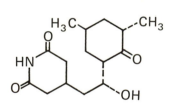

Decamethonium $(CH_3)_3\overset{+}{N}-(CH_2)_{10}-\overset{+}{N}(CH_3)_3$

Diisopropylfluorophosphonate

$$F-\underset{\underset{OCH(CH_3)_2}{|}}{\overset{\overset{OCH(CH_3)_2}{|}}{P}}\rightarrow O$$

Dithiothreitol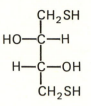

DOPA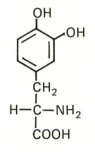

Dopamine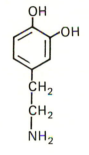

Edrophonium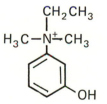

Epinephrine   (adrenaline)

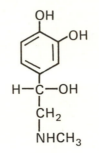

Eserine   (physostigmine)

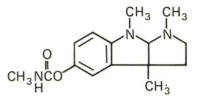

Gamma-aminobutyric acid
(GABA)

$$H_2NCH_2CH_2CH_2COOH$$

Glutamic acid

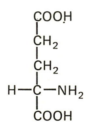

Glycine·

Guanosine-3′, 5′-phosphate   (cGMP)

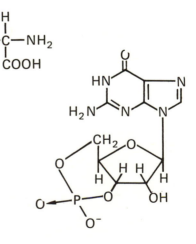

612

Hemicholinium (HC-3)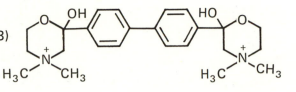

Hexamethonium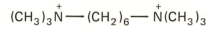

5-hydroxytryptamine (serotonin)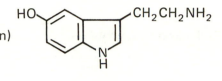

Muscarine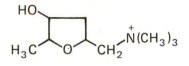

Nicotine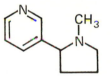

Norepinephrine (noradrenaline)

**Octopamine**

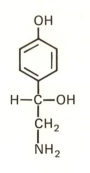

**Perhydrohistrionicotoxin**

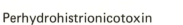

**Phentolamine**

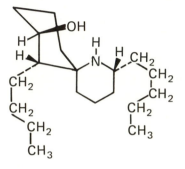

**Picrotoxin**

    A molecular compound containing equimolar and separable picrotin (which is pharmacologically inactive) and picrotoxinin (which is the active principle).

**Picrotoxinin**

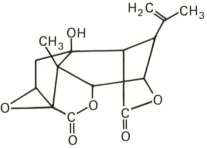

**Reserpine**

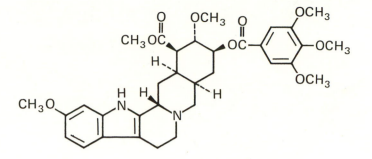

**Theophylline**

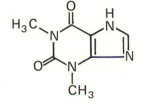

**Vinblastine**

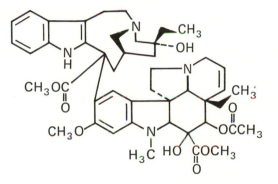

**Xylocaine**

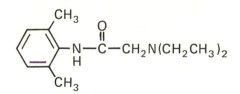